Sports Medicine
in Primary Care

Sports Medicine in Primary Care

EDITED BY

Rob Johnson, MD

Director, Primary Care Sports Medicine
Department of Family Practice
Hennepin County Medical Center
Minneapolis, Minnesota

W.B. SAUNDERS COMPANY
A Harcourt Health Sciences Company
Philadelphia London New York St. Louis Sydney Toronto

W.B. SAUNDERS COMPANY
A Harcourt Health Sciences Company

The Curtis Center
Independence Square West
Philadelphia, Pennsylvania 19106

Library of Congress Cataloging-in-Publication Data

Sports medicine in primary care / edited by Rob Johnson.

p.   cm.

ISBN 0–7216–7871–8

1. Sports medicine.   2. Primary care (Medicine)   I. Johnson, Rob, M.D.
  [DNLM: 1. Athletic Injuries.   2. Primary Health Care.   3. Sports
  Medicine.   QT 261   S7652 2000]

RC1210.S74   2000   617.1′027—dc21

DNLM/DLC   99–37693

Editor: Raymond R. Kersey
Development Editor: Dave Kilmer
Production Manager: Norman Stellander
Project Manager: Edna Dick
Illustration Coordinator: Robert Quinn

SPORTS MEDICINE IN PRIMARY CARE   ISBN 0–7216–7871–8

Printed in the United States of America.

Last digit is the print number: 9   8   7   6   5   4   3   2   1

To my best friend,

Bonnie Young Johnson,

who has tolerated and supported all the time I've dedicated to the practice and teaching of sports medicine.

Contributors

Stephen R. Bindner, B.S., M.D.
Staff Physician, Minnesota Health Family
Physicians P.A., Maplewood, Minnesota
The Exercise Prescription: Adult

Mark Bouchard, M.D.
Associate Clinical Professor, Department of
Family Medicine, University of Vermont School
of Medicine, Burlington, Vermont; Assistant
Director, Family Practice Residency, Maine
Medical Center, Portland, Maine
*Essential Points of the Musculoskeletal Exam:
The Focused History and the Focused Exam*

Janus D. Butcher, M.D.
Associate Clinical Professor, University of
Minnesota, Duluth; Staff Physician, Department
of Orthopedics, St. Mary's Duluth Clinic, Duluth,
Minnesota
Return to Play

William Dexter, M.D., FACSM
Associate Professor, Department of Family
Medicine, University of Vermont School of
Medicine, Burlington, Vermont; Director, Sports
Medicine, and Assistant Director, Family Practice
Residency, Maine Medical Center, Portland,
Maine
*Essential Points of the Musculoskeletal Exam:
The Focused History and the Focused Exam*

Scott Escher, M.D.
Adjunct Professor and Clinical Faculty,
University of Wisconsin-La Crosse; Staff
Physician, Department of Family Medicine and
Section of Sports Medicine, Gundersen Lutheran
Medical Center, La Crosse, Wisconsin
*Advising the Athlete on Nutrition and
Supplements*

BJ Garlick, P.T., E.M.T.
Senior Physical Therapist, Hennepin County
Medical Center, Minneapolis, Minnesota
Office-Based Rehabilitation

Rosemary Greenslade, M.D., M.S.
Physician in Private Practice, Mesa Occupational
and Sports Medicine, Farmington, New Mexico
Preparticipation Evaluation: Adult Assessment

David J. Gronski, M.D.
Clinical Assistant Professor, Department of
Family Medicine, University of Wisconsin-
Madison, Madison, Wisconsin
Injuries to the Upper Extremity

Rob Johnson, M.D.
Director, Primary Care Sports Medicine,
Department of Family Practice, Hennepin County
Medical Center, Minneapolis, Minnesota
*Principles of Training; Chest Injuries; The
Mature Athlete*

Todd L. Kanzenbach, M.D.
Associate Member of Graduate Faculty,
Minnesota State University; Staff and Team
Physician, Minnesota State University Student
Health Services, Mankato, Minnesota
The Exercise Prescription: Youth and Adolescent

Michele LaBotz, M.D.
Sports Medicine Fellow, James A. Taylor Student
Health Service, University of North Carolina at
Chapel Hill, Chapel Hill, North Carolina
Special Issues of Young and Adolescent Athletes

**Constance M. Lebrun, M.D.C.M., M.P.E.,
C.C.F.P.**
Assistant Professor, School of Kinesiology,
Faculty of Health Sciences; Department of Family
Medicine, Orthopedics, and Director, Primary
Care Sport Medicine, Fowler-Kennedy Sport
Medicine Clinic, 3M Centre, University of
Western Ontario, London, Ontario, Canada
Special Issues of the Female Athlete

Jim Macintyre, M.D., M.P.E., FACSM
Co-director, Primary Care Sports Medicine
Fellowship, University of Utah/The Orthopedic

Specialty Hospital; Clinical Assistant Professor, Department of Family and Preventive Medicine, Adjunct Associate Professor, Department of Dance, School of Fine Arts, University of Utah; Director, Primary Care Sports Medicine, The Orthopedic Specialty Hospital, Salt Lake City, Utah
Injuries to the Lower Extremity

Mark McGrail, M.D.

Family Physician, Blanchfield Community Hospital, Fort Campbell, Kentucky
Return to Play

James M. Moriarity, M.D.

Team Physician, University of Notre Dame, Department of Athletics, Notre Dame; Staff Physician, St. Joseph Medical Center, South Bend, Indiana
Risk of Exercise; The Athlete with Medical Problems: The Diabetic Athlete

Patrick Morris, M.D.

Fairview Lakes Regional Health Care, Rush City Area Clinic, Rush City, Minnesota
Genitourinary Problems

Mark W. Niedfeldt, M.D.

Assistant Professor, Departments of Family and Community Medicine, Orthopaedic Surgery, and Cell Biology, Neurobiology, and Anatomy, Medical College of Wisconsin, Milwaukee, Wisconsin
The Athlete with Medical Problems: The Hypertensive Athlete; The Asthmatic or Allergic Athlete; The Athlete with Heart Disease; The Athlete with Chronic Obstructive Pulmonary Disease; Seizure Disorders and Athletics; The Role of Exercise and Athletics in Anxiety and Depression; The Athlete with Infectious Disease

Bobbi (Roberta) Prigge, M.D.

Staff Physician, St. Mary's Duluth Clinic-Ely, Ely, Minnesota
Preparticipation Evaluation: Youth and Adolescent: History

Margot Putukian, M.D., FACSM

Director, Primary Care Sports Medicine and Team Physician, Penn State University, University Park; Assistant Professor, Internal Medicine,

Orthopedics and Rehabilitation, Hershey Medical Center, Hershey, Pennsylvania
Evaluation of Minimal Brain Injury

Jeff Radakovich, M.D.

Assistant Director, Athletic Medicine, Washington State University, Pullman, Washington
Gastrointestinal Problems and Abdominal Trauma

Brent S. E. Rich, M.D., ATC

Head Team Physician, Arizona State University, Tempe; Team Physician: 2000 USA Olympic Team and Arizona Diamondbacks; Private Practice, University Sports Medicine, Phoenix, Arizona
Neck and Cervical Spine Injuries

Jane T. Servi, M.D.

Physician in Private Practice, Northern Colorado Orthopedic Associates, Fort Collins, Colorado
Use of Nonsteroidal Anti-inflammatory Drugs and Analgesics

Stephen M. Simons, M.D., FACSM

Co-Director, South Bend Primary Care Sports Medicine Fellowship, Clinical Assistant Professor of Family Medicine, Indiana University School of Medicine; Director of Sports Medicine and Associate Director, Family Practice Residency, St. Joseph's Regional Medical Center, South Bend, Indiana
Injuries to the Lower Extremity

Bryan W. Smith, M.D., Ph.D.

Clinical Assistant Professor of Pediatrics and Orthopaedics, University of North Carolina School of Medicine; Head Team Physician, James A. Taylor Student Health Service, University of North Carolina at Chapel Hill, Chapel Hill, North Carolina
Special Issues of Young and Adolescent Athletes

L. Tyler Wadsworth, M.D.

Medical Director, Sports Medicine Consultants, LLC, St. Louis, Missouri
Joint Aspiration and Injection

Larik Woronzoff, M.D.

Department of Sports Medicine, Hennepin County Medical Center, Minneapolis, Minnesota
Preparticipation Evaluation: Youth and Adolescent: Physical Examination

Craig C. Young, M.D.

Medical Director of Sports Medicine and
Associate Professor, Orthopaedic Surgery and
Community and Family Medicine, Medical
College of Wisconsin; Team Physician,
Milwaukee Brewers, Milwaukee Mustangs Arena
Football Team, U.S. National Snowboard Team;
Company Physician, Milwaukee Ballet,
Milwaukee, Wisconsin
Back Injuries

Preface

Almost one-fourth of all patients seen in the common outpatient practice of primary care physicians present with musculoskeletal complaints. Furthermore, patients with the common problems of hypertension, diabetes, obesity, and other similar problems that fill our offices day after day should be using exercise as a treatment modality.

This text is designed for you, the primary care physician in office practice. It is designed for your easy reference with chapter-to-chapter consistency to more easily access the necessary information to streamline and improve your office practice of exercise and musculoskeletal medicine. The chapter contributors are experienced primary care physicians who are actively practicing sports medicine and primary care in their respective practices. From their training and experience, they have been able to synthesize the practical, historical, and clinical data that will prove most useful to you, the clinician. It is my hope that you will find sports medicine an enjoyable, rewarding aspect of your medical practice.

ROB JOHNSON

Acknowledgments

I would like to recognize all those clinicians involved in sports medicine with special mention to those sports medicine practitioners who found time in their busy clinical and teaching schedules to contribute to this work. These contributors represent the "grass roots" of sports medicine in North America. A special thanks to Bernice Schuster, my assistant and the coordinator of our sports medicine fellowship program. Without her organizational skills and effective communication, this work would not have been completed.

ROB JOHNSON

NOTICE

Medicine is an ever-changing field. Standard safety precautions must be followed, but as new research and clinical experience broaden our knowledge, changes in treatment and drug therapy become necessary or appropriate. Readers are advised to check the product information currently provided by the manufacturer of each drug to be administered to verify the recommended dose, the method and duration of administration, and contraindications. It is the responsibility of the treating physician, relying on experience and knowledge of the patient, to determine dosages and the best treatment for the patient. Neither the publisher nor the editor assumes any responsibility for any injury and/or damage to persons or property.

THE PUBLISHER

Contents

Essential Points of the Musculoskeletal Exam: The Focused History and The Focused Exam

WILLIAM DEXTER, M.D., FACSM
MARK BOUCHARD, M.D.

THE FOCUSED HISTORY

> If you listen to patients, they will tell you what is wrong with them.
>
> *Adapted from Sir William Osler*

As primary care providers, we have all been taught that the patient's history provides nearly all the information one needs to make a diagnosis. The physical exam should be used to confirm one's initial impression. Therefore, the history is perhaps the most crucial part of the patient encounter. There are several points to emphasize about history taking. The clinician should let patients tell their story without interrupting. Listening is a skill most medical providers need to develop; its importance cannot be overemphasized. By asking open-ended questions rather than closed-ended ones, the caregiver will enable the patient to provide greater detail for the history. Finally, summarizing key points of the history with the patient helps to ensure that the details are accurate and to increase rapport.

There are several key questions one must ask during a musculoskeletal history.[1] They can be classified into four categories, whether the problem is an injury or other disorder: patient's age and occupation, onset and duration of the condition, its site and spread, and its symptoms and behavior. Past medical history, family history, social history, and review of systems should be obtained as well.

Age and Occupation

Age is very helpful in narrowing down the differential diagnosis because various conditions predominantly occur in certain age groups. Children and adolescents are more prone to apophysitis due to their rapid growth. Other conditions, such as Legg-Calvé-Perthes disease, Scheuermann's disease, and slipped capital femoral epiphysis, are typically seen in this population. Growth plate–related injuries, such as Salter-Harris fractures and avulsion injuries, are also seen in this age group. Active adults are more prone to overuse injuries. The elderly experience more problems with osteoarthritis, osteoporosis, and malignancies.

The patient's occupation is a key element for several reasons, including risk factors for various injuries, functional limitations, and aggravating factors. For example, heavy labor is associated with low back pain. Assembly line and computer work are often associated with repetitive motion injury. Carpenters and electricians frequently develop overuse syndromes. Determining the patient's handedness is extremely important and should be documented during the encounter. This can be helpful because upper extremity overuse syndromes typically occur on the dominant side.

Other activities, such as hobbies and sports, may play a significant role as well. Certain sports have well-defined injury patterns (Table 1–1). Also, the patient's training patterns as well as level of physical conditioning need to be taken into account. The level at which the athlete com-

Table 1-1
Sports/Activities and Typical Injury Patterns

Sport/Activity	Injury
Baseball	Acromioclavicular and rotator cuff injuries, "Little League elbow"
Bicycling	Ulnar nerve and pudendal nerve compression
Golfing	Hamate fractures and low back pain
Judged sports (gymnastics, skating)	Disordered eating, stress fractures
Martial arts	Avulsion fractures
Repetitive handwork (knitting, crocheting)	Carpometacarpal arthritis
Rugby	Cervical arthritis
Running	Iliotibial band syndrome, plantar fasciitis
Skiing	Thumb ulnar collateral ligament injury, anterior cruciate ligament injury
Soccer	Anterior cruciate ligament injuries, groin injuries
Swimming	Acromioclavicular and rotator cuff injuries
Wrestling	Dislocated elbow, posterior cruciate ligament injury

petes might influence the aggressiveness of the management approach. In terms of hobbies, activities such as dancing, gardening, and knitting have their own inherent injury patterns. All this information is helpful in generating a differential diagnosis.

Nature of Onset and Duration

The patient may present with an acute injury or one that has developed chronically. Acute injury tends to be easier to assess. The key information to elicit is the mechanism of injury. This is one time when precise, close-ended questioning is appropriate. Knowing the timing of the injury is also essential. If the injury has occurred within the past 20 minutes, the patient may still be in the "window" in which localized swelling has not had time to develop and distort the exam. If the injury occurred (days to weeks) before, fractures have begun to form callus and muscles have begun to atrophy.

Injury resulting from chronic trauma is very common. The history should focus on patterns and change—or lack of change. Changes in the patient's training patterns or work habits can predispose to injury. Adoption of new techniques or a sudden increase in the intensity, duration, or frequency of training or work can be detrimental. A lack of a necessary change can also lead to injury. Examples include use of worn-out equipment, such as running shoes with worn soles, and the practice of running on the same terrain (e.g., asphalt) every day. Chronic trauma can be caused

by normal stress to abnormal tissue, such as a poorly rehabilitated injury that is re-injured. It can also be caused by abnormal stress to normal tissue, as in poor mechanics used by a baseball pitcher.

The duration of the condition will also affect the prognosis and the management approach. There is abundant evidence to suggest that inflammatory tendinitis rapidly develops into a condition more aptly termed "tendinosis."[2] This has been characterized as the abnormal response of the body to the initial injury with the laying down of collagen in an abnormal distribution. Typically, collagen in the musculotendinous unit is aligned parallel to the force vector that the unit provides. In tendinosis, the collagen is laid down haphazardly. This may predispose the involved site to persistent irritation and thus tenderness and pain. Tendinosis that has persisted for months to years may require a very aggressive approach.

Lastly, determining if there have been any prior injuries is helpful in delineating whether patients have any pre-existing conditions placing them at risk. Any specific injuries that might predispose to further injury (e.g., a poorly rehabilitated right ankle leading to favoring of the left ankle and a resultant overuse injury) should be ascertained. Any treatments that have been attempted since the occurrence of the injury should be noted, along with their effectiveness.

Site and Spread

Locating the site of the injury is crucial when taking a history. Having the patient describe where the pain is located and whether it "moves" or travels is helpful. Multiple affected areas may point toward a more systemic process such as inflammatory arthritis or diffuse myopathy. One should ask if the pain radiates. Neuropathic pain tends to follow a dermatomal distribution. Being familiar with dermatomal and myotomal distributions (or at least having access to diagrams showing them) is essential as well. Pain generally refers distally (e.g., hip pathology presenting as knee pain). Also, the more severe the pain, the greater the likelihood that the pain may refer to another area. Always remember to ask about and examine one joint above and one below the area in question.

Symptoms and Behavior

Finally, the symptoms and behavior of the condition need to be evaluated. One method is to determine any functional limitations in terms of the patient's job, hobbies, athletic pursuits, and activities of daily living (ADLs). Have the patient describe what aggravates the pain. Questions about specific activities such as stair climbing, sitting, standing, bending, and running can point to specific areas to be investigated. For example, anterior knee pain associated with climbing down stairs is often indicative of patellofemoral syndrome. Heel pain associated with running may indicate plantar fasciitis. Rating the severity of the pain on a scale of one to ten is helpful only in following the patient's progress. It is unreliable in specifying the actual severity of pain due to the variability of each patient's experience of pain.

The timing of the pain is also an important consideration. Is it constant or intermittent? If intermittent, is it cyclical or irregular? Does it occur with activity or afterward? Does it occur at rest? Pain at night may indicate tumor. Pain or stiffness in the morning is more consistent with an inflammatory process (e.g., rheumatoid arthritis or plantar fasciitis). A grading scale (Table 1–2) for overuse syndromes has been developed.[3] Its simple approach enables the user to easily establish the grade of the injury and thus guide the approach toward management.

Any changes in the characteristics of the pain are helpful when eliciting a history. Note any increase or decrease in the intensity along with any change in the frequency. The quality of the pain can help determine what type of pathology is present. A dull, achy pain is more indicative of muscle or bone pathology. A sharp or shooting pain could be nerve or bone related. Determining if a change was in response to a certain treatment modality is important in guiding therapy.

Associated symptoms need to be investigated. Fevers and chills could be associated with infections such as osteomyelitis, cellulitis, and infectious arthritis. Swelling, color change, and temperature change of the area in question should be ascertained. Finally, the patient should be asked if any numbness, tingling, or weakness is present that might suggest neurologic impairment.

Questions should always be asked concerning whether the patient has experienced any locking, popping, or giving way of the joint in question. Popping is usually significant only if it is associated with pain— "painful popping." Giving way can be due to a mechanical cause (e.g., ligamentous instability), to weakness, or to pain.

Medical, Surgical, Family, and Social History

The past medical history should be screened for arthritides and other connective tissue disorders.

Table 1–2
Grading System for Overuse Syndromes and Management

	Symptoms/Signs	Management
Grade I	Pain after exercise, soreness; vague, hard to distinguish or localize, exam not helpful	Appropriate training and equipment
Grade II	Pain late in exercise and following, still often vague. More localized on exam	Modify training, technique, and equipment. Address mechanics, add relative rest (25% decrease in activity—frequency, duration, or intensity)
Grade III	Pain in middle of exercise, affecting performance; self-modifying of activity, quite focal exam, tender and specific	Decrease activity by 50–75%, consider one week off
Grade IV	Unable to compete; quite painful, pain at rest, atrophy develops	Complete rest, alternative exercise

Chronic underlying diseases such as diabetes, peripheral vascular disease, inflammatory bowel disease (IBD), and stroke predispose to the development of certain musculoskeletal disorders. For example, IBD is associated with arthropathies, diabetes with Charcot joints, and stroke with joint contractures. Current medications can exacerbate musculoskeletal pathology (e.g., loop diuretics exacerbate gout, and statins exacerbate myopathy). Any past surgeries should also be noted.

The patient's psychological and social history is a vital element of the history-taking process. Knowing an athlete's "state of mind" is key in achieving an effective plan for a quick and safe return to play. Chronic pain states are frequently associated with depression that may improve with antidepressant therapy. One should investigate any substance use, including alcohol, tobacco, illicit drugs, and supplements (steroids, creatine, and the like). The living situation as well as current stressors should be screened for. It is surprising how often neck and back pain stem from or are exacerbated by stress in a patient's life.

The family history, while focusing on musculoskeletal diseases primarily, should also include questions about other diseases such as diabetes, IBD, and cancer. Finally, a thorough review of systems may help to narrow the focus in the differential diagnosis. For example, renal colic, hepatitis, endometriosis, and an abdominal aortic aneurysm can all cause back pain.

THE FOCUSED MUSCULOSKELETAL EXAM

> Diagnosis is simply a matter of applying one's anatomy.
>
> *James Cyriax*

General Concepts

The cornerstone to a good exam is ensuring that the patient is relaxed. Findings can be subtle. The anatomy or injured area must be visible; therefore, the patient should be suitably disrobed. Use of shorts and sleeveless shirts is invaluable. In order to perform an adequate musculoskeletal examination, the examiner needs to be comfortable touching and manipulating the patient. Establishing trust with patients through reassurance will help. Letting them know what is being examined and why, as well as describing the findings, help to establish this trust. Always try to examine the uninvolved side first. Painful movements should be performed last. Make sure to remind the patient that the examination may cause symptoms to flare for a day or so. Develop a plan for treatment (medications, modalities) if this occurs.

The patient's history is influential in deciding whether a general or a more focused examination needs to be performed. A uniform, consistent approach promotes a thorough and complete exam. It also helps organize one's thoughts during the documentation process.

Basic biomechanics must be taken into account. A musculotendinous unit's origin and insertion determine its function. The number of joints the unit crosses is also significant. For example, the gastrocnemius crosses both the ankle and the knee, whereas the soleus crosses only the ankle. The action and counteraction of a pair of musculotendinous units (e.g., hamstrings versus quadriceps) helps to maintain "balance" across a particular joint. If one group is overdeveloped as compared with the other, a pathologic condition may develop in the weaker group. One example is the typical overdevelopment of the calf muscle group as compared with underdevelopment of the anterior compartment of the leg, leading to shin splints. Finally, certain muscle groups have dual actions. For example, the rectus femoris crosses two joints and thus can have two actions, i.e., flexing the knee and extending the hip.

Another significant concept is the theory of the kinetic chain. The entire body is linked kinetically from head to toe. Thus, a disturbance in one area can create disorders in a remote area. For example, a pitcher who has weak gluteus maximus muscles may tire after a few innings and not rotate his trunk enough in order to face the plate as he had before tiring. In order to compensate, he must use either the shoulder or elbow to deliver the ball with the appropriate vector toward the plate. This may place additional stress on these areas with possible resultant rotator cuff tendon damage.

In order to adequately diagnose and treat musculoskeletal conditions, one must understand the kinetic chain involved for each patient. Ideally, observing the athlete or worker in action helps to clarify any weaknesses in the chain that may need to be corrected. For example, if the pitcher in the above example does not strengthen the gluteal muscles, he will develop recurrent shoulder or elbow problems despite appropriate therapy to these areas.

The exam can be broken down into the following elements: observation and palpation, range of motion testing, neurovascular exam, special tests, and laboratory and radiologic testing.

Observation

General aspects of the patient that should be observed include body size, body habitus, posture, and stance. Movements such as gait, handshaking, standing, and sitting are informative. The patient's willingness to participate in the exam should be assessed. Items to be observed include gross deformity, asymmetry, swelling, atrophy, and skin changes, including color, texture, and scarring.

Deformity and asymmetry may be secondary to congenital anomalies, recent or past trauma, or destructive arthritides. Swelling is typically characterized as diffuse or localized. Localized swelling of a joint suggests an effusion, hemarthosis, or pyarthrosis. Generalized swelling of a limb may suggest a major infection, tumor, compartment syndrome, or lymphatic or venous obstruction. Atrophy suggests either disuse secondary to pain or denervation of the affected structures. Focal superficial bruising suggests trauma, whereas large ecchymoses might indicate significant tissue disruption (ligament, bone, and muscle). Diffuse bruising or bleeding could indicate coagulopathy. Redness and edema suggest an inflammatory response to trauma or infection.

Palpation

Skills involved in palpation are often overlooked and underutilized. Tremendous amounts of information can be determined by palpating the affected tissues. Tenderness, tissue tension, temperature, and texture should be evaluated through palpation. Tenderness may be graded as follows:

Grade I	Complains of pain
Grade II	Complains of pain and winces
Grade III	Complains of pain and withdraws
Grade IV	Won't allow palpation

Tissue tension helps one assess the tone of the soft tissues and to monitor for edema. Texture can be described as normal, full, or ropy. Fullness is suggestive of an edematous process. Ropiness is more suggestive of chronic spasm and inflamma-

tion. Finally, temperature changes may help to pinpoint a pathologic condition if it is localized. A diffuse increase in warmth occurs in inflammatory processes. Coolness can occur in reflex sympathetic dystrophy or an ischemic extremity.

Crepitus is another finding indicative of a possible pathologic condition and is elicited when a joint undergoes range of motion (ROM) (see below). Although it is fairly nonspecific, it may be associated with tendinitis, synovitis, and degenerative cartilage changes. Finally, hyperesthesia experienced by the patient during palpation indicates a neurologic process.

Range of Motion Testing: Active, Passive, Resisted

ROM testing is a crucial step in the musculoskeletal exam. There is usually a limitation to ROM in most cases when a pathologic condition exists. Active range of motion (AROM) should be evaluated first. Typical values of ROM for all joints should be known for comparison. Table 1–3 shows normal ROM values of each joint. Passive ROM (PROM) can be tested once the patient is at the end of AROM. Precise documentation is a must when measuring ROM. This will enable the examiner to determine whether the patient's condition is worsening or improving.

One should note whether the AROM is full or limited as well as whether the motion is smooth. The patient's willingness to perform this movement should be assessed. Pain and its location in the ROM should be noted. AROM evaluates contractile and inert tissue such as ligaments, joint capsules, bursae, cartilage, and neurovascular elements. A small degree of motion that is associated with a large amount of pain indicates an irritated joint.

Passive ROM testing should be performed at the end of the active range. It stresses the noncontractile tissues about the joint and is not always necessary if the AROM of the joint in question is full. The patient should be relaxed; any pain, limitation, and "end feel" should be noted. Typically, the end feel of a joint is springy with a hard end point. However, different joints have different end feel characteristics. The springy feel is due to stretch of ligaments and the hard end point is bone abutting bone. Abnormal end feel can be described as being springy without a hard end point or a hard end point without a

Table 1–3
Normal ROM Values of the Musculoskeletal System

Shoulder	Abduction	180°	Hip	Abduction	45–50°
	Adduction	45°		Adduction	20–30°
	Flexion	180°		Flexion	120°
	Extension	45°		Extension	30°
	Int. rotation	90°		Int. rotation	35°
	Ext. rotation	90°		Ext. rotation	45°
Elbow	Flexion	135°	Knee	Flexion	130°
	Extension	0–5°		Extension	10°
	Supination	90°		Int/Ext rotation	10°
	Pronation	90°	Ankle	Dorsiflexion	20°
Wrist	Ulnar deviation	30°		Plantar flexion	50°
	Radial deviation	20°		Inversion	30°
	Flexion	80°		Eversion	20°
	Extension	70°	Forefoot	Abduction	10°
Metacarpophalangeal	Flexion	90°		Adduction	20°
	Extension	30–45°	1st Metatarsophalangeal	Flexion	45°
Proximal interphalangeal	Flexion	100–120°		Extension	70–90°
	Extension	0°	Cervical spine	Flexion	45°
Distal interphalangeal	Flexion	45–80°		Extension	55°
	Extension	10°		Lateral bending	40°
				Rotation	70°
Thumb/Metacarpophalangeal	Flexion	50°	Lumbosacral spine	Extension	30°
	Extension	0°		Lateral bending	35°
Thumb/Interphalangeal	Flexion	90°		Rotation	30°
	Extension	20°			
Thumb	Abduction	70°			
	Adduction	0°			

preceding springy feel. The former could be associated with spasm or internal derangement and the latter with an intra-articular loose body.

The pathologic conditions noted in ROM testing can be described under two broad categories: capsular and noncapsular patterns. The capsular pattern is usually seen with intra-articular degenerative or inflammatory changes. It is accompanied by a hard end feel. Each joint has a characteristic capsular pattern, i.e., the hip joint develops decreased internal rotation. There will also be pain or limitation or both on PROM testing.

The noncapsular pattern describes limitation in ROM of a joint other than as described in the capsular pattern. An abnormal end feel is usually noted. Three conditions are usually associated with this type of motion restriction: intra-articular derangements (cartilage, ligamentous tears, bony fractures), ligamentous adherences (adhesive capsulitis), and extra-articular causes (bursitis and musculotendinous tears).

Finally, resisted ROM testing stresses the contractile tissues and their attachments. If performed correctly, it should remove any effects of joint involvement from the exam, and determine if there is damage to the contractile tissues (muscles, tendons, and teno-osseous junction). The test should evaluate for any pain as well as muscle strength. The test should be performed while the joint is in a neutral position and an isometric contraction should be held for approximately 5 seconds. A judgment of whether there is real weakness rather than "give way" weakness may be difficult to make.

Neurovascular Exam

A complete neurovascular exam in the area in question as well as distally is always indicated. Muscle strength, as already noted, should be assessed. The dermatomal distribution of nerves needs to be known for the sensory exam. Two-point discrimination is the most sensitive test, especially on the digits. However, light touch is an adequate screening tool for most areas. Lastly, deep tendon reflexes should be evaluated.

Special Tests

There are numerous special musculoskeletal tests that can be used to help in diagnosis. They focus primarily on ligamentous stability, cartilage derangement, and functional testing. Below are some descriptions of several special tests for the shoulder, elbow, wrist and hand, cervical spine, hip and pelvis, knee, and ankle joints. Tests for other body regions can be found in other chapters.

Shoulder Exam

SUPRASPINATUS TEST

Abduct the shoulder to 90 degrees, move the arm forward to 30–45 degrees, internally rotate ("empty can" sign), and resist upward motion. Some clinicians believe that the supraspinatus can be tested in the same position but without internal rotation. A positive test produces pain with resisted abduction. See Figure 1–1.

IMPINGEMENT TESTS

First Test Passively, forward flex the shoulder to 180 degrees. A positive test yields pain in the shoulder.

Second Test Passively, forward flex the shoulder and elbow to 90 degrees and internally rotate the shoulder. A positive test yields pain in the shoulder. See Figure 1–2.

TEST OF ANTERIOR INSTABILITY

Anterior Drawer With the patient either sitting or supine, grasp the head of the humerus and move forward in the glenoid while stabilizing the acromion with the other hand. Up to 25 percent anterior motion is commonly normal. To determine relative instability, compare with the uninvolved shoulder. See Figure 1–3.

Apprehension Test Abduct the shoulder and flex the elbow to 90 degrees. Externally rotate the shoulder. A positive test occurs when pain or apprehension results from provocation. Apprehension usually occurs following a dislocation or subluxation. If the injury has been chronic or atraumatic, the pain signifies anterior instability caused by a forward glide of the humeral head. See Figure 1–4.

Relocation Test (Neer's Test) Perform the apprehension test with the patient in the supine position. When external rotation causes pain, press down on the humeral head. A positive test occurs if pain lessens (humeral head is returned to normal position in glenoid). See Figure 1–5.

TESTS OF POSTERIOR INSTABILITY

Posterior Drawer Similar to anterior drawer but compare motion in a posterior direction.

Crossed Adduction Test Flex the shoulder to 90 degrees and adduct. A positive test occurs when motion causes pain or subluxation of the posterior shoulder. See Figure 1–6.

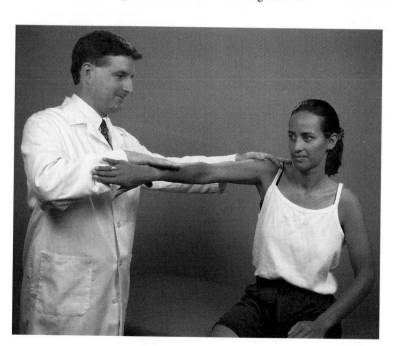

Figure 1–1. Supraspinatus test—indicative of supraspinatus tendinitis.

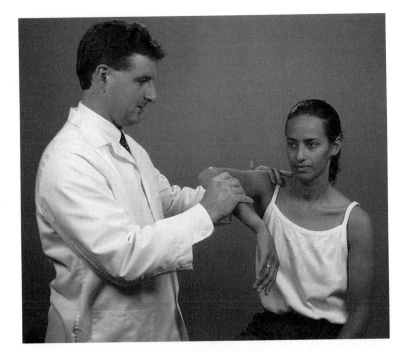

Figure 1-2. Impingement test—indicative of subacromial impingement and associated bursitis.

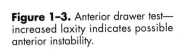

Figure 1-3. Anterior drawer test—increased laxity indicates possible anterior instability.

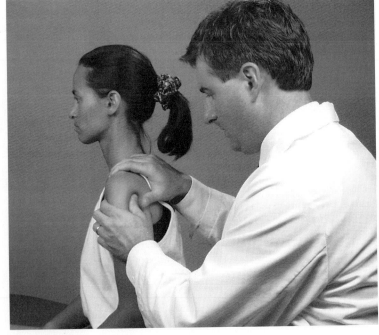

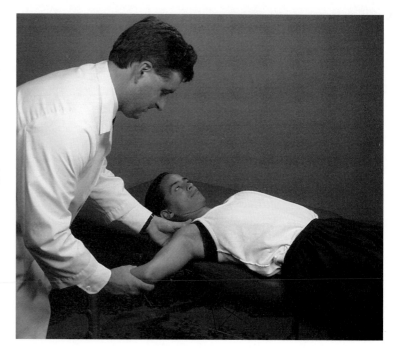

Figure 1–4. Apprehension test—pain and apprehension also indicate possible anterior instability.

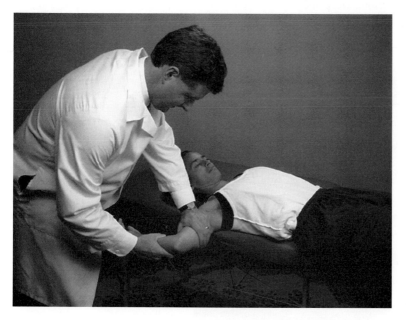

Figure 1–5. Relocation test—decreased pain indicates possible anterior instability.

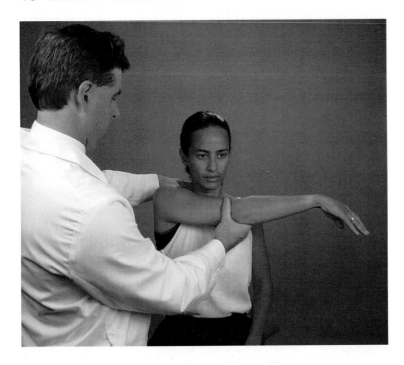

Figure 1–6. Crossed adduction test ("scarf sign")—posterior shoulder pain indicates possible posterior instability. It is also a test for acromioclavicular (AC) arthritis or sprain.

TEST OF INFERIOR INSTABILITY

Pull the arm directly downward. A positive test occurs when the sulcus appears inferior to the acromion ("sulcus sign"). See Figure 1–7.

TEST FOR ACROMIOCLAVICULAR SPRAIN OR ARTHRITIS

Perform an adduction test as described for posterior instability. The test is positive when pain localizes to the acromioclavicular (AC) joint; also known as a positive "scarf sign."

TESTS FOR BICIPITAL TENDINITIS

Yergason's Test With the arm adducted, the examiner should resist both elbow flexion and external rotation. A positive test occurs when pain localized to the bicipital groove or the longhead

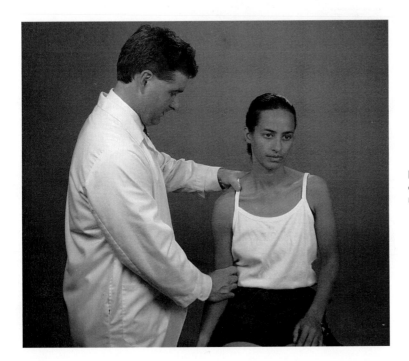

Figure 1–7. "Sulcus sign"—if sulcus appears, indicates possible inferior instability.

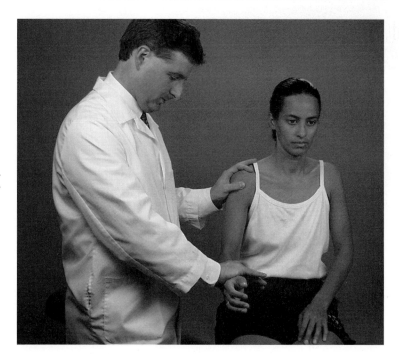

Figure 1–8. Yergason's test—indicates bicipital tendinitis or subluxation.

of the biceps subluxes from the humeral groove. See Figure 1–8.

Speed's Test Place the arm in a neutral, adducted position. Palpate the longhead of the biceps in the bicipital groove. Alternate internal and external rotation. A positive test occurs when pain is reproduced as the longhead passes beneath the examiner's fingers. See Figure 1–9.

TESTS OF LABRAL INJURY

O'Brien's Test Flex shoulder to 90 degrees, adduct shoulder about 30 degrees. Internally rotate the shoulder and resist flexion. Then return the shoulder to neutral rotation and resist flexion. A positive test occurs when pain is present with internal rotation but absent in a neutral position. See Figure 1–10.

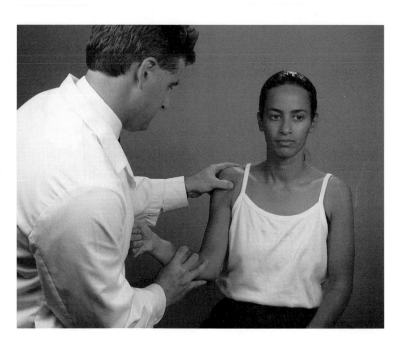

Figure 1–9. Speed's test—indicates bicipital tendinitis.

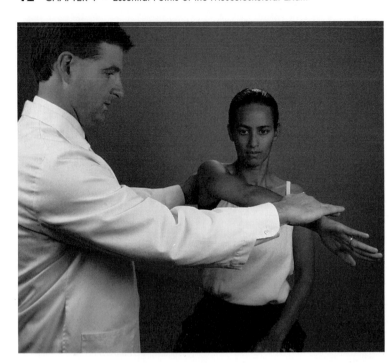

Figure 1-10. O'Brien's test—suggests a superior labrum anterior posterior (SLAP) lesion of the superior labrum.

Clunk Test With the patient in either the upright or supine position, apply an axial compressive load to the humerus and move the humerus across the front of the body. A positive test occurs when either a mechanical "clunk" is felt or pain is provoked by motion. See Figure 1–11.

Crank Test Abduct the shoulder to 135 degrees. Apply an axial compressive load to the humerus and internally/externally rotate the shoulder. A positive test occurs when pain or clunking of the labrum is provoked by the maneuver. See Figure 1–12.

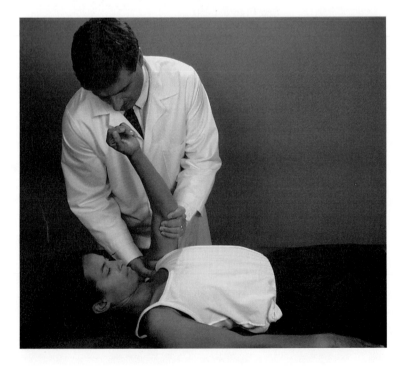

Figure 1-11. Clunk test—suggests a labral injury.

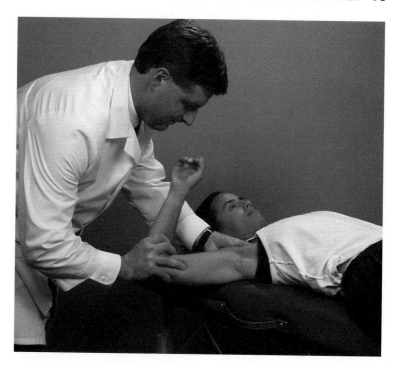

Figure 1-12. Crank test—also suggests a possible labral injury.

TEST FOR INFRASPINATUS AND TERES MINOR INJURY

With the arm adducted, flex the elbow and resist external rotation. A positive test occurs when pain in the posterior shoulder is provoked by the maneuver. See Figure 1–13.

TEST FOR SUBSCAPULARIS INJURY

With the arm adducted, flex the elbow and resist internal rotation. A positive test occurs when pain is elicited in the anterior shoulder. See Figure 1–14.

TESTS FOR ROTATOR CUFF TEAR

"Drop Arm" Test Abduct the shoulder to 180 degrees. Slowly lower the arm to side. A positive test occurs when the shoulder abruptly drops from 120 to 80 degrees.

Resisted Shoulder Abduction Abduct the shoulder to 90 degrees. Have the patient resist your attempt to lower the arm. A positive test occurs when the patient is able to offer no resistance. The painful shoulder will resist briefly, then "give." The torn rotator cuff "gives" immediately. See Figure 1–15.

Elbow

TEST OF LATERAL STABILITY

With the elbow flexed a few degrees, valgus stress tests the integrity of the ulnar collateral ligament. Varus stress across the elbow tests the radial collateral ligament complex. Compare with the other side. Laxity and pain indicates a ligament sprain. Figure 1–16 illustrates valgus stress.

TEST FOR LATERAL EPICONDYLITIS

Resisted wrist extension should cause pain that localizes to an area just distal to the lateral epicondyle. See Figure 1–17.

Wrist and Hand

TEST FOR NAVICULAR FRACTURE ("anatomic snuffbox")

Pain with palpation in the area just dorsal and distal to the radial styloid process indicates a possible navicular fracture that should be splinted or casted. See Figure 1–18.

TEST FOR de QUERVAIN'S TENOSYNOVITIS (Finkelstein's test)

Have the patient make a fist with the thumb tucked inside the other fingers. While stabilizing the fore-

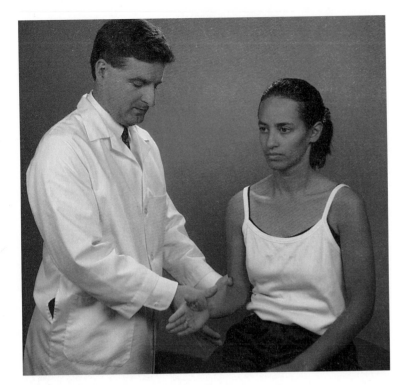

Figure 1-13. Resisted external rotation—suggests injury to the infraspinatus and/or teres minor.

Figure 1-14. Resisted internal rotation—suggests injury to the subscapularis.

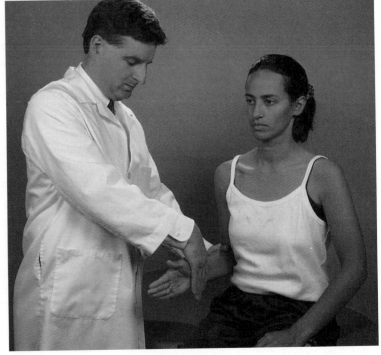

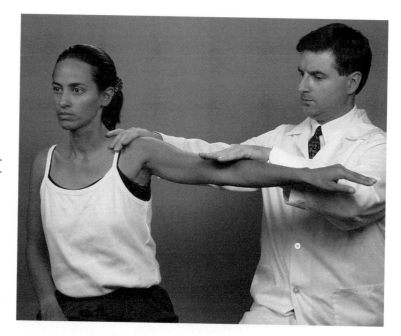

Figure 1-15. Resisted abduction—points to injury to the supraspinatus.

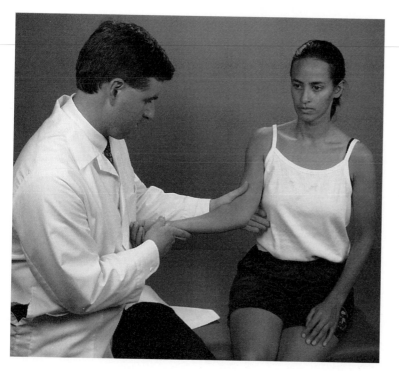

Figure 1-16. Valgus stress—laxity and pain suggest an ulnar collateral ligament (UCL) injury.

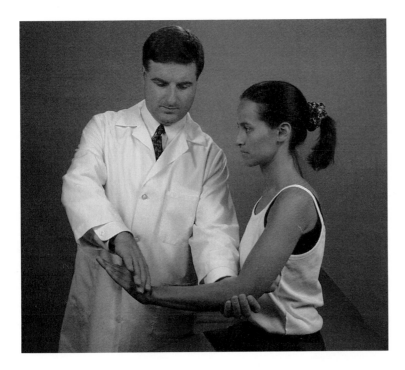

Figure 1-17. Resisted wrist extension—pain at lateral epicondyle suggests lateral epicondylitis.

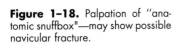

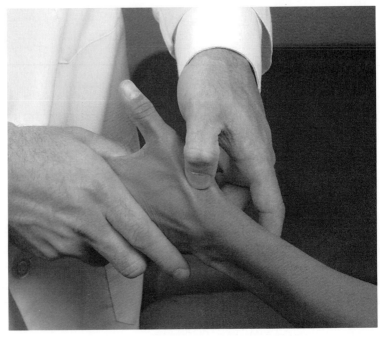

Figure 1-18. Palpation of "anatomic snuffbox"—may show possible navicular fracture.

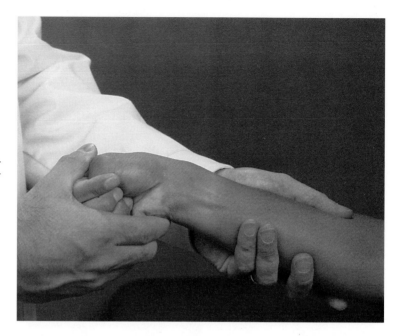

Figure 1–19. Finkelstein's test—suggests de Quervain's tenosynovitis.

arm with one hand, ulnar deviate the wrist with the other hand. Pain is suggestive of tenosynovitis of the abductor pollicis longus and extensor pollicis brevis tendons. See Figure 1–19.

TESTS FOR CARPAL TUNNEL SYNDROME

Tinel's Sign Tap over the volar carpal ligament (the "roof" of the tunnel). If there is pain or numbness in the medial nerve distribution, the test is positive. See Figure 1–20.

Phalen's Test Flex the wrist maximally and hold for at least 60 seconds. A positive test occurs with pain or numbness in the median nerve distribution. See Figure 1–21.

Cervical Spine

TEST FOR NERVE ROOT COMPRESSION (Spurling's maneuver)

Have the patient rotate head to symptomatic side with slight neck extension. Then compress cervical spine by pressing down on top of the patient's head. If pain or numbness appears in a dermatomal distribution, the test is considered suggestive of nerve root compression. See Figure 1–22.

TEST FOR THORACIC OUTLET SYNDROME (Adson's test)

The patient's radial pulse is palpated with one hand. The arm is then abducted, extended, and externally rotated. While the pulse is still being palpated, the patient is asked to take a deep breath and turn his/her head *toward* the arm being tested. A positive test will yield a diminished pulse. See Figure 1–23.

Hip and Pelvis

TEST OF GLUTEUS MEDIUS MUSCLE (Trendelenburg test)

Stand behind the standing patient and observe the sacral dimples overlying the posterior superior iliac spines. Have the patient stand on one leg. If the pelvis on the unsupported side remains neutral or descends, the test is suggestive of a weak gluteus medius on the unsupported side. See Figure 1–24.

TEST FOR ILIOTIBIAL BAND TIGHTNESS (Ober's test)

The patient lies on the uninvolved side. Keep the hip in neutral flexion, abduct the hip, and flex the knee to 90 degrees. Release the abducted leg. If the hip remains abducted, the test is positive; this is suggestive of a contracted or tight iliotibial band. See Figure 1–25.

TEST OF THE SACROILIAC JOINT (Faber's test)

With the patient supine, place the hip of the affected side (side of the low back pain) in the

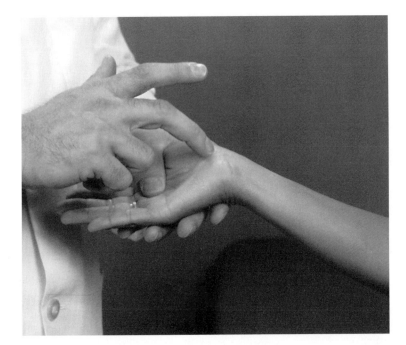

Figure 1-20. Tinel's sign—indicative of carpal tunnel syndrome.

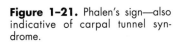

Figure 1-21. Phalen's sign—also indicative of carpal tunnel syndrome.

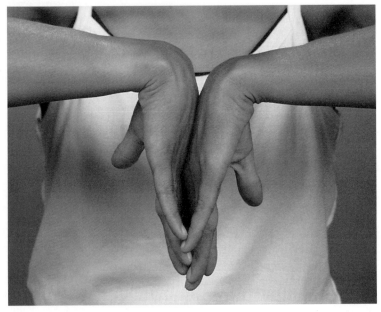

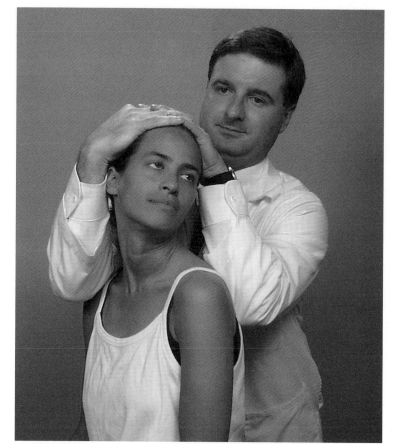

Figure 1-22. Spurling's maneuver—suggestive of cervical nerve root compression.

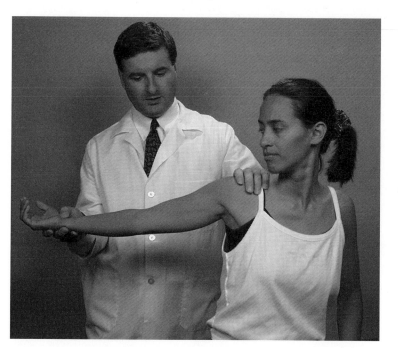

Figure 1-23. Adson's test—indicates thoracic outlet syndrome.

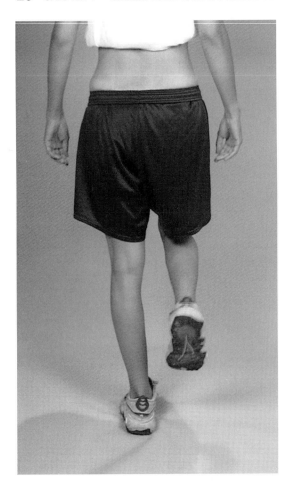

Figure 1-24. Trendelenburg test—indicates weakness of gluteus medius muscle.

Figure 1-25. Ober's test—indicates tight iliotibial band.

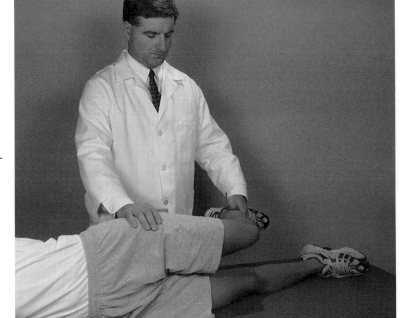

following positions: flexion, abduction, and external rotation. The legs should be in the shape of a "figure of four." Then place one hand on the opposite anterior superior iliac spine and the other on the involved knee. Apply pressure on the knee along with counterpressure at the contralateral anterior superior iliac spine (ASIS). A positive test will produce increased pain in the low back on the involved side. See Figure 1–26.

Knee

MEDIAL/LATERAL STABILITY TEST

Valgus Stress Test Knee is flexed 30 degrees. Tests medial collateral ligament (MCL) stability and status. See Figure 1–27.

Varus Stress Test Knee is flexed 30 degrees. Tests lateral collateral ligament (LCL) stability and status. See Figure 1–28.

ANTERIOR CRUCIATE LIGAMENT STABILITY TESTS

Lachman's Test Position the knee at 10 to 20 degrees of flexion. Fix the femur with one hand and pull the tibia forward with the other. Note the presence or absence of an "end point." A positive

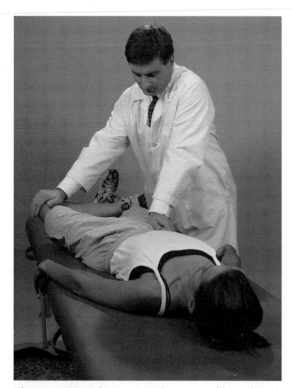

Figure 1–26. Faber's test—indicates possible ipsilateral sacroiliac dysfunction.

Lachman's occurs when the tibia moves forward without a discernible end point and suggests a tear of the anterior cruciate ligament. The test is most effective in an acute or subacute situation. See Figure 1–29.

Anterior Drawer Position the knee at 90 degrees of flexion. Sit on the patient's foot and pull the tibia forward. Note the presence or absence of an end point. Forward movement of the tibia without an end point is a positive test and suggests a complete anterior cruciate ligament tear. The test is more likely to be useful in a chronic situation. See Figure 1–30.

Pivot Shift Position the knee in extension with the tibia in internal rotation. Apply an axial load and valgus stress while moving the knee from flexion to extension. A positive test occurs if the tibia abruptly shifts or jerks into place (tibia is reduced) at about 30 degrees of flexion. A positive test suggests an absent anterior cruciate ligament. See Figure 1–31.

POSTERIOR CRUCIATE LIGAMENT STABILITY TESTS

Posterior Drawer Position the knee at 90 degrees of flexion. Push the tibia in a posterior direction. A positive test occurs when the tibia moves posteriorly without an end point.

Posterior Sag The tibial tubercle sags in comparison with the uninvolved side. May compare with both hips and knees flexed to 90 degrees.

TESTS FOR MENISCAL INJURY

Palpate along both medial and lateral joint lines.

McMurray's Test Position the knee in maximum flexion. Internally and externally rotate the tibia. Note the location of pain. Externally rotate the tibia and move the knee from flexion to extension with varus stress. Medial joint line pain suggests medial meniscus injury. See Figure 1–32. Next, internally rotate tibia and move knee from flexion to extension with valgus stress. Lateral joint line pain suggests lateral meniscus injury. See Figure 1–33.

TESTS OF EXTENSOR MECHANISM

Apprehension Test Flex the knee slightly. Push the patella laterally. A positive test occurs when patient withdraws or becomes "apprehen-

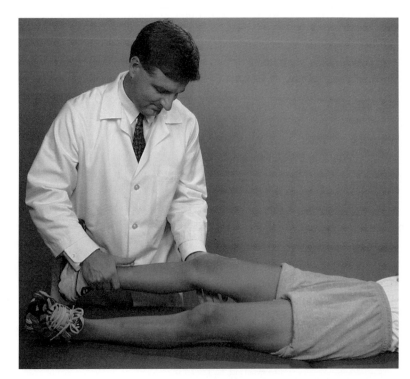

Figure 1-27. Valgus stress—pain and laxity indicates MCL injury.

Figure 1-28. Varus stress—pain and laxity indicates LCL injury.

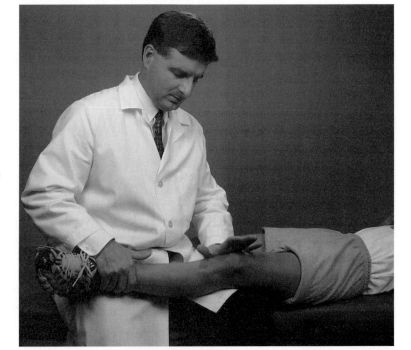

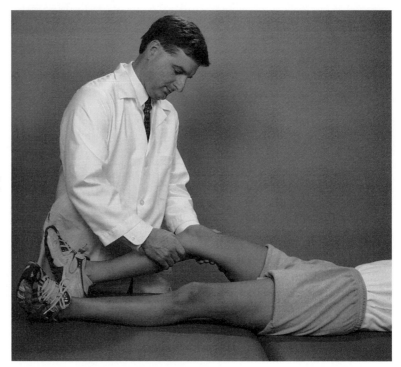

Figure 1-29. Lachman's test—pain and laxity indicates anterior cruciate ligament injury.

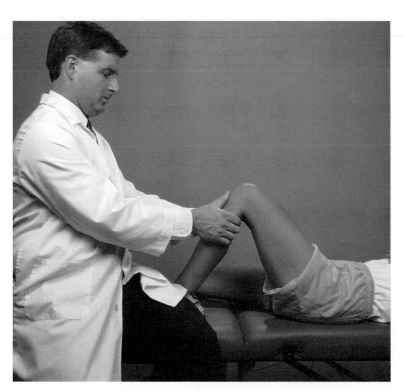

Figure 1-30. Anterior drawer test—pain and laxity indicates anterior cruciate ligament injury.

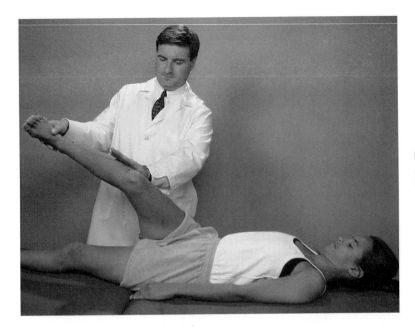

Figure 1–31. Pivot shift test—shows possible anterior cruciate ligament insufficiency.

sive." Suggests recent patellar subluxation/dislocation. See Figure 1–34. Palpate along the medial and lateral faces of patella. Pain suggests patellofemoral injury or inflammation.

Pseudocompression Test/Compression ("Grind") Test Position knee in extension. Push the patella down into femoral groove. A positive test occurs when pain is caused by this maneuver. If no pain, have patient cautiously contract quads.

A positive test with this maneuver causes pain. See Figure 1–35.

Ankle

TALAR TILT

Invert the ankle to end ROM and compare with the uninvolved side. Laxity suggests insufficiency of the lateral ankle ligament complex. See Figure 1–36.

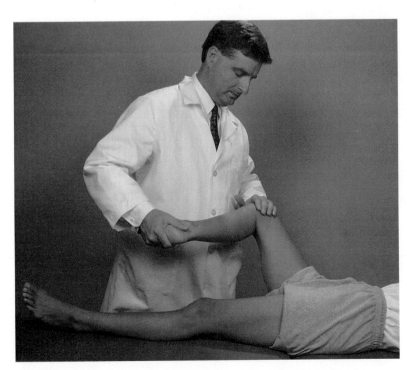

Figure 1–32. McMurray's test—external tibial rotation and varus stress indicates medial meniscal injury.

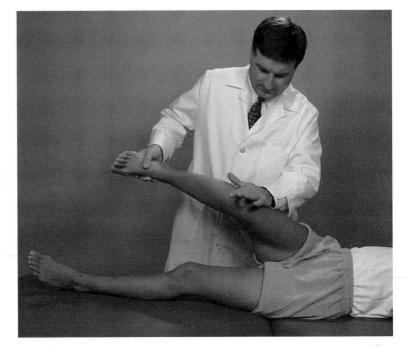

Figure 1-33. McMurray's test—internal tibial rotation and valgus stress are indicative of lateral meniscal injury.

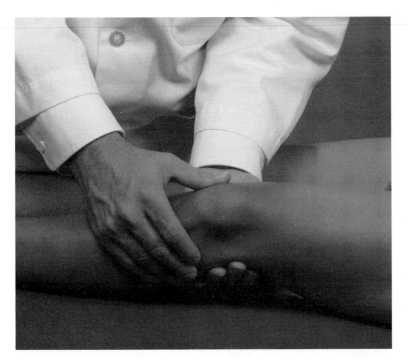

Figure 1-34. Apprehension test—indicates possible recent patellar subluxation or dislocation.

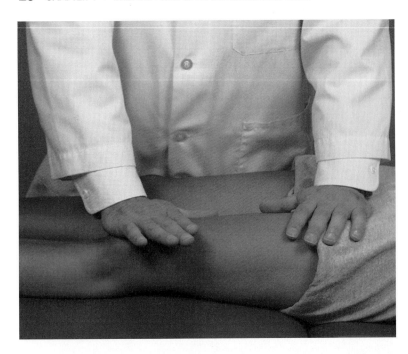

Figure 1–35. Pseudocompression/Grind test—indicates probable patellofemoral syndrome.

ANTERIOR DRAWER

The examiner cups the heel in one hand and the same forearm controls the position of the foot. Fix the tibia with the other hand and pull the heel forward. Movement of the foot forward on the tibia represents a positive test. When the test is positive, this indicates a tear of the anterior talofibular ligament. See Figure 1–37.

EXTERNAL ROTATION TEST

Position the ankle in the neutral position. Grasp the medial aspect of the foot and ankle, fix the tibia, and rotate the foot externally. A positive test occurs when this maneuver causes pain at the site of the syndesmotic ligaments (tibiofibular ligament) and represents a "high sprain." See Figure 1–38.

TEST FOR ACHILLES' TENDON RUPTURE (Thompson's test)

Place the patient in the supine position. Squeeze the calf of the affected side. In a positive test, ankle plantar flexion is not produced. See Figure 1–39.

Radiographic and Laboratory Testing

Radiologic testing does merit special mention. Bone radiographs are usually the initial step if after the physical exam the diagnosis is in question or a bony pathologic condition is likely. One should have a standard routine for evaluating bone radiographs. It is usually better to look at the "big picture," i.e., to view the radiograph in a general way and then to focus on specifics. The name, date, body area, and the number of views should be noted and documented.

Specifics that should be delineated on a radiograph include bony shape, size, and contour. Bony alignment, bone texture (osteoporosis, osteopetrosis, and Paget's disease) and new bone formation (periosteal and exostoses) should be noted. Close-up examination of the radiograph can be performed by either examining the entire circumference of the bones or checking for common pathologic findings or anatomic derangements (joint margins, joint space, ligamentous attachments).[4]

Laboratory evaluation will depend on the clinical presentation. Common tests for ruling out inflammatory arthritis include antinuclear antibody (ANA), rheumatoid factor, and erythrocyte sedimentation rate (ESR). If an infectious process is being considered, a white blood cell count with differential, ESR, and blood culture is required. Synovial fluid should be sent for white blood cell count with differential, red blood cell count, aerobic culture, and crystal analysis. If myopathy is in the differential, creatine kinase and aldolase levels should be obtained. These tests are basic aids for formulating a differential diagnosis.

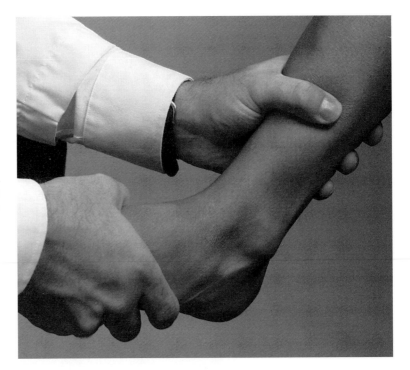

Figure 1-36. Talar tilt test—increased laxity and pain suggests lateral ankle ligament insufficiency.

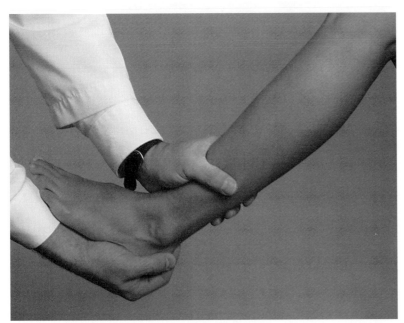

Figure 1-37. Anterior drawer test—increased laxity indicates anterior talofibular ligament injury.

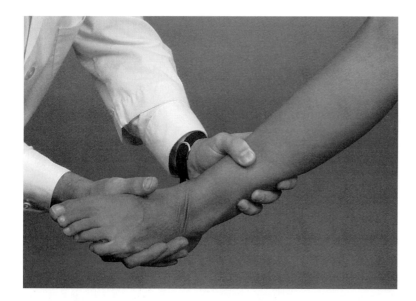

Figure 1–38. External rotation test—pain points to syndesmotic ligament injury ("high ankle sprain").

Figure 1–39. Thompson's test—lack of ankle plantar flexion indicates torn Achilles' tendon.

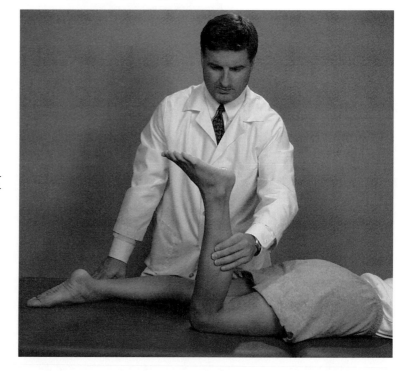

Key Points

- History is crucial. Use open-ended questions when possible.
- Occupation, sports, hobbies, functional limitations, predisposing factors need to be determined.
- Is the injury acute or chronic?
- The kinetic chain is important in understanding the etiology of the injury and in preventing recurrence.
- Knowledge of anatomy is vital in delineating a patient's injury.

ACKNOWLEDGMENT

All pictures are courtesy of Maine Medical Center, Portland, ME, Audiovisual Department and Lawrence Groton, photographer.

REFERENCES

1. Cyriax JH, Cyriax PJ: Cyriax's Illustrated Manual of Orthopaedic Medicine. Oxford; Butterworth-Heinemann, 1996.
2. Nirschl RP: Elbow Tendinosis/Tennis Elbow. Clinics in Sports Medicine 1992, Vol. 11, No. 4.
3. Puffer JA, Zachazewski JE: Management of overuse injuries. Am Fam Physician 38:225–232, 1988.
4. McRae R: Clinical Orthopedic Examination. New York, Churchill Livingstone, 1990.

Chapter 2 | Preparticipation Evaluation

I *Youth and Adolescent: History*

BOBBI (ROBERTA) PRIGGE, M.D.

The screening preparticipation examination primarily emphasizes the cardiac and musculoskeletal assessment in an effort to decrease the chance of injury and death during sports participation. Although the incidence of sudden death in high school athletes is low—estimated to be between 1 in 100,000 and 1 in 300,000—the death of a seemingly healthy young person is a devastating event. Unfortunately, there is no definitive way to identify the athlete at risk for sudden death, but preparticipation screening can identify some athletes at risk for injury, illness, or death. Approximately 7.6 percent of athletes screened require further evaluation, and approximately 1.3 percent of all potential athletes are restricted from participation.[1] Many athletes who are not cleared for one sport may be allowed to participate in other sports.

There are numerous recommendations about the adequate frequency and extent of evaluation necessary to clear an athlete for a particular sport. These recommendations vary from a complete evaluation prior to the start of each new season (i.e., multiple examinations each year for athletes in more than one sport), to annual examinations, to complete examinations with each new level of play (e.g., junior high, high school, college). Many advocate for the latter, along with a review of the medical history and interval injuries on an annual basis. There is no clear consensus on the most appropriate interval for screening. Currently, requirements are dictated by each state's high school governing organization. Some sports organizations also have specific requirements for how frequently the preparticipation evaluation should be conducted.

The preparticipation evaluation (PPE) allows physicians a unique opportunity to prevent injury and help athletes prepare for competition. At first glance, the PPE may seem like a mundane task of filling out paperwork to meet the requirements of state or sport organizations. However, if the physician focuses on the goals of the PPE and the opportunity it provides to make a significant impact on the lives and success of these athletes, it can be an enjoyable and rewarding experience for both athlete and physician.

GOALS

The goals of the PPE are to:

1. Identify any medical or musculoskeletal problems that may contribute to illness, injury, or death
2. Identify factors that may predispose the athlete to injury
3. Meet medical and legal requirements of states, sport organizations, or insurance companies

Although the PPE is not meant to take the place of routine health care for student athletes, it is often the only time many of them will see a physician. In fact, studies have shown that many athletes and parents plan to have the PPE be the athlete's only health care provider contact.[1, 2] Therefore, if time allows, secondary goals of the preparticipation evaluation should address issues of health care maintenance and counseling regarding risky behaviors. Many health care providers use this opportunity to discuss tobacco, alcohol, and drug use and sexual activity.

TIMING AND FORMAT

Ideally, the timing of the PPE is 6 to 8 weeks before the season starts. This allows time for evaluation, treatment, and rehabilitation, prior to the start of practice, of any condition identified during the screening examination. Many schools prefer to evaluate athletes involved in fall sports the preceding spring, before school is dismissed for the summer.

Two formats are used for the PPE. The first is the traditional office-based examination, which allows for continuity of care and ease of referral for further evaluation, if necessary. Athletes are more likely to discuss sensitive issues in this type of setting, especially if the examiner is the athlete's primary care provider. The PPE can be a part of the athlete's more comprehensive health care in this setting. Some drawbacks to this format include cost and time. Furthermore, some physicians have less experience in sports medicine and in detecting musculoskeletal abnormalities.

The other format is a multiple station format, which allows for the screening of many athletes efficiently and cost effectively by making use of a variety of providers at different stations. Athletic trainers, physical therapists, or coaches can test strength, flexibility, and body composition. Ancillary personnel can assist with height, weight, blood pressure, and vision screening. A physician reviews the medical history. Other physicians can conduct the medical and musculoskeletal evaluations. Finally, a physician reviews the findings from the various stations to determine if clearance can be given or if further evaluation is necessary. The down side of this format is that it often lacks continuity as well as privacy and the opportunity and time to discuss sensitive concerns.

HISTORY TAKING

The history component of the PPE is very important. Just as in other medical evaluations, the history often gives clues to the diagnosis. Approximately 78 percent of the problems requiring restriction and 74 percent that require further evaluation are identified in the history.[1] An effective way of obtaining a history is through a health questionnaire that the athlete can fill out and then review with the physician. Having the questionnaire available ahead of time so the athlete and parent can fill it out together improves the accuracy of the information.

The actual questions will vary depending on the questionnaire used but should address some basic categories. The following sections will briefly discuss each of the categories and will be followed by a list of possible questions. A good example of a questionnaire can be found in the monograph *Preparticipation Physical Examination,* 2nd edition, published by The Physician and Sportsmedicine and endorsed by the American Academy of Family Physicians, American Academy of Pediatrics, American Medical Society for Sports Medicine, American Orthopaedic Society for Sports Medicine, and American Osteopathic Academy of Sports Medicine.[3]

Underlying Medical Conditions

Underlying medical conditions may influence the athlete's ability to participate in athletics. In other instances a history of a chronic medical condition may put the athlete at risk for other problems, such as heat illness. In both cases, it is helpful for coaches, trainers, and team physicians to be aware of such conditions when working with the athlete. For example, a history of seizure disorder or the loss of one eye, or some other paired organ, may place the athlete at increased risk in certain sports. It is helpful for the coach, team physician, and trainer to know about a history of diabetes or seizure disorder in case an emergency event should happen during practice or competition. The athlete can be asked specific questions to elicit the history of a chronic problem. Asking about previous hospitalizations or surgery is meant to trigger the athlete's and parents' memory regarding any significant medical conditions. A history of prescription or over-the-counter medication use may disclose a chronic medical problem that the athlete might otherwise forget to mention. Certain medications (e.g., anticholinergics, beta-blockers, decongestants, diuretics) put athletes at increased risk for heat illness. Identifying this risk ahead of time allows for education of the athlete, parents, and coaches about heat illness prevention as well as the signs and symptoms of heat injury. The following questions may be useful:

Have you had any injuries or illnesses since your last examination?

Do you have any chronic medical problems or illnesses?

Have you ever had surgery?

Have you ever been hospitalized?

Do you take any medications (prescription or over the counter)?

Do you take any supplements or vitamins?

Do you have any problems with your vision?

Do you wear glasses or contact lenses?

Do you use any other protective or corrective equipment (for example, hearing aid or retainer)?

Cardiac Disease

Cardiac disease, primarily structural disease, is the most common cause of nontraumatic sudden death in young athletes. Careful attention to any symptoms suggestive of heart disease is one of the priorities of the health history. Unfortunately, most of the young athletes who die suddenly will not have any symptoms prior to their death. Only 18 percent of athletes, in one study, had any cardiovascular symptoms in the 36 months preceding death.[4] Important symptoms to consider in the history include syncope or near-syncope, chest pain on exertion, dyspnea on exertion, and palpitations or skipped heart beats. The most common cardiac condition that can lead to sudden death in young athletes is hypertrophic cardiomyopathy. This is followed by coronary artery abnormalities, ruptured aortic aneurysms (usually in association with Marfan syndrome), myocarditis, valve problems such as aortic stenosis, and atherosclerotic coronary artery disease (uncommon unless in the setting of familial hyperlipidemia).[4] A family history of premature sudden cardiac death is important to elicit because many of these problems have a genetic component. The American Heart Association believes that the PPE, with careful attention to the history, and cardiac examination are the best available and most practical approach to screening for cardiac disease.[5]

Relevant questions include the following:

Have you ever passed out while exercising?

Have you ever felt dizzy while exercising?

Have you ever had chest pain during exercise?

Have you ever been told you have high blood pressure or a heart murmur?

When exercising do you get tired more quickly than your friends?

Do you ever feel as if your heart is racing or skipping beats?

Has anyone in your family died suddenly before age 50? Before age 35?

Asthma and Allergies

Asthma and allergies can significantly impair an athlete's performance. Making sure that these conditions are optimally treated before the start of the season is in the best interest of the athlete. Although it is the responsibility of the athlete to have appropriate medications available during workouts and competition (for example, albuterol inhaler, EPI pen [epinephrine injection 1:1000]), many trainers, coaches, and team physicians will want to know of these conditions so they can also have appropriate medications available. Many athletes with exercise-induced asthma are undiagnosed. Asking about wheezing and coughing with exercise or dyspnea on exertion can help identify athletes with undiagnosed exercise-induced asthma.

Have you ever been diagnosed with asthma?

Do you have any allergies (medication, food, insect bites/stings, hayfever)?

Do you ever wheeze or cough during or after exercise?

When exercising do you get short of breath more than your friends?

Concussion or Neurologic Symptoms or Injury

Some neurologic conditions (for example, cervical stenosis or transient quadriparesis not adequately evaluated) may limit an athlete's participation in certain sports. Therefore, a review of neurologic injury is warranted. Furthermore, athletes who have had a concussion are at increased risk of a second concussion. The PPE can be a time to educate athletes about the signs and symptoms of minimal brain injury (MBI). If there is a history of MBI, further questioning can be done to evaluate the extent of injury (What type of symptoms did you have? How long did they persist? What were you told about further participation in contact sports?). A history of multiple concussions warrants further evaluation prior to clearance for contact sports. A history of a recent concussion warrants further questioning to determine that recovery is complete and that it is safe for the athlete to return to practice and competition.

Have you ever had a head injury or concussion?

Have you ever been unconscious or knocked out?

Have you ever had a seizure?

Have you ever had a burner, stinger, or pinched nerve?

Have you ever had numbness or tingling in your arms, hands, or feet?

Musculoskeletal Injuries

It is important to ensure adequate rehabilitation after an injury. If an athlete returns to participation without appropriate rehabilitation, he/she may be at risk for reinjury or secondary injury of another area. Ideally the PPE allows assessment of rehabilitative status prior to the start of the season. Asking about any special equipment is meant to lead to further questioning if the athlete has equipment but does not specify a history of injury to that area.

Have you ever had a sprain or strain?
Have you ever had a fracture or dislocation?
Do you wear any special equipment or braces (neck roll, knee brace, ankle brace, orthotics)?

Dermatologic Conditions

There are some dermatologic conditions that are spread among athletes, especially athletes in contact sports or who compete on mats (wrestling, gymnastics). Athletes with such conditions are not allowed to compete while the rash is in a contagious state unless adequate occlusion is maintained to prevent transmission. It is to the athlete's advantage to have any such lesions treated prior to the start of the season.

Do you have any skin problems currently (for example, rash, itching, fungal infection)?

Heat Illness

A history of prior heat illness is a risk factor for further heat injury. Because of the potential life-threatening nature of heat illness it is important to educate athletes about the signs and symptoms of heat injury and the steps that can be taken to prevent heat illness.

Have you ever had a heat injury, heat exhaustion, or heat stroke?
Do you get ill when you exercise in the heat?

General Health

Because the PPE often serves as the athlete's only contact with a physician and to avoid outbreaks of measles, it is important to ensure that immunizations are up to date.

When was your last tetanus, measles, mumps, rubella (MMR), hepatitis B immunization?

The Female Athlete Triad

An association between amenorrhea, eating disorders, and decreased bone density has been well documented in female athletes. Disordered eating is a very common problem in athletes. There are also concerns about weight loss tactics used by wrestlers. The following questions have been shown to be good screening tools for these problems:

What is the most you have weighed in the last year? The least? What is your ideal weight?
How old were you when you first started your menstrual periods?
How many periods did you have in the last year?

Other Health Concerns

This allows the athlete an opportunity to address any concerns about his/her health and often can be a tool to address some sensitive issues such as sexual activity and drug and alcohol use.

Do you have any particular concerns you would like to discuss?
Do you feel stressed?

It is important to remember that the PPE is a screening tool and a starting place for sports clearance. If any issues are raised on the history questionnaire that cannot be adequately evaluated with further questioning or during the physical examination, then further evaluation will be required. Having the athlete follow up with his/her primary physician or return at another time for further evaluation are appropriate options.

REFERENCES

1. Goldberg B, Saraniti A, Witman P, et al: Pre-participation sports assessment: An objective evaluation. Pediatrics 66(5):736–745, 1980.

2. Krowchuck D: The preparticipation athletic examination: A closer look. Pediat Ann 26(1):37–47, 1997.
3. American Academy of Family Physicians, American Academy of Pediatrics, American Medical Society for Sports Medicine, et al: Preparticipation Physical Evaluation, 2nd ed. Minneapolis, McGraw-Hill, 1996.
4. Maron BJ, Shirani J, Poliac L, et al: Sudden death in young competitive athletes. JAMA 276(3):199–204, 1996.
5. Maron B, Thompson P, Puffer J, et al: Cardiovascular preparticipation screening of competitive athletes. Circulation 94:850–856, 1996.

II *Youth and Adolescent: Physical Exam*
LARIK WORONZOFF, M.D.

Of the many parts of the preparticipation physical examination, the most important assessments involve the musculoskeletal and cardiac systems.[1] Musculoskeletal injuries are the most common sports-related injuries, and cardiac problems are the most common cause of exertional sudden death in athletes.

VITAL STATISTICS

Height and weight should be recorded. Physicians should be aware of potential weight issues attendant upon certain sports, from the well-known excessive weight loss in sports such as gymnastics and wrestling to the lesser-noted excessive weight gain in sports such as football.

Blood pressure and heart rate must be determined. Blood pressure should be measured with an appropriately sized cuff. Significant hypertension may be present if the following age-dependent values are exceeded:

- 6 to 9 years: 122/78 mm Hg
- 10 to 12 years: 126/82 mm Hg
- 13 to 15 years: 136/86 mm Hg
- Over 16 years: 140/90 mm Hg[2]

If blood pressure is elevated, a second measurement should be obtained after the patient rests quietly for 10 to 15 minutes. A careful history, with special attention to use of caffeine, nicotine, and medications, should be obtained.[1] If the blood pressure continues to be elevated, the athlete must

be reassessed at a future time or seen by his/her primary physician.

EYES

Visual acuity should be checked with a Snellen eye chart. Vision should be 20/40 or better in each eye with or without corrective lenses.[3] Anisocoria (unequal pupils) should be noted, especially if the athlete participates in contact or collision sports.[1] If an athlete is blind or has very poor vision in one eye, he/she should be counseled on the risks of participation and encouraged to use protective eyewear.[1, 3]

EARS, NOSE, AND THROAT

A general examination of ears, nose, and throat is sufficient unless abnormalities are noted, or the sport dictates a more specialized examination. The physician should be aware of specific findings that may signal the presence of disorders more prevalent in certain athletes. Examples include oral ulcers, gingival hyperplasia, and enamel erosion in bulimia (more common in gymnasts), the high arched palate of Marfan syndrome (more common in basketball and volleyball players), and oral lesions, including leukoplakia, in smokeless tobacco users (more common in baseball players).[1, 3]

CARDIAC FUNCTION

Radial and femoral pulses should be palpated, noting rhythm and strength. Absent or diminished femoral pulses may indicate coarctation of the aorta. The heart should be auscultated and any murmurs, extra heart sounds, abnormal beats, or abnormal rhythms noted. Murmurs should arouse suspicion if greater than II/VI (louder than S_1 and S_2), diastolic, or holosystolic.[2] Murmurs should also be auscultated using different techniques to screen for hypertrophic cardiomyopathy. Any murmur that gets louder with a Valsalva maneuver or quieter with techniques that increase left ventricular end-diastolic pressure (squatting) should arouse suspicion, and the athlete should be considered for echocardiogram and/or referral to a cardiologist.[3] Midsystolic murmurs have been noted in 30 to 80 percent of athletes, and third and fourth heart sounds (S_3 and S_4) are also heard in 50 percent of athletes.[4] Arrhythmias are occasionally heard and should be further evaluated with an electrocardiogram.[3]

PULMONARY FUNCTION

This part of the examination should include inspection for asymmetry and auscultation for wheezes, crackles, or rubs. This is an excellent time to discuss smoking issues.

ABDOMEN

The physician should inspect the abdomen for asymmetry or scars. Palpation should be performed, searching for hepatosplenomegaly, masses, rigidity, and tenderness.

GENITOURINARY EVALUATION

In screening PPEs, the genitalia are usually examined in men only.[3] The physician should note single or undescended testes, testicular masses or irregularities, and hernias.[3] Athletes with a single testicle should be counseled about risks and the need for protection, especially if they will be involved in contact or collision sports. Delayed development should be addressed in any female with delayed menarche (over 16 years old) or any male without secondary sexual characteristics by the age of 18.

MUSCULOSKELETAL SYSTEM

If there is no history of musculoskeletal injury, a general examination of the major joints (neck, back, shoulder, elbow, wrist, hip, knee, ankle) will suffice.[4] This general examination should include inspection for contour and symmetry, palpation, strength testing, and range of motion testing.[3] An example of an orthopedic screening examination is given in Table 2–1. If a history of injury is given, or if an abnormality is discovered during the general examination, a more detailed musculoskeletal examination should be performed. Also, the clinician may consider doing detailed musculoskeletal examinations for certain sports, such as shoulder examinations in throwers and swimmers or knee examinations in jumpers and football players.[4] Detailed musculoskeletal examinations for all asymptomatic athletes is time-consuming and produces a very low yield.[3]

NEUROLOGIC ASSESSMENT

A normal musculoskeletal screening examination obviates the need for a complete neurological ex-

Figure 2–1. The general musculoskeletal screening examination consists of the following: (1) inspection, athlete standing, facing toward examiner (symmetry of trunk, upper extremities); (2) forward flexion, extension, rotation, lateral flexion of neck (range of motion, cervical spine); (3) resisted shoulder shrug (strength, trapezius); (4) resisted shoulder abduction (strength, deltoid); (5) internal and external rotation of shoulder (range of motion, glenohumeral joint); (6) extension and flexion of elbow (range of motion, elbow); (7) pronation and supination of elbow (range of motion, elbow and wrist); (8) clench fist, then spread fingers (range of motion, hand and fingers); (9) inspection, athlete facing away from examiner (symmetry of trunk, upper extremities); (10) back extension, knees straight (spondylolysis/spondylolisthesis); (11) back flexion with knees straight, facing toward and away from examiner (range of motion, thoracic and lumbosacral spine; spine curvature; hamstring flexibility); (12) inspection of lower extremities, contraction of quadriceps muscles (alignment, symmetry); (13) "duck walk" four steps (motion of hip, knee, and ankle; strength; balance); (14) standing on toes, then on heels (symmetry, calf; strength; balance). (From Preparticipation Physical Evaluation, 2nd ed. The Physician and Sportsmedicine, a division of the McGraw-Hill Companies, Minneapolis, MN. Copyright © 1997, the McGraw-Hill Companies.)

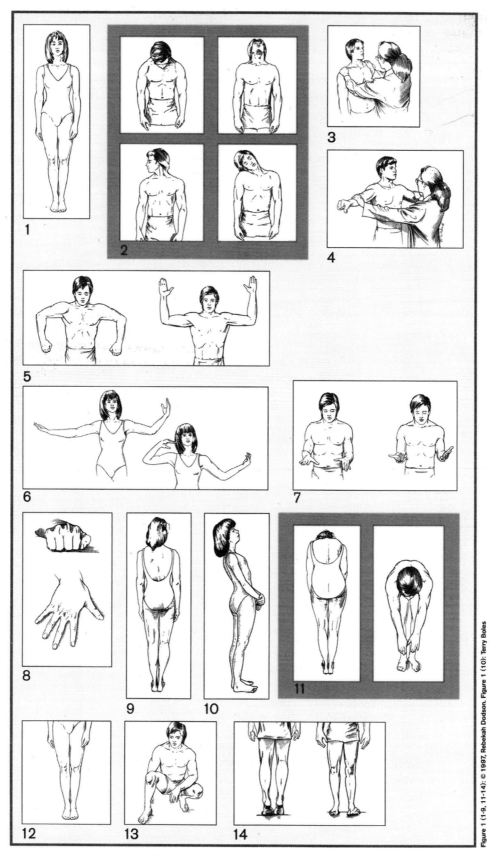

Figure 2–1. *See legend on opposite page*

Figure 1 (1-9, 11-14): © 1997, Rebekah Dodson. Figure 1 (10): Terry Boles

Table 2–1
The Two-Minute Orthopedic Examination

Instructions	Points of Observation
Stand facing examiner	Acromioclavicular joints, general habitus
Look at ceiling, floor, over both shoulders; touch ears to shoulders	Cervical spine motion
Shrug shoulders (examiner resists)	Trapezius strength
Abduct shoulders 90 degrees (examiner resists at 90 degrees)	Deltoid strength
Full external rotation of arms	Shoulder motion
Flex and extend elbows	Elbow motion
Arms at sides, elbows flexed 90 degrees; pronate and supinate wrists	Elbow and wrist motion
Spread fingers; make fist	Hand or finger motion and deformities
Tighten (contract) quadriceps; relax quadriceps	Symmetry and knee effusion; ankle effusion
"Duck walk" four steps (away from examiner with buttocks on heels)	Hip, knee, and ankle motion
Back to examiner	Shoulder symmetry, scoliosis
Knees straight, touch toes	Scoliosis, hip motion, hamstring tightness
Raise up on toes, raise heels	Calf symmetry, leg strength

Source: Sports Medicine: Health Care for Young Athletes, 2nd ed. American Academy of Pediatrics, Elk Grove Village, IL, 1991. Used with permission of the American Academy of Pediatrics.

amination.[3, 4] A history of a neurologic injury or problem, however, warrants further investigation. For example, in an athlete with a history of recurrent "burners" or "stingers" (neurapraxia of the brachial plexus due to compression or traction injury that is common in football), the clinician should check Sperling's test and perform a thorough upper extremity neurologic examination.

SKIN

The skin examination should include inspection for rashes, lesions, and infestations, particularly those that appear contagious or malignant.

OPTIONAL EVALUATIONS

Many aspects of the PPE are often included but can be considered optional. Body composition is sometimes checked using skin-fold measurement or submersion in water. Tanner stage for boys is used by some to assess physical maturity of the athlete. Its need has been questioned because athletes are grouped by age in athletics, not by physical maturity. Maturity is not used as a guideline for participation in collision or contact sports; however, the physician may choose to counsel physically immature athletes accordingly.[2] Fitness level (strength, flexibility, speed, agility, balance, endurance, power) can be checked if resources are available. Laboratory tests (for example, urinalysis, hemoglobin) are needed only if clinically indicated.[2, 5] Routine laboratory tests have been shown to be of little value.[2]

REFERENCES

1. Myers A, Sickles T: Preparticipation sports examination. Primary Care 25(1):225–236, March 1998.
2. Johnson RJ: The sports qualifying screening evaluation. Minnesota Fam Physician 14(2):11–14, Summer 1991.
3. Preparticipation Physical Evaluation Task Force: Preparticipation Physical Evaluation, 2nd ed. Minneapolis, The Physician and Sportsmedicine, McGraw-Hill, 1997.
4. Smith DM: The preparticipation physical exam. *In* Mellion MB, Walsh WM, Shelton GL (eds): The Team Physician's Handbook. Philadelphia, Hanley & Belfus, 1996.
5. Bratton RL: Preparticipation screening of children for sports. Sports Med (5): 300–307, Nov. 24, 1997.

III *Adult Assessment*
ROSEMARY GREENSLADE, M.D., M.S.

EXERCISE AND CARDIAC EVENTS: RISKS AND BENEFITS

Among people older than 35, probably 95 percent of exercise-related cardiac deaths are due to underlying coronary artery disease. Many reports of cardiovascular events during exercise have appeared in the medical and lay literature, suggesting that strenuous physical activity may precipitate myocardial infarction or sudden cardiac death in this age group.[1]

Although the risk of a serious cardiovascular event during exercise is low, it is higher during exercise than during sedentary activities. The overall risk/benefit ratio for a physically active lifestyle is favorable. A study by Siscovick et al.[2] found that the risk of exercise death actually decreases as people are more active, expressing the importance of exercise in primary prevention.

There is no evidence that exercisers with a healthy cardiovascular system are at risk of sudden cardiac death. It is important to emphasize that only people with underlying heart disease are at risk of an exercise-related cardiac event. Therefore, to identify people at risk for exercise-related cardiovascular complications, it is necessary to first identify those patients with underlying heart disease. Herein lies the dilemma.

The Exercise Stress Test: A Diagnostic Dilemma

Although the graded exercise stress test is considered the most valuable and practical tool for detecting coronary artery disease in symptomatic patients with chest pain, its diagnostic value for asymptomatic patients has been questioned.[3] For this group of individuals, the test has low sensitivity (many with disease will be missed) and poor specificity (many false-positive results). Even more important is a screening tool's positive predictive value. For exercise testing, this means the probability that an asymptomatic patient who tests positive will actually have the disease (coronary artery disease). Values as low as 21 percent have been reported in the literature,[4] and it appears that most in whom tests are positive do not have significant coronary artery disease.

The graded exercise test's poor performance as a screening tool may be due to the current concept that the degree of coronary narrowing is not necessarily related to the risk of sudden death. Critical lesions with 70 percent or greater occlusion frequently develop collaterals and the myocardium has adapted to the associated ischemia. The most dangerous lesions are those that are 30 to 60 percent occluded and develop fissures and abruptly rupture. Because only half of those who experience sudden cardiac death during exercise have prodromal symptoms, the most effective use of time and money may be educating patients about what heart disease feels like and alerting them to any unusual discomfort between their earlobes and umbilicus.

The Exercise Stress Test: Alternative Uses

Many have proposed that the exercise stress test be used as a maximal exercise tolerance evaluation.[3, 5] Several practical applications for testing asymptomatic adults are possible, including patient motivation to begin and or maintain an exercise program, fitness determination and risk assessment for this undertaking, as well as direct measurement of maximal heart rate and/or maximal oxygen consumption. The latter two variables can be used to calculate heart rate training intensity zones, which can be programmed into portable wrist heart rate monitors. Pulse and blood pressure response can be used to assess future risk of hypertension. Viewing the maximal exercise tolerance test as another risk factor for coronary artery disease allows physicians to reassure patients about the likelihood of a benign prognosis for an uneventful test, especially if they were able to attain their maximum predicted heart rate. It would be advisable to avoid labeling test results as either positive (coronary artery disease is present) or negative (coronary artery disease is not present) and instead to view the test as establishing and encouraging safe exercise parameters. This approach would avoid the tendency to create "cardiac cripples"[3] who abstain from exercise because of a "positive" test result. Also, those with a negative result will not be given a false sense of security and the impression that they have no risk.

PREPARTICIPATION SCREENING

Because no set of guidelines on exercise testing and participation can cover every individual patient scenario and because there is disagreement about the indications for exercise testing, the American College of Sports Medicine has provided some general guidance, which is summarized in Table 2–2 and in the following discussion.[6]

Healthy Individuals

Healthy individuals with no known or apparent underlying disease can begin a *moderate*-intensity (40 to 60 percent $\dot{V}O_{2\ max}$) exercise program such as walking, without a medical examination or exercise testing as long as they begin exercising slowly, progress gradually, and are alert to worrisome symptomatology. The individual should be able to sustain this level of moderate-intensity exercise comfortably for up to 60 minutes. *Vigorous* exercise (above 60 percent $\dot{V}O_{2\ max}$) is described as being a challenge, 13 or greater on the RPE (rating of perceived exertion) Borg scale of 20, and results in significant increases in heart rate and ventilatory rate. The level of intensity can be maintained only for approximately 15 to 20 minutes by an untrained individual. For men age 40 or above and women age 50 or above, a medical examination and physician-supervised maximal exercise test are recommended before a vigorous exercise program is begun. A submaximal test up to 75 percent of age-predicted maximal heart rate in apparently healthy patients of any age can be done without physician-supervision by well-trained or certified individuals. As already discussed, the information gathered and physiologic parameters measured from a maximal exercise test can still be very useful in helping these patients establish their target heart rate training zone and also monitor safe progression toward higher intensity zones.

Higher Risk Patients

Higher risk individuals include those with two or more of the following major coronary risk factors:

Table 2–2
Guidelines for Exercise Testing and Participation

	Apparently Healthy		Higher Risk*		
	Younger ≤40 years (men) ≤50 years (women)	Older	No Symptoms	Symptoms	With Disease†
Medical examination and diagnostic exercise test recommended prior to:					
Moderate exercise‡	No	No	No	Yes	Yes
Vigorous exercise#	No	Yes	Yes	Yes	Yes
Physician supervision recommended during exercise test:					
Submaximal testing	No	No	No	Yes	Yes
Maximal testing	No	Yes	Yes	Yes	Yes

*Persons with two or more risk factors or symptoms (see text).

†Persons with known cardiac, pulmonary, or metabolic disease.

‡Moderate exercise (exercise intensity 40 to 60% $\dot{V}O_{2\ max}$)—Exercise intensity well within the individual's current capacity and can be comfortably sustained for a prolonged period of time, i.e., 60 minutes, slow progression, and generally noncompetitive.

#Vigorous exercise (exercise intensity > 60% $\dot{V}O_{2\ max}$)—Exercise intense enough to represent a substantial challenge and which would ordinarily result in fatigue within 20 minutes.

Note: The "no" responses in this table mean that an item is not necessary. The "no" response does *not* mean that the item should not be done. A "yes" response means that an item is recommended.

Source: American College of Sports Medicine: Guidelines for Exercise Testing and Prescription, 4th ed. Philadelphia, Lea & Febiger, 1991, Table 1–3.

- Diagnosed hypertension
- Serum cholesterol at or above 240 mg/dl
- Cigarette smoking
- Diabetes mellitus (patients with insulin-dependent diabetes mellitus [IDDM] for longer than 15 years, or who are over age 30 and patients with non–insulin-dependent diabetes mellitus [NIDDM] over age 35 should be classified under "with disease" on Table 2–2).
- Family history of coronary or other atherosclerotic disease in parents or siblings prior to age 55.

Higher risk individuals also include those with metabolic disease (diabetes, thyroid, renal, and liver disease) and symptoms suggestive of cardiopulmonary disease including the following:

- Anginal type pain or discomfort in the chest, jaw, or arms
- Shortness of breath with mild exertion
- Dizziness or syncope
- Orthopnea or paroxysmal nocturnal dyspnea
- Palpitations or tachycardia
- Claudication
- Known heart murmur

An exercise test is recommended for higher risk patients of any age before starting a vigorous program and a maximal test for these patients should be physician supervised. For those patients with risk factors or disease who are symptom-free, moderate exercise may be undertaken gradually without a medical evaluation or an exercise test. These patients should monitor themselves for worrisome symptoms, which would warrant further evaluation. As discussed earlier, symptom-free patients may opt for exercise testing to establish target heart rate training zones, which are more accurately calculated with direct measurement of maximal heart rate.

Patients With Disease

A complete medical evaluation and stress testing prior to starting any exercise program is recommended for all patients with known cardiopulmonary, vascular, or metabolic disease. For primary care physicians doing exercise stress testing on lower risk patients, these individuals may warrant referral to a cardiologist, especially those with high risk of acute cardiovascular disease and possible death (unstable angina, recent myocardial infarction, cardiomyopathy, and the like). Several conditions (left bundle branch block, Wolf-Parkinson-White syndrome, pacemaker patients) preclude reliable diagnostic electrocardiographic information from exercise testing.[6] In patients with disease it is important to assess the safety of vigorous exercise, measure functional capacity to monitor progress, and use the stress test diagnostically to establish prognosis and need for further evaluation.

SUMMARY

Exercise stress testing is often used inappropriately as a screening device for cardiovascular disease in healthy, asymptomatic people, but this should not preclude its use for fitness assessment and exercise prescription in all groups of patients.

REFERENCES

1. Franklin S, Blaior H, Thompson VC: Exercise and cardiac complications: Do the benefits outweigh the risks. Physician Sports Med 22(2): 56–68, 1994.
2. Siscovick DS, Weiss HS, Fletcher RH, et al: The incidence of primary cardiac arrest during vigorous exercise. New Engl J Med 311(14): 874–877, 1984.
3. Johnson R: Assessing cardiac risk with exercise test. Your Patient and Fitness 7(1): 6–13, 1993.
4. Froehlicher VF, Maron B: Exercise testing and ancillary techniques to screen for coronary heart disease. Prog Cardiovasc Dis 14:261–274, 1981.
5. Thompson PD, Sherman C: Cardiovascular screening, tailoring the preparticipation exam. Physician Sports Med 24(6):47–106, 1996.
6. American College of Sports Medicine: Guidelines for Exercise Testing and Prescription, 4th ed. Philadelphia, Lea & Febiger, 1991.

Chapter 3 | The Exercise Prescription

I *Youth and Adolescent*
TODD L. KANZENBACH, M.D.

Physical fitness is very important to cardiovascular health, weight control, and prevention of certain diseases such as hypertension, diabetes mellitus, and hypercholesterolemia. Hypertension, diabetes mellitus, and hypercholesterolemia are more prevalent in obese patients and are important risk factors in coronary heart disease. Children are no exception; it follows that we should encourage good fitness traits at a young age. Studies show that over the last 30 years obesity in children has been steadily increasing, with a 54 percent increase in children ages 6 to 11 and a 39 percent increase in youth ages 12 to 17.[1] Many believe this increase is due to an increase in sedentary activities (for example, watching television, spending time on computers, playing computer games) and a decrease in physical activity. A national survey in 1984 found that approximately 50 percent of children, grades 5 through 12, were not participating in adequate physical activity as defined by the American College of Sports Medicine (ACSM). It is reasonable to assume that cardiovascular disease, diabetes mellitus, and other obesity-related diseases might increase in the future, as sedentary children become sedentary adults. It is then reasonable to assume that improving physical activity at a young age can lead to decreased illness in adulthood.

For children who are active, it is important to note that pediatric sports programs are increasing steadily. There are approximately 30 million children ages 6 to 21 involved in competitive sports, with younger children participating in major competitions. These facts, along with the motivation of potentially making large amounts of money in sports (even if this is unlikely), the number of sports programs is expected to increase.[2] However, it is crucial to realize that children are not miniature adults and would not necessarily benefit from the same exercise programs as adults.

EXERCISE AND ILLNESS

As children mature into adults, heart disease and diabetes become more prevalent, partly because of decreasing physical activity as they get older. It has been proved that physical inactivity is the most predictive single risk factor for heart disease in Americans than any other single risk factor.[3] Poor physical fitness has been found to be a factor in adult diseases such as coronary heart disease and diabetes mellitus, but fatty plaques have been found at autopsy even in the arterial walls of children and adolescents.[1] A recent study that evaluated childhood activity over the last 55 years showed that poor physical fitness combined with obesity in adolescence was a stronger predictor of an increased mortality rate from all causes, especially heart disease, than poor physical fitness and obesity in adulthood.[1]

EXERCISE AND TRAINING

Once a child is determined to be at high risk for coronary heart disease or presents with the intention to exercise, it is important that the care provider take into account the physiology of the child athlete. Children experience an increased metabolic cost during exertion, compared to adults, which results from an increased respiratory rate, more oxygen consumption per kilogram of body weight, and a higher stroke volume than an adult. Children have lower anaerobic capabilities, resulting from a decreased ability to utilize muscle glycogen and produce lactate.[4] They cannot generate the same amount of energy as adults can for similar activities. But, despite this deficit, children recover from anaerobic activity more quickly and also have less severe effects from strenuous activity compared with adults, due mainly to decreased lactate production. Children are, on the other hand, similar to adults with respect to aerobic capacity. It is crucial to know that children can also have problems with thermoregulation. They are not as efficient at cooling as adults; they sweat less and have a higher threshold for sweating.

Strength training is another fitness issue that

may be encountered by the physician. Strength training in children is controversial because the concept is not as well established in children as in adults. Studies have shown, however, that a well-structured program may be beneficial. As children grow, their strength increases and actually parallels their growth. As they train, they may experience an increase in strength but do not usually develop increased muscle hypertrophy or lean body mass. The pubescent's increase in strength usually is a result of myogenic adaptations (increased contractile proteins and enlarged and thickened connective tissue). The prepubescent child develops strength from neurogenic adaptations (improved recruitment of motor units, improved motor skills, and decreased inhibition). The neurogenic adaptations usually are better developed through lighter weights and increased repetitions.[4] Although strength parallels growth, the growing spurt does have its drawbacks. As the skeleton grows, the soft tissues (muscles, ligaments, and tendons) lag behind in their growth, leaving the child with poor flexibility and coordination. These facts, along with the risk of injury while weightlifting, make it imperative that the child receive appropriate instruction and supervision.

The risks of physical inactivity and disease prevention, as well as the difference between children and adults, have been discussed. The real challenge in designing an exercise program is finding an exercise regimen that is enjoyable and appealing to children.

EXERCISE AND TREATMENT

The importance of getting children to become more active has brought out recommendations from many organizations, including the following from the major medical organizations that have posted official statements.

The American Academy of Family Physicians (AAFP) and U.S. Preventive Services Task Force recommends that all patients, parents and children, receive exercise education and counseling on disease prevention.

The American Academy of Pediatrics (AAP) recommends the following assessment at each visit:

- Infancy: Parents are questioned about their child's motor development and activities.

Also, parents are encouraged to be role models for their children by participating in regular exercise.

- Preschool: Parents should encourage and support physical activity that is appropriate for the age group and developmental level of the child.
- School age: Physicians should encourage and advise the child to participate in regular physical activity and refrain from passive activities (i.e., television and video games). (Tables 3–1 and 3–2.)
- Adolescence: Perform routine sports preparticipation visits and encourage activity at other patient visits.

The ACSM recommends that health care professionals become more involved in promoting increased physical activity for children and youth. It also recommends that children engage in 20 to 30 minutes of physical activity each day to promote good health.[5] As children reach adulthood, the recommendations change slightly to recommending at least 30 minutes of cumulative activity of "perceived" moderate intensity most days of the week, preferably every day.[6]

The American Medical Association (AMA) recommends that adolescents receive annual counseling about exercise and its benefits.

These recommendations may appear simple and general, but physicians need to keep exercise

---

Table 3–1
Guidelines for Training a Child Athlete

Training sessions, 2 to 3/week
  Warm up (decreased risk of injury)
  Stretching
  Resistance/endurance exercise
  Fun/skill activity
Stretching
Cool down (increased lactate clearance during active recovery)
Adult prescriptions for aerobic exercise and strength training can be used (avoid extremes in exercise duration and intensity)
Avoid
  Prolonged monotonous activities
  Anaerobic training (concentrate on skill and movement patterns for anaerobic sports, such as basketball and soccer)
  High heat and humidity
  Be conservative, prescribe an easily tolerable program
  Have a high index of suspicion for injury
  Note any pain, especially back pain

Source: Cook PC, Leit ME: Issues in the pediatric athlete. Orthop Clin North Am 26(3):453–464, July 1995.

Table 3-2
Sample Strength Training Protocol

Determine appropriate starting weight
    Start with light weights and low repetitions
    Work on form and proper technique before progressing
      in the program
    Adjust weight until it can be lifted properly 10 times
      before fatigue occurs
Training
    1 or 2 sets of 10 to 15 repetitions with 2 to 3 rest
      periods two to three times per week
Increase weight
    When repetitions can be completed without fatigue and
      with good form
    Small, manageable increase in weights
    After 1 to 3 months of consistent training (2 or 3 days/
      week), add a third set of 10 to 15 repetitions

Source: Data from Grana WA: Strength training. *In* Stanitski CL, DeLee JC, Drez D Jr (eds): Pediatric and Adolescent Sports Medicine. Philadelphia, W.B. Saunders, 1994.

principles in mind when counseling patients. In fact, in one study, 4 out of 5 patients responding had never been told to exercise by their physician at patient visits. Physicians should advise and encourage physical activity at every opportunity.[7]

These activities should be enjoyable and fun for children in order for them to start and continue participation. It is imperative that the emphasis be on generally being active and not on doing "exercises." Preschool children generally are active enough and need only a safe environment and encouragement but not necessarily structure. The care provider should emphasize activities that can be continued through adulthood, such as tennis, hiking, swimming, canoeing, and bicycle riding, instead of merely emphasizing the "traditional" team sports activities.

Children with disabilities and disorders should be encouraged to participate in appropriate activities. Guidelines have been published by several committees and associations (Tables 3–3 and 3–4).

CONCLUSION

Decreased physical activity in children is an enormous health problem, and there is evidence it may be worsening. Evidence of atherosclerosis has been found in children, and it is thought that the incidence of diseases such as coronary heart disease, diabetes, and hypertension may be significantly reduced if children become more physically active. While encouraging such activity, do not think of children as "small adults"—their

Table 3-3
Medical Conditions Affecting Sports Participation

Condition	May Participate
Atlantoaxial instability (instability of the joint between first and second cervical vertebrae) *Explanation:* Athlete needs evaluation to assess risk of spinal cord injury during sports participation.	Qualified Yes
Bleeding disorder *Explanation:* Athlete needs evaluation.	Qualified Yes
Cardiovascular diseases	
Carditis (inflammation of the heart) *Explanation:* Carditis may result in sudden death with exertion.	No
Hypertension (high blood pressure) *Explanation:* Those with significant essential (unexplained) hypertension should avoid weight and power lifting, body building, and strength training. Those with secondary hypertension (hypertension caused by a previously identified disease) or severe essential hypertension need evaluation. Reference 4 defines significant and severe hypertension.	Qualified Yes
Congenital heart disease (structural heart defects present at birth) *Explanation:* Those with mild forms may participate fully; those with moderate or severe forms, or who have undergone surgery, need evaluation. Reference 3 defines mild, moderate, and severe disease for the common cardiac lesions.	Qualified Yes
Dysrhythmia (irregular heart rhythm) *Explanation:* Athlete needs evaluation because some types require therapy or make certain sports dangerous, or both.	Qualified Yes
Mitral valve prolapse (abnormal heart valve) *Explanation:* Those with symptoms (chest pain, symptoms of possible dysrhythmia) or evidence of mitral regurgitation (leaking) on physical examination need evaluation. All others may participate fully.	Qualified Yes

Table 3–3
Medical Conditions Affecting Sports Participation *Continued*

Condition	May Participate
Heart murmur *Explanation:* If the murmur is innocent (does not indicate heart disease), full participation is permitted. Otherwise the athlete needs evaluation (see discussion under congenital heart disease and mitral valve prolapse).	Qualified Yes
Cerebral palsy *Explanation:* Athlete needs evaluation.	Qualified Yes
Diabetes mellitus *Explanation:* All sports can be played with proper attention to diet, hydration, and insulin therapy. Particular attention is needed for activities that last 30 minutes or longer.	Yes
Diarrhea *Explanation:* Unless disease is mild, no participation is permitted, because diarrhea may increase the risk of dehydration and heat illness (see discussion under Fever).	Qualified No
Eating disorders Anorexia nervosa Bulimia nervosa *Explanation:* These patients need both medical and psychiatric assessment before participation can be allowed.	Qualified Yes
Eyes Functionally one-eyed athlete Loss of an eye Detached retina Previous eye surgery or serious eye injury *Explanation:* A functionally one-eyed athlete has a best corrected visual acuity of <20/40 in the worse eye. These athletes would suffer significant disability if the better eye was seriously injured as would those with loss of an eye. Some athletes who have previously undergone eye surgery or had a serious eye injury may have an increased risk of injury because of weakened eye tissue. Availability of eye guards approved by the American Society for Testing Materials (ASTM) and other protective equipment may allow participation in most sports, but this must be judged on an individual basis.	Qualified Yes
Fever *Explanation:* Fever can increase cardiopulmonary effort, reduce maximum exercise capacity, make heat illness more likely, and increase orthostatic hypotension during exercise. Fever may rarely accompany myocarditis or other infections that may make exercise dangerous.	No
Heat illness, history of *Explanation:* Because of the increased likelihood of recurrence, the athlete needs individual assessment to determine the presence of predisposing conditions and to arrange a prevention strategy.	Qualified Yes
HIV infection *Explanation:* Because of the apparent minimal risk to others, all sports may be played that the state of health allows. In all athletes, skin lesions should be properly covered, and athletic personnel should use universal precautions when handling blood or body fluids with visible blood.	Yes
Kidney: absence of one *Explanation:* Athlete needs individual assessment for contact/collision and limited contact sports.	Qualified Yes
Liver: enlarged *Explanation:* If the liver is acutely enlarged, participation should be avoided because of risk of rupture. If the liver is chronically enlarged, individual assessment is needed before collision/contact or limited contact sports are played.	Qualified Yes
Malignancy *Explanation:* Athlete needs individual assessment.	Qualified Yes
Musculoskeletal disorders *Explanation:* Athlete needs individual assessment.	Qualified Yes

Table continued on following page

Table 3–3
Medical Conditions Affecting Sports Participation *Continued*

Condition	May Participate
Neurologic	Qualified Yes
History of serious head or spine trauma, severe or repeated concussions, or craniotomy.	
Explanation: Athlete needs individual assessment for collision/contact or limited contact sports, and also for noncontact sports if there are deficits in judgment or cognition. Recent research supports a conservative approach to management of concussion.	
Convulsive disorder, well controlled	Yes
Explanation: Risk of convulsion during participation is minimal.	
Convulsive disorder, poorly controlled	Qualified Yes
Explanation: Athlete needs individual assessment for collision/contact or limited contact sports. Avoid the following noncontact sports: archery, riflery, swimming, weight or power lifting, strength training, or sports involving heights. In these sports, occurrence of a convulsion may be a risk to self or others.	
Obesity	Qualified Yes
Explanation: Because of the risk of heat illness, obese persons need careful acclimatization and hydration.	
Organ transplant recipient	Qualified Yes
Explanation: Athlete needs individual assessment.	
Ovary: absence of one	Yes
Explanation: risk of severe injury to the remaining ovary is minimal.	
Respiratory	Qualified Yes
Pulmonary compromise including cystic fibrosis	
Explanation: Athlete needs individual assessment, but generally all sports may be played if oxygenation remains satisfactory during a graded exercise test. Patients with cystic fibrosis need acclimatization and good hydration to reduce the risk of heat illness.	
Asthma	Yes
Explanation: With proper medication and education, only athletes with the most severe asthma will have to modify their participation.	
Acute upper respiratory infection	Qualified Yes
Explanation: Upper respiratory obstruction may affect pulmonary function. Athlete needs individual assessment for all but mild disease (see discussion under Fever).	
Sickle cell disease	Qualified Yes
Explanation: Athlete needs individual assessment. In general, if status of the illness permits, all but high exertion, collision/contact sports may be played. Overheating, dehydration, and chilling must be avoided.	
Sickle cell trait	Yes
Explanation: It is unlikely that individuals with sickle cell trait (AS) have an increased risk of sudden death or other medical problems during athletic participation except under the most extreme conditions of heat, humidity, and possibly increased altitude. These individuals, like all athletes, should be carefully conditioned, acclimatized, and hydrated to reduce any possible risk.	
Skin: boils, herpes simplex, impetigo, scabies, molluscum contagiosum	Qualified Yes
Explanation: While the patient is contagious, participation in gymnastics with mats, martial arts, wrestling, or other collision/contact or limited contact sports is not allowed. Herpes simplex virus probably is not transmitted via mats.	
Spleen: enlarged	Qualified Yes
Explanation: Patients with acutely enlarged spleens should avoid all sports because of risk of rupture. Those with chronically enlarged spleens need individual assessment before playing collision/contact or limited contact sports.	
Testicle: absence of or undescended	Yes
Explanation: Certain sports may require a protective cup.	

Source: Used with permission from the American Academy of Pediatrics, Committee on Sports Medicine and Fitness. Medical conditions affecting sports participation. Pediatrics 94(5):757–760, 1994.

Table 3–4
Classification of Sports by Contact

Contact/Collision	Limited Contact	Noncontact
Basketball	Baseball	Archery
Boxing*	Bicycling	Badminton
Diving	Cheerleading	Body building
Field hockey	Canoeing/kayaking (white water)	Bowling
Football	Fencing	Canoeing/kayaking (flat water)
Flag	Field	Crew-rowing
Tackle	High jump	Curling
Ice hockey	Pole vault	Dancing
Lacrosse	Floor hockey	Field
Martial arts	Gymnastics	Discus
Rodeo	Handball	Javelin
Rugby	Horseback riding	Shot put
Ski jumping	Racquetball	Golf
Soccer	Skating	Orienteering
Team handball	Ice	Power lifting
Water polo	Inline	Race walking
Wrestling	Roller	Riflery
	Skiing	Rope jumping
	Cross-country	Running
	Downhill	Sailing
	Water	Scuba diving
	Softball	Strength training
	Squash	Swimming
	Ultimate frisbee	Table tennis
	Volleyball	Tennis
	Windsurfing/surfing	Track
		Weightlifting

*Participation not recommended.

Source: Used with permission from the American Academy of Pediatrics, Committee on Sports Medicine and Fitness. Medical conditions affecting sports participation. Pediatrics 94(5):757–760, 1994.

physiology is different, their emotions and motivation are different, they respond to exertion differently, and they are more prone to injury during puberty. Although our society strongly encourages competitive sports, it is important that the activities for the majority of children and adolescents are encouraged more for enjoyment, physical fitness, and disease prevention than for competition.

REFERENCES

1. U.S. Public Health Service: Physical activity in children. Am Fam Physician 50(6):1285–1288, Nov. 1, 1994.
2. Dyment PG (ed): Sports Medicine: Health Care for Young Athletes, 2nd ed. Chapter 11, Epidemiology and prevention of sports injuries. American Academy of Pediatrics, Elk Grove Village, IL, 1991, pp. 146–171.
3. Healthy People 2000: National Health Promotion and Disease Prevention Objectives. Washington, D.C., Dept. of Health and Human Services, Public Health Service, 1990. DHHS Publication No. (PHS) 91-50213.
4. Cook PC, Leit ME: Issues in the pediatric athlete. Orthop Clin North Am 26(3):453–464, July 1995.
5. American College of Sports Medicine: Physical fitness in children and young. Med Sci Sports Exerc 20:422–423, 1988.
6. Pate RR, Pratt M, et al: Physical activity and public health. A recommendation from the Centers for Disease Control and Prevention and the American College of Sports Medicine. JAMA 273:402–407, 1995.
7. Shephard RJ: Fitness of a nation: Lessons from the Canada Fitness Survey. New York, S. Karger, 1986, pp. 133–181.

II *Adult*
STEPHEN R. BINDNER, M.D.

Society has changed dramatically in the last 100 years. Along with all the great technological and medical advancements has come a shift in lifestyles and employment, changing from heavy labor to service industries, which are for the most part sedentary. The average person in Western society is eating better and becoming overall less active. This trend has led to epidemic levels of obesity and all the associated diseases that follow. In order to consider the component of the exercise prescription this chapter will first outline the key aspects of the problem and then discuss some of the strategies for bringing a change in the quality of patients' lives.

MAJOR ILLNESSES AND EXERCISE

Vascular System

Cardiovascular disease, which is still the number one cause of death in the industrialized world, can be attributed to many factors. One reason stems from the eating habits of modern society, which too often include high-fat meals and snacks with large portions. This trend, along with often-stressful schedules, sedentary jobs, and leisure inactivity, has contributed to rising rates of obesity. Of all the things that contribute to heart disease, inactivity and obesity are the most pertinent to this chapter. Studies have shown that inactivity and obesity put patients at risk for sudden cardiac death, atherosclerosis, hypertension, and stroke.[1]

Inactivity by itself without considering obesity accounts for doubling the risk of coronary artery disease.[2] With up to 60 percent of the U.S. population being inactive, this risk factor is more prevalent than smoking, hypertension, and elevated cholesterol. Just as inactivity contributes to cardiovascular disease, increased activity has been found to prevent and modify pervasive atherosclerosis.[1] Part of this effect is due to an increase in heart size and function and increased coronary vessel size with formation of collateral vessels. Exercise has also been found to decrease systolic blood pressure,[3] decrease low-density lipoprotein cholesterol levels, and increase high-density lipoprotein cholesterol levels.[4, 5]

One of the concerns with using exercise to treat cardiovascular disease or just encouraging a healthy lifestyle is the risk of sudden cardiac death. Death from exercise in adults under the age of 30 is most commonly due to hypertrophic cardiomyopathy. Sudden cardiac death after the age of 30 is overwhelmingly due to coronary artery disease. People who are mostly sedentary and exert themselves only periodically are at the greatest risk of sudden cardiac death. By developing an active lifestyle, people lessen their risk of sudden cardiac death overall, although they are at risk while they are exercising. But because the time spent at that level of exertion is minimal, the overall risk is lower.[6]

The points to emphasize with patients regarding increasing their physical activity are that it will reduce the risk of an early death, reduce risk of atherosclerosis and heart disease, lessen chances of angina, prevent and treat hypertension, and improve blood lipid profiles.

Osteoarthritis

The major factors that contribute to osteoarthritis are genetics, obesity, a history of joint injury, neurologic deficits, abnormal joint kinetics or anatomy, and muscle weakness. There is a stronger association with arthritis and being overweight in women.[7] A twin study revealed a 9 to 13 percent increased risk for osteoarthritis for every kilogram increase in weight.[8] Obviously, many factors can combine to increase the chance of an individual developing osteoarthritis and of its being severe. For example, a lineman from the NFL who has had meniscal injuries in his youth, has been overweight his whole life, and has adopted a sedentary lifestyle later in life will be at increased risk for osteoarthritis.

Many patients have concerns that repetitive impact exercises such as running will cause joint degeneration. However, both animal studies and human studies of long distance runners have shown that the activity actually stabilizes the articular cartilage matrix and strengthens the muscles that provide shock absorption for the joint. On the other hand, sports that involve torsional forces and high impact are more likely to increase the chance of developing osteoarthritis. These factors should be considered when individualizing an exercise prescription. Exercises that involve low torsion and impact are walking, using stationary exercise equipment, and swimming. Examples of moderate impact activity are downhill skiing, running, aerobics, in-line skating, and weight lifting. The court, field, and racquet sports along with water skiing, and competitive running are in the class of high-impact sports.

Diabetes Mellitus

The most important fact to remember about diabetes is that exercise equals insulin. This fact is important as we consider how diabetes has become more prevalent in our society and when we try to treat elevated blood sugar levels. Obesity is a problem associated with type II diabetes. Type II diabetes is thought to involve abnormalities in insulin secretion, absorption, and sensitivity along with abnormalities in glucose secretion from the liver. Inactivity and associated obesity are thought to contribute to less responsiveness of the beta cells of the pancreas to stimulation by increased serum glucose and to the decrease in insulin receptors on target cells that are responsible for transporting glucose into the cells. Studies have shown that the risk of getting diabetes increases by 25 percent for every unit over a body mass index of 22 kg/m^2. Also, it is a major risk factor if the weight is concentrated in the abdominal region.[1]

If the efforts of physicians and their patients to prevent type II diabetes have failed, then once it occurs, it is important to include exercise as part of a treatment plan. Exercise is helpful in both the acute response, acting like insulin in transporting glucose into the cells,[9] and the chronic adaptation phase, which leads to weight loss. In non–insulin-dependent type II diabetics not on oral hypoglycemics, exercise cannot be overdone with regard to problems with hypoglycemic reactions. However, in the diabetic on an oral agent or insulin, care must be taken not to vary the exercise program too much and to include more frequent monitoring of blood sugar levels.

Cancer

The risk of developing breast cancer decreases by 60 percent in women who are physically active.[10]

Many of the other associations with activity and cancer are through the link of obesity. Multiple studies have revealed a correlation between obesity and colon cancer (in men and women), breast cancer, endometrial cancer, and gallbladder cancer.[11]

Psychological Disorders

At the foundation of many of the psychological problems related to obesity is the Western ideal of being thin. It is ironic that in this environment obesity rates have increased. Some of the fall-out of this problem is disordered eating behaviors such as binge eating, anorexia nervosa, and abnormal purging behavior seen in bulimia nervosa. Much of this stems from the population's attempt to conform to an image of thinness and from a lower regard for health. Unrelated to the thin obsession, it is important to recognize obesity and lack of activity as markers for diseases such as depression and schizophrenia. Often it is necessary to treat the depression to be successful in treating the obesity. Overall, patients who exercise will find an improved quality of sleep, less depression, improved cognitive functioning, improved stress management, and overall improved self-esteem whether they have a diagnosed mental problem or just suffer from the stresses of daily life.

Weight Management and Obesity

When discussing obesity in the United States, the focus often is on weight. Some patients refuse to be weighed when they check in for an office visit. Other patients claim they would rather smoke cigarettes than have to deal with the dreaded weight gain. However, it is more important to emphasize the need for physical activity and its benefits than to dwell on pounds. In general, it is the goal of the physician to help patients become more healthy by halting weight gain, increasing their amount of activity, and promoting a low-fat diet.

There are many ways to advise patients on weight loss or obesity. The simplest way is to use height and weight tables that give a general range of an "ideal weight." The fault in these tables is the lack of consideration of genetic body type and body composition. Recently, the standard for defining what is considered being overweight has changed. In the recent report from the NIH, *Clinical Guidelines on the Identification, Evaluation, and Treatment of Overweight and Obesity in Adults,*[1] the threshold for being overweight was lowered to a body mass index (BMI) of 25. The BMI gives a general reference range for weight based on height. It is calculated as weight (in pounds) divided by the height (in inches) squared. This fraction is multiplied by the constant 704.5. Any number under 18.5 is considered underweight, 18.5 to 24.9 is normal, 25 to 29.9 is overweight, 30 to 39.9 is obesity, and any number greater than 40 is morbid obesity. Again, this tool correlates without regard to body type or percentage of lean muscle mass. However, these tables and calculations are useful when counseling those who are chronically inactive in whom the excess weight can often be inferred to be excess fat.

The next most simple and useful tool that is underutilized in the doctor's office is checking waist circumference. The measurements determined from the NIH data set an increased relative risk and morbidity for waist circumference greater than 40 inches in men and 35 inches in women. These measurements are most useful in counseling patients in the BMI range of 25 to 35 kg/m².

The most accurate way to assess for obesity is to determine the percentage of body fat. The general accepted standards for men are 20 to 25 percent fat as borderline obese, and anything greater than 25 percent fat as obese. For women, the numbers are 30 to 35 percent for borderline obese and greater than 35 percent for obese. The methods for calculating these measurements are many. The gold standard has long been the use of measuring body weight while immersed in water and comparing this to the scale weight. Then, correcting for the density of water and the air in the gastrointestinal tract and lungs, the volume of the body is calculated and is compared to standards of body composition. The most widely used tool in health clubs, training rooms, and physician offices is the fat caliper. This tool measures skin folds from multiple sites. These numbers are plugged into standardized equations along with the measured weight, yielding a percentage fat composition. The accuracy of this method is ±3 percent. The accuracy varies with the skill of the examiner. A newer form of measurement that is being used in health clubs is an infrared tool that calculates total body composition based on a biceps measurement of reflected electromagnetic radiation. Some other tools are bioelectric impedance, magnetic resonance imaging, and other complex radiographic techniques that are not as cost effective as the other techniques available.

One of the new controversies in the field of weight management is the concept of the fat and fit. The argument is based on the premise that much of the data for obesity does not take into account activity level. Some preliminary data from Dr. Steven Blair, Director of Epidemiology and Clinical Applications at the Cooper Institute for Aerobics Research, has shown that men who were fat and aerobically fit had lower death rates than men with normal weights who were inactive. From this it is reasonable to emphasize to inactive, obese patients that the first step in healthy living is to be active. If they then build on this base and balance increased energy expenditure with calorie restriction, the fat (and weight) will come off.

When counseling patients who have both a higher than normal amount of lean muscle mass and adipose tissue for their particular BMI, it is useful to calculate the ideal body weight based on an ideal percentage of body fat for their particular lean muscle mass (Table 3–5).

FORMULATING THE PRESCRIPTION

The first part of this chapter has discussed reasons why an exercise prescription is necessary. This next section will dwell on the prescription itself, that is, the actual behavior patients might adopt to live healthier lives. This prescription will entail recommendations regarding aerobic training, resistance training, flexibility, and weight control.

For a long time the American College of Sports Medicine (ACSM) and the American Heart Association recommended a minimum of 20 minutes of aerobic exercise 3 times a week raising

Table 3–5
Calculating Desired Body Weight

Step 1 100% − fat % = lean body weight percentage
Step 2 Body weight × lean body weight percentage = lean body weight
Step 3 100 − desired percentage body fat = desired lean body weight percentage
Step 4 Lean body weight/desired lean body weight percentage = desired body weight

the heart rate up to 70 to 85 percent of the age-adjusted maximum heart rate. In 1996, the NIH and ACSM released new recommendations.[12] After examining the bulk of relevant literature regarding physical activity and cardiovascular health, they concluded that the goal for both children and adults should be to accumulate 30 minutes of physical activity per day, most days of the week. This change in thinking suggests this activity need not occur in one sitting or be in the form of running, biking, or swimming. Activity can be accumulated through two 10-minute walks and 10 minutes of gardening, for example. The thought behind this approach is that it might encourage people who hesitate to exercise to begin performing the bare minimum of activity that is thought to give cardiovascular benefit.

There is still benefit with the old recommendations in that the more vigorous the activity, the better the cardiovascular health. HDL cholesterol will increase and blood pressure will decline. The new guidelines are a way of encouraging those who are inactive to find simple ways to change. The key to the guidelines is to assess where a patient's activity level is, what the outcome is that you are trying to produce, and what can be done to alter activity for the better. For example, a 50-year-old male with a family history of heart disease, borderline hypertension, and a BMI of 31 who already fulfills the 30-minutes-a-day requirement might benefit from the next step of adding vigorous exercise 20 minutes 3 times a week.

The aforementioned patient brings up the question of when it is necessary for patients to consult a physician before starting an activity program. Data from the ACSM (1991) states that if someone will be performing activity that will keep the heart rate under 60 percent of the maximum heart rate, medical clearance is probably not necessary.[13] This recommendation presumes the activity is undertaken gradually, does not involve competition, and is within the patient's capability. However, if more vigorous activity is desired, then certain people should be evaluated. This group includes men over 40, women over 50, and anyone with a major cardiovascular risk factor: hypertension, diabetes mellitus, hyperlipidemia, family history of early cardiac death or atherosclerosis, and cigarette smoking. The usual tool of medical clearance is the stress ECG with or without echocardiography. Second and third benefits of doing a stress test are that the information is useful when developing the specifics of the prescription and

it serves as a tool for motivation by measuring progress.

A discussion of aerobic fitness would not be complete without mentioning some of the specific tools for measuring aerobic activity. Aerobic capacity is the maximum capability of the body to transport and utilize oxygen. Aerobic exercise uses large muscle groups in a continuous and rhythmic manner. Oxygen uptake is defined as the $\dot{V}O_2$ = heart rate × systemic vascular difference (arterial − venous oxygen) with the $\dot{V}O_{2\,max}$ being the maximum capability of the oxygen transport system. Measuring the $\dot{V}O_{2\,max}$ can be a guide for assessing a patient's cardiovascular fitness, although it is used mainly for athletes and research purposes and is impractical for the general population.

The next easiest tool for measuring exercise intensity is the heart rate. The maximum heart rate is found by subtracting the subject's age from 220. The target heart rate is then a percentage of the maximum heart rate, with different ranges for different levels of training intensity. These calculations are useful when guiding the intensity of workouts for cardiovascular fitness (short bouts of 70 to 85 percent intensity) of calorie and fat burning (long bouts at 50 to 65 percent intensity).

The easiest tool for guiding exercise intensity is perceived exertion. This method requires people to rate their exercise or activity on a scale of easy to very hard. It has been found that if someone exercises at a certain intensity and assigns a subjective value (a rating of that perceived exertion), the level of perceived exertion is accurately reproduced at a subsequent exercise bout. If one matches a desired heart rate with that exertion level on a stress test, the patient is able to duplicate that level of exertion when exercising independently in a wide variety of activities.

Often when primary care physicians develop an exercise prescription, they concentrate only on aerobic fitness. Although this aspect is the most important, it is not the only concern. Most jobs in modern society do not require significant strength or use of most major muscle groups. Just as automobiles have eliminated walking as a source of remaining fit, so has the sedentary employment of most U.S. citizens weakened the musculoskeletal system. The benefits of strength training include increasing muscle mass for increased calorie expenditure,[14] decreased bone loss in women after menopause, a favorable effect on lipid profiles, possible reduction in resting blood pressures, and increased insulin sensitivity and glucose tolerance. Just as with other forms of increased activity there is improved self-esteem and confidence. And last, for the elderly, there is improved function with a decrease in falls and fewer fractures when a fall does occur.

The amount of strength training to provide the preceding benefits is not the same as needed to "bulk up" for competitive sports participation. All that is needed is a twice-weekly regimen that uses all the major muscles. Each session should include two sets of exercises for each muscle group. Each set should consist of 8 to 12 repetitions at a load to challenge and fatigue the muscle. It is not necessary to do multiple exercises for the same muscle group, although it is reasonable to provide variety to minimize boredom.

Many hesitate to start a program for a variety of reasons (Table 3–6). It is important to counsel patients that they should not expect huge muscle gains from this limited workout. The initial increases in strength in the first month of a program are due to neurologic adaptation of the neuromuscular system and improved recruitment of motor units.

The third area that deserves mentioning is flexibility and stretching. These are important in preventing injuries while exercising and performing various activities of daily life. It is best to stretch after the muscles have been warmed up to minimize injury risk. It is also vital to do long controlled stretches without bouncing. Bouncing (ballistic stretch) can cause tearing of the muscle tissue.

Table 3–6
Common Excuses for Not Exercising and Possible Solutions

Excuses	Solutions
I don't know how	Personal trainer
	Community center classes
	Learn from friends
	Watch instructive video tapes
I may get injured	Lift with a friend and spotter
I don't like free weights	Use machines
I don't like gyms	Purchase second hand equipment
I can't afford it	Make weights out of household products
It's boring	Lift with a friend
	Lift while watching TV or listening to music

GIVING THE PRESCRIPTION

No matter how convinced doctors are of the benefits, the key to a successful exercise program is getting the patient to accept the need for change. The first step is to assess the patient's current activity level and the willingness to change. A good resource for patients is the book *Changing for Good* by James Prochaska, John Norcross, and Carlo DiClemente. If the patient is in a *precontemplation phase* and satisfied with the inactive status, it is important to review the facts of how changes in activity will be of benefit. Many people enter the contemplation phase with the sole purpose of losing weight. This goal then becomes an important part of the plan. It is important in these patients to emphasize the dual role of increased activity and decreased food consumption as the best way to lose pounds and keep them off.

The next phase is the *preparation phase,* in which the patient actually develops a plan to make the necessary changes. This is a good time to introduce the mnemonic of IFIT, which stands for *in*dividuality, *f*requency, *in*tensity, and *t*ime. When starting someone on an exercise program, it is most important to understand the patient's individual history, goals, and previous failures. This information facilitates a focused plan.

The next step is establishing frequency. In someone who has always been relatively inactive, it is first necessary to develop a routine. Once a daily routine is established, the patient can start increasing the duration of the exercise. When that is accomplished, an increase in intensity may be implemented to reduce monotony and increase the cardiovascular benefit.

A valuable supplement to this phase is the use of a journal. People who log their exercise and correlate the activity with their diet typically do a better job. It allows them to see how well they are balancing energy in and energy out. This is also useful in the next phase of action as the plan evolves to fit the patient's changing goals. Last, program maintenance ensures that the patient accept the changes as part of his/her identity.

Another model for encouraging activity is an adaptation of the diet pyramid—the exercise pyramid, introduced by Jane Norstrom (Fig. 3–1). The exercise pyramid involves promoting good activities and limiting inactivity. It advocates establishing a base of activity. Once the base is established more activities are added for variety, fun, and improved benefit.

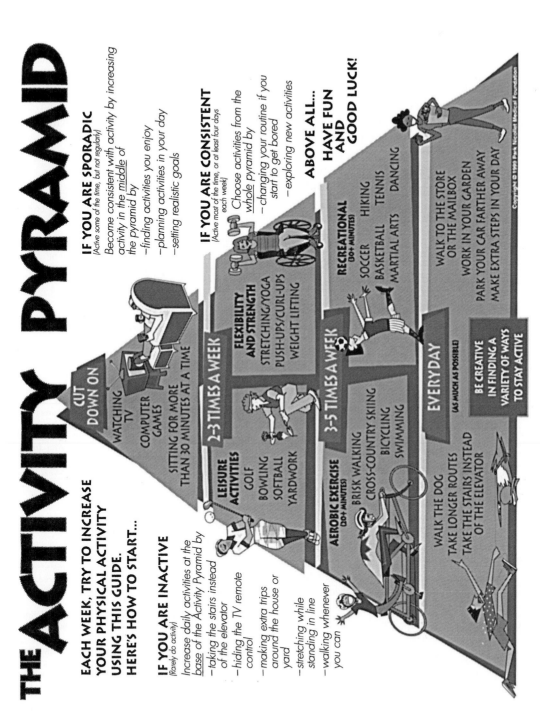

THE ACTIVITY PYRAMID

EACH WEEK, TRY TO INCREASE YOUR PHYSICAL ACTIVITY USING THIS GUIDE. HERE'S HOW TO START...

IF YOU ARE INACTIVE
(Rarely do activity)

Increase daily activities at the base of the Activity Pyramid by
– taking the stairs instead of the elevator
– hiding the TV remote control
– making extra trips around the house or yard
– stretching while standing in line
– walking whenever you can

IF YOU ARE SPORADIC
(Active some of the time, but not regularly)

Become consistent with activity by increasing activity in the middle of the pyramid by
– finding activities you enjoy
– planning activities in your day
– setting realistic goals

IF YOU ARE CONSISTENT
(Active most of the time, or at least four days each week)

Choose activities from the whole pyramid by
– changing your routine if you start to get bored
– exploring new activities

ABOVE ALL...
HAVE FUN AND GOOD LUCK!

CUT DOWN ON
WATCHING TV
COMPUTER GAMES
SITTING FOR MORE THAN 30 MINUTES AT A TIME

2-3 TIMES A WEEK

FLEXIBILITY AND STRENGTH
STRETCHING/YOGA
PUSH-UPS/CURL-UPS
WEIGHT LIFTING

LEISURE ACTIVITIES
GOLF
BOWLING
SOFTBALL
YARDWORK

3-5 TIMES A WEEK

AEROBIC EXERCISE
(20+ MINUTES)
BRISK WALKING
CROSS-COUNTRY SKIING
BICYCLING
SWIMMING

RECREATIONAL
(20+ MINUTES)
SOCCER   HIKING
BASKETBALL   TENNIS
MARTIAL ARTS   DANCING

EVERYDAY
(AS MUCH AS POSSIBLE)
WALK THE DOG
TAKE LONGER ROUTES
TAKE THE STAIRS INSTEAD OF THE ELEVATOR
WALK TO THE STORE OR THE MAILBOX
WORK IN YOUR GARDEN
PARK YOUR CAR FARTHER AWAY
MAKE EXTRA STEPS IN YOUR DAY

BE CREATIVE IN FINDING A VARIETY OF WAYS TO STAY ACTIVE

Figure 3–1. Park Nicollet exercise pyramid. (From Park Nicollet HealthSource, Minneapolis, Minnesota. Copyright © 1999, Park Nicollet Medical Foundation.)

One of the first things to mention when giving an exercise prescription is to make a distinction between exercise and activity. Most people still have the impression that changing their activity level must entail an "exercise program" in which they must run laps around the track or sit on a boring stationary bicycle staring at a wall. The first hurdle is to emphasize the need to limit habits of inactivity.

One of the worst forms of inactivity is watching television. The odds of being overweight are 4.6 times greater for children who watch more than 5 hours of television per day compared with those who watch less than 2 hours per day.[15] One of the paradoxes in modern society is the advertising of fast, convenient, and high-calorie fatty foods by professional athletes urging the public to "supersize" it. Although professional athletes who are 7 feet tall and burn 6000 calories a day may be able to eat that type of diet, the general population is getting fatter by the day.

The reasons for patients to exercise are well established. The trick is convincing patients of the importance of activity for overall health. Once convinced, they need help to start, build, and maintain a program. The basic principles are to start slow, individualize, tap into social support (buddy system, significant other, employer), advocate planning and logging, and implement aggressive follow-up.

Physicians must be conscious of their personal role in their patients' fitness. What type of role models are they? Do they give the same excuse, claiming, "I'm too busy to exercise?" Do they fall victim to the "eat when you can" philosophy, which usually involves poorly planned, high-fat meals? Physicians also need to be in touch with their attitudes toward sedentary patients. Patients sense disapproval. As with all aspects of medicine, it is important to recognize obesity and its cohort, inactivity, as a disease state and treat it as such.

Physicians also need to be advocates on the local and regional scene to promote physical education in schools, new recreational centers, and bike routes in the community. In some communities physicians lobby for insurance companies to support the preventive aspects of health plans.

Medicine has shown that diligence and persistence can improve health outcomes successfully, as shown by those who targeted heart disease, hypertension, cigarette smoking, and cervical cancer. Rather than feeling hopeless in the "battle of the bulge," physicians who persist and are aggressive in treating inactive patients will see a positive change in their patients' lives.

REFERENCES

1. National Institutes of Health: Clinical Guidelines on the Identification, Evaluation, and Treatment of Overweight and Obesity in Adults. Bethesda, MD, NIH, June 1998.
2. Powell KE, Thompson PD, Caspersen CJ, Kenderick JS: Physical activity and the incidence of coronary heart disease. Ann. Rev. Public Health 8:253–287, 1987.
3. MacMahon S, Cutler J, Brittain E, Higgins M: Obesity and hypertension: Epidemiology and clinical issues. Eur Heart J 8(suppl B):57–70, 1987.
4. King AC, Haskell WL, Taylor CB, et al: Group- vs. home-based exercise training in healthy older men and women. A community based clinical trial. JAMA 266:1535–1542, 1991.
5. Durstine JL, Haskell WL: Effects of exercise training on plasma lipids and lipoproteins. Exerc Sport Sci Rev 22:477–521, 1994.
6. Siscovick DS, Weiss NS, Fletcher RH, Lasky T: The incidence of primary cardiac arrest during vigorous exercise. New Engl J Med 311:874–877, 1984.
7. Felson DT, Anderson JJ, Naimark A, et al: Obesity and knee osteoarthritis. The Framingham study. Ann Intern Med 109:18–24, 1988.
8. Cicuttini FM, Baker JR, Spector TD, et al: The association of obesity with osteoarthritis: A twin study. J Rheumatol 23:1221–1226, 1996.
9. Ivy JL: The insulin-like effect of muscle contraction. Exerc Sports Sci Rev 15:29–51, 1987.
10. Bernstein L, Henderson BE, Hanisch R, et al: Physical exercise and reduced risk of breast cancer in young women. J Natl Cancer Inst 86(18):1403–1408, 1994.
11. Shephard RJ: Exercise in the prevention and treatment of cancer: An update. Sports Med 15(4):258–280, 1993.
12. Physical Activity and Cardiovascular Health. NIH Consensus Statement. 13(3):1–33, Dec. 18–20, 1995.
13. American College of Sports Medicine (1991): Guidelines for Exercise Testing and Prescription, 4th ed. Philadelphia, Lea & Febiger, 1991.
14. Feigenbaum MS, Pollock ML: Strength training: Rationale for current guidelines for adult fitness programs. Phys Sports Med 25(2):44–64, 1997.
15. Gortmaker SL, Must A, Sobot AM: Television viewing as a cause of increasing obesity among children in the U.S., 1986–1990. Arch Pediatr Adolesc Med 150(4):356–362, 1996.

Chapter 4 | Principles of Training

ROB JOHNSON, M.D.

The basis for most athletic and recreational activities is aerobic and anaerobic fitness. Important complements to the aerobic base are strength and flexibility programs. Intuitively, both components should enhance athletic performance, either through bigger, stronger, faster athletes or reduced injury frequency. An understanding of these programs and their implementation is necessary for the clinician who may be asked to evaluate athletes. Knowledge of these training modes is important in understanding the demands of a particular sport in order to appropriately and safely prepare and evaluate the athlete for practice and competition.

This chapter discusses the principles of aerobic, anaerobic, strength, and flexibility training programs. The SAID (specific adaptation to imposed demand) principle governs all physical training. Specific adaptation means that any physiologic change or growth that occurs will be specific to the type of training. The quantity of change that occurs depends on the level of the imposed demand. Thus, the greater the load or the greater the intensity, the greater the change (adaptation).

Any training program should be based on two principles—overload and specificity. *Overload* describes the principle of imposing a greater stress on the body or muscle group than that body part is accustomed to experiencing. Repetitive application of overload is the primary physiologic stimulus for the physiologic system to adapt to and, ultimately, demonstrate physiologic gains.

Specificity means that a specific training regimen results in specific outcomes. Each sport has specific demands that require specific skills. If these skills are not developed, the athlete will not be able to maximize performance. For example, a runner needs to train by running. If he or she chooses to train by swimming, the muscles involved in swimming are those that adapt. Physiologically, training affects either the central component (the heart and lungs) or the peripheral component (the vascular and muscular systems).

The heart and lungs do not discriminate between training by running and training by swimming. They benefit from both training modes. However, the peripheral changes are most affected by the "specificity" of the training mode. Different muscles are used for different activities, such as swimming, running, and biking. Each sport has different requirements and demands for performance and, thus, for training. Let us consider some of the specific capabilities that participants in each sport must develop to some degree.

1. Strength—the ability to produce a maximum force in a single, maximal effort
2. Speed strength—high forces exerted at high speeds
3. Muscular endurance—the ability to perform muscle work over time without fatigue
4. Speed endurance—the ability to produce high forces at high velocities over time
5. Cardiovascular endurance—the ability of the cardiovascular system, lungs, and muscles to transport, deliver, and use oxygen during the performance of work
6. Power—the ability to exert force rapidly
7. Flexibility—the ability to move a joint through a full range of motion (ROM)
8. Metabolic demands—the energy system that is determined to be the primary energy producer for a specific activity or sport.

AEROBIC AND ANAEROBIC TRAINING

For most sports, aerobic conditioning represents the base of the conditioning pyramid upon which all other training and performance rests. The two components of aerobic training are central and peripheral. The central component consists principally of cardiac output: cardiac output (CO) = heart rate (HR) $\times$ stroke volume (SV). The central component of aerobic fitness is the most general in its response to training. Thus, many types of aerobic training will condition the central component. The peripheral component consists of vascular responses, oxygen extraction, and alterations of subcellular components necessary for energy production within specific muscle groups.

A further principle of aerobic and anaerobic conditioning is specificity. A training program should reflect the type of aerobic or anaerobic conditioning that mimics the requirements of the sport of participation. The body's different energy systems can provide short-term energy (under 10 seconds), intermediate energy (10 seconds to 2 minutes), or prolonged energy (2 minutes to several hours). Each energy system must be developed through training to support the sport-specific demands.

The principles of overload and progression apply to both aerobic and anaerobic training. Specific guidelines for initiating exercise can be found in Chapter 3, on exercise prescription.

The key variables in aerobic training are frequency, intensity, and duration. For most, a safe frequency is every other day. As fitness improves, the frequency can be increased. Once the frequency is increased to daily activity, the intensity or duration can be increased. To minimize injury risk or undue fatigue, it is wise to alter only one training variable at a time as one increases the training effort.

Expected improvement in fitness level as measured by maximum oxygen consumption ($\dot{V}O_{2\,max}$) is generally about 20 to 25 percent over the course of 8 to 12 weeks. An individual can reach a genetically determined peak improvement usually over 18 to 24 months.

Each competitive sport has different aerobic requirements. Consequently, the amount of time devoted to aerobic training should be dictated by these demands. For instance, football has minimal aerobic requirements compared with cross-country running or skiing.

To enhance aerobic speed, it is necessary to intersperse brief periods of higher intensity training with periods of recovery. Typical higher intensity periods of activity, or intervals, are measured in seconds to minutes. The recovery intervals are frequently equal to the time of the exercise interval. The number of intervals performed is dictated by the energy demands of the sport. Commonly, intervals will be repeated eight times or more. The training for each sport continues to evolve.

Coaching clinics and professional journals are available to update coaches in training techniques to improve performance for sport. The reader should consult the local coaching staff or coaching journals to refine understanding of sport-specific aerobic and anaerobic training.

STRENGTH TRAINING

The following basic terms apply to the discussion of strength training routines:

1. Concentric muscle contraction—muscle contraction (muscle work) while the muscle shortens.
2. Eccentric muscle contraction—muscle contraction (muscle work) while the muscle lengthens.
3. Isometric muscle contraction—muscle contraction without any associated movement; muscle activity without any ROM. This activity strengthens the muscle at the specific joint angle used during the muscle contraction.
4. Isotonic muscle contraction—muscle activity in which the muscle moves through a full ROM against a fixed resistance or weight.
5. Isokinetic muscle contraction—muscle activity in which the muscle moves through a full ROM against a variable resistance at a fixed speed (angular velocity).
6. Progressive resistance exercise—a program that uses increasing resistance as strength gains are realized.

The next step in developing an effective strength training program is program design. A good program has the following characteristics:

1. Exercises are selected that are appropriate for the specific demands of a particular sport with special emphasis on the muscle groups used in that sport.
2. Each program should include at least one power exercise (power clean, hang clean, snatch, and push press) to improve neuromuscular coordination and power among "power zone" muscles (muscles from the thigh to the ribs).
3. There should be differences in emphases depending on whether it is a pre-, in-, or off-season strength program.

4. The exercise order should progress from exercises with the most intensity to those with the least intensity.

5. Push and pull exercises are alternated (alternating triceps and biceps curls or alternating military presses and lateral pulls).

6. Upper and lower body exercises are alternated (alternating bench press with leg press).

7. Pre- and off-season exercises are done before practice. In-season strength training is done after practice.

Most strength training routines are described in terms of repetitions and sets. Repetitions (reps) represent the number of times a particular exercise is performed before the person rests or initiates the next exercise. A set represents one series of repetitions of a group of exercises followed by rest or another set of exercises. The volume of a particular workout is the number of sets multiplied by the number of repetitions.

Different combinations of sets and numbers of reps can provide a "specific" workout with a predictable result. For instance, to develop power for sprinting or other explosive sports, the athlete should perform 3 to 6 sets of 1 to 3 reps of a particular exercise. The following workouts are specific for providing the given results:

- For muscle strength, perform 3 to 5 sets of 3 to 8 reps.
- For muscle hypertrophy, perform 3 to 6 sets of 8 to 12 reps.
- For muscle endurance, perform 2 sets of 15 to 20 reps.
- For power, perform 3 to 6 sets of 1 to 3 reps.

To determine the resistance or weight to be used for a specific exercise, a percentage of a 1-repetition maximum (1 RM) is typically used. One RM is defined as the maximum weight, or resistance, that can be lifted in a single repetition.

- For muscle strength, the weight should be 80 to 90 percent of 1 RM.
- For muscle hypertrophy, the weight should be 70 to 80 percent of 1 RM.
- For muscle endurance, the weight should be 60 to 70 percent of 1 RM.
- For power, the weight should be about 80 percent of 1 RM.

The amount of rest between sets can also lead to specific muscle development. To develop strength and power, rest 2 to 4 minutes between sets. For muscle endurance, 30 seconds of rest between sets is effective. Finally, if muscle hypertrophy is the goal, rest should be between 30 seconds and 2 minutes between sets. To make strength gains, most experts recommend two to four workouts per week.

The purpose of strength training is to improve athletic performance and reduce injuries, although the data to support the benefit of either to athletes is unclear. Performance criteria as they relate to strength training are not easily measured. For power sports, size induced by strength training seems to be important.

The relationship between injury and strength training has been evaluated. Studies are conflicting, with some showing no difference in injury frequency between strong and weak subjects and some showing a slightly increased injury risk in the stronger group. In some studies, agonist/antagonist muscle imbalances have demonstrated increased injury frequency when "normal" ratios are not maintained. Other studies fail to support this contention. Right/left imbalances have suggested greater injury risk in the hamstrings and increased sprains and strains in lower extremities. Despite the varying results of these studies, most clinicians and therapists think that there is an advantage conferred on those who perform sport-specific strength training.

FLEXIBILITY TRAINING

Flexibility decreases with age. How much flexibility reduces injury rate or increases performance is, like strength training, uncertain. Nevertheless, stretching has been incorporated into most fitness programs. There is little doubt of the value of stretching for those who have experienced soft tissue injuries. Soft tissue injury results in decreased motion about the injured joint. Therefore, rehabilitation must reestablish normal motion to facilitate the athlete's return.

Principles

Simply stated, stretching is increasing the length of a tissue. Flexibility training, then, is a program that is designed to increase the range of motion about a joint. Two types of stretches are described. The *elastic* stretch causes a temporary increase in the length of a tissue that returns to its normal length when the stretching stress is removed. A *plastic* stretch results in a more permanent increase in tissue length. This lengthening remains after the stretching stress is eliminated. With each stretch, both plastic and elastic elements are affected. Because plastic elements remain lengthened, stretching that affects these elements should be emphasized. Low force loads over longer periods of time most effectively result in plastic deformation, the desired effect.

The effects of stretching are local. Only the tissues that are stretched make the adaptations. Consequently, stretching must be performed for each specific joint to improve the range of motion about each joint.

Stretching with elevated muscle-tendon temperatures increases the plastic effects. The best way to elevate the temperature is through muscle activity. Stretching should not be done to a cold muscle. Stretching just after awakening is also unwise because muscles are particularly tight after sleep. The most effective stretch is performed after about 5 to 10 minutes of activity or at the completion of a workout.

The greatest effect on flexibility is movement patterns. If one's activity is typified by limited range of motion, adaptive shortening is likely to occur. The greatest loss of flexibility occurs in the first 2 weeks after cessation of movement activities or stretching. Beyond 4 weeks, flexibility losses are minimal. Measurable effects of any flexibility program may take at least 4 weeks after the initiation of a program.

Techniques

Many techniques have been described for stretching. Most athletic trainers and physical therapists have their preferred stretching routines. Generally, the scientific data support the use of a *static* stretch to develop flexibility. That is, slowly stretching the muscle-tendon unit to mild discomfort (traction) and holding that stretch for a given duration. Current research suggests holding a stretch for 30 seconds, relaxing for 5 to 10 seconds, and repeating the stretch at least 3 times. Holding the stretch less than 30 seconds is not as effective. Holding a stretch longer than 30 seconds fails to produce any significant flexibility gains.

A variation of flexibility training frequently employed by physical therapists and athletic trainers is proprioceptive neuromuscular facilitation (PNF), or stretch-contract-relax. PNF is performed with an assistant. The joint is stretched to the end ROM and held for 5 to 30 seconds. In this position, the agonist muscle (muscle being stretched) is isometrically contracted for an equal length of time, followed by a relaxation cycle of 5 to 10 seconds. The entire stretch-contract-relax cycle is then repeated several times. Further refinement of PNF involves the addition of an isometric contraction of the antagonist muscle. A ballistic (bouncing) stretch is seldom recommended because jerky movements have an injury potential and fail to significantly alter the plastic elements of soft tissues. Finally, each sport has different flexibility requirements, some placing a greater emphasis on flexibility and some requiring greater ROM at a specific joint.

Flexibility and Injury

The studies regarding flexibility and injury have been remarkably conflicting. Although some have shown that "tight" athletes are more often injured, other studies have found no relationship between flexibility and injury risk. Others have shown injury trends in those athletes at both extremes of flexibility—too tight or too loose. As in strength training, right-left imbalances in flexibility might be more predictive of injury. Strength and flexibility differences/imbalances related to prior injury may be an independent risk factor for future injury.

PLYOMETRICS

A popular form of training for improving athletic performance in many sports is plyometrics (commonly referred to as "plyos"). Plyometrics is the use of countermovement to overload the muscular system, as in jumping. This form of overload results in specific adaptations. A popular example of plyometrics is depth jumping. In this technique, the athlete drops from an elevated surface. Immediately upon landing, the athlete performs a maximal vertical jump.

The Theory

Plyometrics is a hybrid of eccentric and concentric activity that loads both elastic and contractile

Table 4–1
Sample Grading System for Muscle Function Parameters

Sport	Flexibility	Strength	Power	Anaerobic	Aerobic
Football	3	4	4	3	2
Running backs	3	4	4	4	3
Basketball	3	3	4	4	4
Baseball	3	3	4	4	2
Tennis	4	2	3	4	3
Swimming	4	4	2	2	4
Sprints	4	4	2	4	2
Distance running	3	2	2	2	4
Sprinting	3	3	3	4	2
Golf	3	4	4	2	1
Soccer	3	2	3	4	4
Ice hockey	2	3	4	4	3
Volleyball	3	2	4	4	2
Bicycling	3	3	4	3	4
Skiing	3	3	4	3	2
Cross country skiing	2	3	3	3	4

Key: 4 = essential for optimum performance of a sport or function (e.g., aerobic endurance for distance running or strength for football); 3 = synergistic for optimum performance of a sport or function (e.g., anaerobic endurance in bicycling or speed in basketball); 2 = necessary at a certain level, usually for injury prevention (e.g., strength in tennis or flexibility in cross country skiing); 1 = minimal, but a small amount required to support performance in the sport (e.g., aerobic endurance in golf).

Utilization: Use this table to profile each sport regarding key performance parameters. Then design the training program and practice sessions based on the individual sport's profile.

Source: Adapted from Kibler W, Ben MD: The Sport Preparticipation Fitness Examination. Champaign, IL: Human Kinetics Pubs, 1990.

components of the muscle. The reactive properties of the muscle are maximized in the activity that switches rapidly from negative work to positive work. The activation of the stretch reflex in switching from negative to positive work contributes to the improvement of muscular force generation through the combined effects of a voluntary muscle contraction and an involuntary muscle contraction triggered by the stretch reflex.

The role of stored elastic energy is also exploited in this activity. Any muscle that contracts immediately after being stretched generates a greater force than a muscle that is not pre-stretched.

The Research

Subjects who performed plyometric exercises accelerated faster, did more work in less time, generated more power, and were more efficient than athletes who trained without plyometrics. The question of whether fast-twitch or slow-twitch fibers gained more from this training has not been answered conclusively.

Technique

Depth jumping was previously mentioned as an example of plyometric training. Depth jumping

from 30 to 40 inches has resulted in maximal speed in switching from negative to positive work. Depth jumps of 20 inches have been effective in increasing strength and motor performance. Other plyometric techniques include hopping, bounding, leg tuck jumps, and a growing list of newer exercises. Weighted medicine balls are popular forms of upper extremity plyometric training. Both power and speed sports and endurance sports now employ various forms of plyometric training. The author's personal experience suggests that injudicious use of plyometric training can significantly increase the risk of soft tissue injury.

For further information regarding training programs, helpful sources include a local high school or college conditioning coach, a trained professional at a local health club or YMCA, or a professional certified by the National Strength and Conditioning Association (NSCA).

SUGGESTED READINGS

Baechle TR: Preseason strength training. *In* Mellion M, Walsh WM, Shelton GL (eds): The Team Physician's Handbook, Philadelphia, Hanley & Belfus, 1996, pp. 132–142.
Blanke D: Preseason conditioning: Flexibility. *In* Mellion M, Walsh WM, Shelton GL (eds): The Team Physi-

cian's Handbook. Philadelphia, Hanley & Belfus, 1996, pp. 143–149.

Knapik JJ, Jones BH, Harris JM: Strength, flexibility and athletic injuries. Sports Med 14(5):277–288, 1992.

Latin RW: Preseason conditioning: Aerobic power. *In* Mellion M, Walsh WM, Shelton GL (eds): The Team Physician's Handbook. Philadelphia, Hanley & Belfus, 1996, pp. 125–131.

Lundin P, Berg W: A review of plyometric training. National Strength Conditioning Assoc J 13(6):22–29, 1991.

Murray J, Karpovich PV: Weight Training in Athletics. Englewood Cliffs, NJ, Prentice-Hall, 1983.

Novich MM, Taylor B: Training and Conditioning of Athletes. Philadelphia, Lea & Febiger, 1983.

Strength and Conditioning: The Professional Journal of the National Strength and Conditioning Association. *(Editor's Note: This is a continuing, receivable subscription. Each issue has specific programs for a variety of sports. I recommend, for those interested, subscribing to this journal for regular updates in strength, conditioning, and flexibility.)*

Chapter 5 | Advising the Athlete on Nutrition and Supplements

SCOTT ESCHER, M.D.

Athletes work on more than endurance, strength, and flexibility when trying to improve their performance. They also strive to optimize nutrition in order to train and compete at the highest level possible. Many athletes also use nutritional supplements and medications in their pursuit of excellence. This chapter discusses basic nutritional practices used in sports as well as ergogenic aids.

GENERAL NUTRITION

Carbohydrates, fats, and protein are the three basic dietary components. Each component plays a distinct role in an athlete's nutritional milieu at different times in the training cycle. Fluid replacement is another important, although often overlooked, component of nutrition in athletes and nonathletes.

Carbohydrates

Carbohydrates and fats supply the energy utilized during athletic activity. The American Dietetic Association recommends that 50 to 55 percent of an athlete's total daily calories come from complex carbohydrates and that an additional 10 percent come from simple sugars. Two mechanisms supply glucose to the working muscle during exercise. Carbohydrate stored in muscle as glycogen is one source of glucose. Liver glycogen is also broken down and enters the blood stream, where it is taken up by the muscle. When the available glycogen is exhausted, the athlete must slow down physical activity. The point at which the available glycogen is depleted is called "hitting the wall" or "bonking" by athletes. Increasing the body's glycogen stores before exercise or supplying car-

bohydrate during exercise will delay glycogen depletion and may improve endurance. Methods to achieve this are discussed later in this section.

Protein

Protein is used to build and rebuild muscle. Very little is utilized for energy during exercise in most athletes. The current recommended dietary allowance (RDA) for protein in the human diet is 0.8 g/kg/day. Nitrogen balance studies have shown that both male and female athletes need more than the RDA of protein in their diet. Endurance athletes need 1.2 to 1.4 g/kg/day, and strength athletes need 1.4 to 1.8 g/kg/day to maintain nitrogen balance. This represents a 50 to 225 percent increased protein need over RDA levels. By following the recommendation of taking 10 to 15 percent of dietary calories in the form of protein, athletes usually meet this increased need for protein. Consider that 3000 calories a day is a modest intake for most athletes; 15 percent of this would be 112.5 g of protein per day, or 1.6 g/kg in a typical 70-kg athlete. Some athletes will not meet these protein needs because of poor food choices or because of the unique demands of their sports. Athletes such as wrestlers and gymnasts may use a calorie-restricted diet and may not meet their protein needs. In these athletes, supplemental protein may be beneficial.

Some athletes supplement their protein requirement with amino acids in the belief that individual amino acids are more beneficial than amino acid macromolecules (dietary protein). Some studies have shown that amino acids increase the body's natural secretion of growth hormone. Most studies show no benefit in using amino acids over dietary protein or protein supplements.

Fats

Fats are an important source of energy for the working athlete. Even athletes with very low fat stores have enough fat reserves to complete all but the most arduous multiday athletic events. It has been suggested that endurance athletes can improve performance by using a high-fat diet. Although elevated free fatty acids in the serum can allow for glycogen sparing (which permits the athlete to exercise longer before running out of glycogen), most studies do not show improved performance in endurance athletes on high-fat diets.

Fluid Replacement

Fluids are often the forgotten piece of the athlete's nutritional puzzle. Fluid is necessary to help the athlete maintain body temperature. Muscle is only about 25 percent energy efficient, meaning that approximately 75 percent of the energy expended during exercise is given off as heat. The body must disperse this energy or it will soon become hyperthermic. The most efficient means of dispersing this heat in the majority of environmental conditions is through perspiration. Athletes can lose up to 1.8 liters of water per hour in perspiration. If the athlete starts out an exercise session in a dehydrated condition or does not replace fluid at a sufficient rate, performance suffers. As little as 2 percent dehydration impairs heat tolerance. If blood is shunted to the skin to facilitate heat loss, less is available to bring oxygen and other nutrients to the working muscle. Thirst is a late sign of dehydration and thus is a poor mechanism for gauging fluid status. Athletes need to take in fluid before they become thirsty in events that last longer than 45 minutes or performance can suffer. The athlete should attempt to ingest about 8 ounces of fluid for every 15 minutes of endurance activity.

Pre-event Nutrition

The pregame meal should be chosen to attempt to optimize carbohydrate stores and fluid levels in the athlete. This meal should be individualized for each athlete. For obvious reasons, it is not wise to experiment with pregame nutrition on the day of an important competition. Each athlete should test a particular meal during training before using it preceding an important event. For most athletes a meal high in complex carbohydrate and low in fat approximately 4 hours before the event is optimal. A small serving of pasta or pancakes can effectively meet this requirement. The carbohydrate will provide energy during the event. Fat can slow digestion and lead to feeling sluggish or cause gastrointestinal problems during competition. The athlete should avoid carbohydrate in the hour before an event. This can cause insulin to be elevated at the beginning of an event and thereby lower available blood glucose levels transiently at the start of competition. Drinking 500 ml of fluid 1 to 2 hours before the event will help to optimize fluid status in combination with the above recommendation of 8 oz every 15 minutes.

Glycogen loading is a method endurance athletes, such as marathon runners and triathletes, use to increase the muscle glycogen levels above normal before an event. Typically, a glycogen-loading regimen consists of a glycogen-depleting activity about 1 week before the race. In the past this was followed by 3 days of a high-protein, low-carbohydrate diet to further deplete glycogen. In the final 3 days before competition, the athlete would then consume a diet consisting of at least 70 percent carbohydrate. Many athletes do not tolerate the low carbohydrate portion of this cycle and become lethargic and irritable. Studies have shown that athletes who skip the low carbohydrate portion of the earlier regimen and simply eat a high carbohydrate diet in the three days before competition have glycogen levels nearly as high as those achieved with the classic glycogen loading regimen but without the associated problems.

Nutrition During Athletic Participation

Fluid replacement is the most important aspect of nutrition during an event. In events lasting more than 45 minutes, the athlete should attempt to balance fluid loss with replacement. Without adequate fluid replacement, the athlete has more difficulty with heat dissipation. As more blood is diverted to the skin for heat dissipation, less is available for the working muscle.

In events lasting longer than 45 to 60 minutes, carbohydrate intake can supply energy to the muscles, allowing them to exercise longer before depleting the stored muscle and liver glycogen. Many athletes do not tolerate solids during exercise. Most athletes do tolerate carbohydrate-containing liquids. Fluids containing 4 to 8 percent carbohydrate in solution are absorbed as quickly as water alone, allowing the athlete to rehydrate as well as spare glycogen. Gatorade is one readily available solution containing carbohydrates for endurance athletes. Athletes should test their tolerance of carbohydrate replacement drinks before using them in competition.

Athletes who engage in "ultra" events, which can last for several hours, run the risk of hypernatremia or hyponatremia. The sodium concentration of sweat is lower than that of blood. Although uncommon, prolonged sweating without fluid replacement can cause hypernatremia. If athletes replace their fluid loss with water alone, they can dilute the remaining sodium, causing hyponatremia. Thus, most athletic fluid replacement solutions do contain sodium for palatability and to reduce the risk of hyponatremia.

Post-event Nutrition

After a practice or a game an athlete needs to replenish fluid and glycogen. Replacing fluid is easy. The athlete should drink noncaffeinated, nonalcoholic liquids in amounts that will bring body weight back to pre-event weight or produce pale, dilute urine.

Replenishing glycogen is also relatively simple. The athlete needs to ingest carbohydrates. The body manufactures glycogen best when fed within 2 hours of exercise. Thus, athletes should attempt to ingest approximately 100 g of carbohydrate within 2 hours of exercise. This can be as simple as eating a bagel with juice or two pancakes with syrup. Complex carbohydrates replenish glycogen better in the long run than simple sugars. Athletes can tire more quickly in successive bouts of exercise if they do not replenish glycogen each day.

In the past, athletes took salt tablets to avoid dehydration. This practice is discouraged today. Athletes get enough sodium in their diet and in replacement drinks to replace that lost in perspiration. The extra sodium in salt tablets may simply increase the need for water in an already dehydrated athlete.

PERFORMANCE-ENHANCING AGENTS

Athletes seek to improve performance through better nutrition and training techniques. Some athletes attempt to enhance their performance with ergogenic aids. Athletes have been experimenting with ergogenic aids for centuries. The Greek Olympians ate lion hearts for courage. In the modern Olympics, a cyclist died from a strychnine overdose in the early 1900s. (In low doses, strychnine is a central nervous system stimulant.) Urine drug testing was implemented in Mexico City in 1968, and numerous Olympic athletes have tested positive for banned substances since. Both the NCAA (National Collegiate Athletic Association) and the IOC (International Olympic Committee) have a list of prohibited substances. Each has a hotline for athletes, coaches, and physicians to call if they have a question about a particular agent. The arm of the NCAA charged with enforcement of drug testing is the National Center for Drug-Free Sport. The phone number is (816) 474-8655 and the website is www.drugfreesport.com. The U.S. Olympic Committee hotline number is 1-800-233-0393 or 1-888-233-0393, and their Internet site is www.olympic-usa.org. The NCAA also puts out *The Athletic Drug Reference,* which answers many commonly asked questions about ergogenic aids and lists thousands of drugs, noting their status as banned or accepted by the USOC or the NCAA.

Numerous substances have been purported to be ergogenic aids. Some may indeed improve certain aspects of performance, while others have, at best, a positive placebo effect. Only those substances proved to improve performance are banned. For many years the IOC did not test for recreational drugs if they were not believed to improve performance, but it may be reversing this position. The NCAA does test for recreational drugs. The following portions of this chapter give an overview of banned ergogenic aids and discuss some of the alleged ergogenic aids that are not banned but are often used by athletes.

Banned Performance-Enhancing Agents

There are several categories of banned substances. Each category is discussed briefly.

Stimulants

Stimulants can be divided into four categories: (1) psychomotor substances, (2) sympathomimetic amines, (3) clenbuterol, and (4) caffeine. Amphetamines and cocaine are psychomotor substances that have been used by athletes to delay fatigue. They were used by football players in the 60s to bring about a rage state. Psychomotor substances increase heart rate, blood pressure, and metabolic rate. They can cause tremor, anxiety, and insomnia, and may make it difficult to dissipate the heat generated during exercise. Most studies have shown no improvement in sporting activities in athletes using psychomotor substances.

Pseudoephedrine, phenylpropanolamine, and ephedrine are some of the most commonly available sympathomimetic amines. These substances are available over the counter in cold and allergy preparations. The sympathomimetic amines are similar to the psychomotor substances in terms of effects and side effects. Anxiety is more problematic with the sympathomimetic amines.

Clenbuterol is a beta-2 agonist that was originally used as a partitioning agent in livestock. Partitioning agents increase muscle weight and decrease fat weight. Clenbuterol is used by strength athletes as an alternative to anabolic androgenic steroids. Several swimmers were found to have clenbuterol in their systems in the 1992 Olympic Games. Beta-2 agonists have been shown to improve strength and power in humans in some studies.[3]

Caffeine, a ubiquitous stimulant, is unique in that it is the only substance that is banned above a certain concentration in the urine. The NCAA bans caffeine levels above 15 µg/ml, and it is banned above 12 µg/ml by the IOC. It would take 4 to 8 cups of coffee over 1 hour to reach the 12 µg/ml level. Caffeine increases the availability of free fatty acids and may spare glycogen in endurance athletes. It also may increase the force of muscular contraction.

Anabolic Androgenic Steroids

Anabolic androgenic steroids (AAS) have been used since the 1950s. They were initially used by weight lifters in Eastern Europe. Currently, AAS are used illegally in sports in which size and strength are at a premium, such as football and the field events in track. Some endurance athletes use AAS, in the belief that they will help them recover quicker after hard workouts.

AAS are related to the male sex hormone testosterone. Each of the various AAS have differing half-lives and degrees of anabolism (muscle building) and androgenicity (sexual characteristics). Athletes use different forms of AAS in 6- to 12-week cycles. They often "stack" two or more AAS during different phases of their cycle. It is difficult to study the effect of AAS in athletes because many are illegal without a doctor's prescription and some athletes take dosages up to eight times the recommended physiologic doses. It is difficult to perform a good controlled study at these levels. Studies have shown that AAS in conjunction with proper diet and exercise will help increase strength and muscle mass. The increased mass lasts for at least 5 months. AAS have not been shown to improve performance in endurance sports.

AAS have numerous side effects. Psychological effects include increased depression and hypomania as well as numerous reports of increased aggression in AAS users. AAS, especially oral formulations, have detrimental effects on the liver, causing elevated liver functions as well as liver tumors. Female users can develop clitoromegaly, hirsutism, or male pattern baldness and may demonstrate other male sex characteristics, such as a deeper voice. Males can develop gynecomastia. In adolescents AAS can cause precocious puberty or premature physeal closure as well as other side effects.

Beta Blockers

Beta blockers are banned in the shooting sports such as riflery and archery because of their tremor-reducing effects. Beta blockers probably diminish performance in aerobic athletes.

Alcohol

Alcohol is similar to beta blockers in that it is banned only in the shooting events because of its tremor-reducing properties.

Diuretics

Diuretics are banned because they artificially reduce weight, which is important in sports that have weight requirements, such as wrestling or weight lifting. Diuretics are also used to dilute the urine in order to illicitly pass urine drug tests.

Peptide Hormones and Analogues

Peptide hormones are the body's messengers to distant sites of action. They have only recently become available in amounts that athletes could use for ergogenic purposes through genetic engineering. When derived from human or animal sources, they were prohibitively expensive

Human Growth Hormone Growth hormone (GH) is used by some athletes to increase body mass and strength. Endogenous GH is released by the anterior pituitary gland and acts on the body through the effect of somatomedins. GH increases protein synthesis and bone growth. If the growth plate is still open, the bone increases in length as well as width. No studies have shown increased strength in trained athletes who take GH supplements. Excess GH has numerous side effects, including acromegaly, which is also seen in people with pituitary tumors. Other side effects include glucose intolerance, myopathy, arthritis, and hypothyroidism. At the present time it is impossible to separate endogenous from exogenous GH with urine drug testing. Some athletes see GH as an alternative to AAS without the risk of testing positive for a banned drug.

Erythropoietin and Blood Doping Erythropoietin (EPO) is a hormone produced by the kidneys that activates red blood cell (RBC) production in the marrow. This hormone effectively increases the hemoglobin concentration in the blood stream for up to 120 days, which is the life cycle of an RBC. "Blood doping" increases hemoglobin concentration by another means. In blood doping, the athlete is given RBCs via transfusion of autologous or homologous blood. Increased hemoglobin will allow more oxygen to be delivered to the working muscle. Studies on the effect of blood doping and EPO use have shown increased $\dot{V}o_{2\ max}$, or an increase in the athlete's ability to utilize oxygen. Specifically this translates into faster times in endurance races for runners, cross-country skiers, and other aerobic athletes. Athletes with higher hemoglobin concentrations also have less of a problem with heat build-up during exercise. With higher hemoglobin levels these athletes can get the needed amount of oxygen to working tissue using less blood, allowing more blood to the periphery for heat dissipation. Several members of the U.S. Olympic bicycling team in 1982 admitted to blood doping. Currently it is not possible to detect blood doping or tell exogenous from endogenous EPO with urine testing.

Side effects of increased hemoglobin concentrations include the risk of blood sludging and vascular occlusion, especially when dehydrated.

Transfusion-related conditions such as transfusion reactions, thrombophlebitis, hepatitis, and HIV are also risks in blood doping. Blood pressure also increases more at a specific work load in athletes given EPO than in those who do not take it.

Luteinizing Hormone, Follicle-Stimulating Hormone, and Chorionic Gonadotropin This group of hormones act on the testicles to produce testosterone. Athletes typically use these compounds to induce production of testosterone in their atrophic testicles after they have been on a cycle of AAS. AAS use commonly causes the testicles to atrophy via negative feedback inhibition. The effects and side effects are similar to those of AAS, as noted previously. Most athletes do not use these hormones for their anabolic effects because they have more pronounced side effects than do the AAS.

Narcotics

Narcotics are banned by the IOC, but most are allowed by the NCAA in limited amounts.

Corticosteroids

The IOC allows topical corticosteroids. With medical justification, inhaled and local corticosteroid injections are also allowed. Other modes of delivery of this group of medications are limited by the IOC. The NCAA allows corticosteroid use.

Local Anesthetics

The IOC allows local anesthetics only when an athlete is given prior authorization for medically justified reasons.

Beta-2 Agonists

These agents are allowed in inhaled form only. The IOC allows use of only albuterol, terbutaline, and salmeterol. This category is limited because these agents may be ergogenic in the same way as another beta-2 agonist, clenbuterol.

Urine Manipulation

Chemical manipulation of the urine with substances such as diuretics is banned, as they may help to circumvent results of urine drug testing. Physical manipulation of the urine is also banned.

Many stories abound about athletes substituting another person's urine for their own.

Possible Performance-Enhancing Agents

Athletes have tried numerous substances in the quest for improved performance. Most substances involved in the biochemistry of energy production have been utilized in an attempt to improve performance. These compounds are too numerous to discuss in this chapter. Some of the more common ergogenic aids that are not currently banned are discussed briefly.

Creatine

Creatine use may increase the levels of creatine phosphate (CP) in the cell. CP contains a high-energy phosphate bond that regenerates ATP (adenosine triphosphate) from ADP (adenosine diphosphate). ATP is the common source of energy to working muscle. Athletes who engage in high-intensity anaerobic activities can exercise at highest intensity for a few more seconds if their creatine phosphate levels are high. After the body uses up all the pre-existing ATP and CP, the lactic acid cycle becomes the dominant means of supplying energy to the maximally stimulated muscle. Performance degrades quickly when lactate accumulates in muscle.

Several studies have shown improvement in short, high-intensity activities with creatine.[4, 5] The athletes showing the most improvement are those with the lowest levels of CP before supplementation. These athletes typically have lower protein diets or are vegetarians. Athletes using creatine often gain weight, although it is not known if this is truly increased muscle. Typically, strength or anaerobic athletes use creatine. Anecdotally, some athletes who use creatine have problems with cramping, muscle strains, and heat illness.

Creatine is not a muscle builder. It is an energy source that permits more intense training.

Bicarbonate

Bicarbonate loading attempts to increase the body's ability to buffer lactic acid production in vigorously working muscle. The bicarbonate buffers the acidity of increased lactic acid at maximal exertion. With decreased acidity the muscle can continue to exercise longer before fatigue ensues. Some studies have shown improved times in activities which are predominantly anaerobic, such as running 800 meters or less.[6–8] Gastrointestinal distress often limits use of bicarbonate loading.

Phosphate

The ingestion of phosphate is known as phosphate loading. Increased levels of phosphate may increase the levels of 2,3-diphosphoglycerate (2,3-DPG) in RBCs. Increased 2,3-DPG shifts the oxygen dissociation curve to the right, and more oxygen is then delivered to the working muscle at a given oxygen tension. Training at altitude also increases 2,3-DPG. Some studies have shown improved performance in athletes engaged in mainly aerobic sports who have ingested excess phosphate.[9, 10] Gastrointestinal upset is also the main problem with phosphate loading.

Vitamins and Minerals

Vitamin and mineral supplementation is common in athletes; it is believed that 30 to 80 percent of athletes fortify their diets in this way. No studies have shown conclusively that vitamin or mineral supplementation in nondeficient athletes improves performance. Some athletes with restricted or poor diets may note improved health and performance with vitamin and mineral use.

CONCLUSION

Proper nutrition is a relatively easy way to optimize athletic performance. A registered dietitian can aid the athlete in individualizing the diet to meet nutritional needs. Many competitors also use supplements and ergogenic aids in their pursuit of optimal performance with varied success.

REFERENCES

1. Clark N: Nancy Clark's Sports Nutrition Guidebook. Champaign, IL, Human Kinetics, 1997.
2. Fuentes RJ, Rosenberg JM, Davis A (eds): Athletic Drug Reference '96. Durham, NC, Clean Data, Inc., 1996.
3. Martineau L, Horan MA, Rothwell NJ, et al: Salbutamol, a β_2-adrenoreceptor agonist, increases skeletal muscle strength in young men. Clin Sci 83:615–621, 1992.
4. Juhn MS, Tarnopolsky M: Oral creatine supplementation and athletic performance: a critical review. Clin J Sport Med 8:286–297, 1998.

5. Noonan D, Berg K, Latin RW, et al: Effects of varying dosages of oral creatine relative to fat-free body mass on strength and body composition. J Strength Cond Res 12(2):104–108, 1998.
6. Goldfinch J, McNaughton L, Davies P: Induced metabolic alkalosis and its effects on 400-m racing time. Eur J Appl Physiol 57:45–80, 1988.
7. Wilkes D, Gledhill N, Smyth R: Effect of acute induced metabolic alkalosis on 800-m racing time. Med Sci Sports Exerc 15(4):277–280, 1983.
8. Kozak-Collins K, Burke ER, Schoene RB: Sodium bicarbonate ingestion does not improve performance in women cyclists. Med Sci Sports Exerc 26(12):1510–1515, 1994.
9. Cade R, Conte M, Zauner C, et al: Effects of phosphate loading on 2,3-diphosphoglycerate and maximal oxygen uptake. Med Sci Sport Exerc 16(3):263–268, 1984.
10. Duffy DJ, Conlee RK: Effects of phosphate loading on leg power and high intensity treadmill exercise. Med Sci Sport Exerc 18(6):674–677, 1986.

Chapter 6 | Office-Based Rehabilitation

BJ GARLICK, P.T., E.M.T.

Health care providers encounter patients with a wide variety of sports injuries. It may be a 6-year-old with wrist pain from a fall in her soccer game or a center for a high school football team whose ankle is swollen to the size of the football. It may even be a 76-year-old with shoulder pain who is trying to break his age group record at the state master's swim meet. One thing that is typical in injured athletes is their desire to be better now! Should the young girl with a greenstick fracture be allowed to play? Can the center play in next week's game? How soon can the swimmer resume the crawl stroke after an injection for his bursitis? It is the care provider's responsibility to help athletes reach their goals while respecting the body's healing time restraints and following sound rehabilitation principles. This chapter addresses these principles.

It is important to remember the goals of sports medicine: (1) to prevent injuries and (2) to facilitate the *safe* return of the injured athlete to the previous level of activity as quickly as possible.[1] A large survey showed that 65 percent of family physicians performed preparticipation examinations for school or community leagues, and 45 percent served as team physicians for one or more sports.[2] This study emphasizes the impact of sports medicine on medical practice. Doctors, physical therapists, athletic trainers, and other care providers involved in the care of athletes need to understand the principles of sports medicine to aid in the prevention of injuries and to treat the athletes who do become injured.

One of the key elements in injury prevention is the athlete's preseason physical condition. Some athletes will use their sports season to get into shape. This practice is not advisable because it leaves the athlete prone to injury, especially in the first few weeks of the season. The preseason physical and screening is ideally done 2 to 3 months before the sport season begins. Old injuries, muscle imbalances, lack of flexibility, and decrease in balance and proprioception can be evaluated and, if necessary, can be corrected before the season starts (see Chapter 2).

Another key element in injury prevention is to ensure proper rehabilitation once an injury has occurred. Some athletes may attempt to return to their sport without clearance. In these situations, established guidelines and communication between athletes, medical personnel, parents, and coaches are important in determining when athletes may return to play. In some cases athletes may be allowed to practice on a limited basis as long as the coach and other players are alerted to the limitations. For example, the injured center may practice snapping the ball to the quarterback and the punter yet be restricted from blocking until cleared. When is the athlete able to return to full practice? This is the question everyone asks. Specific criteria must be established and met before the athlete can safely return to full practice. It is then up to the coach to decide if the athlete is ready to compete.

The first step in a successful sports medicine rehabilitation program is an accurate diagnosis. The care provider may be present at the sporting event and may witness the injury. Or the athlete may consult the care provider, seeking help. The mechanism of injury is a valuable piece of information because it can aid in identifying the injured structures. The injury may be microtraumatic or macrotraumatic. *Macrotrauma* is the injury resulting from a single event; *microtrauma* describes an overuse injury that occurs over time.[3, 4] A thorough evaluation will ensure an accurate diagnosis, which allows a proper rehabilitation program to be established. The evaluation needs to encompass observation as well as objective measurements. Watch how the athlete walks, moves, and holds himself or herself in a resting position. It is important to compare injured and noninjured sides for deformity, atrophy, changes in skin color, and swelling. The clinician should test strength, measure range of motion (ROM) both actively and passively, and measure circumference for atrophy or inflammation. Ligaments can be stressed to determine laxity. If the lower extremity is involved, single leg balance should be assessed with eyes open and eyes closed. Palpate for temperature differences, muscle splinting, tenderness, crepitus, deformity, and thickness around a joint.

Once the dysfunctions are listed, the athlete is informed of the diagnosis, and goals are established; a treatment plan is outlined, and the athlete's role is made clear. The general rule in rehabilitation is that the rehabilitation time is double the immobilized time.[5] Therefore, it is important that athletes receive an immediate appointment with the primary caregiver directing their rehabilitation.

Successful rehabilitation depends on many factors, and an ideal progression is outlined as follows:

> Early intervention
> Identify injured structures
> > How severe?

What stage of healing?
How is the injury affecting function?
Goal-oriented treatment plan
> Short-term and long-term goals are established from problem list discovered from evaluation
Education of the athlete
Functional reassessment
> Know the biomechanics and skills needed for the sport
Safe return to sports activity

GOALS OF REHABILITATION

In sports medicine, it is not necessary to wait for the injury to heal before beginning rehabilitation. Treatment is aimed at restoring function while the healing process continues. Treatment can begin right in the office, and patients will need to begin a home program as well, especially if entry into physical therapy is delayed for a few days.

The goals of rehabilitation are as follows:

> Minimize the inflammatory response
> Protect the injured structures
> Control pain

Table 6–1
Characteristics and Clinical Signs of the Stages of Inflammation, Repair, and Maturation of Tissue

	Acute Stage Inflammatory-Reaction	Subacute Stage Repair and Healing	Chronic Stage Maturation and Remodeling
CHARACTERISTICS	Vascular changes Exudation of cells and chemicals Clot formation Phagocytosis, neutralization of irritants Early fibroblastic activity	Removal of noxious stimuli Growth of capillary beds into area Collagen formation Granulation tissue Very fragile, easily injured tissue	Maturation of connective tissue Contracture of scar tissue Remodeling of scar Collagen aligns to stress
CLINICAL SIGNS	Inflammation Pain before tissue resistance	Decreasing inflammation Pain synchronous with tissue resistance	Absence of inflammation Pain after tissue resistance
PHYSICAL THERAPY TREATMENT APPROACH	Control effects of inflammation: Modalities Immobilization Cautious gentle movement	Prevent or minimize contracture and adhesion formation: Gentle active movement, gradually increasing in intensity and range	Restore function: Progressive stretching, strengthening, and functional exercises

Source: Kisner C, Colby LA: Therapeutic Exercise: Foundations and Techniques. Philadelphia, F.A. Davis, 1990, p. 215.

Restore ROM, strength, flexibility, speed, agility, power, endurance, and proprioception

Maintain cardiorespiratory fitness

Restore balance and proper gait for walking, running, sprinting

Restore skills needed for sports competition

Keep the athlete focused and motivated

Initial care of traumatic injuries is started immediately, with the goal of preventing edema and hemorrhage, which result in pain, muscle spasm, and loss of motion.[5] The inflammation in the injured limb can also cause neuromuscular inhibition and muscle weakness.[1] Inflammation is a natural response to trauma and is necessary to start the repair process, but left unchecked, the inflammatory response can lengthen the time necessary for a positive outcome. There is no known way of speeding up the body's natural healing process, but healing can be optimized by following more progressive healing guidelines, especially by using less immobilization. It has been reported that muscle strength may decrease up to 17 percent within the initial 72 hours of immobilization.[4]

Initially sprains, strains, and contusions are treated with PRICE,[5-7] or *p*rotection, *r*est, *i*ce, *c*ompression, and *e*levation. Protection of the injured structures is accomplished with splints, slings, braces, taping, and crutches. If the athlete is limping, crutches will assist with ambulating. Rest means active rest. The noninjured structures and the cardiovascular system need to be maintained in top physical condition. The injured structures are taken through range of motion exercises as guidelines permit. Ice is the first step in treating any kind of trauma. Ice reduces the tissue damage, decreases the amount of hemorrhage, and minimizes muscle spasm. Ice also helps reduce pain and inflammation. Ice is applied for 20 minutes or less and should not be applied directly to the skin except with ice massage. Caution should be used if ice is applied over major subcutaneous nerves, especially in athletes with little subcutaneous fat.[8] Crushed ice conforms to contours of the body more easily than ice cubes; for home use, a bag of frozen vegetables or a slush ice bag works well. The basic recipe for a home slush ice bag is 5 oz. of water to every 1 oz. of rubbing alcohol in a plastic freezer bag.

Compression is used to help reduce inflammation. It is also an effective means of stopping hemorrhage. Compression creates a pressure gradient around blood vessels so that the pressure is greater on the outside of the blood vessels to help stop plasma seepage. Compression is accomplished with an Ace bandage wrap, or an elastic sleeve; the Tubigrip elastic sleeve is easier to apply and allows the athlete to wear a shoe. It can also be worn with the stirrup types of supports. The combination of ice and compression is achieved with the Cryocuff and Cryotemp devices.

An injured limb that is in a dependent position can be very painful. Elevation of the injured limb promotes better circulation by helping to decrease pooling of blood and stimulating venous return. The higher the elevation, the more effective the reduction in swelling.[1] Elevation works best if the limb is positioned above the heart. At night, pillows can be used to raise the limb, or the foot of the bed can be elevated by placing a phone book or brick under each leg of the bed. This allows the athlete to sleep supine, prone, or on one side without pillows interfering with mobility. When the ankle is elevated, the knee should be supported to prevent hyperextension.

TREATMENT OF SOME COMMON INJURIES

Strains

A strain happens if a muscle or tendon is overstretched or subject to a contractile force that exceeds its capability. Strains are broken down into three different classifications:

1. First-degree strain (mild strain)—tear of a few muscle or tendon fibers, mild pain and swelling, strong but painful muscle contraction.

2. Second-degree strain (moderate strain)—tearing of a moderate number of muscle or tendon fibers; a moderate amount of pain, swelling, and disability; weak and painful muscle contraction. An irregularity or depression may be palpated.

3. Third-degree strain (severe strain)—complete rupture of the muscle tendon unit; extremely weak or unable to contract muscle; pain and swelling may be minimal to severe; may require surgery.

Sprains

Ligaments help stabilize the joints through a full ROM. They have sensory functions in providing protective reflexes and joint proprioception.[9] A ligamentous sprain occurs when a joint is forced beyond its normal range. The athlete may or may not hear a pop at the time of injury. Sprains are classified as follows:

1. Grade I (mild sprain)—a few torn fibers, no instability, minimal pain, minimal swelling, localized tenderness, joint stiffness, minimal bruising.

2. Grade II (moderate sprain)—more swelling, limited ROM, some joint instability, more bruising.

3. Grade III (severe sprain)—total rupture of ligaments, joint instability, profuse swelling, bruising, and hemarthrosis.

For both sprains and strains, early intervention would be as follows:

Stage 1
    Treatment: PRICE principles
        Avoid positions of stress to injured structures
        Passive ROM within limits of pain
        Gentle isometric exercises
        Maintain strength of surrounding structures
        Maintain cardiovascular endurance
Stage 2
    Treatment: PRICE principles continue
        Gradually progress from PROM (passive range of motion) to AAROM (active assisted range of motion) to AROM (active range of motion) within pain-free guidelines
        Increase the resistance with isometric exercise
        Isotonic exercises started
        Proprioception exercises started
Stage 3
    Treatment: As full ROM is achieved and flexibility is restored, resistance can be increased
        Proprioception exercises progress
        Speed, power, and endurance exercises
Stage 4
    Treatment: Sport-related skills
        Proprioception drills for neural protection are very important to avoid reinjury

Treatment of Ankle Sprains

Stage 1: PRICE
    Athlete is limping; crutches issued, feather to partial weight bearing
    Stirrup type of orthosis issued
    Gentle ROM exercises instructed within pain-free range
    Submaximal isometrics within pain-free ROM
    Do ROM exercises, 10 reps each, every hour during the day
    Instructed in alphabet tracing with toes
    Towel stretch for gastrocnemius-soleus, 1 minute, for 3 to 5 reps
    Ice applied for 15 to 20 minutes every few hours
    Tubigrip measured for proper compression for circumference of ankle. Felt horseshoe pads will offer compression around the malleoli. This can be inserted under the Tubigrip.
    AROM (active range of motion) to the knee instructed
    Straight leg raises all four directions (hip flexion, abduction, adduction, and extension), 4 or 5 sets of 10
    Upper body ergometer for cardiovascular exercise
Stage 2
    Continue PRICE principles
    Full AROM of ankle is obtained
    Multiple-angle isometrics (every 15 degrees of available motion)
    Light weights or elastic resistance exercises started
    Sitting proprioception exercises: At home use a square board (12 to 14 inches) over a dowel or baseball bat and rock heel to toe, side to side.

Healing Time Frame

During the rehabilitation process there should be no increase in pain or inflammation. Ice is used after exercise. There is no set timetable in progression from Stage 1 to Stage 2, and so on. Thus, it's preferable for stage 1 to take 5 days rather than increase the athlete's pain and symptoms so that there is a smooth progression from one phase to another. The SAID principle (specific adaptations to imposed demands) must be stressed in the rehabilitation process so that the athlete can return safely to his/her sport.[1] An important question to ask the athlete is, "Do you *trust* your ankle (or whatever part is injured)?" Sometimes there is so much psychological pressure from other sources to return to play that a more reliable response is obtained with that question rather than, "Do you feel ready to play?"

OVERUSE INJURIES

When an athlete's training does not allow sufficient rest and recovery, the constant repetitive stress placed on ligaments, tendons, joints, and bone can lead to injury. These nonacute injuries are often described as microtraumatic overuse injuries. It is important to find the causes of the overuse and correct them. The problem often has been progressing for weeks to months before the athletes seek help. Athletes need to be educated about these causative factors and ways of correcting them.

The rule of "too" applies here: too much exercise done too hard, too soon, too much, too frequently, with muscles that are too tight, too weak, too tired, or too stressed. Contributing factors are training errors, lack of strength, lack of flexibility, inadequate recovery, or faulty biomechanics. The causes of the overuse injury must be discovered and corrected. For example, if malalignment is a problem—which is common in the lower extremity—orthotics may be indicated.

Treatment begins with ice and rest. Rest may be active rest, such as cutting the exercise load in half, or doing some type of cross training to maintain conditioning without stressing the injured structures. Exercise treatment is designed to stimulate the tissues via concentric (muscle shortening) and eccentric (muscle lengthening) work, with emphasis on the eccentric exercises. This work will focus on increasing muscle length, load, and speed. Increasing resting length on the muscle-tendon unit will decrease strain during joint motion. Progressively increasing resistance will increase the tensile strength of the tendons. Increasing speed of movement would also increase the load on the tendon.[10] Controlled eccentric training produces hypertrophy of the muscle and tendon, which results in the capacity to transmit more force. This is thought to decrease the risk of injury. When returning to full activity, the athlete must perform proper warm-up and stretching, and maintain adequate hydration to ensure viable ground substance within the tendon.[11]

With overuse injuries in the lower extremities, decreased flexibility must be addressed. For example, with Achilles tendinitis and plantar fasciitis, stretching the calf (gastrocnemius and soleus)

Table 6-2
Staging of Tendinitis and Overuse Syndrome

Grade	Symptoms	Treatment
I	Pain only after activity Does not interfere with performance Often generalized tenderness Disappears before next exercise session	Modification of activity Assessment of training pattern Possibly NSAIDs
II	Minimal pain with activity Does not interfere with intensity or distance Usually localized tenderness	Modification of activity Physical therapy; NSAIDs; consider orthotics
III	Pain interferes with activity Usually disappears between sessions Definite local tenderness	Significant modification of activity Assess training schedule Physical therapy; NSAIDs*; consider orthotics
IV	Pain does not disappear between activity sessions Seriously interferes with intensity of training Significant local sign of pain, tenderness, crepitus, swelling	Usually need to temporarily discontinue aggravating motion Design alternate program May require splinting Physical therapy and NSAIDs
V	Pain interferes with sport and activities of daily living Symptoms often chronic or recurrent Signs of tissue changes and altered associated muscle function	Prolonged rest from activity NSAIDs plus other medical therapies† Consider splint or cast Physical therapy May require surgery

*In some circumstances, injection of steroids into the tendon sheath may be considered, along with other medications such as heparin.
†Occasionally, systemic steroids are used with appropriate reference to the benefit/risk ratio.
Source: Reid DC: Sports Injury Assessment and Rehabilitation. New York, Churchill Livingstone, 1992, p. 80.

muscles with the slant board gives the athlete a solid end point. An easy way to fashion a slant board at home is by placing a 3-inch phone book or brick under a 12- to 14-inch board. It is important to stretch with the subtalar joint in its neutral position to effectively stretch the muscle. This is achieved by slightly toeing in or supinating the foot. The stretch should start at 30 seconds and build up to 2 to 3 minutes.

Stress Fracture

If the overuse injury affects bone, a stress fracture may result. A stress fracture causes localized tenderness, possible localized edema, pain with activity, and possible increased pain at night when at rest. Pain on percussion of the bone and increased pain with a tuning fork test may help raise the suspicion of a stress fracture.[12] Therapeutic ultrasound will also elicit pain at the stress fracture site. X-rays taken in the early stages are often negative, so if there is a high suspicion of stress fracture, it should be treated as such. Stop the activities that are causing the pain. Immobilization is not recommended, as it will lengthen the rehabilitation time by causing muscle atrophy.

Treatment for a stress fracture usually involves activities that will maintain the athlete's cardiovascular status without adding stress to the injured bone. Water running in the deep end of a swimming pool with a life vest is a good alternative for a runner. Garrick advises the 10-day absolute pain-free rule before activities are gradually resumed. He also advocates cycling for rehabilitation for its decreased weight bearing, concentric muscle activity (less stress to healing bone), and general aerobic benefits.[5] A pneumatic leg brace worn with tibial stress fractures allows return to full, unrestricted pain-free activity significantly sooner than traditional treatment.[13]

Patellofemoral Injuries

It appears that every anterior knee pain is now called patellofemoral syndrome. A very careful evaluation is needed for accurate diagnosis and to determine whether the cause is malalignment, overuse, tendinitis, or an apophysitis.

Treatment of such injuries is as follows:

1. PRICE principles to eliminate inflammation, effusion, and pain because these symptoms selectively inhibit the VMO (vastus medialis obliquus)
2. Taping/bracing for patella malalignment
3. Orthotics for lower extremity malalignment
4. Flexibility of lateral retinacular structures, iliotibial band, hamstrings, and gastrocnemius
5. Strengthen VMO and its timing of firing; improve VMO/VL (vastus lateralis) ratio to 1:1[14]
6. Strengthen gluteal muscles and emphasize proper alignment for weight-bearing exercises[15]

There should be less than 10 percent difference between lower extremities for ROM, strength, and flexibility. The primary care physician needs to approve the athlete's return to play.

Table 6–3
Fat Pad Irritation and Patellar Tendinitis: Signs and Symptoms

Fat Pad Irritation	Patellar Tendinitis
Tenderness at inferior patella	Tenderness at inferior patella
"Puffy" knees	Knees not "puffy"
Pain exacerbated by:	Pain exacerbated by:
Prolonged standing	Jumping
Negotiating stairs	Mid to full squat
Hyperextended/locked back knees	Straighter quadriceps (Q) angle (<15 degrees for
Pain when going up stairs as weight-bearing leg	females, <12 degrees for males)
extends, when acute	Pain when at ¾ to full squat; pain on jumping
Pain reproduced on extension or on overpressure	No pain on extension or on overpressure
Tenderness at inferior pole	Tenderness at inferior pole
Posterior displacement of inferior pole	No displacement of inferior pole

SHOULDER INJURIES

Assessment

In the evaluation and treatment of shoulder injuries one must remember the glenohumeral joint does not act in isolation but is part of the shoulder complex. The shoulder complex comprises the glenohumeral joint, the acromioclavicular joint, the sternoclavicular joint, and the sternothoracic articulation. Cervical problems may also cause shoulder pain and weakness, and therefore, cervical involvement must be ruled out as the cause of shoulder symptoms. The shoulder complex is subject to overuse, trauma, fractures, dislocations, and laxity. The evaluation must identify the injured soft tissues or the type of joint problem so that an appropriate treatment plan can be established. The soft tissues of the shoulder complex provide both static and dynamic stability; therefore, the evaluation must identify if there is loss of ROM from weakness, tissue inflexibility, capsular adhesions, force couple imbalances, or abnormal joint mechanics. The evaluation of the shoulder must also include examination of the scapula, which provides the origin of the rotator cuff muscles and positions the glenoid for efficient glenohumeral rotation. It also provides the proximal stability for upper extremity mobility. The scapula also functions to position the muscles for eccentric contraction, an action in which the muscles "brake" the acceleration phase of throwing, or decelerate the shoulder.

Treatment

The goals of treatment of shoulder overuse, microtrauma, or rotator cuff injury initially are to decrease the pain and inflammation, prevent rotator cuff muscle atrophy from muscle reflex inhibition, and decrease the effects of immobilization.[16] In the rehabilitation process, it is important to consider the vascularization of the rotator cuff and biceps tendons. When the arm is in the dependent neutral position and when the arm is adducted,

---

Table 6–4
Checklist for Discharge from Sports Physical Therapy: Lower Extremity Injuries

Anthropometric Measurements	Parameters		Functional Rehab	
	———— ————		1. Toe/heel raises	————
	———— ————		2. Jog slowly, straight	————
	———— ————		3. Jog faster	————
	———— ————		4. Jog faster: stop & start	————
Pain	———— ————		5. Run on track	————
AROM	———— ————		6. Sprinting	————
PROM	———— ————		7. Jog figure 8s	————
Biomechanical corrections	———— ————		8. Run figure 8s	————
Assistive devices (taping, braces)	———— ————		9. Cariocas	————
Flexibility			10. Cutting—½ speed	————
Achilles/gastrocnemius/soleus	———— ————		11. Cutting—full speed	————
Hamstrings	———— ————		12. Distance, running	————
Low back	———— ————		13. Continue wt. tr.	————
Abductors	———— ————		14. Return—drills	————
Adductors	———— ————		15. Return—non-contact	————
Iliotibial band	———— ————		16. Return—practice	————
Hip flexors	———— ————		17. Return—competition	————
Rectus femoris	———— ————		18. Isokinetic tests	————
Quadriceps	———— ————		Functional tests (sport-specific)	————
Strength quads	———— ————		1 month	
hams	———— ————		6 months ————————————	
Power quads	———— ————		12 months ————————————	
hams	———— ————			
Power quads	———— ————			
hams	———— ————			
Endurance	———— ————			
Kinesthetic proprioceptive tests	———— ————			
Functional jump/hop tests	———— ————			

Source: Davies GJ: A Compendium of Isokinetics in Clinical Usage and Rehabilitation Techniques, 4th ed. Onalaska, WI, S&S Publishers, 1992, p. 278.

filling of the blood vessels is diminished, reducing the blood supply for nutrition and oxidation necessary for healing.[17] Thus, it is important to maintain slight abduction of the arm at rest and during rotator cuff exercises.

In the early phase of rehabilitation, emphasis is on restoring ROM to the shoulder, both actively and passively. If there are capsular restrictions, joint mobilization is indicated and is especially important in restoring inferior humeral glide to prevent further impingement in the overhead position. Passive static stretches with cuff weights or a cane to stretch the tight muscles is important in the initial stage. Correct shoulder mechanics must be carefully observed to ensure that the supraspinatus is working correctly to depress and stabilize the humeral head with ROM, or exercises and stretching could lead to further impingement. Scapular stabilization exercises are performed with glenohumeral ROM. In the early stages, care is needed to avoid increasing the pain. Use of ice is recommended after exercises.

Return-to-play guidelines for upper extremities are as follows:

No pain
Passive ROM and active ROM within 10 percent or less of normal limits
Flexibility within 10 percent of normal limits
Sensation normal
Kinesthesia is intact (kinesthesia is the ability to perceive the extent and direction of motion)
Reflexes test normal
Manual muscle test 5/5
Proper ratio of shoulder strength internal rotation/external rotation (IR/ER) 3:2, extension/flexion (E/F) 5:4, adduction/abduction 2:1[16, 18]
Physician's release to play

LOW BACK PAIN

In sports activity about 10 percent of injuries involve the back. Most are self-limiting and are never treated.[3] Those injured patients who do seek help need a thorough evaluation to determine an accurate diagnosis. This process is often not easy because of the multitude of structures that can cause pain. (It is also important to ask if the athlete has had this problem before to rule out too early a return to sports before adequate recovery.)

Table 6–5
Conservative Management for Shoulder Impingement

Warm up with Codman's and capsular stretch
Transverse friction massage for tendinitis
1. Range of motion two times a day if ROM is limited.
2. Strengthening exercises are done in pain-free ROM only; if isotonic exercise not tolerated, then isometrics are utilized.
3. Scapular stabilization exercises, as follows:
   A. Scapular retraction done actively
   B. Scapular retraction done with rubber tubing resistance
   C. Prone shoulder extension
   D. Prone shoulder horizontal abduction
   E. Standing weight shift through arms with hands on tabletop
   F. Wall push-ups
   G. Proprioception exercises (1) with scapula pinched and down, shoulder flexed about 80 degrees with hand on ball against the wall, roll ball clockwise and counter clockwise; and (2) kneeling on floor, hands on balance board, shift weight through arms to move board clockwise and counterclockwise
4. Isotonic strengthening done with free weights (shoulder internal rotation, and adduction may be done with elastic resistance) starting with ¼-inch bands and building up to 50 repetitions, then progressing to ½ inch, 1 inch, etc. All exercises are done in proper alignment with the lifting motion done to the count of 3 and lowering to a count of 6. Apply ice after exercise for 20 minutes. Exercises A through E should be emphasized.
   A. Shoulder abduction in the "empty can" position
   B. External rotation done in side-lying position
   C. External rotation done prone with elbow at shoulder height
   D. Internal rotation done while side-lying on involved side
   E. Shoulder adduction done while standing with body rotated 90 degrees from door, involved side toward the door with rubber resistance from top of door
   F. Shoulder flexion to 90 degrees, thumb faces forward
   G. Shoulder abduction to 90 degrees, thumb faces up
   H. Shoulder extension done prone or standing bent at waist
   I. Horizontal adduction done supine
   J. Horizontal abduction done prone, thumb faces up
   K. Shoulder elevation or shrugs
   L. Shoulder depression done by arm chair press-ups
   M. Push-ups start with wall push-up, progress to table top, knees, then toes

Data from Andrews JR, Wilk KE. The Athlete's Shoulder. New York, Churchill Livingstone, 1994; and Buss D, Swanson K: Shoulder Protocol. University of Minnesota.

There are many sports that place rotatory forces, compressive forces, repetitive loading, or stressful positioning on the spine. Understanding the biomechanics and stresses of the sport will aid in identifying the possible cause of the low back pain and in determining when the athlete will be able to return to the sport. Did trauma cause this injury or did it develop slowly? Are there signs and symptoms of a musculoskeletal disorder or disk problem?

Treatment in the acute phase is to ice, educate, motivate, and keep the patient moving. Patients *must* take an active role in their rehabilitation. Athletes are shown different positions to use to decrease stress and pain. If they have a lateral shift, they are taught to correct for it. The lateral shift, or "protective scoliosis," often occurs when disk material moves posterolaterally, causing a disk bulge or herniation. The shift or curve appears much higher in the spine than the injured level, and the trunk appears to be off center. Nine out of ten subjects exhibit a lateral shift away (contralateral) from the painful side, and the incidence of sciatica and neurologic deficit is higher in those with a shift toward the painful side (ipsilateral).[19] Neutral spine positions are taught. Gentle ROM exercises are done to achieve extension, flexion, or a combination, depending on the diagnosis. Stabilization exercises are taught early in the process. Early involvement in aerobic exercise that does not stress the back (pool, upper body ergometer, and the like) is very important to maintain conditioning.

Athletes must have a good ROM and normal strength of upper and lower abdominals, back musculature, and hips. Athletes must be able to do their sport drills and skills without pain. They must restore and maintain flexibility to back and hip musculature. They must restore their speed, power, endurance, coordination, and proprioception of torso and hips.

SUMMARY

This chapter has been an attempt to educate the primary caregiver in the initial steps in sports rehabilitation. A full rehabilitation program is required to restore the muscles and joints to optimal function, or the athlete is at risk for reinjury. Manual therapy, especially joint mobilization, was not discussed but is an important component in restoring full physiologic ROM and accessory movements. Proprioceptive neuromuscular facilitation (PNF), another manual therapy technique, uses the body's natural patterns of movement to restore strength, flexibility, and coordination. Other techniques such as open- or closed-chain exercises, plyometrics, and isokinetic exercises are discussed elsewhere. Modalities were not emphasized, yet they, too, are used in the rehabilitation process. The reader should consult the references for further information.

Let's return to the three athletes from the first paragraph. The 6-year-old was allowed to play soccer when the cast was removed and she had recovered full functional use of her upper extremity. The football player was able to return to full practice within 6 days if wearing an ankle support. The coach decided he was ready to play. The master swimmer took almost 7 weeks to recover from the bursitis, which resulted from the supraspinatus tendinitis he had acquired from a rapid increase in training distance.

Injuries are a part of sports activities. Athletes come to us seeking help. When all the members of the sports medicine team work together and use sound rehabilitation principles, a successful outcome can be achieved.

REFERENCES

1. Prentice WE: Rehabilitation Techniques in Sports Medicine. St. Louis, Mosby, 1994.
2. Mellion MB (ed): Office Management of Sports Injuries and Athletic Problems. St. Louis, Mosby, 1988.
3. Sallis RE, Massimino F (eds): ACSM Essentials of Sports Medicine. St. Louis, Mosby, 1997.
4. Kibler WB, Herring SA, Press JM, Lee PA: Functional Rehabilitation of Sports and Musculoskeletal Injuries. Gaithersburg, Aspen, 1998.
5. Garrick JG, Webb DR: Sports Injuries: Diagnosis and Management. Philadelphia, W.B. Saunders, 1990.
6. Mellion MB: Sports Medicine Secrets. Philadelphia, Hanley & Belfus, 1993.
7. Booher JM, Thibodeau GA: Athletic Injury Assessment. St. Louis, Mosby, 1994.
8. Covington DB, Bassett FH III: When cryotherapy injures: the danger of peripheral nerve damage. Physician Sports Med 21(3):78–93, 1993.
9. DeLee JC, Drez D Jr (eds): Orthopaedic Sports Medicine Principles and Practice. Philadelphia, W.B. Saunders, 1994.
10. Curwin S, Standish WB: Tendonitis: Its Etiology and Treatment. Lexington, MA, Collamore Press, 1984.
11. Timm KE: 16th Annual Sports Medicine Physician-Therapist Team Concept Conference, Dallas, TX, Nov. 3–5, 1995.
12. Irvin R, Iversen D, Roy S: Sports Medicine Prevention, Assessment, and Rehabilitation of Athletic Injuries. Boston, Allyn & Bacon, 1998.
13. Swanson EJ Jr, et al: The effects of a pneumatic leg brace on return to play in athletes with tibial stress fractures. Am J Sports Med 25(3):322–328, May–June, 1997.
14. Eiland G: 16th Annual Sports Medicine Physician-Therapist Team Concept Conference, Dallas, TX, Nov. 3–5, 1995.

15. Grelsamer R, McConnell J: The Patella: A Team Approach. Gaithersburg, Aspen, 1998.
16. Davies GJ: A Compendium of Isokinetics in Clinical Usage and Rehabilitation Techniques, 4th ed. Onalaska, WI, S&S Publishers, 1992.
17. Andrews JR, Wilk KE: The Athlete's Shoulder. New York, Churchill Livingstone, 1994.
18. Ivey FM, Jr: Evaluating acute knee injuries. Am Fam Physician 25(2):122–129.
19. McKenzie R: Mechanical Diagnosis and Therapy. Part A: The Lumbar Spine Course Notes. Course Syllabus. University of Minnesota, Minneapolis, Sept. 1996.
20. Buss D, Swanson K: Shoulder Protocol. University of Minnesota.

Chapter 7 | Return to Play

JANUS D. BUTCHER, M.D.
MARK McGRAIL, M.D.

Determining when to allow an athlete to resume training and competition following an injury is one of the most crucial and difficult functions of the team physician. With a few notable exceptions (for example, following traumatic brain injury and anterior cruciate ligament reconstruction), there are no specific or structured guidelines to direct the treating physician. A thorough understanding of the mechanics, physiology, pathoanatomy, and healing principles in injured tissues is essential to making appropriate decisions regarding return to play.

Although it is impractical (if not impossible) to provide specific guidelines governing the return to play for all athletic injuries in all sports, several general principles can be applied to guide this decision:

1. Injured tissue must be returned to preinjury levels of function, or to a point at which participation will not result in reinjury. This level is generally measured as full, pain-free range of motion and normal strength (greater than 80 percent of the uninjured side).

2. Associated dynamic and static stabilizing tissue should be adequately retrained through strengthening, flexibility, and proprioceptive rehabilitation.

3. Technique and equipment factors that may have contributed to the initial injury must be addressed.

4. When appropriate, functional bracing, taping, and orthotics are employed.

5. A sport-specific return to activity program is constructed and supervised utilizing physical therapists, athletic trainers, and coaches. This program should begin with basic skills (e.g., straight-line running) with increasing complexity until the athlete is able to accomplish all tasks specific for the sport. Because the treatment plan and return-to-play program

must be individualized for each athlete, no one program is appropriate for all athletic injuries.

Although there are important differences between acute and overuse injuries, which will be discussed below, these general guidelines apply to both types of injury.

In a sense, the planning for return to participation in sport begins with the initial injury evaluation. This is particularly true in high-level collegiate or professional athletes in whom even a minor injury can have significant individual and team ramifications. The athletic trainer or sideline physician must first recognize that an injury has occurred (typically an injury is obvious, but many athletes will try to hide their injury to continue to play), and the athlete should be removed from play for further evaluation.

Frequently, the physician will feel pressure from the athlete, coaches, parents, or the community to allow continued play or an early return to play. This decision may be further complicated by input received from the athlete's own physician or specialist whose opinion differs from that of the team physician. However, the decision regarding when to allow the athlete to return to play following injury is the responsibility of the team physician. This decision is, of course, made with the input of the coaches, trainers, therapists, and other health care providers, but final clearance rests with the team physician. There may be times when a compromise is appropriate. For instance, a collegiate track athlete with an overuse injury who wants to run in the last event of his/her career may be allowed to run that race. In making these decisions, the physician must weigh the risks and benefits to the individual and discuss them with the athlete to allow the athlete to make an informed decision.[1] However, if there is significant risk to the athlete's well-being from continued play, it rests on the team doctor to hold the athlete from participation. This decision should be based on clinical, ethical, and medicolegal grounds.[1]

Each tissue involved in sports injury has unique properties affecting the reparative process. These differences govern the appropriate treatment approach, healing time, and eventual return to play. A basic understanding of these principles will assist in predicting the time required to return the athlete to full participation. Details regarding specific injuries can be found in the other chapters of this text; the following is a general discussion regarding tissue injury.

ACUTE INJURIES

Muscle

The most common mechanisms resulting in acute muscle injuries are direct blows and excessive tension. Direct trauma frequently leads to local cellular damage and hemorrhage but may result in complete disruption of the muscle unit. Tension injuries can be caused by passive stretching or more commonly through an eccentric overload of the activated muscle.[2] These injuries typically result in tearing at the musculotendinous junction.

Treatment of these types of injuries is approached through balancing protection from excessive tension (short-term immobilization and avoidance of weight bearing) with rehabilitation exercises. Studies have shown that early range of motion exercises and strengthening will speed recovery following muscle injury.[2] The typical time from injury to return to play depends on site and severity of injury but typically ranges from 10 days to 6 weeks.[3]

Tendon

Most sports-related tendon injuries arise from excessive strain related to either an acute macrotraumatic event, or more commonly repetitive microtrauma (see later discussion regarding overuse injuries). Tissue healing following acute tendon injury is generally discussed in three phases[4]: (1) the acute inflammatory phase is characterized by clot formation and the inflammatory cascade, which provide the framework and cellular constituents for later repair; (2) the reparative phase is directed by tissue macrophages and marked by neovascularization and collagen production by fi-

broblasts; and (3) in the remodeling or strengthening phase the extracellular matrix becomes organized with complete collagen maturation, usually occurring within 4 months.

The time to complete repair is dictated by the extent of injury and the specific tissue involved. Typically, the acute phase is measured in days, the reparative phase in weeks, and the strengthening phase in months. Similar to the management of muscle injuries, early mobilization of injured tissue appears to facilitate the healing process. This must be balanced with the need to rest the tissue and prevent further injury.

Ligament

Ligamentous injuries occur when the normal range of motion of a joint is exceeded, resulting in abnormal stretch of the ligament. These types of injuries are often classified as grade 1 injury (ligamentous stretch without tear), grade 2 (a partial tear), and grade 3 (complete rupture of the ligamentous structure).

The process of ligament healing is similar to that described for tendons. Because of the relative avascularity of these tissues, the time required for complete repair can be quite protracted. Also, in spite of adequate therapy, permanent joint laxity following such injury is common.

Because the healing process can be prolonged, athletes will frequently complain of pain even when all evidence of acute injury has resolved. However, with these injuries, the athlete frequently can return to play before complete healing has occurred by utilizing a functional brace or taping to protect the joint from excessive motion. Although many ligaments will heal if protected from repeat injury, others (such as the anterior cruciate ligament) will not heal in any meaningful sense. These cases may be managed through rehabilitation of the dynamic stabilizing structures (muscles and tendons) and functional bracing or may require surgical therapy if instability persists.

An athlete with a low-grade ligamentous injury may be able to return to play very quickly if adequate bracing can be achieved. More significant injuries, such as a complete rupture of the medial collateral ligament, may require 4 to 12 weeks of therapy for the athlete to regain joint stability.[5] The primary late complaint following ligamentous injury is instability. Athletes with significant instability following adequate rehabilitation and bracing should be referred for possible surgical treatment.

Bone

Acute injuries to bone range from a simple contusion to overt fractures. Acute fractures are common in collision and high-velocity sports, although they can occur in any activity. The majority of fractures are treated initially with splinting (until swelling subsides) followed by a period of cast immobilization. For fractures that require closed reduction, a plaster or fiber glass cast may be used in the initial management. The length of immobilization is determined by several factors, including the patient's age, fracture type, location, and required activity during treatment. The clinician should consult the relevant literature to determine the appropriate treatment of the specific fracture.

The typical immobilization period ranges from 1 month (e.g., uncomplicated fracture in a young patient) to 3 months or more (e.g., scaphoid fracture), with 4 to 6 weeks being typical. A playing cast may be utilized for some upper extremity fractures in sports that do not require finger dexterity in the injured hand. Early surgical fixation has been advocated for certain fractures (e.g., scaphoid and proximal fifth metacarpal fractures) in order to dramatically reduce the immobilization time and speed the return to play[6] for high-level athletes who require the full use of the hand. A period of aggressive rehabilitation is typically required following casting to restore the preinjury range of motion and strength prior to resuming competition.

OVERUSE INJURIES

A majority of sports-related injuries and pain complaints arise from repetitive microtrauma. The most commonly involved tissues in these overuse injuries are tendon and bone. Overuse injuries are particularly problematic in the competitive athlete because both players and coaching staffs tend to minimize their significance and thus allow continued abuse. As a result, these athletes often present to the physician after a prolonged period of "playing through" the pain. The evaluation and treatment of these conditions are further complicated because the presenting symptom is frequently a

Table 7-1
Intrinsic and Extrinsic Factors Contributing to Overuse Injuries

Intrinsic factors	
Muscle strength imbalances	Physical fitness
Poor flexibility	Weight
Knee malalignment	Personality
Abnormal foot biomechanics	Age
Systemic diseases	Gender
Extrinsic factors	
Type of activities chosen	Training methods
Shoes and other foot wear	Health habits
Equipment deficiencies	(smoking, diet)
Training surfaces	Environmental conditions

manifestation of an occult problem such as a remote biomechanical abnormality or technique deficiency. This has been described as the concept of "victims and culprits," wherein the pain complaint is the victim and the occult cause is the culprit.[7] The contributing "culprits" are often discussed in terms of intrinsic or extrinsic factors (Table 7–1). Intrinsic factors refer to anatomic and functional deficiencies or imbalances that result in abnormal stresses being applied to normal tissue. Extrinsic factors generally refer to training errors, equipment deficiencies, and poor playing surfaces.

In addressing the athlete's problem, the treating physician must not only promote healing of the injured tissue but also investigate, identify, and correct these causative factors before the athlete's return to participation.

GENERAL REHABILITATION PRINCIPLES

Returning the injured athlete to competition usually involves a step-wise progression through a rehabilitative process, with the end goal being resumption of participation at the preinjury level of play. Although several models have been used,[3, 8] the following five-step progression is fairly representative. The key to the successful and expedient return to sport is to tailor the program to each athlete based on the injury, the chosen sport, psychosocial influences, and comorbid conditions. It is essential to employ a team approach, including physical therapists, athletic trainers, and coaches, in this recovery. The broadly labeled phases of treatment are listed in Table 7–2.

Acute Treatment and Evaluation This phase is the time immediately following the injury and

Table 7–2
Five-Step Return-to-Play Rehabilitation Program

1. Acute injury treatment
   Key points: Immobilization protection
   Provide adequate analgesia
   Make accurate anatomic diagnosis
2. Promote optimal healing
   Key points: Protection
   Early mobilization
   Active rest (maintain fitness)
3. Functional rehabilitation
   Key points: Balanced flexibility and strengthening program
   General aerobic and strength training
4. Sports-specific retraining
   Key points: Progression of running and strength
   Skill retraining
   Technique coaching
5. Return to play
   Key points: "Objective" rehabilitative goals met
   Functional bracing and taping employed
   Continued technique coaching

is characterized by acute swelling, bleeding, and tissue destruction. The goals in the immediate treatment stage are to prevent further injury, provide adequate analgesia, and establish an accurate diagnosis. Typically, the acronym PRICEMM is used to describe the treatment modalities in this step (Table 7–3).[8] Protection is provided through the temporary use of full or partial immobilization, which typically includes casting (in a fracture), an immobilizer (in an acute knee injury), or a functional brace (in an ankle sprain). Each injury or injury location requires a specific brace to appropriately balance protection and early rehabilitation (Table 7–4). Functional bracing has been shown to dramatically decrease the time to return to play.[9]

Although no conclusive benefit has been shown for the use of nonsteroidal anti-inflammatory drugs (NSAIDs) in the healing of tissues, these medications do often provide pain relief.

Table 7–3
PRICEMM Treatment for Acute Injuries

Protection
Relative rest
Ice
Compression
Elevation
Medications
Modalities

Acetaminophen or narcotic pain medications may also be appropriate options, depending on the type and severity of the injury.

It is crucial to accurately diagnose the type and extent of injury as well as any associated occult injuries in the first few days following the event. Diagnosis frequently is not possible immediately following the injury because of swelling and pain. In these cases it is usually appropriate to protect the injury and reevaluate in 2 to 3 days. A careful neurovascular examination must be performed, and radiographs are obtained to ensure that no fracture is present before the athlete is released. If an early diagnosis is necessary to direct treatment, more sophisticated imaging techniques such as magnetic resonance imaging, computed tomography, or bone scintigraphy may be useful. If the protection and reevaluation option is appropriate, frequent follow-up must be assured.

Promoting Optimal Healing Following the initial treatment stage, which typically lasts a few days, the next goal is to promote optimal healing by protecting and rehabilitating the injured tissue while maintaining aerobic and strength conditioning. Although resting the injured tissue is vital to allow proper healing, early controlled mobilization facilitates recovery in most soft-tissue injuries. This early mobilization limits strength losses (strength may decrease by up to 20 percent in one week of complete immobilization) and maintains range of motion.[3] In the early phase of treatment, this is best accomplished by therapist- or trainer-supervised passive and active range of motion exercises using pain as the guide for progression. Physical modalities such as ultrasound, phonophoresis, electrical stimulation, and iontophoresis are also useful in promoting healing.[10]

Aerobic capacity and strength should be maintained as much as possible throughout the injury period through cross-training (stationary bike, running in a swimming pool, and other activities) and weight machines. Initiating this early may be very beneficial to the athlete's emotional state by encouraging participation in the treatment process.[11]

Functional Rehabilitation As the injury resolves, specific attention must be paid to strengthening both the injured tissues and the associated dynamic supporting structures. Often tissues that were not involved in the initial injury will be weakened through immobilization or reflex inhibition. Functional rehabilitation is aimed at neuro-

Table 7–4
Typical Bracing Options for Injuries

Injury	Brace
Hand	
Ulnar collateral ligament	Thumb spica splint/cast
Scaphoid fracture	Thumb spica cast (short or long arm)
De Quervain's tenosynovitis	Thumb spica splint
Wrist	
Dorsal wrist sprain	Neutral wrist splint
Radius fracture	ORIF or muenster cast
Shoulder	
Dislocation	Immobilizer (after reduction)
Acromioclavicular separation	Sling
Clavicle fracture	Immobilizer, sling, or figure-of-eight sling
Knee	
Medial collateral ligament	Hinged knee brace, MCL brace
Anterior cruciate ligament	Derotation brace, ACL brace
Meniscal tear	Hinged knee sleeve (?)
Ankle and lower leg	
Achilles tendinitis	3/8″ heel lift, cam walker boot
Lateral ankle sprain	Functional brace, taping
Anterior ankle sprain	Functional brace, taping
Shin splints	Orthotics, tibial sleeves, taping
Posterior tibialis tendinitis	Short leg cast (foot inverted), cam walker with arch support
Foot	
Plantar fasciitis	Viscous heels, rigid heel cups, arch supports, tension night splints
Turf toe	Rigid plantar toes extension (Morton's brace), taping
Anterior tibialis tendinitis	Cam walker, short leg cast

muscular retraining, strengthening of injured and associated supporting tissues, and restoration of normal joint motion. This stage of treatment is primarily accomplished through self-directed exercise with supervision from the trainer and therapist. Physical therapy modalities (ice, ultrasound, massage, phonophoresis, iontophoresis) continue to be useful in providing analgesia and anti-inflammatory effects.

Sport-Specific Retraining In most cases, the pain associated with an injury will significantly diminish before the athlete's rehabilitative process is complete. The athlete is usually motivated to return to the sport as soon as possible and is at risk for reinjury if not appropriately prepared to participate in the sport. It is important therefore to retrain athletes in the specific activities associated with their sport prior to resumption of regular participation. Typically this begins with running drills, plyometrics, and specific technique coaching (throwing, swimming, and the like) done in a noncompetitive supervised setting. The goal of this stage of rehabilitation is to develop the specific neuromotor coordination required to perform all the tasks involved in their sport.

Several objective criteria have been proposed to determine when it is safe to resume sport partic-ipation. The most commonly cited criteria are the return of full range of motion of the injured joint and 80 to 90 percent of the muscular strength (measured isometrically or isotonically in comparison with the uninvolved side), and an ability to accomplish all sports-specific skills/demands.[8] Although these provide relatively objective criteria for the team physician, it is clear that more specific guidelines are needed.[1] This is an area of active interest in the sports medicine literature, and specific treatment protocols are being published regularly.

Return to Athletics and Sports When the athlete has healed (determined by using the preceding criteria and the resolution of pain with activity) and adequately regained the sports-specific skills, he/she should be gradually returned to full practice. In the early practice sessions, particular attention should be directed at using appropriate technique and ensuring that prescribed bracing or protective gear is being used properly. To minimize the risk of reinjury, it is often necessary to provide a very specific training and practice schedule for the athlete during the transition back to full participation. If the rehabilitation period has been brief, the athlete can make the transition back to competition quickly. For those with a prolonged rehabilitation, a stepped transition with very deliberate increases in participation should be constructed. For instance, the track athlete recovering from a lower leg stress fracture may need specific instructions regarding weekly mileage increases, intensity, and rest days.

Many injuries are season-ending or even career-ending. In these cases it is particularly important to be realistic with the athlete in setting the goals for recovery and return. In cases in which the rehabilitation will encompass the off-season, the athlete must be instructed in the risk of reinjuries and recreational injuries. Structured rehabilitation may be difficult to continue during school breaks when the athlete does not have access to the training room. Here again, specific instructions should be given to the athlete, and the use of a physical therapist outside the school should be considered.

Developing the Specific Program

Each injured athlete requires a rehabilitation and return to play program tailored to the specific injury, taking into account the level of participation, athletic goals, psychologic state, and comorbid medical conditions. Typically, the progression of the rehabilitation program is based on symptomatology and functional improvement. Seldom, if ever, is it based on time. This program should be monitored directly by the athletic trainer or physical therapist with frequent follow-up with the team physician. The treatment options, goals, and general time line to recovery should be discussed with the athlete at each visit. Communication between members of the treatment team, the athlete, the parents (when appropriate), and coaches is vital to reach the treatment goals. Involvement of specialists such as sports psychologists, physiologists, dietitians, and other medical subspecialists should be encouraged when appropriate.

An example of this approach can be seen in the endurance runner who develops tibial stress fractures. This condition may require a fairly protracted period of active rest with the use of long leg air stirrup braces, cam walker boot, or even casting. During this time of immobilization, alternative activities (such as use of a ski machine, running in a swimming pool, or cycling) would be encouraged to maintain cardiovascular conditioning. As the athlete's symptoms diminish, a balanced strengthening and stretching program would be initiated to correct underlying biomechanical deficiencies that led to the injury. In addition, the athlete should be evaluated for orthotics and proper running shoes to correct abnormal foot biomechanics.

When the symptoms have resolved and the injury has healed, a graduated running program is instituted, beginning with a jog/walk for short distances every other day and then increasing this as tolerated. For many competitive athletes this program must be even more specific in outlining exact distances allowed, frequencies, and the progression schedule. In this area, the athletic trainer is a key member of the treatment team. Other risk factors for the development of this injury may need to be investigated. For instance, the female athlete presenting with this injury should be questioned regarding diet, depressive symptoms, and menstruation to rule out the possibility of the female athlete triad. Overall, the time for symptom resolution and return to play in this athlete may be 4 weeks to 3 months, depending on the severity of the stress reaction.

At the other end of the spectrum are the minor injuries that are treated with limited time away from the sport. An example is a soft tissue contusion in an upper extremity in a hockey player that does not affect his play. These athletes may miss little or no participation time and can treat the injury while continuing to participate actively in their sport. This discussion relies heavily on the experience and comfort of the team physician and trainers who determine when it is safe for the athlete to continue to play with an injury.

PSYCHOLOGICAL ASPECTS OF ATHLETIC INJURY

The psychological impact of an injury is often overlooked, yet it can have a profound impact on the athlete's rehabilitation and return to play. It is common for injured athletes to experience anger, depression, anxiety, lower self-esteem, and other emotional or psychosomatic symptoms as a result of the injury and subsequent exclusion from their sport. This emotional response is typically proportional to the degree of injury and can result in significant psychological dysfunction in the athlete.[12]

The team physician, trainers, and coaches must be aware of these complications of sports injury and be prepared to refer the athlete to the appropriate providers when necessary. Screening tools such as the Beck Depression Inventory or profile of mood states (POMS) may be useful in screening for these problems in injured athletes.

Several psychological interventions have been found to have a positive effect on rehabilitation and eventual return to play. These methods include relaxation, healing imagery, positive self-talk, and goal setting, among others.[11] In injured athletes with more serious psychiatric sequelae, the early involvement of a mental health provider is crucial to recovery. It is important in these athletes to evaluate for suicide ideation or intention and to intervene immediately if the individual is at risk.

REFERENCES

1. Mitten MJ, Mitten RJ: Legal considerations in treating the injured athlete. J Orthop Sports Phys Ther 21(1):38–43, 1995.
2. Garrett WE: Muscle strain injuries: Clinical and basic aspects. Med Sci Sports Exerc 22(4):436–443, 1990.
3. Herring SA: Rehabilitation of muscle injuries. Med Sci Sports Exerc 22(4):453–456, 1990.
4. Leadbetter WB: Cell-matrix response in tendon injury. Clin Sports Med 11(3):533–578, 1992.
5. Reider B: Medial collateral ligament injuries in athletes. Sports Med 21(2):147–156, 1996.
6. Rettig AC, Kollias SC: Internal fixation of acute stable scaphoid fractures in the athlete. Am J Sports Med 24(2):182–186, 1996.
7. Macintyre JG, Lloyd-Smith DR: Overuse injuries. *In* Renstrom PA (ed): Sports Injuries: Basic Principles of Prevention and Care. Boston, Blackwell Scientific Publications, 1993, pp. 139–160.
8. O'Connor FG, Howard TM, Fieseler KM, Nirschl RP: Managing overuse injuries: A systematic approach. Phys Sports Med 25(5):88–113, 1997.
9. Swenson EJ, DeHaven KE, Sebastianelli WJ, et al: The effect of pneumatic leg brace on return to play in athletes with tibial stress fractures. Am J Sports Med 25(3):322–328, 1997.
10. Rivenburgh DW: Physical modalities in the treatment of tendon injuries. Clin Sports Med 11(3):645–659, 1992.
11. Smith AM: Psychological impact of injuries in athletes. Sports Med 22(6):391–405, 1996.
12. Smith AM, Scott SG, O'Fallon WM, Young ML: Emotional responses of athletes to injury. Mayo Clin Proc 65:38–50, 1990.

Chapter *8*

Use of Nonsteroidal Anti-inflammatory Drugs and Analgesics

JANE T. SERVI, M.D.

Nonsteroidal anti-inflammatory drugs (NSAIDs) are among the most commonly used medications in the United States. Annual worldwide sales are estimated at $1 billion.[1] Their easy accessibility as over-the-counter medication contributes to their popularity. They are utilized in sports medicine to control pain, thereby allowing early return to activity that speeds healing, and to decrease inflammation, which presumably helps to speed healing directly.[1] These two mechanisms assume that postinjury inflammation of itself is bad; however, some believe that inflammation may be good for the healing process and should not be suppressed.[1]

MECHANISM OF ACTION

Trauma ruptures cell walls. The intracellular contents that leak out are broken down by the enzyme cyclooxygenase to prostaglandins, leukotrienes, and other components of the inflammatory process.[2] Prostaglandins promote vasodilatation, chemotaxis, and increased vascular permeability, thereby playing a role in the acute inflammatory response to injury.[3] Additionally, prostaglandins enhance bradykinin, a substance that stimulates the formation and release of more prostaglandins.[3] Prostaglandins also sensitize nerve endings, making nerve fibers fire more aggressively and at a lower stimulus than they would normally fire.[2]

Arachadonic acid is converted to various prostaglandins by the enzymatic action of cyclooxygenase. NSAIDs exert their anti-inflammatory and analgesic effect by blocking this reaction.[3, 4] Aspirin acetylates cyclooxygenase, thereby irreversibly inhibiting the formation of prostaglandins. Other NSAIDs reversibly inhibit cyclooxygenase by competitive inhibition.[3] Other mechanisms by which NSAIDs may work include inhibition of superoxide generation in neutrophils, inhibition of phospholipase C in mononuclear cells, inhibition of neutrophil aggregation, inhibition of neutrophil and monocyte migration, inhibition of phosphodiesterase, inhibition of peripheral lymphocyte responses to mitogen stimulation, inhibition of lipoxygenase, inhibition of leukotriene production, and proliferation of B and T cells.[3, 4]

PHARMACOLOGY

NSAIDs may be classified according to chemical structure or half-life (Tables 8–1 and 8–2). To reach a "steady state," 5 half-lives of the particular NSAID are necessary. For instance, if the NSAID has a half-life of 4 hours, 5 doses, or 20 hours, are necessary to reach the steady state, provided that dosage is regular. For the longer-acting NSAIDs, serum concentrations may continue to rise for several weeks, even after 5 half-lives have been exceeded.[3] For the NSAIDs with longer half-lives, serum concentrations tend to remain stable between doses, once the steady state has been reached. For NSAIDs with half-lives less than or equal to 4 hours, serum levels fluctuate between doses.[3]

Generally, NSAIDs are metabolized by the liver, and excreted by the kidneys. If hepatic or renal insufficiency exists, NSAIDs should be used cautiously, and if they are used, the dose should be reduced by one-third to one-half.

ADVERSE EFFECTS OF NSAIDS

Although use of NSAIDs is beneficial in sports medicine, their use is also associated with adverse

Table 8–1
Nonsteroidal Anti-inflammatory Drugs by Class

Carboxylic Acids
Proprionic Acid Derivatives
  Flurbiprofen (Ansaid)
  Ibuprofen (various brand names, e.g., Advil, Nuprin)
  Ketoprofen (Orudis, Oruvail)
  Naproxen (Naprelan, Naprosyn)
  Oxaprozin (Daypro)
Salicylates
  Acetylsalicylic acid (aspirin)
  Salsalate (various brands, e.g., Disalcid)
  Choline or magnesium salicylate (Trilisate)
Phenylacetic Acids
  Diclofenac sodium (Voltaren)
  Diclofenac potassium (Cataflam)
Fenamates
  Meclofenamate sodium (Meclomen)
  Mefenamic acid (Ponstel)
Indoles
  Indomethacin (Indocin)
  Sulindac (Clinoril)
  Tolmetin sodium (Tolectin)
Pyranocarboxylic acid
  Etodolac (Lodine)

Nonacids
Naphthylalkanone
  Nabumetone (Relafen)
Enolic Acids
Oxicams
  Piroxicam (Feldene)
Pyrazoles
  Ketorolac tromethamine (Toradol)
Benzene Acetic Acids
Bromobenzyl Monosodium Salt
  Bromfenac sodium (Duract)
Combination Product
Phenylacetic Acid and Prostaglandin E$_1$ Analogue
  Diclofenac sodium and misoprostol (Arthrotec)
Cox-2 Inhibition
Diaryl Substituted Pyrazole
  Celecoxib (Celebrex)
Diaryl Substituted Furanone
  Rofecoxib (Vioxx)

effects. Up to one-half of patients taking NSAIDs will have an adverse event, and 1 to 2 percent of these reactions may be serious.[1] Adverse effects of NSAIDs tend to be dose-related, with the most common adverse reactions involving the gastrointestinal (GI) tract. GI side effects may consist of dyspepsia, nausea, heartburn, constipation, and other minor side effects. More serious side effects consist of gastric and duodenal ulcerations, GI bleeding or perforation, and mucosal injury to the small or large intestines. These reactions are partly attributed to the inhibition of prostaglandin synthesis, which results in decreased endogenous mucosal protection.[3] NSAIDs may also exert an effect on cell metabolism, cell adhesion, and the interaction between epithelial cells and the mucosal inflammatory and immune responses in the GI tract.[3] NSAIDs may activate quiescent inflammatory bowel disease.[4] The prevalence of adverse reactions to NSAIDs increases with increasing age (over age 65), past history of ulcer disease, alcohol abuse, and simultaneous use of another NSAID, anticoagulant, or a corticosteroid.[2–4] One study using endoscopic observation showed a 6.7 percent

Table 8–2
Classification of NSAIDs by Half-Life

Short (<4 hours)	Intermediate (4–12 hours)	Long (>12 hours)
Bromfenac sodium	Celecoxib	Nabumetone
Diclofenac potassium	Diflunisal	Oxaprozin
Diclofenac sodium	Etodolac	Piroxicam
Diclofenac sodium and misoprostol	Indomethacin	Rofecoxib
Diclofenac sodium-XR	Ketoprofen, extended release	
Ibuprofen	Ketorolac	
Ketoprofen	Naproxen	
Meclofenamate sodium	Naproxen sodium	
Tolmetin sodium	Sulindac	

incidence of gastric ulceration and a 1.4 percent incidence of duodenal ulceration after ingestion of NSAIDs for 7 days.[3] Studies have also indicated that as many as 30 percent of NSAID users will develop gastroduodenal ulcers.[5] GI side effects can be minimized by choosing nonacetylated salicylates, using the lowest effective dose, taking medication with food, and using concurrently with misoprostol (Cytotec), sucralfate (Carafate), H_2-receptor antagonists, or omeprazole (Prilosec).[3]

It is estimated that up to 5 percent of patients receiving NSAIDs will develop renal complications.[6] NSAID-induced renal adverse effects include electrolyte imbalance and allergic interstitial nephritis.[3] Inhibition of prostaglandins is the underlying mechanism for electrolyte imbalance and occurs more frequently in volume-depleted patients and those with underlying renal insufficiency or hypoalbuminemia.[3, 4] Interstitial nephritis results in acute renal failure. Fenoprofen accounts for the majority of these very rare and unpredictable cases.[3, 4] Chronic and severe renal disease is a contraindication for NSAID therapy.

Hepatic toxicity associated with NSAID use results in an asymptomatic elevation of serum transaminase levels, which reverses upon discontinuance of the medication. Sulindac and diclofenac may produce a higher incidence of hepatitis compared with ibuprofen and ketoprofen, which pose the lowest risk.[3, 4] Profound hepatotoxicity is uncommon. High-risk patients include those with a history of hepatitis, cirrhosis, or alcoholism.[7]

NSAIDs may also have hematologic adverse effects, including inhibition of platelet aggregation, agranulocytosis, and aplastic anemia. Whereas nonacetylated salicylates and nabumetone have little effect on platelet function, many NSAIDs reversibly inhibit platelet aggregation by inhibiting cyclooxygenase.[3] Aspirin irreversibly inhibits platelet aggregation. Phenylbutazone and indomethacin are associated with an increased frequency of agranulocytosis and aplastic anemia compared with other NSAIDs.[3, 4]

Rarely, NSAID use can exacerbate bronchial asthma, especially in those with the triad of asthma, nasal polyps, and aspirin intolerance. Other adverse effects include CNS and pulmonary side effects and cutaneous reactions.[3] Side effects as a result of NSAID use are often unpredictable. One NSAID, ketorolac tromethamine (Toradol), is indicated only for short-term use (5 days) to minimize potential side effects.

DRUG INTERACTIONS

Blood pressure should be monitored in patients taking NSAIDs concurrently with antihypertensives, especially angiotensin-converting enzyme (ACE) inhibitors and β-adrenergic blockers. NSAIDs interfere with antihypertensive treatment through their effects on volume and prostaglandin-dependent vascular and renal function.[4] Lithium and phenytoin levels should be followed when used simultaneously with NSAIDs. Blood sugar levels should be checked in those taking NSAIDs and oral hypoglycemic agents simultaneously. Anticoagulants may interact with NSAIDs.

USE OF NSAIDS IN THE ATHLETIC SETTING

The net result of a traumatic injury to an athlete is pain. The objective in treating an injury is to enhance the healing process, not necessarily removing the pain that bars the athlete from activity. However, when pain and inflammation management are provided, an injury prognosis can be improved through early entry into the rehabilitation phase.

There is not general consensus, however, on the use of anti-inflammatory medications. Some care providers believe that such use is unnecessary and counterproductive and that blocking prostaglandins actually delays healing. Some think that an attempt to change the natural response to an injury is misguided, while others believe that we also need to address the psychosocial response to injury.[3]

Proponents of early NSAID use cite experimental studies that report ibuprofen given prophylactically and therapeutically is effective in reducing delayed-onset muscle soreness and improving muscular performance when compared with placebo and control subjects. Another study shows that anti-inflammatory medications may prevent weakening of the muscle-tendon unit in the early postinjury period and increase maximum failure load of the tissue in the late postinjury period. Another study indicates that these drugs temporarily increase the strength of healing dense fibrous tissue. Many attribute the beneficial effect of NSAIDs after soft tissue injury to their analgesic effects, allowing for early range of motion.[3]

Others believe there is no advantage to the use of NSAIDs in the early setting, citing experimental research that anti-inflammatory medication may interfere with early repair phase when macrophages are mobilized to remove cellular debris, erythrocytes, and fibrin clot. Macrophage inhibition could delay muscle regeneration. The significance of altered chondrocyte function on cartilage has not yet been determined, although one animal study states that salicylates and several other NSAIDs suppress proteoglycan biosynthesis in normal and degenerating articular cartilage.[3, 5] One animal study also demonstrated a retarded fracture healing rate associated with ibuprofen and indomethacin use.[9] Indomethacin suppressed the expression of insulin-like growth factor-1 messenger RNA in callus after femoral fracture in rats.

From a psychosocial standpoint, many athletes feel social or self-imposed pressure to return to the competitive arena as quickly as possible after an injury, and some become psychologically depressed or demoralized if they are withheld from their activity. These athletes may look for a "quick fix" in the form of a pill. If they are able to dampen their pain response from injury, they believe that they have achieved a "cure." However, when the pain quotient has been decreased or removed, often the remainder of the treatment protocol (ice, range of motion, stretching, strengthening, and proprioceptive retraining) gets neglected and appropriate rehabilitation is never achieved. One of the goals in the treatment of an athletic injury should be enlisting the athlete in an active, rather than passive, treatment program.

There are many variables to consider with the use of NSAIDs, including the time to onset of action, ease of compliance, cost, the patient's prior experience with specific NSAID use, adverse drug reactions, drug-drug interactions, and acute or chronic injury.

There are a multitude of NSAIDs on the market; thus, it is not always possible to predict which one a given individual will respond best to, and there is no evidence that any of these drugs is any more efficacious across the board than any of the others.[3]

It is considered pragmatic to start with the older NSAIDs first, as they tend to be cheaper and better studied. If the first NSAID does not work (it takes about five consecutive doses of a drug to reach optimal effective levels), it is advisable to try a different agent from another chemical family (see Table 8–1).

General rules for NSAID prescription include choosing less expensive options if they are effective, utilizing the lowest dose that is effective for relieving pain and inflammation, considering patient compliance when deciding on frequency of dosage, and keeping in mind the side effect profile. NSAIDs have an analgesic ceiling; therefore, taking more than the recommended dose will not decrease pain, but it will increase the risk of side effects.[3] This precaution is particularly important in the elderly, who have changes in metabolism, renal function, and blood pressure. Shorter acting (more frequent dosing) agents may be more effective for acute injury, whereas compliance is improved with longer acting NSAID use in chronic injury.

In patients with increased symptoms of gastroesophageal reflux disorder secondary to peptic ulcer disease, NSAIDs may carefully be combined with H_2 blockers, misoprostol (Cytotec), diclofenac/misoprostol (Arthrotec), or omeprazole (Prilosec). NSAIDs containing sodium may exacerbate hypertension and NSAIDs may reduce efficacy of antihypertensives, especially ACE inhibitors and β-adrenergic blockers. Blood pressure should be monitored with simultaneous use. Low-dose aspirin therapy for cardiovascular prophylaxis should not affect NSAID use.

OTHER ANALGESICS

Acetaminophen (e.g., Tylenol) is an analgesic and an antipyretic. It produces its analgesic effect by elevation of the pain threshold and antipyresis through action on the hypothalamic heat-regulating center.[10] Acetaminophen is equal to aspirin in analgesic effectiveness and is unlikely to produce many of the side effects associated with aspirin and NSAIDs. It is indicated for temporary relief of minor muscular aches including those associated with bursitis, neuralgia, sprains, and overexertion.[10] Massive overdosage may be associated with hepatotoxicity.

Muscle relaxants are utilized when pain is present secondary to muscle spasm or in the treatment of painful muscle strains. Muscle relaxants are centrally acting agents that do not directly relax tense skeletal muscles in humans.[11] The mode of action of muscle relaxants on relieving acute muscle spasm of local origin has not been established, but it may be related to their sedative properties. The use of muscle relaxants is indicated as an adjunct to rest, physical therapy, and other measures for the relief of discomfort associated with acute, painful musculoskeletal conditions.[11] Because of their sedative properties, their use may be beneficial in those who are experiencing a sleep disturbance secondary to the pain from their injury. Users should be warned that there may be impairment in physical and mental abilities.

Narcotics have limited use for most sport injuries. Short-term use for extremely painful conditions (fractures, postoperatively, and some acute injuries) should not be withheld. The risk of developing addiction in a patient taking narcotics for analgesia is minimal, less than 0.5 percent.[3]

Tramadol hydrochloride (Ultram) is a centrally acting synthetic analgesic. It is indicated for management of moderate to moderately severe pain. Its mode of action is not completely understood. It has at least two complementary mechanisms of action: binding of parent and metabolite to μ-opioid receptors and weak inhibition of reuptake of norepinephrine and serotonin.[12] Adverse events are similar to those of an opioid: dizziness, somnolence, nausea, constipation, sweating, and pruritus.[12] There is less respiratory depression associated with tramadol use than with opioids. The seizure threshold is lowered in those with seizure disorders, and physical dependence is observed in patients who have been previously dependent on other opioids. Withdrawal symptoms can occur upon abrupt discontinuance of tramadol. Tramadol does have the potential to cause psychic and physical dependence of the morphine type.

Corticosteroid injections, when used properly, have potential benefits that outweigh their side effects. Steroid use is associated with problems when too large a dose is used, an inappropriate drug is chosen, injections are administered too frequently, or poor injection technique allows spread of the drug to adjacent tissue.[13]

There are no guidelines referring to the frequency of corticosteroid injections. Safety can be maximized if only three to four injections are given to an area or joint in a 1-year span. If the first injection does not resolve the pain, the second can be given within 1 to 6 weeks from the first.

Only corticosteroids with a large anti-inflammatory (glucocorticoid) and low fluid balance effect (mineralocorticoid) are useful in treating musculoskeletal problems.[13] Steroids also differ in the potency of their anti-inflammatory effect and in their duration of action within tissues.

Steroids are indicated when treating an inflammatory process. The larger the dose, the greater the systemic effect. Systemic effects include flushing and menstrual irregularity, rare impaired glucose tolerance, osteoporosis, psychological disturbance, steroid arthropathy, muscle atrophy and myopathy, immunosuppression, and adrenal suppression. Local side effects include infection, subcutaneous atrophy, tendon rupture, skin atrophy, depigmentation, and discoloration.

CONCLUSION

Most patients will recover from an injury whether or not a NSAID is utilized in the treatment process. NSAIDs clearly offer an analgesic effect, which is the most common reason for their use. Short-term studies suggest that in patients treated with an NSAID, healing was slightly more rapid, inflammation was slightly decreased, and return to practice was occasionally quicker than for those receiving a placebo.[1] Although there is no dispute of the important role that prostaglandins play in the biochemical reaction of inflammation, it can be questioned whether, if the body's natural response to injury is inflammation, suppression of this response by NSAIDs hastens the healing process. It has not been established that inflammation is a harmful response to injury, so perhaps this response should not be chemically altered. Although prostaglandins of the E series participate in the pain response and increase vascular permeability, prostaglandins in the F series may be involved in enhancing the formation of ground substance and thereby favor wound healing.[15] NSAID use may adversely affect injury outcome, when suppression of the pain response leads to a more deleterious injury (for example, shin splint progression to stress fracture.) Because NSAID ingestion is associated with many adverse events, it is important that the sports medicine practitioner decide on utilization of NSAIDs on an individual basis, weighing the risks and the benefits of NSAID use and taking into account each individual, injury, and situation. NSAID value is clearly maximized when these drugs are used in conjunction with relative rest, ice, compression, elevation, and rehabilitation.

REFERENCES

1. Weiler JM: Medical modifiers of sports injury—the use of nonsteroidal antiinflammatory drugs (NSAIDs) in sports soft-tissue injury. Clin Sports Med 11(3):625–644, 1992.

2. Thornton JS: Pain relief for acute soft-tissue injuries. Physician Sportsmed 25(10):108–114, 1997.

3. Hannah G: Nonsteroidal anti-inflammatory drugs. *In* Andrews JR, et al (eds): Injuries in Baseball. Philadelphia, Lippencott-Raven, 1998, pp. 431–435.

4. Furst DE: Are there differences among nonsteroidal antiinflammatory drugs? Arthritis Rheum 37(1):1–9, 1994.

5. Gomes JA, Roth SH, Zeeh J, et al: Double-blind comparison of efficacy and gastroduodenal safety of diclofenac/misoprostol, piroxicam and naproxen in the treatment of osteoarthritis. Ann Rheum Dis 52:881–885, 1993.

6. Schnitzer TJ: NSAIDs in orthopaedic practice: Management guidelines for arthritis patients. Contemp Orthop 30(5):383–389, 1995.

7. Amadio P, Cummings DM, Amadio PB: NSAIDs revisited: Selection, monitoring, and safe use. Postgrad Med 101(2):257–271, 1997.

8. Brandt KD, Palmoski MJ: Effects of salicylates and other nonsteroidal anti-inflammatory drugs on articular cartilage. Am J Med 77:65–69, 1984.

9. Altman RD, Latta LL, Keer R, et al: Effect of nonsteroidal antiinflammatory drugs on fracture healing: A laboratory study in rats. J Orthop Trauma 9(5):392–400, 1995.

10. Physicians' Desk Reference for Nonprescription Drugs, 13th ed. Montvale, NJ, Medical Economics, 1992, pp. 591–592.

11. Physicians' Desk Reference, 51st ed. Montvale, NJ, Medical Economics, 1997, p. 2782.

12. Physicians' Desk Reference, 50th ed. Montvale, NJ, Medical Economics, 1996, p. 1585.

13. Saunders S, Cameron G: Corticosteroids in injection. *In* Techniques in Orthopaedic & Sports Medicine, 1st ed. London, W.B. Saunders, 1997, pp. 1–5.

14. Walsh WM, Hald RD, Peter LE: Musculoskeletal injuries in sports. *In* Mellion MB, Walsh WM, Shelton GC (eds): The Team Physician Handbook. Philadelphia, Hanley & Belfus, 1990, p. 254.

15. Calabrese LH, Ronney TW: The use of nonsteroidal anti-inflammatory drugs in sports. Phys Sportsmed 14(2):89–97, 1986.

Chapter 9 | Evaluation of Minimal Brain Injury

MARGOT PUTUKIAN, M.D., FACSM

Minimal brain injury or concussion is common in sports, yet accounts for some of the most devastating injuries that we see. Although this type of injury occurs commonly, much is still unknown about its pathophysiology, proper diagnosis, and treatment, as well as the natural history of traumatic brain injury. Much of this information has been based on opinions and experience rather than clinical research. The goal of this chapter is to present the spectrum of head injuries that occur in sports, with emphasis on minimal brain injury, and the evaluation and treatment of these injuries, along with a discussion of some of the return-to-play decisions that need to be made. Although many of these answers are yet to be formulated, an understanding of the complexities of brain injury and how they relate to participation in sports can provide the physician with important tools with which to manage athlete patients.

Most head injuries that occur in the athletic realm are minor when compared with the spectrum of head injuries that occur in high-velocity motor vehicle accidents. Despite this, it is important to remember that severe injuries can occur on the athletic field and, along with repetitive injuries, can have serious, longstanding sequelae. Vascular injuries, some of which can rapidly expand and/or can occur in association with skull fractures, must be recognized early. Cervical spine injuries can also accompany head injuries and must be considered in every athlete who sustains a head injury. In addition, when an athlete sustains a second brain injury before completely recovering from a first injury, the "second impact syndrome,"[1] including brain edema and even death, can result. Finally, the "postconcussive syndrome," with longstanding symptoms after minimal brain injury, can have a significant impact on activities outside the sport and may have serious long-term sequelae.

Along with the concerns for the short- and long-term consequences of acute minimal brain injury, there is also some concern for an athlete who sustains repetitive head injuries. This risk is paramount in the sport of boxing, where the goal of the sport is to knock an opponent unconscious with repetitive blows to the head. The cumulative brain injury that occurs has been termed the "punch drunk" syndrome, or posttraumatic encephalopathy, and there is concern that this may be a precursor for dementia or Alzheimer's disease.[2–4] Soccer is another sport in which repetitive head injury can result because of the sport-specific skills of heading, or using the head to propel the ball (discussed later). Whether soccer poses a risk for cumulative damage has not been studied, and is very controversial.

The natural history of head injury in sports and the significance of cumulative injury remain unclear, and many mild head injuries continue to go undetected. The medical support staff available often varies at different levels of participation, underscoring the need to educate athletes, parents, coaches, and athletic trainers so that head injuries are detected and treated. It remains common for athletes to continue playing despite symptoms because of an expectation that this is "part of the game." McLatchie[5] found that in 544 rugby athletes 56 percent had sustained at least one head injury associated with amnesia afterward. For 58 players, the posttraumatic amnesia lasted more than an hour, and yet only 38 players were brought to a hospital for treatment.

EPIDEMIOLOGY OF HEAD INJURY IN SPORTS

Many head injuries, especially in the younger age group, go undetected; therefore, the exact incidence is unknown. Often athletes will not report symptoms, either because they take them lightly and feel they are an accepted element of participation or because they fear being taken out of the game if they admit injury. Many athletes are evaluated on the sidelines and not referred for further evaluation, again leading to an underreporting of the true incidence of minor head injury.

The National Head Injury Foundation reports that sports cause 18 percent of minor head injuries, compared with 46 percent from motor vehicle accidents, 23 percent from falls, and 10 percent from assaults. Sports caused 3 to 10 percent of the roughly 500,000 hospital admissions due to traumatic brain injury in 1984.[6] Head injury accounts for 4.5 percent of all high school sports injuries and 19 percent of all nonfatal injuries in football.[7, 8] There is a 15 to 20 percent risk for head injury per season at the high school level, with 200,000 of these injuries occurring annually[9, 10] and an average of eight deaths in head-injured football players per year.[11]

At the National Collegiate Athletic Association (NCAA) level, the use of the Injury Surveillance System (ISS) was developed in 1982 and has proved to be instrumental in careful assessment of assessing injury epidemiology. The Committee on Competitive Safeguards and Medical Aspects of Sports within the NCAA utilizes the data from the ISS to consider implementation of new rules to prevent and reduce injuries. The injury definition utilized by the ISS is one of time lost from participation, and, more important, the data provide a denominator of athlete exposure so that a true injury incidence can be determined.

The NCAA data for 1984–1991 demonstrate that head concussions account for 1.8 to 4.5 percent of total injuries, with an incidence of injury of 0.11 to 0.27 injuries per 1000 athlete exposures. This compares with an injury rate of 0.06 to 0.55 per 1000 athlete exposures and 1.6 to 6.4 percent in 1995–1996. Some of these data are presented in Tables 9–1 through 9–3. From these collegiate data, ice hockey has the highest percentage of total injuries attributed to head injuries, followed by football, field hockey, women's lacrosse, and men's soccer. Injury rates in sports with and without head protection differ less than might be expected, such that ice hockey, football, and men's lacrosse head injury rates are comparable to those in men's and women's soccer and field hockey. Concussion rates are the highest in football, with ice hockey, men's and women's soccer, field hockey, and men's lacrosse just behind.

In all but four sports from the 1984–1991 data, player contact is the primary mechanism of injury. Contact with the stick is the primary mechanism in field hockey, and contact with the ball accounted for the mechanism most commonly in baseball, softball, and women's lacrosse. Careful assessment of injury data can be very useful in determining the risk for injury in particular sports, as well as looking for ways in which injuries can be prevented. Determining the mechanism of injury is obviously an important part of this assessment. Looking at how concussion rates have changed over time within a sport can also provide information related to rule changes. An increase within a particular sport in the concussion injury rate may also be due to an increased awareness and thus an increased ability to detect these head injuries that probably would have been missed in the past. An increase in the number of athletic trainers and physicians attentive to medical needs of athletes can also explain a reported increase in injury rates within a particular sport. Given that the symptomatology for head injury is often subtle, it is understandable that many types of injuries that in the past were ignored or undetected are now under more careful scrutiny and are now reported.

Table 9–1
Frequency of Concussions as a Percentage of All Game Injuries 1989–1998

Head Protection Required		No Head Protection	
Ice hockey*	7.5%	Women's lacrosse*	8.5%
Men's lacrosse*	5.2%	Women's soccer	6.5%
Football*	4.5%	Men's soccer	5.4%
Spring football	3.9%	Field hockey	5.2%
Softball	3.6%	Women's basketball	4.9%
Baseball	2.7%	Men's basketball	3.1%

*Sport requires mouth guard.

Table 9–2
Concussion Injuries per 1000 Athletic Exposures, 1989–1998

Head Protection Required		No Head Protection	
Football*	1.8	Wrestling	1.2
Ice hockey*	1.4	Men's soccer	1.1
Men's lacrosse*	0.8	Women's soccer	1.1
Spring football	0.4	Women's lacrosse*	0.6
Softball	0.2	Field hockey	0.5
Baseball	0.2	Women's basketball	0.4
		Men's basketball	0.3

*Sport requires mouth guard.

It is important when looking at any epidemiologic data that any other selection biases are also accounted for. In the NCAA ISS data it is therefore important to consider the population being assessed and the level of competition. It is also important to consider the information retrieval system in place at all the various institutions and the inherent weaknesses of the data because of these systems. Gender issues as well as sport-specific issues may affect the data as much as the level of the athlete being assessed.

It is important that epidemiologic data be used to help make decisions to maintain safety without significantly changing the sport. For example, some have proposed that head injuries in women's lacrosse and field hockey can be reduced by the use of helmets in these sports. However, the data do not necessarily support a rule change in that the concussion injury rate is fairly low; one might accept more of an argument for helmets with shields to prevent facial lacerations, nasal fractures, and dental injuries. In addition, would adding helmets to these sports change the sport in such a way as to have a negative consequence? Would athletes be more aggressive and feel more invulnerable and thus be at greater risk for head and neck injuries as a result? These questions are important to consider when evaluating and interpreting injury data.

In ice and field hockey, the use of helmets resulted in a decreased incidence of head injury.[14, 15] Football has seen a significant decrease in head injuries between the period 1965–1974 compared to 1975–1984,[16] with a decrease since 1976 of

Table 9–3
NCAA Head Injury, Concussion, and Neck Injury Rate, 1984–1991

Sport	Head Injury		Concussion‡		Neck Injury	
	IR*	%†	IR	%	IR	%
SPORTS WITH NO HEAD PROTECTION						
Field hockey	0.23	4.5	0.20	3.8	0.05	1.0
Women's lacrosse	0.17	4.1	0.16	3.9	0.03	0.7
Men's soccer	0.31	4.0	0.25	3.2	0.03	0.4
Women's soccer	0.29	3.7	0.24	2.8	0.08	1.0
Women's basketball	0.16	3.1	0.15	3.0	0.05	0.9
Men's basketball	0.14	2.5	0.12	2.1	0.04	0.8
Wrestling	0.28	2.9	0.20	1.8	0.51	5.4
SPORTS WITH HEAD PROTECTION						
Ice hockey	0.30	5.4	0.25	4.5	0.09	1.7
Football	0.29	4.5	0.27	4.1	0.28	4.2
Men's lacrosse	0.22	3.2	0.19	3.0	0.12	1.7
Women's softball	0.11	2.9	0.11	2.9	0.06	1.6
Baseball	0.09	2.8	0.07	2.1	0.01	0.3

*Injuries expressed as IR (injury rate), which equals injuries per 1000 athlete exposures.
†Injuries are expressed as percentage of all reported injuries.
‡Concussions are a subset of all head injuries.

roughly 50 percent.[17] These improvements have been credited to rule changes prohibiting spearing and to changes in helmet designs. In ice hockey there has been great debate over whether helmets have indeed changed the game, with one study demonstrating that in 75 percent of 246 head injuries the mechanism was violence unrelated to the on-ice activities (high sticking, deliberate pushing, fistfights).[18] This would suggest that in order to decrease head injuries in hockey, more attention should be placed on rule enforcement and control of the game, with use of protective equipment being perhaps less important.

For the sports of baseball and softball, the helmeting of athletes is an important and unintrusive method of providing protection from head injuries. Helmets have been shown to be effective in reducing injury,[19] and because the mechanism of head injury is contact with the ball,[20] using a helmet while at bat is appropriate. Because of the nature of both these sports, the use of a helmet also does not interrupt or change the way the sport is played in any appreciable way.

Probably the best example of how a helmet can decrease the trauma and death associated with head injury is recreational bicycling. Bicycling is a high-risk activity because the rider's surface is often pavement, and collisions sometimes involve motor vehicles being driven at high speeds. It has been estimated that there is a 50 percent chance of head injury due to a fall, and that if the bicyclist is riding at 20 miles per hour, a fall can be fatal.[21] Bicycle injuries account for 1300 deaths annually, and many of these are due to head injuries.[22] An approved bicycle helmet has been shown to decrease the risk of brain injury by 88 percent.[22] Other than comfort and the low cost of an appropriate helmet, there is excellent evidence to support the value of wearing a helmet for bicycling.

The NCAA injury data demonstrate that head injuries and concussions are clearly important injuries for both helmeted and nonhelmeted athletes. The long-term sequelae and associated injuries that occur in conjunction with head injuries indicate the importance of management for these injuries. Thus, health care professionals must understand the spectrum of head injuries and how they present in the athletic realm. The care of the head-injured athlete should be well planned and organized so that an emergency care plan is easier to carry out calmly. The intent of this chapter is to outline some basics related to head injury, how

to treat such injuries, and some of the complications, and finally implications for future research.

DEFINITIONS

Two general types of head injuries are often described: focal brain injury and diffuse brain injury. Focal injuries include subdural and epidural hematomas, cerebral contusions, and intracranial hemorrhages, both subarachnoid and intracerebral. Focal injuries often occur as a result of blunt trauma, with both loss of consciousness (LOC) and/or focal deficits. Although less common than diffuse brain injury, focal injuries can occur in the realm of athletics. When focal injuries are associated with focal deficits or LOC, they are less likely to go undetected. However, focal injuries sometimes present with more subtlety. Early detection and treatment of these injuries are important and may mean the difference between life and death.

FOCAL BRAIN INJURIES

In a subdural hematoma, blood accumulates in the subdural space, generally as a result of disruption of the low-pressured venous system. The athlete often is unconscious and may or may not present with focal deficits and a slow deterioration in mental status. Subdural hematomas are further defined as simple or complex, the complex form being associated with cerebral contusion or brain edema and swelling. Simple subdural hematomas do not involve either condition and have an associated mortality rate of 20 percent. Complex subdural hematomas are associated with a mortality rate higher than 50 percent. Figures 9–1 and 9–2 show examples of a subdural hematoma.

The age of the patient can affect how subdural hematomas present themselves clinically. In an older patient, the normal, age-related cerebral atrophy allows for a larger potential subdural space, and therefore these athletes may not have significant brain injury.[23] In the younger athlete, the potential space is much smaller, and therefore, a smaller amount of bleeding will cause symptoms. In addition, the symptoms in younger athletes may be due to compression of normal brain tissue, and not necessarily to the focal deficits seen with the space-occupying presentation in the older athlete.[24]

Epidural hematomas are generally due to the

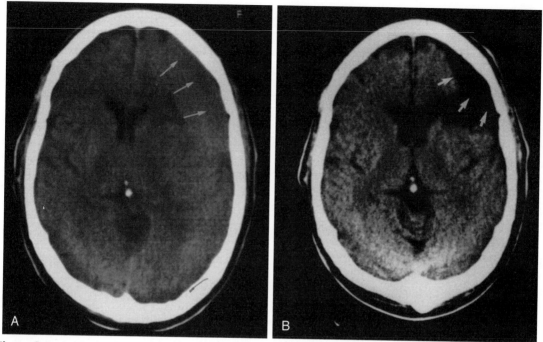

Figure 9–1. *A,* CT scan demonstrating an isodense subdural hematoma (*arrows*). *B,* Postoperative CT scan demonstrating chronic subdural fluid collection (*arrows*) in the region where the previous isodense subdural hematoma was identified (see *A*). Note that there is a focal area of decreased density in the underlying brain cortex, consistent with posttraumatic encephalomalacia. (From Rizzo M, Tranel D: Head Injury and Postconcussive Syndrome. New York, Churchill Livingstone, 1995, p. 75.)

disruption of the high-pressured arterial system, usually the middle or other meningeal arteries. The accumulation of blood into the epidural space therefore occurs rapidly, and in the classic form, epidural hematomas present with an initial LOC, then recovery with a lucid interval. This interval is followed by headache, deteriorating mental status and eventual LOC, pupillary abnormalities

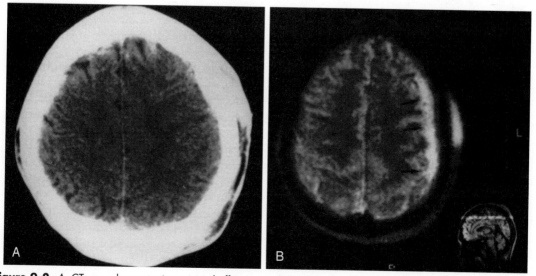

Figure 9–2. *A,* CT scan demonstrating minimal effacement of the cortical sulci on the left and adjacent superficial soft tissue injury. *B,* Axial MRI (TR2000, TE45) obtained at the same time as *A.* Note the subdural hematoma on the left (*arrows*), which is isodense on the CT scan. (From Rizzo M, Tranel D: Head Injury and Postconcussive Syndrome. New York, Churchill Livingstone, 1995, p. 75.)

(pupil dilated unilaterally, ipsilateral to clot), decerebrate posturing, and contralateral motor weakness.[25] Unfortunately, only one third of patients present in this classic manner[24] (Fig. 9–3).

Hemorrhage, intracerebral hematoma, and cerebral contusions generally cause headache, confusion, and posttraumatic amnesia, often without LOC. When a hemorrhage occurs on the surface of the brain (in the subarachnoid space) it is termed subarachnoid, whereas if it is located within the substance of the brain it is termed intracerebral. Cerebral contusions and hemorrhage can be associated with complications, including hydrocephalus and changes related to mass effect.

Several diagnostic imaging studies can be utilized to demonstrate the abnormalities associated with traumatic brain injury, including most commonly computed tomographic (CT) scanning, magnetic resonance (MR) imaging, and electroencephalography (EEG).[26–31] In a study of patients with severe closed head injuries in whom LOC was persistent and intensive care admission was required, 88 percent demonstrated abnormalities on MR imaging, and the degree and duration of brain injury related to the depth of the brain lesion on MR imaging.[32]

CT scanning and MR imaging are both useful in diagnosing epidural and subdural hematomas, although CT is often preferred because it is better at detecting bony abnormalities as well as blood in the acute setting. MR imaging may be better at detecting subtle injuries; this is especially true when the study is obtained more than 48 hours after the injury.[33–35] Although MR imaging may demonstrate a greater volume of injury than a CT scan of the same injury, those lesions that require surgical intervention are detected by CT scanning.[36] Emergent neurosurgical consultation is warranted for hematomas when they are detected, and if surgical evacuation is warranted, the time between injury and treatment may be essential in terms of prognosis and return to function.

DIFFUSE BRAIN INJURIES

Diffuse brain injuries represent the other main subset of brain injuries that occur and by definition are not associated with focal intracranial pathology. Diffuse brain injury represents a continuum of progressively more severe brain dysfunction, depending on the extent of structural or anatomic disruption. Nonstructural brain injuries are the least severe because anatomic integrity is well

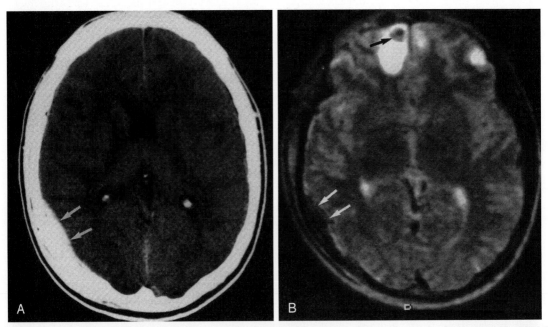

Figure 9–3. *A,* CT scan demonstrating a focal epidural hematoma (*arrows*). *B,* Axial T$_2$-weighted MRI (TR2000, TE105) obtained at the same time as the CT scan in *A.* Note the appearance of the epidural hematoma (*white arrows*), which is of decreased signal intensity. There is also a focal acute right frontal hematoma (*black arrow*) with adjacent edema. A smaller left frontal contusion is also present. This was not identified by CT. (From Rizzo M, Tranel D: Head Injury and Postconcussive Syndrome. New York, Churchill Livingstone, 1995, p. 77.)

maintained. Cerebral concussion is often considered in this category, although as will be discussed, concussion can also be associated with structural diffuse brain injury.

Structural diffuse brain injuries are the most severe diffuse brain injuries and are therefore at the other end of the clinical spectrum, being associated with anatomic disruption. Diffuse axonal injury is generally associated with prolonged brain injury and coma with LOC that often lasts longer than 6 hours. Neurologic, psychological, and personality deficits are common complications of diffuse axonal injury, occurring because of the axonal disruption in the white matter of the brain stem and cerebral hemispheres.

Cerebral concussion was defined as early as 1966 as "a clinical syndrome characterized by immediate and transient impairment of neurologic function secondary to mechanical forces."[37] Concussion may or may not involve LOC and/or memory dysfunction. Confusion and amnesia are the hallmarks of concussion, although a variety of symptoms may occur. Table 9–4 presents symptoms of head injuries; however, determining the severity of injury generally depends on whether LOC occurs and how long it persists, as well as other measures of consciousness and mental functioning.

Cerebral concussion is the most common head injury that occurs in the realm of athletics, and in comparison to the spectrum of head injuries that occur in motor vehicle and other high-velocity injuries, tends to be mild. Although it is uncommon to see focal injuries or significant anatomic disruption in the athletic setting, it is certainly essential that all injuries are taken seriously; there is no such thing as a minor head injury. Mild injuries can be associated with significant morbidity and even death, and many of the complications can affect basic functions that transcend all aspects of daily life. These minimal traumatic brain injuries are the focus of the remainder of this chapter.

MECHANISMS AND PATHOPHYSIOLOGY OF HEAD INJURY

Understanding the different mechanisms and pathophysiology of head injury in sport is useful in predicting the extent of injury and outcome.[38–40] This information may also supply health care pro-

Table 9–4
Signs and Symptoms of Cerebral Concussion

Loss of consciousness (LOC)
Confusion
Posttraumatic amnesia (PTA)
Retrograde amnesia (RGA)
Disorientation
Delayed verbal and motor responses
Inability to focus
Headache
Nausea/vomiting
Visual disturbances (photophobia, blurry vision, double vision)
Disequilibrium
Feeling "in a fog," "zoned out"
Vacant stare
Emotional lability
Dizziness
Slurred/incoherent speech
Excessive drowsiness
Symptoms consistent with postconcussive syndrome
   Loss of intellectual capacity
   Poor recent memory
   Personality changes
   Headaches
   Dizziness
   Lack of concentration
   Poor attention
   Fatigue
   Irritability
   Phonophobia/photophobia
   Sleep disturbances
   Depressed mood
   Anxiety

viders with tools to make interventions that may eventually decrease or prevent head injuries. Extensive research has been devoted to the pathophysiology of head trauma, and it is an area of research that continues to expand.

Research models have demonstrated that anatomic disruption occurs with diffuse brain injury. Axonal and myelin sheath disruption occurs throughout the white matter of the hemispheres and brain stem, as well as petechial hemorrhages in periventricular regions, and chromatolysis and cell loss occur throughout the cortical gray matter and brain stem nuclei.[41–44] Gross atrophy can result with repetitive injury.[45] In athletics, acceleration and impact forces tend to be the same, and thus these mechanisms can be thought of similarly.[46] When the force is rotational, the resultant shearing forces are substantial, and it is thought that this mechanism accounts for more severe structural injuries.[40, 46, 47] The reader is referred to a recent review of the neuropathology of traumatic brain injury[23] for more extensive information.

The three basic mechanisms that occur in head injuries related to sport include the stationary head hit with a forceful blow (impact or compressive force), the moving head that hits a nonmoving object (accleration or tensile force), and the head being struck parallel to its surface (shearing or rotational force). Impact forces—for example, when a football lineman is struck on the head—can be considered "coup" injuries, in which the brain surface lying beneath the impact area is the maximal area of injury. Acceleration injuries, such as when a soccer player dives to the ground and strikes his/her head, can be considered "contrecoup" injuries because the area of maximal injury is on the opposite side of the area struck. Shearing injuries occur with any rotational force, the clearest example occurring when a boxer is struck by a hook punch. More than one mechanism can occur in a specific injury pattern—for example, an acceleration force along with a rotational force—with more severe cumulative damage.[48] Understanding the mechanisms can help predict injury severity as well as predict the area of maximal injury.

In a simplistic approach, if one considers that the brain tissue is floating within the container of the skull in the cerebrospinal fluid (CSF) that protects and provides nutrients, these mechanisms of injury make sense. When the head accelerates in one direction, the brain itself lags behind and ultimately moves toward the back of the skull, making the CSF layer thinner at that area. If the head then strikes an object—whether it is fixed or moving—the brain tissue is least protected at the area opposite to where the head strikes, producing the contrecoup injury. Within the skull, the bony ridges and dura mater brain attachments (falx cerebri, tentorium cerebelli) are areas at increased risk.[49] These fixed structures act in many ways like a reef against which the delicate brain matter can smash in the setting of head trauma. Understanding these structural limitations can also help the examiner predict which part of the brain is likely to be injured.

When considering the biomechanical forces that may affect injury severity, the state of the neck musculature becomes important. Applying Newton's second law, in which mass × acceleration = force (or acceleration = force / mass), if the neck musculature is rigid when the head is struck, the forces imparted to the head may be less than if the neck musculature is not rigid. When the neck muscles are rigid, the mass of the head takes on an approximation of the mass of the body. The higher the mass, the higher the force needed to create the same acceleration. If the neck muscles are not rigid, then the mass is smaller, and the forces that strike the head do so with greater acceleration, with the potential for greater brain injury. This makes inherent sense in that athletes such as soccer and football players will state that they feel less head and neck pain if they strike the ball with proper technique and stabilization of their head than if they are struck without warning. This observation implies that proper technique in these sport-specific skills (heading in soccer, tackling in football) as well as strengthening of the neck musculature may have a role in minimizing severity of injuries.

An area of research that is new and exciting involves the neurochemical and neurometabolic changes that occur with concussive brain injury. There may be a disruption in the way in which cells utilize oxygen when ionic fluxes (due in part to the release of excitatory amino acids such as glutamine) occur in response to brain injury.[50, 51] With a concussive injury, cells that are not mechanically disrupted are thus exposed to these ionic fluxes in the setting of an increased need for glycolysis. Glucose metabolism has been shown to be increased in an animal model following brain injury using[^{14}C]2-deoxy-D-glucose autoradiography.[52, 53] Concurrently, the blood flow to the cerebrum is diminished,[54] which leads to a mismatch between the glucose demand and availability, which can ultimately result in cell dysfunction and possibly an increased risk for a second insult.[55]

This animal research has been validated in humans as well with an increased cerebral glucose metabolism noted after brain injury occurring as a result of ionic shifts.[56] Changes that occur include alterations in potassium, glutamine, and calcium, as well as a decrease in cerebral blood flow, and oxidative metabolism. These changes have been demonstrated using [^{18}F]fluorodeoxyglucose–positron emission tomography (FDG-PET) scanning studies in severely brain-injured patients.[56, 57]

EVALUATION OF THE BRAIN-INJURED ATHLETE

It is essential that the evaluation and management of a potentially brain-injured athlete be complete, well organized, and carried out by qualified medical personnel. The evaluation includes a thorough history, complete neurologic evaluation with particular attention to the mental status, and determination of cognitive functioning. Careful and close follow-up of these athletes is crucial to determine when they can return to play. These decisions are often quite difficult and require an individualized approach that takes into account several factors. Concern for repetitive injury as well as postconcussive sequelae is also a factor.

In the initial evaluation, there should also be high suspicion for associated injuries, including cervical spine injuries and skull fractures. The athlete should be asked if there is any head or neck pain and, if so, to describe it. For athletes evaluated on the field or court, neck pain should be treated as an unstable cervical spine injury until proved otherwise, and these athletes merit spine boarding and cervical immobilization. For the helmeted athlete, leave the helmet in place unless an airway needs to be secured and the mask cannot be cut away.[58] If the athlete does not have neck pain and does not have a tender cervical spine, he/she may be safely transferred to the sidelines for further questioning.

The history is extremely important in determining the level of cognitive functioning that athletes have, as well as determining the memory of the events before and after the injury. It is extremely helpful to ask athletes pertinent questions regarding the specifics of the event such as who they were playing, what the team was wearing, what the special plays and the score were, what happened after they were hit, who were some of their teammates, and what was for dinner the night before. This provides the examiner with an idea of the athlete's orientation as well as the level and degree of memory retrieval and information processing. In the office setting, this information may be more difficult to ascertain, but an effort should be made to find out as much as possible regarding the exact events that took place. It is also important to determine if there was a witnessed period of unconsciousness. Obviously, teammates or family members who are present can help in validating information as well as providing as much information as possible.

Some of the most useful questions that can be asked at the site of the injury include more sophisticated sport-specific questions that pertain to anterograde and retrograde memory. Asking athletes about events prior to the game or during practice tests their ability to remember events prior to the injury (retrograde memory). Having the coach or teammate ask the athlete, "What do you do on the 'special' play?" can determine whether the athlete is able to remember information learned prior to his/her injury (recall of information learned). Asking the athlete to remember five objects presented at the time of examination and then asking the athlete to name them 5 minutes later test the ability to remember new learned information (anterograde memory). All this information can help determine the severity of injury. In addition, when there is a significant injury, it serves the dual purpose of convincing coaches and family members that the athlete cannot return to the event.

The symptoms that can occur with minor brain injury are varied and, along with disturbances in memory and consciousness, can include headache, nausea, vomiting, tinnitus, "feeling in a fog," and imbalance. Special attention should be paid to visual disturbances, any motor or sensory deficits, or other focal deficits. Asking about previous head and neck injuries is also essential, and as much specific information as possible should be obtained. This information is also important when deciding about a return to participation.

When an athlete is seen in the office setting, it is sometimes difficult to get a detailed history. For complicated injuries in which prolonged LOC has occurred, the Glasgow Coma Scale (GCS) has been an excellent predictor for long-term morbidity and death (see Table 9–5). In the athletic setting, more serious injuries may be associated with an abnormal GCS score. These results are well established universally. The GCS is a universal brain injury scoring system with accurate prognostic value. If the GCS is greater than 11, more than 90 percent of patients will have complete recovery, whereas if the GCS is less than 5, 80 percent of patients will die or remain in a vegetative state.[49]

After the athlete's orientation is assessed, the remainder of the physical examination targets neurologic abnormalities. Visual-field deficits, pupillary abnormalities, and extraocular movements as well as other cranial nerve deficits are evaluated. Motor examination, sensory examination, and cerebellar examination of the lower and upper extremities as well as reflexes are carefully noted.

Associated injuries, such as cervical spine injuries or skull fractures should also be assessed. If one sees any evidence for skull fracture (Table 9–6), then a CT scan should be obtained immedi-

Table 9-5
Glasgow Coma Scale

Parameter	Score*
Eye opening	
Eyes open spontaneously	4
Eyes open to verbal command	3
Eyes open only with painful stimuli	2
No eye opening	1
Verbal response	
Oriented and converses	5
Disoriented and converses	4
Inappropriate words	3
Incomprehensible sounds	2
No verbal response	1
Motor response	
Obeys verbal commands	6
Response to painful stimuli (upper extremities)	
Localizes pain	5
Withdraws from pain	4
Flexor posturing	3
Extensor posturing	2
No motor response	1

*Total score = eye opening score + verbal response score + motor response score. The lower the score, the poorer the prognosis.
Source: Cantu RC, Micheli J (eds.): Guidelines for the Team Physician, 2nd ed. Philadelphia, Lea & Febiger, 1991.

ately. In addition, if cervical spine tenderness is present, appropriate radiographs should be obtained, with additional testing as indicated.

Sustained LOC and any evidence of focal deficits require evaluation by some type of brain imaging. Often, CT scanning is the initial study obtained because it is better at demonstrating acute hemorrhage and subtle skull fractures. MR imaging can be useful if the time elapsed from injury is more than 48 hours. It is also more sensitive at detecting subtle areas of contusion or hemorrhage.

Careful monitoring of the head-injured athlete is necessary, regardless of the initial management. It is important that the athlete, parents, coaches, and trainers be all aware of symptoms to watch for as well as guidelines regarding management of pain. Aspirin and even anti-inflammatory medications should be avoided early, as well as narcotics and alcohol. Acetaminophen is often used in the semiacute setting for headache relief, although care should be taken in terms of its use.

Any new symptoms should be noted and the athlete who continues to have symptoms or develops new symptoms should not be allowed to return to participation. These symptoms include even a "mild headache." Athletes should report when symptoms have disappeared and when they feel they are 100 percent back. Further management decisions can then be made, including return to participation or keeping the athlete out of activity for a certain interval of time. These specific return-to-play decisions must be individualized and will be discussed later in further detail.

COMPLICATIONS AND SEQUELAE OF BRAIN INJURY

Although the most common brain injuries that occur in the athletic setting are minor, it is important to be aware of the sequelae and complications that can occur, especially in the setting of recurrent injury. Cervical spine and skull fractures, which deserve special attention, have already been mentioned. In addition, posttraumatic seizures, second impact syndrome, and the postconcussive syndrome can all occur in the setting of minor brain injury. It is important that the athlete, coach, and parents understand the significance of head injuries such that these complications can be

Table 9-6
Signs of Skull Fracture

Sign	Interpretation
Battle's sign	Postauricular hematoma
Rhinorrhea	CSF leaking from the nose
Otorrhea	CSF leaking from the ear canal
Raccoon eyes	Periorbital ecchymosis due to leakage of blood from anterior fossa into periorbital tissues
Hemotympanum	Blood behind the eardrum
Cranial nerve injuries	Especially involving the facial nerve
Palpable malalignment of calvarium	Skull fracture

Source: Cantu RC, Micheli J (eds.): Guidelines for the Team Physician, 2nd ed. Philadelphia, Lea & Febiger, 1991.

avoided if possible and detected early if they do occur.

Skull fractures are often associated with underlying brain injury, as well as focal deficits and sometimes seizure activity. When a skull fracture is present, the risk for underlying intracranial hemorrhage is estimated as 20 times higher than if a head injury occurs without skull fracture.[59] With skull fracture, infection is also another significant concern and may result from open transmission of organisms from the skin and the environment directly into the brain and surrounding tissues, with life-threatening consequences.

As mentioned previously, it is important to assess for cervical spine injuries when the head injury occurs. Cervical spine injuries occur in 5 to 10 percent of severe head injuries.[60] Radiographs are important for the acute injury, and repeat radiographs should be considered if symptoms persist. If there are no symptoms or if neurologic symptoms related to the cervical spine abate and radiographs are normal, MR imaging should be obtained to better assess the soft tissue structures or occult fracture.

Seizures can occur in association with head injury roughly 5 percent of the time, with the majority occurring within the first week of trauma. Most often, these occur in association with a skull fracture or intracranial hemorrhage. In children under age 16 years, seizures are less likely in association with a depressed skull fracture than in their adult counterparts. Posttraumatic epilepsy is more likely in individuals who develop seizures within the first week of injury, have posttraumatic amnesia (PTA) for longer than 12 hours, have intracranial hemorrhage, or in whom any neurologic deficit is present after injury. Having a normal EEG does not predict whether an individual will develop posttraumatic seizure.[61] For a complete discussion of whether an athlete with epilepsy should participate in sports with a risk of head injury, the reader is referred elsewhere.[62]

Postconcussive syndrome is also a potential sequel of brain injury and can be described as a constellation of symptoms that can be quite disabling for the athlete. Persistent headaches, irritability, fatigue, vertigo, imbalance, visual disturbances, sleep disturbances, inability to concentrate, and emotional lability are all symptoms described in postconcussive syndrome. The presentation of these symptoms is often variable, with regard to both onset as well as persistence. MR imaging or CT scanning as well as other studies should be considered to rule out intracranial lesions. There is considerable debate as to whether LOC or PTA has any relationship to the development of postconcussive syndrome.[63] In addition, it is sometimes difficult to differentiate postconcussive syndrome from persistent symptoms after an acute injury. Trauma-induced migraine can also present similarly and is difficult to differentiate from both persisting acute symptoms and postconcussive syndrome.

In 1994, criteria for postconcussive syndrome were presented in the Diagnostic Statistical Manual (DSM-IV) of the American Psychiatric Association based on recommendations from Brown[64] (Table 9–7). The criteria include LOC, PTA for over 12 hours, and seizure activity within 6 months of injury, but many clinicians believe that they are too strict. Many physicians use the diagnosis of postconcussive syndrome whenever patients have typical symptoms and signs after sustaining head trauma, even if the injury appears minimal.

Table 9–7
Proposed Criteria for Postconcussive Syndrome

A. History of head injury that includes at least two of the following:
  1. Loss of consciousness for 5 minutes or more
  2. Posttraumatic amnesia of 12 hours or more
  3. Onset of seizures (posttraumatic epilepsy) within 6 months of head injury

B. Current symptoms (either new symptoms or substantially worsening pre-existing symptoms) to include
  1. At least the following two cognitive difficulties
    a. Learning or memory (recall)
    b. Concentration
  2. At least three of the following affective or vegetative symptoms
    a. Easy fatiguability
    b. Insomnia or sleep/wake cycle disturbances
    c. Headache (substantially worse than before injury)
    d. Vertigo/dizziness
    e. Irritability and/or aggression on little or no provocation
    f. Anxiety, depression, or lability of affect
    g. Personality change (e.g., social or sexual inappropriateness, child-like behavior)
    h. Aspontaneity, apathy

C. Symptoms associated with a significant difficulty in maintaining premorbid occupational or academic performance or with a decline in social, occupational, or academic performance

Source: Brown SJ, Fann JR, Grant I: Postconcussional disorder: Time to acknowledge a common source of neurobehavioral morbidity. J Neuropsychiatry Clin Neurosci 6:15, 1994.

The treatment of postconcussive syndrome and trauma-induced migraine is very difficult and often incorporates a multidisciplinary approach, including psychotherapy, medications, biofeedback, and physical therapy. The neurochemical changes that occur in acute injury most likely are the same ones that may explain the pathogenesis of posttraumatic headache and migraine. There are changes in electrolytes, excitatory amino acids, serotonin, catecholamines, and endogenous opioids, impaired glucose utilization, and neuropeptides.[65] The most common medications utilized in treatment are the beta blockers and tricyclic antidepressants. The management of these problems is discussed in further detail elsewhere.[66–68]

One of the most troubling complications of brain injury is the second impact syndrome (SIS) described by Saunders[1] and Schneider.[69] The term second impact syndrome describes fatal brain swelling and edema that occurs when an athlete sustains a second head impact before completely recovering from an initial head injury. Symptoms from the first injury may be as mild as a headache, and the impact may be as mild as a blow to the chest that snaps the head back.[49] SIS has been reported in both adults and children,[70, 71] and after the second impact, collapse and death generally follow within seconds to minutes.

The exact pathophysiology of SIS appears to be related to an increased sensitivity of the vasculature within the brain after the first injury. Dysfunction in the autoregulation of the cerebral vasculature occurs with the second impact, with resultant vascular congestion and increased intracranial pressure. Herniation of the brain and brain stem results in coma and respiratory failure.[72] SIS underscores the importance of preventing athletes with a head injury from returning to the sport until they are completely asymptomatic at rest as well as exertion.

Recurrent head trauma and chronic traumatic encephalopathy (CTE) can also be a complication of brain injury. CTE is thought to occur as a result of cumulative effect of multiple blows to the head with premature loss of normal central nervous system function. It has been described in boxers despite no loss of consciousness, and it is difficult to predict which athletes will develop symptoms. It is unclear whether it is possible to predict the number of blows that can be sustained before CTE and brain dysfunction will occur.[73]

CLASSIFICATION SYSTEMS

There are several classification systems in the literature[73–78] for head injury, and most also include return-to-play guidelines. Most of the head injuries that occur in the realm of sport are mild injuries. Differentiating mild from more severe head injuries remains difficult, and return-to-play decisions is one of the most important roles for the team physician. The goal is to return athletes to activity as soon as possible, yet not before complete recovery. Many factors must be considered, including the athlete's previous history, the severity of the injury, and the sport.

More important than following any particular classification system is understanding the importance for individualizing treatment for the head-injured athlete. The classification systems to date are based on clinicians' judgments and opinions, and are not based on long-term prospective data in athletes. There is some merit in understanding the various classification systems that have been proposed, and most of them use LOC, retrograde and anterograde memory disturbances, and symptoms or physical findings to define the severity of injury. Several classification systems are outlined in Table 9–8.

With the classification systems that have already been outlined, the same athlete can be "graded" differently. For example, for an athlete with significant retrograde amnesia (RGA) and posttraumatic amnesia but no loss of consciousness,[48] classifications would include a Torg IV, Nelson III, Cantu II, or Colorado Medical Society III. Given this disparity, it is more useful to use descriptive terms such as LOC, RGA, and PTA as well as symptoms and physical findings. Although the classification systems have their own merit, the consistency with which one system is used is likely to be more important than the specific classification chosen. Physicians, athletic trainers, and emergency room and consulting physicians should be clear as to which classification system, if any, they are accustomed to using.

RETURN-TO-PLAY DECISIONS

Once the acute management of the brain-injured athlete has been addressed, the next controversial decision involves determining when that athlete can return to sports activities. This decision is

Table 9–8
Classification Systems and Return-to-Play Guidelines

Torg: Grades of Cerebral Concussion, 1982

I. Short-term confusion, no LOC, no amnesia
II. Confusion + amnesia, no LOC, + PTA
III. Confusion + amnesia, no LOC, + PTA, + RGA
IV. +LOC (immediate transient), + amnesia (PTA, RGA)
V. +LOC (paralytic coma) → coma vigil, respiratory arrest
VI. +LOC (paralytic coma) → death

Nelson: Classification of Concussion, 1984

0. No complaints initially, + subsequent complaints of HA, difficulty with sensorium
I. +stunned or dazed, no LOC or amnesia, clears quickly (<1 min)
II. HA, cloudy sensorium (>1 min), no LOC, + amnesia
III. +LOC (<1 min), not comatose, grade II symptoms during recovery
IV. +LOC (>1 min), not comatose, grade II symptoms during recovery

Cantu Grading System for Concussion, 1986

I. Mild: no LOC, PTA <30 min
II. Moderate: + LOC <5 min, or PTA >30 min but <24 hr
III. Severe: +LOC >5 min, or PTA >24 hr

Colorado Medical Society: Guidelines for the Management of Concussion in Sport, 1991

I. Confusion without amnesia, no LOC
   - Remove from contest.
   - Examine immediately and every 5 min for the development of amnesia or postconcussive syndrome at rest and with exertion.
   - Permit return to contest if amnesia does not appear and no symptoms appear for at least 20 min.
II. Confusion with amnesia, no LOC
   - Remove from contest and disallow return.
   - Examine frequently for signs of evolving intracranial pathology.
   - Reexamine the next day.
   - Permit return to practice after 1 full week without symptoms.
III. +LOC
   - Transport from field to nearest hospital by ambulance (with cervical spine immobilization if indicated).
   - Perform thorough neurologic evaluation emergently.
   - Admit to hospital if signs of pathology are detected.
   - If findings are normal, instruct family for overnight observation.
   - Permit return to practice only after 2 full weeks without symptoms.

American Academy of Neurology, 1997

I. Transient confusion, no LOC, concussion symptoms or mental status abnormalities that resolve in <15 min.
   - Remove from contest.
   - Examine immediately and at 5-min intervals for development of mental status abnormalities or postconcussive symptoms at rest and with exertion.
   - May return if abnormalities and symptoms clear within 15 min.
   - A subsequent grade I concussion in same contest eliminates player from contest, returning only if asymptomatic after 1 week at rest and upon exertion.
   - Following subsequent grade III concussion athlete should be withheld from play for a minimum of 1 asymptomatic month. MD may elect to extend that period beyond 1 month, depending on clinical evaluation and other circumstances.
   - CT or MRI recommended for athletes whose HA or other associated symptoms worsen or persist for longer than 1 week.
   - Any abnormality on CT or MRI consistent with brain swelling, contusion, or other intracranial pathology should result in termination of the playing season for that athlete, and return to play in the future should be seriously discouraged in discussions with the athlete.

Cantu Guidelines: Return to Play After Concussion

Grade I
- *First concussion:* May return to play if asymptomatic (no HA, dizziness, impaired orientation, concentration, or memory loss during rest and exertion) for 1 week.
- *Second concussion:* Return to play in 2 weeks if asymptomatic at that time for 1 week.
- *Third concussion:* Terminate playing season; may return to play next season if asymptomatic.
Grade II
- *First concussion:* May return to play if asymptomatic for 1 week.
- *Second concussion:* Remove from play for a minimum of 1 month; athlete may return to play then if asymptomatic for 1 week; consider terminating playing season.
- *Third concussion:* Terminate playing season; athlete may return to play next season if asymptomatic.
Grade III
- *First concussion:* Remove from play for a minimum of 1 month; athlete may then return to play if asymptomatic for 1 week.
- *Second concussion:* Terminate playing season; athlete may return to play next season if asymptomatic.

Table continued on following page

Table 9–8
Classification Systems and Return-to-Play Guidelines *Continued*

Colorado Medical Society Guidelines: Return to Play

II. Transient confusion, no LOC, concussion symptoms or mental status abnormalities that last >15 min.
  - Remove from contest, no return that day.
  - Examine on site frequently for signs of evolving intracranial pathology.
  - Reexamine athlete following day.
  - Neurologic examination by MD 1 week after asymptomatic before return.
  - CT or MRI if HA or other symptoms worsen or persist for more than 2 weeks.
  - Following a subsequent grade II concussion, return to play deferred until symptom-free at rest and with exertion for at least 2 weeks.
  - Terminating season of play is mandated by any abnormality on CT or MRI consistent with brain swelling, contusion, or other intracranial pathology.
III. Any LOC, either brief (seconds) or prolonged (minutes)
  - Transport from field to ER by ambulance if unconscious or worrisome signs appear.
  - Consider cervical spine immobilization.
  - Thorough neurologic examination emergently, including appropriate neuroimaging procedures.
  - Admit if any signs of pathology or mental status abnormalities exist.
  - If normal evaluation, may send athlete home.
  - Neurologic status should be assessed daily thereafter until all symptoms have stabilized or resolved.
  - Prolonged LOC, persistent mental status alterations, worsening symptoms, or abnormalities on neurologic examination requires urgent neurosurgical evaluation or transfer to trauma center.
  - After brief (seconds) grade III concussion, the athlete should be held out until asymptomatic for 1 week at rest and upon exertion.
  - After prolonged (minutes) grade III concussion, athlete should be withheld from play until asymptomatic for 2 weeks at rest and upon exertion.
  Grade I
  - *First concussion:* Remove athlete from contest. Examine immediately and every 5 min for the development of amnesia or postconcussive symptoms at rest and with exertion. May return to contest if amnesia does not appear and no symptoms appear for at least 20 min.
  - *Second concussion:* If in same contest, eliminate from competition that day; otherwise, treat as grade I.
  - *Third concussion:* Terminate playing season. No contact sports for at least 3 months, and then only if asymptomatic at rest and exertion.
  Grade II
  - *First concussion:* Remove from contest and disallow return. Examine frequently for signs of evolving intracranial pathology. Reexamine the next day. May return to practice after 1 full week without symptoms.
  - *Second concussion:* Defer return to play for 1 month. Termination of playing season considered.
  - *Third concussion:* Termination of playing season mandated.
  - *Note:* Terminate playing season at any stage if any abnormality appears on CT/MRI studies.
  Grade III
  - *First concussion:* Transport from field by ambulance (with cervical spine immobilization if indicated) to nearest hospital. Thorough neurologic evaluation is performed emergently. Hospital confinement is indicated if signs of pathology are detected. If findings are normal, give instructions to family for overnight observation. Athlete may return to practice only after 2 full weeks without symptoms; no contact allowed. Return to full contact activity at 1 month only if athlete has been asymptomatic at rest and exertion for at least 2 weeks.
  - *Second concussion:* Playing season terminated (also terminate if any abnormality appears on CT/MRI). Return to contact sports should be seriously discouraged.

Key: LOC, loss of consciousness; PTA, posttraumatic amnesia; RGA, retrograde amnesia; HA, headache; CT, computed tomography; MRI, magnetic resonance imaging.

essential in sports such as football, ice hockey, wrestling, martial arts, boxing, rugby, and soccer, in which the risk of head injury and significant contact is high. In addition, other activities such as equestrian sports, motorcycle, automobile, and boat racing, and sky diving also have an inherent risk for head trauma that must be taken into account.

Most of the classification systems discussed earlier also include return-to-play guidelines,[73–77] which again are not based on long-term prospective data and thus remain guidelines. Many factors must be considered in the decision to return an athlete to participation, including the specific injury and clinical course, past history, complications, and the athlete's readiness to return. Careful assessment and close follow-up are essential. Although there may be some complaints about keeping an athlete out of play too long, the physician bears the brunt of the responsibility for allowing an athlete to return to activity too early.

The decision to return an athlete to sports activity after focal and structural diffuse brain injury is difficult, made without prospective long-term data in athletes, and thus often is based on personal opinion and judgment. Injuries included here are all types of intracranial hemorrhage (epidural, subdural, and intracerebral hematoma, and subarachnoid hemorrhage) as well as SIS and diffuse axonal injury. Cantu has recommended that athletes with any of these lesions can return to play as long as they do not have (1) persistent postconcussive symptoms, (2) permanent central neurologic sequelae (organic dementia, hemiplegia, homonymous hemianopia), (3) hydrocephalus, (4) spontaneous subarachnoid hemorrhage from any cause, or (5) symptomatic neurologic or pain-producing abnormalities around the foramen magnum.[49] In addition, if any athlete has had surgical intervention for any of these problems, serious consideration must be given to their return to contact sports. The surgical procedure is believed to produce some subdural scarring, which can theoretically produce additional tethering forces within the calvarium. Cantu has recommended that athletes with focal or diffuse brain lesions who have not had surgery or any of the contraindications just listed may return to activity one full year after neurologic recovery.[49]

As discussed earlier, the brain injury that occurs in the athletic setting is often mild, and studies such as MR imaging, CT, and EEG are often normal despite significant abnormalities in mental function. For many parents and athletes, it is incomprehensible that an athlete who cannot remember his/her name or the date or events before and after the injury will have normal studies. Without abnormal findings, it is difficult for the health care provider to determine when the athlete is truly back to "normal." In addition, the situation is quite different from that of an injury such as an ankle sprain, for which returning an athlete to play at 80 percent with taping and bracing may pose risks that a health care provider may be willing to take.

Probably the safest ultimate guideline in making the return-to-play decision for the head-injured athlete is never to allow an athlete who is experiencing any symptoms to participate. Once these athletes are completely asymptomatic, it is also important to have them perform an "exercise challenge" in a setting in which there is no risk for head injury in order to assess whether the cardiovascular system can withstand the stress of exertion alone with no recurrence of symptoms. An exercise challenge allows athletes to return to some level of activity without further risk of rein-

jury or cumulative injury and in most situations allows them to return to some sport-specific activities as well. Once they can tolerate this without any symptoms, they can continue to progress with sport-specific skills until contact is allowed and finally full return to participation. It is important to "progress" athletes as they are comfortable, and protecting them from contact can fulfill the physician's responsibility yet still allow the athlete to be at practice and remain an integral part of the team.

It is imperative that the physician discuss the rationale behind holding the athlete out of activity with the athlete as well as the parents and coaches. It is also essential that athletes, parents, and coaches understand the importance of reporting any new symptoms. Explaining the risks of recurrent injury and the SIS can be useful. It is also helpful to explain that athletes who have had a concussion appear to be at a greater risk of sustaining another concussion than someone who has never had a concussion.[8, 79] Although the exact risk is difficult to quantify, it certainly diminishes as time passes. The guidelines for return to play that exist provide a template for determining when it is reasonable to allow athletes with different severities of injury to return. Important in the discussion between the physician and the athlete is whether the athlete is at all apprehensive about returning to participation. In some situations the athlete may not feel ready to participate, and if these questions are not asked, the athlete may be apprehensive and thus be at potential risk for additional injury.

For both the assessment and recovery phases of minimal brain injury, neuropsychological testing has been shown to be quite useful.[80–82] Neuropsychological testing involves tests that provide a reliable assessment and quantification of brain functioning by examining brain-behavior relationships. These measurements assess memory recall, attention and concentration, problem-solving abilities, visual tracking, reaction time, and speed of information processing as well as other measures of cognitive function. A variety of different tests are available, many of which are well validated. The research using neuropsychological testing specifically with an athletic population is impressive.[32, 48, 83, 84] Neuropsychological testing has gained recent attention, and as research evolves with its use, methods of treating head injuries and return-to-play issues may change in the future.

Neuropsychological testing is one example of

some of the newer ways to evaluate head injury. With a battery of these tests performed before the season is under way, a "baseline" of function in these various realms of cognitive function is obtained. If the athlete subsequently sustains a head injury, additional testing can be obtained and then compared with the baseline studies. Limitations currently include the time and cost of testing, as well as the normal "learning curve" that occurs with repetitive testing. In addition, it is important currently that these tests be interpreted by qualified neuropsychologists, which may limit their application. Despite these limitations, neuropsychological testing remains useful in detecting mild head injuries[36, 80–82, 84–86] and in assessing acute and chronic effects, and may be more sensitive than classical testing in assessing cognitive function.[48, 83]

The use of neuropsychological testing in conjunction with MR imaging and CT scanning in brain-injured patients has been studied.[36] When 20 mild or moderate head-injured patients were evaluated with all three tests, investigators found that MR imaging detected more intracranial lesions than did CT scanning (though none requiring surgical intervention), and neuropsychological testing during hospitalization in the acute phase revealed deficits that correlated to the location and size of lesions on MR imaging. Follow-up testing at 1 and 3 months after injury revealed improvements in memory and cognition that mirrored a decreased lesion size.

In a study of United States college football players, Alves demonstrated no deficits in cognitive function in athletes after an initial head injury, but if a second injury occurred soon after, deficits in cognitive function became apparent.[83] Other preliminary research has demonstrated deficits after mild head injury compared with baseline preseason testing despite normal CT and MR imaging.[87] Those data also demonstrated that head injuries that are more severe (based on clinical classification) are associated with a higher percentage of abnormal tests, and persistence below baseline values for a longer time.

The deficits in neuropsychological testing often resolve over time, yet until recently, the lack of baseline testing has made their application difficult. Different athletes have different abilities and thus will have different results on the various tests based on their strengths and weaknesses in various aspects of cognitive function. In addition, different head injury patterns may result in different patterns of dysfunction. Both of these factors illustrate the importance of individual baseline testing.

Postural sway testing has been another area of head injury research that may prove useful in the clinical setting. Postural stability testing has been compared with a small battery of cognitive tests and found to reveal deficits in head-injured athletes 1 day after injury, whereas the cognitive tests remained unchanged.[88] The postural tests remained abnormal 3 to 5 days after the injury, although the differences were no longer statistically different. These studies raise some interesting questions. Are the differences seen in postural sway or neuropsychological tasting of clinical significance, or are they too sensitive in the assessment of brain injury? At what point are athletes able to protect themselves from further injury such that even though they are not at 100 percent, they can still participate safely? We are less willing to take risks in the brain-injured athlete, yet the objective of many sports medicine physicians is to return athletes to play as soon as possible without putting them at undue risk for further injury or long-term complications. These questions are the most important ones facing the health care provider taking care of the head-injured athlete.

New diagnostic imaging studies are also being utilized in the assessment of brain injury, including near-infrared spectroscopy,[89, 90] single photon emission computed tomography (SPECT),[91, 92] magnetic resonance angiography,[93] and diffusion-weighted MR imaging.[94] How these new studies will change the way in which head-injured athletes are assessed in the future remains an exciting area of research. These tests are noninvasive, may correlate with the neurochemical and metabolic changes that occur with head injury, and may be more sensitive than MR imaging and CT, which seem to be superior in detecting focal brain lesions. The research in all these areas can only expand the knowledge base and improve the manner in which brain-injured athletes are managed.

SPORT-SPECIFIC CONCERNS

With a few sports, some interesting questions arise when considering brain injury. The evaluation and management of many head-injured athletes are similar, but in these few sports special concerns exist because of the nature of the sport. Boxing and soccer are two sports that merit special attention.

Boxing

Although a full discussion of the concerns regarding head injury in boxing is not possible in this chapter, the very nature of boxing involves the objective of striking the competitor with multiple blows to the head until he is rendered unconscious. Recent reviews have discussed the cumulative effects of boxing on brain function.[95] Chronic brain injury can result from the cumulative effects of boxing, first termed the "punch drunk syndrome" in 1928[96] and later termed "dementia pugilistica"[97] or "chronic progressive traumatic encephalopathy."[98] This syndrome occurs in 9 to 25 percent of professional boxers, and there appears to be a correlation with the number of fights boxers participate in and the length of their career.[98] Cerebellar, pyramidal, extrapyramidal, and occasionally cognitive and personality abnormalities can be present. The changes do not usually present until approximately 16 years of boxing and they progress slowly.[95]

MR imaging, CT, and EEG studies have been used to assess boxers and have demonstrated abnormalities, compared with control subjects, thought to be correlated with cumulative brain injury.[100, 101] Studies have demonstrated cerebral atrophy,[101, 102] and in one study of 338 active professionals, 7 percent of CT scans were abnormal and 22 percent were borderline.[100] This study also found a correlation between abnormal CT scan and a history of knockout or technical knockouts. There has been some controversy, however, in that another retrospective study of soccer players, boxers, and track and field athletes did not show any abnormalities in EEG, CT, and MR imaging as well as neuropsychological tests.[95] More prospective studies are needed to assess the cognitive abnormalities associated with the cumulative trauma of boxing.

There has been an attempt to protect boxers from cumulative and repetitive brain injury, with certain states being more proactive than others. In New York State, mild concussions result in a mandatory 45-day suspension, moderate concussions result in a 60-day suspension, and a 90-day suspension along with a normal CT and EEG studies are required after a severe concussion.[103]

These guidelines are in place to protect the boxer from repetitive injury, and yet more data are needed to regulate the sport at a national level.

Soccer

Soccer is the other sport in which the sport-specific skills involved may put the athlete at risk for cumulative brain injury. Striking the ball with the head is a sport-specific skill unique to soccer, and recently, a debate has started over whether the repetitive heading may be similar to the repetitive blows incurred in boxing. Although this suggestion has created some controversy, there are no well-controlled prospective data to support these claims.

Heading technique is often compared to a catapult wherein the upper and lower extremity go into extension prior to impact, then forcefully contract so that the ball is struck as the trunk goes into flexion. As skill and technique improve, the neck muscles are kept rigid as the head strikes the ball,[103] decreasing the angular acceleration of the head and ultimately decreasing the risk of head and neck injury.[104] In younger players, there may be an increased risk for injury due to improper technique in a setting in which the neck musculature may not be well developed.

In a typical male European soccer player's career, 2000 blows to the head are sustained during approximately 300 games.[31] When the ball is kicked, it travels at an average speed of 14.4 km per hour and from 10 meters away, has an average impact speed of 116 km per hour, although at full force this can reach up to 200 km per hour.[106, 107] The ball-skull contact lasts from 1/63 to 1/128 second, and the longer the ball is in contact with the head, the lesser the impact forces will be. These repetitive forces have raised concern for cumulative brain injury.

Sortland in 1982 reported degenerative changes in the cervical spine in 40-year-old soccer players equivalent to those expected in 50- to 60-year-olds.[108] In a study of Norwegian players, CT scanning showed cerebral atrophy, which was most often seen in players that considered themselves "typical headers."[31] Finally, in an EEG study of soccer players, changes were seen in players that had acute or chronic complaints secondary to heading.[108] Many of these studies have methodological flaws including no control groups, no control group for acute head injuries, and no control group for comparison to alcohol use or motor vehicle accidents.

In a study referred to earlier that used EEG, MR imaging, and CT scanning as well as neuropsychological testing, no abnormalities were noted in soccer players and boxers who were compared with control track athletes.[95] In another recent well-controlled study of U.S. National Team male soccer players compared with track and field athletes, no significant difference in MR imaging results were demonstrated. More prospective research is needed to address whether the changes that may occur in soccer are due to repetitive heading or to other aspects of the sport.

Soccer is different from boxing in terms of the biomechanics involved with heading a soccer ball and being repetitively hit on the head. The acceleration forces (units of gravity, or g) in soccer are much less than boxing; $20g$ versus $100g$.[110] In addition, the forces that occur in soccer are generally linear, with rigidity supplied by the contraction of the neck, trunk, and hip musculature. In boxing, the forces are generally rotational, creating more shearing forces and resultant brain injury[30] (Figs. 9–4 and 9–5). There are times in soccer play that the ball may strike the head when the athlete is not expecting it, and thus the soccer player may be at risk if the technique is not correct.

Head injuries in collegiate soccer players have been demonstrated to occur at a fairly high rate. When these data are scrutinized, the injuries are found to occur as a result of contact with another player, the ground, or the goal posts. The head

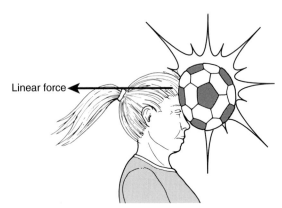

Figure 9–5. Soccer heading typically produces linear force to head. (From Garrett WE Jr, et al (eds): The U.S. Soccer Sports Medicine Book. Baltimore, Williams & Wilkins, 1996, p. 198.)

injuries that occur in soccer are generally mild concussions. There is a paucity of data that are well controlled or prospective in nature, and none that demonstrate that heading the ball leads to cumulative brain injury. In a pilot study with collegiate men and women soccer players at Penn State University,[111] no acute effects of heading were seen as measured by neuropsychological testing before and after a typical session. More long-term, well-controlled, prospective data are needed.

CONCLUSION

Traumatic brain injury in sport is not uncommon and has significant morbidity and mortality associated with it. The spectrum of injury varies from the mild injury that allows an athlete to return to play 20 to 30 minutes later to the severe injury with a potential for fatal consequences. The medical team taking care of athletes must understand the complexity of brain injury and be well prepared to systematically manage these injuries. Once an athlete has sustained a potential head injury, care must be taken to exclude cervical spine or associated skull fractures, and additional diagnostic testing may be necessary to exclude focal intracranial injuries or associated injuries. Careful management and follow-up are essential, and return-to-play decisions can be difficult.

New techniques and tools to assess minimal brain injury are on the horizon and may change the manner in which these injuries are treated. These tools may be more sensitive in assessing cognitive function and may prove to be a useful

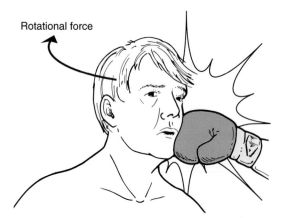

Figure 9–4. Punching impact in boxing often produces rotational force. (From Garrett WE Jr, et al (eds): The U.S. Soccer Sports Medicine Book. Baltimore, Williams & Wilkins, 1996, p. 197.)

part of the preparticipation physical examination. More long-term prospective studies are needed in the athletic setting to better assess the natural history of head injury and to understand the complexities of injury recovery that may guide return-to-play decisions. With more of this information, the health care management for these complex injuries will improve.

REFERENCES

1. Saunders RL, Harbaugh RE: The second impact in catastrophic contact-sports head trauma. JAMA 252:538–539, 1984.
2. Spear J: Are footballers at risk for developing dementia? Int J Geriatric Psychiatry 10:1011–1014, 1995.
3. Mayeux R, Ottman R, Tang MX, et al: Genetic susceptibility and head injury as risk factors for Alzheimer's disease among community-dwelling elderly persons and their first degree relatives. Ann Neurol 33:494–501, 1993.
4. Mortimer JA, French LR, Hutton JT, et al: Head injury as a risk factor for Alzheimer's disease. Neurology 35:264–266, 1985.
5. McLatchie G, Jennett B: ABC of sports medicine. Head injury in sport. Br Med J 308:1620–1624, 1994.
6. Kraus JF: Epidemiology of head injury. In Cooper PR (ed): Head Injury, 2nd ed. Baltimore, Williams & Wilkins, 1987, pp. 1–19.
7. Garrick JG, Requa RK: Medical care and injury surveillance in the high school setting. Phys Sports Med 9:115, 1981.
8. Gerberich SG, Priest JD, Boen JR, et al: Concussion incidence and severity in secondary school varsity football players. Am J Public Health 73:1370–1375, 1983.
9. Buckley WE: Concussions in college football. Am J Sports Med 16:1, 1988.
10. Wilberger JE: Minor head injuries in American football. Sports Med 15:5, 1993.
11. Torg JS, Vegso JJ, Sennett B: The National Football Head and Neck Injury Registry: 14 year report on cervical quadriplegia, 1971–1984. JAMA 254:3439, 1985.
12. Bruce DA, Schut L, Sutton LN: Brain and cervical spine injuries in children and adolescents. Primary Care 11(1):175–194, 1984.
13. Zariczny B, Shattuck LJ, Mast TA, et al: Sports related injuries in school age children. Am J Sports Med 8:318–324, 1980.
14. Hodgson VR: National operating committee on standards for athletic equipment. Football helmet certification program. Med Sci Sports 7:225–232, 1975.
15. Bishop PJ: Impact performance of ice hockey helmets. Safety Res 10:123–129, 1978.
16. Mueller FO, Blyth CS: Fatalities from head and cervical spine injuries occurring in tackle football: 40 years' experience. Clin Sports Med 6:185–196, 1987.
17. Cantu RC, Mueller F: Catastrophic spine injury in football 1977–1989. J Spinal Dis 3:227, 1990.
18. Pforringer W, Smasal V: Aspects of traumatology in ice hockey. J Sports Sci 5:327–336, 1987.
19. Goldsmith W: Performance of baseball headgear. Am J Sports Med 10(1):31–37, 1982.
20. National Collegiate Athletic Association: Injury Surveillance 1983–91. Overland Park, KS, Randall Dick, 1992.
21. Greensher J: Non-automotive vehicle injuries in adolescents. Pediatr Ann 17:114–121, 1988.
22. Graham DI: Neuropathology of head injury. In Narayan RK, Wilberger JE Jr, Povlishock JT (eds): Neurotrauma. New York, McGraw-Hill, 1996, pp. 46–47.
23. Graham DI: Neuropathology of head injury. In Narayan RK, Wilberger JE Jr, Povlishock JT (eds): Neurotrauma. New York, McGraw-Hill, 1996, pp. 46–47.
24. Bruno LA, Gennarelli TA, Torg JS: Management guidelines for head injuries in athletics. Clin Sports Med 6:1, 1987.
25. Warren WL, Bailes JE: On the field evaluation of athletic head injuries. Clin Sports Med 17(1):13–26, 1998.
26. Borczuk P: Predictors of intracranial injury in patients with mild head injury. Ann Emerg Med 25:731–736, 1995.
27. Davis RL, Mullen N, Makela M, et al: Cranial computed tomography scans in children after minimal head injury with loss of consciousness. Ann Emerg Med 24:640–645, 1994.
28. Hoffman JR: CT for head trauma in children. Ann Emerg Med 24:713–715, 1995.
29. Jordan BD: Head injury in sports. In Jordan BD, Tsairis P, Warren R (eds): Sports Neurology. Gaithersburg, Aspen, 1990.
30. Lampert PW, Hardman JM: Morphological changes in brains of boxers. JAMA 251(20):2676–2679, 1984.
31. Tysvaer AT, Storli OV, Bachen NI: Soccer injuries to the brain: A neurologic and electroencephalographic study of former players. Acta Neurol Scand 80:151–156, 1989.
32. Levin HS, Williams D, Crofford MJ, et al: Relationship of depth of brain lesions to consciousness and outcome after closed head injury. J Neurosurg 69(6):861–866, 1988.
33. Mittl RL, Grossman RI, Heihle JF, et al: Prevalence of MR evidence of diffuse axonal injury in patients with mild head injury and normal CT findings. Am J Neuroradiol 15:1583–1589, 1994.
34. Gentry LR, Godersky JC, Thompson B, et al: Prospective comparative study of intermediate field MR and CT in the evaluation of closed head trauma. Am J Neuroradiol 150:673, 1988.
35. Jenkins A, Teasdale G, Hadley DM, et al: Brain lesions detected by magnetic resonance imaging in mild and severe head injuries. Lancet 2:445–446, 1986.
36. Levin HS, Amparo E, Eisenberg JM, et al: Magnetic resonance imaging and computerized tomography in relation to the neurobehavioral sequelae of mild and moderate head injuries. J Neurosurg 66:706–713, 1987.
37. Report of the Ad Hoc Committee to Study Head Injury Nomenclature. Proceedings of the Congress of Neurological Surgeons in 1964. Clin Neurosurg 12:386–394, 1966.
38. Ryan AJ: Protecting the sportsman's brain. Br J Sports Med 25(2):81–86, 1991.
39. Macciocchi SN, Barth JT, Littlefield LM: Outcome after mild head injury. Clin Sports Med 17(1):27–36, 1998.
40. Elson LM, Ward CC: Mechanisms and pathophysiology of mild head injury. Semin Neurol 14:8–18, 1994.
41. Adams H, Mitchell DE, Graham DI, et al: Diffuse brain damage of immediate impact type. Its relationship to "primary" brain stem damage. Brain 100:489–502, 1977.
42. Adams H, Mitchell DE, Graham DI, et al: Diffuse brain damage of immediate impact type. Its relationship to "primary" brain stem damage. Brain 100:489–502, 1977.
43. Peerless SJ, Rencastle NB: Shear injuries of the brain. Can Med Assoc J 96:577–582, 1967.
44. Chason JL, Hardy WG, Webster JE, et al: Alterations in cell structure of the brain associated with experimental concussion. J Neurosurg 15:135–139, 1958.
45. Hugenholtz H, Richard MT: Return to athletic competition following concussion. Can Med Assoc J 127:827–829, 1982.

46. Ommaya AK: Head injury mechanisms and the concept of preventative management: A review and critical synthesis. J Neurotrauma 12:527–546, 1996.

47. Ommaya AK, Gennarelli TA: Cerebral concussion and traumatic unconsciousness. Correlation of experimental and clinical observations in blunt head injuries. Brain 97:633–654, 1974.

48. Putukian M, Echemendia RJ: Managing successive minor head injuries: Which tests guide return to play? Physician Sports Med 24(11):25–38, 1996.

49. Cantu RC, Micheli J (eds): American College of Sports Medicine's Guidelines for the Team Physician. Philadelphia, Lea & Febiger, 1991.

50. Katayama Y, Becker DP, Tamura T, et al: Massive increases in extracellular potassium and the indiscriminate release of glutamate following concussive brain injury. J Neurosurg 73:889–900, 1990.

51. Katayama Y, Cheung MK, Alves A, et al: Ion fluxes and cell swelling in experimental traumatic brain injury: The role of excitatory amino acids. In Hoff JT, Betz AL (eds): Intracranial Pressure. VII. Berlin, Springer, 1989, pp. 584–588.

52. Yoshino A, Hovda DA, Katayama Y, et al: Hippocampal CA3 lesion prevents the post-concussive metabolic derangement in CA1. J Cereb Blood Flow Metab 11(suppl 2):S343, 1991.

53. Yoshino A, Hovda DA, Kawamata T, et al: Dynamic changes in local cerebral glucose utilization following cerebral concussion in rats: Evidence of a hyper- and subsequent hypometabolic state. Brain Res 561:106–119, 1991.

54. Yamakami I, McIntosh TK: Alterations in regional cerebral blood flow following brain injury in the rat. J Cereb Blood Flow Metab 11:655–660, 1991.

55. Jenkins LW, Moszynski K, Lyeth BG, et al: Increased vulnerability of the mildly traumatized rat brain to cerebral ischemia: The use of controlled secondary ischemia as a research tool to identify common or different mechanisms contributing to mechanical and ischemic brain injury. Brain Res 477:211–224, 1989.

56. Hovda DA, Lee SM, Smith ML, et al: The neurochemical and metabolic cascade following brain injury: Moving from animal models to man. J Neurotrauma 12(5):143–146, 1995.

57. Bergsneider M, Hovda DA, Shalmon E, et al: Cerebral hyperglycolysis following severe traumatic brain injury in humans: a positron emission tomography study. J Neurosurg 86:241–251, 1997.

58. Kleiner DM, Cantu RC: Football Helmet Removal, American College of Sports Medicine, Current Comment. Indianapolis, IN, Lippincott Williams & Wilkins, 1996.

59. Edna TH: Acute traumatic intracranial hematoma and skull fracture. Acta Chir Scand 149:449–451, 1983.

60. Marion DW: Head injuries. In Fu FH, Stone DA (eds): Sports Injuries; Mechanisms, Prevention, Treatment. Baltimore, Williams & Wilkins, 1994, pp. 813–831.

61. Henderson JM, Browning DG: Head trauma in young athletes. Med Clin North Am 78(2):289–303, 1994.

62. Cantu RC: Epilepsy and athletics. Clin Sports Med 17(1):61–69, 1998.

63. Bornstein RA, Miller HB, van Schoor JT: Neuropsychological deficit and emotional disturbance in head-injured patients. J Neurosurg 70:509–513, 1989.

64. Brown SJ, Fann JR, Grant I: Postconcussional disorder: Time to acknowledge a common source of neurobehavioral morbidity. J Neuropsychiatry Clin Neurosci 6:15–22, 1994.

65. Packard RC, Ham LP: Pathogenesis of post traumatic headache and migraine: A common headache pathway? Headache 37(3):142–152, 1997.

66. Rizzo M: Overview of head injury and postconcussive syndrome. In Rizzo M, Tranel D (eds): Head Injury and Postconcussive Syndrome. New York, Churchill Livingstone, 1996, pp. 1–18.

67. Truncosco JC, Gordon B: Neuropathology of closed head injury. In Rizzo M, Tranel D (eds): Head Injury and Postconcussive Syndrome. New York, Churchill Livingstone, 1996, pp. 47–56.

68. Barcellos S, Rizzo M: Post-traumatic headaches. In Rizzo M, Tranel D (eds): Head Injury and Postconcussive Syndrome. New York, Churchill Livingstone, 1996, pp. 139–175.

69. Schneider RC: Head and Neck Injuries in Football. Baltimore, Williams & Wilkins, 1973.

70. McQuillen JB, McQuillen EN, Morrow P: Trauma, sports, and malignant cerebral edema. Am J Forensic Med Pathol 9:12–15, 1988.

71. Bruce DA, Alavi A, Bilaniuk L, et al: Diffuse cerebral swelling following head injuries in children: the syndrome of "malignant brain edema." J Neurosurg 54:170–178, 1981.

72. Cantu RC: Second-impact syndrome. Clin Sports Med 17(1):37–44, 1998.

73. Quality Standards Subcommittee, American Academy of Neurology, Practice Parameter: The management of concussion in sports (summary statement). Neurology 48:581–585, 1997.

74. Cantu RC: Return to play guidelines after a head injury. Clin Sports Med 17(1):45–60, 1998.

75. Colorado Medical Society: Guidelines for the Management of Concussion in Sports. Denver, Colorado Medical Society, Sports Medicine Committee, May 1990 (revised May 1991).

76. Nelson WE, Jane JA, Gieck JH: Minor head injury in sports: A new classification and management. Physician Sportsmed 12(3):103–107, 1984.

77. Torg JS: Athletic Injuries to the Head, Neck, and Face. St. Louis, Mosby–Year Book, 1991.

78. Kelly JP, Rosenburg JH: Diagnosis and management of concussion in sport. Neurology 48:575–580, 1997.

79. Zemper E: Analysis of cerebral concussion frequency with the most commonly used models of football helmets. J Athletic Training 29(1):44–50, 1994.

80. Abreau F, Templer DI, Schuyler BA, et al: Neuropsychological assessment of soccer players. Neuropsychology 4:175–181, 1990.

81. Rimel RW, Giordani B, Barth JT, et al: Disability caused by minor head injury. Neurosurgery 9(3):221–228, 1981.

82. Rimel RW, Giordani B, Barth JT, et al: Moderate head injury: Completing the clinical spectrum of brain trauma. Neurosurgery 11(3):344–351, 1982.

83. Alves WM, Rimel RW, Nelson WE: University of Virginia prospective study of football-induced minor head injury: Status report. Clin Sports Med 6(1):211–218, 1987.

84. Tysvaer AT, Lochen EA: Soccer injuries to the brain; a neuropsychologic study of former soccer players. Am J Sports Med 19(1):56–60, 1991.

85. McLatchie G, Brooks N, Galbraith S, et al: Clinical neurological examination, neuropsychology, electroencephalography and computed tomographic head scanning in active amateur boxers. J Neurol Neurosurg Psychiatry 50:96–99, 1987.

86. Porter MD, Fricker PA: Controlled prospective neuropsychological assessment of active experienced amateur boxers. Clin J Sports Med 6:90–96, 1996.

87. Putukian M, Echemendia RJ, Phillips TG: Neuropsychological Baseline Testing in the Management of Head Injured College Athletes: The Penn State Concussion Program. Presented at the American Medical Society

for Sports Medicine Annual Meeting, Colorado Springs Colorado, April 6, 1997.

88. Guskiewicz KM, Riemann BL, Perrin DH, et al: Alternative approaches to the assessment of mild head injury in athletes. Med Sci Sports Exerc 27(7):213–221, 1997.

89. Kirkpatrick PJ: Use of near-infrared spectroscopy in the adult. Philos Trans R Soc Lond B Biol Sci 352(1354): 701–705, 1997.

90. Robertson CS, Gopinath SP, Chance B: A new application for near-infrared spectroscopy: Detection of delayed intracranial hematomas after head injury. J Neurotrauma 12(4):591–600, 1995.

91. Masdeu JC, Abdel-Dayem H, Van Heertum RL: Head trauma: Use of SPECT. J Neuroimaging 5(suppl 1):S53–57, 1995.

92. Lewis DH: Functional brain imaging with cerebral perfusion SPECT in cerebrovascular disease, epilepsy, and trauma. Neurosurg Clin North Am 8(3):337–344. 1997.

93. James CA: Magnetic resonance angiography in trauma. Clin Neurosci 4(3):137–145, 1997.

94. Ono J, Harada K, Takahashi J, et al: Differentiation between dysmyelination and demyelination using magnetic resonance diffusional anisotropy. Brain Res 671(1):141–148, 1995.

95. Haglund Y, Eriksson E: Does amateur boxing lead to chronic brain damage? A review of some recent investigations. Am J Sports Med 21:97–109, 1993.

96. Martland HS: Punch drunk. JAMA 91:1103–1107, 1928.

97. Millspaugh JA: Dementia pugilistica. US Naval Med Bull 35:297, 1937.

98. Critchley M: Medical aspects of boxing, particularly from a neurological standpoint. Br Med J 1:357–362, 1957.

99. Mortimer JA: Epidemiology of post-traumatic encephalopathy in boxers. Minn Med 68:299–300, 1985.

100. Jordan B, Zimmerman R: Computed tomography and magnetic resonance imaging comparisons in boxers. JAMA 263:1670–1674, 1990.

101. Jordan B, Jahre C, Hauser A, et al: CT of 338 active professional boxers. Radiology 185:509–512, 1992.

102. Bogdanoff B, Natter H: Incidence of cavum septum pellucidum in athletes: A sign of boxer's encephalopathy. Neurology 39:991–992, 1989.

103. Wilberger JE Jr, Maroon JC: Head injuries in athletes. Clin Sports Med 8:1, 1989.

104. Burslem I, Lees A: Quantification of impact accelerations of the head during the heading of a football. *In* Reilly T, Lees A, Davids K, et al (eds): Science and Football: Proceedings of the First World Congress of Science and Football. London, E&FN Spon Ltd., 1987, pp. 243–248.

105. Tysvaer AT: Head and neck injuries in soccer. Impact of minor trauma. Sports Med 14(3):200–213, 1992.

106. Schneider PG, Lichte H: Untersuchungen zur Groesse der Krafteinwirkung beim Kopfballspiel des Fussballers. Sportarzut Sportmed 26:10, 1975.

107. Smodlaka VN: Medical aspects of heading the ball in soccer. Physician Sportsmed 12(2):127–131, 1984.

108. Sortland O, Tysvaer AT, Storli OV: Changes in the cervical spine in association football players. Br J Sports Med 16:80–84, 1982.

109. Jordan SH, Green GA, Galanty HL, et al: Acute and chronic brain injury in United States National Team soccer players. Am J Sports Med 24(2):205–210, 1996.

110. Green GA, Jordan SE: Chronic head and neck injuries. *In* Garrett WE, Kirkendall DT, Contiguglia SR (eds): The US Soccer Sports Medicine Book. Baltimore, Williams & Wilkins, 1994, pp. 191–204.

111. Putukian M, Echemendia RJ, Mackin S: Acute effects of heading in soccer: A prospective neuropsychological evaluation. Presented at American Medical Society for Sports Medicine Annual Meeting, Nashville, Tennessee, April 5, 1998.

Chapter 10

Neck and Cervical Spine Injuries

BRENT S. E. RICH, M.D., A.T.C.

Assessment and treatment of traumatic neck and cervical spine injuries in sports must be done with great care and concern for the athlete because of the potential for devastating and long-lasting sequelae. Soft tissue injuries, involving the ligamentous structures, along with injuries to the bone elements or spinal cord account for 2 to 3 percent of all sports injuries.[1] Although the vast majority of these injuries resolve in a few weeks, the common occurrence of the minor injury must not allow a cavalier attitude. Neck and cervical spine injuries are most common (70 percent) in aquatic sports (e.g., diving, body surfing, waterskiing), but are also seen in football (7 percent), gymnastics (6 percent), snow sports (5 percent), and wrestling (3 percent), and may occur in any sport.[2]

TYPES OF NECK AND CERVICAL SPINE INJURIES

Injuries in the cervical region are categorized according to the following format:
1. Soft tissue injuries
   a. Cervical sprains
   b. Cervical strains
2. Nerve injuries
   a. Brachial plexus neurapraxia
   b. Transient quadriplegia
   c. Complete or incomplete spinal cord paralysis
3. Cervical spine fractures and dislocations
   a. Posterior element fractures
   b. Anterior element fractures
4. Cervical disk herniations

Soft Tissue Injuries

Presentation and Progression

Cervical sprains and strains are common injuries involving the muscular and ligamentous structures of the cervical spine. Much like the "whiplash" or hyperextension-hyperflexion injuries that are a consequence of motor vehicle accidents, they result from a rapid acceleration/deceleration mechanism. Conversely, there may be no history of traumatic event other than awaking from sleep with pain.

The stiff neck presents with pain and decreased range of motion without neurologic compromise. The paracervical or upper trapezius muscles are involved with localized pain. Symptoms affecting the shoulders, arms, and middle and low back are occasionally present. There may be an associated muscle tension headache but no impairment in cognitive function. Fever or systemic illness does not correlate with an acute strain; however, if these elements are present, the athlete may have an infection, which should be pursued vigorously.

An assessment of motivational factors for recovery is important. The potential for litigation or benefits, either financially or as a release from working, should be determined.

Diagnosis

The history may reveal a traumatic or nontraumatic cause. Diagnosis is confirmed by lack of neurologic involvement (i.e., numbness, tingling) but an impaired range of active or passive range of motion. Pain may be produced by either active or passive attempts to advance beyond the range of motion limits. Palpable tissue texture changes including muscle spasm, tightness, or trigger point tenderness reinforce the diagnosis.

Comparative range of motion from right to left (either sidebending or rotation) will reveal the range of motion normality and abnormality. Forward flexion (chin to chest) and extension may also be limited or cause pain. Radiographs are usually unremarkable. Although they are not always necessary in minor injuries, documented normal films may be beneficial in litigation cases.

Natural History

Most soft tissue injuries resolve within a few weeks of injury. Following injury there may be a "twinge" of pain without initial loss of motion. Gradually, over the next several minutes to hours, the body responds by muscle spasm and "splinting" the area of insult. This results in pain beyond the area of spasm. As time progresses, uninvolved muscles may develop soreness and spasm as they are forced to adapt or compromise. Eventually, the muscles relax as the inflammation resolves and the tissues heal. Without stretching and restrengthening, the involved region may be susceptible to recurrent injury. Although most injuries resolve in several weeks, some individuals complain of persistent pain for several years after injury.[3]

Treatment

Immobilization with a soft cervical collar may be indicated, although use of these devices is not universally accepted.[4] Occasionally, narcotic pain medication is indicated for severe pain. Resting of the muscles may be achieved by using muscle relaxant medication, primarily at night, to restore pain-free and restful sleep. Nonsteroidal anti-inflammatory medications will also influence and decrease the inflammatory cascade.

The steps in the natural progression of soft tissue injury can be changed by the application of physical therapy modalities. Immediate postinjury treatment includes the application of ice to decrease the inflammatory response by limiting the tissue mediators. Gentle traction and therapeutic massage will decrease the painful muscle spasm. Other modalities (i.e., ultrasound, electrical muscle stimulation, deep tissue or trigger point massage, localized heat, or iontophoresis) will aid to decrease the prolonged soreness and restore range of motion. Once range of motion has been reestablished and pain has decreased, strengthening exercises are crucial to finalize treatment and prevent reinjury.

When to Refer

No consultant referrals are necessary for the majority of soft tissue injuries of the cervical spine regions. Usually these are self-limiting conditions that resolve within a few weeks. Referral to physical therapy may be indicated early in the treatment process to promote the resolution of injury. If the condition has not resolved within 8 to 12 weeks, reassessment of the initial diagnosis may be in order and consultation may be necessary if a different cause is determined.

Key Points

- Early ice, rest, and nonsteroidal anti-inflammatory drugs (NSAIDs)
- Restore full range of motion and strength either by a home exercise program or supervised physical therapy
- Determine individual motivation factors and reinforce that most soft tissue injuries are self-limiting

Nerve Injuries

Presentation and Progression

Neurologic injury of the cervical spine ranges from transient to permanent. Because x-ray findings may be negative and nerve conduction studies initially are of limited value, peripheral nerve deficits may be the only objective evidence of a neurologic injury. Therefore, a thorough knowledge of neurologic anatomy is necessary to assess cervical injuries. An accurate evaluation requires an understanding of the brachial plexus and the segmental sensory and motor distribution innervated by the corresponding nerves, along with the deep tendon reflexes (Tables 10–1 to 10–3).

Table 10–1
Upper Extremity Segmental Sensory Distribution

Spinal Nerve	Dermatomal Distribution
C5	Lateral upper arm
C6	Lateral forearm, hand and the radial two digits
C7	Middle finger
C8	Ulnar two digits and medial hand and wrist
T1	Medial forearm

Table 10–2
Upper Extremity Segmental Motor Innervation

Spinal Nerve	Area of Innervation
C5, C6	Deltoid, biceps, brachialis, forearm supinators
C6, C7	Forearm pronators
C7	Triceps and wrist extensors
C8, T1	Intrinsic muscles of the hand

Brachial Plexus Lesions ("Burners") The most common transient neurologic injury involving the neck region is the "burner" or "stinger" syndrome. The "burner," or brachial plexus neurapraxia, involves a stretch or compression injury to the brachial plexus. It is reported to occur in 65 percent of college football players, although one survey reported that only 70 percent of players with this problem report their symptoms to the medical staff.[5] Burners occur most often in football but are also seen in wrestling, hockey, and other sports. The athlete presents with pain in the region of the lateral neck and down the arm to the fingers. Numbness and paresthesia accompany the pain, along with varying degrees of motor weakness involving the shoulder and upper arm musculature.

Transient Quadriplegia and Complete or Incomplete Spinal Cord Paralysis Transient quadriplegia and spinal cord paralysis are very serious career-threatening injuries. Suspicion and recognition are crucial in proper treatment. Therefore, any injured athlete complaining of neck pain, numbness, tingling, or upper or lower extremity weakness—however transient—should be suspected of a spinal cord injury until proved otherwise.[6] If the athlete is unconscious, a severe neck injury should be suspected, and the basics of traumatic care that involves the ABCs (*a*irway management, *b*reathing, and assessing *c*irculation) should be employed.[7] Once the athlete has been

Table 10–3
Upper Extremity Segmental Deep Tendon Reflexes

Spinal Nerve	Reflex
C5	Biceps
C6	Brachioradialis
C7	Triceps

stabilized, determining the disability is the next step. Complete injuries leave the athlete with no motor or sensation below the level of injury, whereas in incomplete injuries some function is preserved. Spinal shock appears as a complete injury but resolves within 24 hours.

Transient quadriplegia involves numbness, burning pain, sensory loss, and weakness or temporary paralysis that resolve in a few minutes.[8] The mechanism of injury involves hyperflexion or hyperextension and axial loading of the cervical spine. Controversy exists as to the exact etiology of this condition, and possible causes include developmental cervical stenosis, congenital fusion, discogenic disease, and cervical instability. The cervical stenosis controversy is beyond the scope of this chapter, but in general, if the bony canal is greater than 15 mm, it is considered normal, but if it is less than 13 mm, it is abnormal.[6] Torg has proposed a mechanism to determine the relationship between cervical stenosis and neurologic injury, but although interesting, the Torg ratio method is not universally accepted.

Diagnosis and Natural History

Evaluation of the athlete with a burner first involves a knowledge of the sport and skill level of the athlete. The unilateral upper limb involvement is a hallmark of the injury. Clancy et al. described a classification system[9] of grades 1 through 3. Grade 1 lesions involved neurapraxia resulting in a temporary conduction block of nerve function. No axonal disruption occurs, but there is loss of selective demyelination of the axon sheath. Most symptoms resolve in minutes but some can last for days to weeks. Grade 2 lesions are axonotmesis injuries lasting at least 2 weeks. There are motor and sensory losses that show on electromyographic (EMG) studies. The epineurium is intact, but the axon is damaged. Although full function is anticipated, growth only occurs at a rate of 1 to 2 mm per day. Grade 3 lesions leave long-lasting or permanent deficits because not only are the axons involved but also the endoneurium is disrupted. Regrowth may be impaired without surgical restoration. EMG changes are positive.

The sideline physical examination confirms a burner. Upper extremity weakness is present but usually resolves in a few minutes. The shoulder abductors and biceps should be examined for C5 nerve root level, the wrist extensors for C6, triceps for C7, and hand intrinsic muscles for C8 to T1. These tests should be compared bilaterally for weakness and can be done without removal of equipment. Sensory parasthesias, though painful and frightening to the athlete, resolve as normal function returns to the injured nerves. Reflexes should be examined for persistent symptoms. If full neck and upper arm range of motion, strength, and sensation return, the athlete may be allowed to return to play. If there are persistent motor or sensory symptoms, return to play should be delayed until these symptoms resolve. The treating physician should be willing to delay return to participation if this is clinically indicated. Additionally, time is needed to investigate the mechanism of injury, duration of symptoms, occurrence of previous injury, active cervical range of motion, and reproduction of symptoms with provocative tests. A thorough postgame or next-day evaluation should be performed if indicated.

Transient quadriplegia should be thoroughly investigated and taken extremely seriously to prevent a devastating result. A full neurologic examination should be performed as well as a complete history, including mechanism of injury, duration of symptoms, and residual effects. Plain radiographs should be obtained and magnetic resonance (MR) imaging, computed tomography (CT) scanning, or electromyelography (EMG) should be employed as indicated to evaluate for bony injury, ligamentous abnormalities, or nerve root or cord compression. Return to participation should be precluded if abnormalities exist. If all of the studies are normal, decision about return to participation should be made on an individual basis with full awareness that permanent neurologic deficits may occur. Consultation with a neurosurgeon should be considered.

Complete paralysis or incomplete paralysis necessitates emergent evaluation and treatment by a neurosurgeon. Surgical intervention should be performed as indicated.

Treatment

Treatment for the majority of burners involves watchful waiting. Cervical spine radiographs (including flexion and extension views) are indicated to evaluate cervical spine abnormalities or foraminal encroachment. MRI or CT is not indicated initially but should be ordered for persistent symptoms. Because EMG abnormalities do not present for at least 2 weeks, those studies should not be

performed initially. Ideally, the EMG should be performed between 2 and 4 weeks if symptoms persist.[10] Postinjury care includes ice application, nonsteroidal anti-inflammatory medications, and gentle massage. Neck strengthening should be employed to prevent reinjury. Proper tackling techniques should be demonstrated and reviewed. The use of protective equipment (i.e., neck rolls, Cowboy collar) is controversial. Use should be individualized but is not universally accepted.

Treatment for spinal cord injury necessitates following an emergency action plan for removing that athlete from the playing surface in such a way that does no further harm. Prior to the sport season the medical staff should practice spine board stabilization so that everyone is familiar with the procedure. Emergency medical technicians or paramedics should be contacted with the emergency medical system (EMS) in the local area. Consultation with qualified consultants should be done with any suspected serious spinal cord injury.

When to Refer

Consultation with a neurologist should be considered for burners that persist for more than several weeks. Because these injuries gradually resolve, patience is indicated. Spinal cord injuries necessitate neurosurgeon evaluation.

Guidelines for Management

For burners, athletes may return to play in the same contest if full range of motion, strength, and sensation return. The athlete should be withheld from play or practice until symptoms have resolved.

If symptoms have completely resolved and the work-up is negative, athletes with transient quadriplegia should be evaluated on an individual basis in regard to return to play in the sport. They must understand the risks involved in further participation. There should be no rush to return these athletes to play until all factors have been evaluated.

Although spinal cord–injured athletes may not participate in the sports in which they became injured, full physical and emotional support should be given to them by all the parties involved with the athlete. Disabled athletes participate in other sports, and these options should be presented to spinal cord–injured athletes as indicated.

Key Points

- Neurologic injuries should never be taken lightly.
- A thorough history and physical examination should be performed followed by serial neurologic examinations.
- Return to play may be instituted for burners if all symptoms abate and full range of motion, strength, and sensation have been restored.
- Transient quadriplegia is a serious condition and may be a precursor to permanent injury if participation is continued.
- Complete or incomplete paralysis obviously precludes further sports participation at the current level.
- Opportunities to continue to be involved in sports should be made available to disabled athletes on an individual basis.

Cervical Spine Fractures and Dislocations

Axial loading is one of the primary mechanisms of injury in cervical spine fractures and dislocations. Such injuries are seen in a multitude of sports, but football, diving, skiing, and rugby are the most common. Cervical spine fractures are classified into posterior and anterior element fractures.

Presentation and Progression

The first step in identification of a cervical spine fracture is the suspicion that one exists. Pain upon palpation with or without neurologic deficit in the upper extremity is the presenting complaint. Like the syndromes mentioned earlier, appropriate precautions must be employed when the athlete is removed from the field of play. Leaving the helmet on is indicated until evaluation in the emergency department and the obtaining of a cross-table lateral x-ray. If a bony abnormality is found on a plain radiograph, CT or MR imaging evaluation is indicated to determine the extent of the bony disruption or spinal cord involvement.

Diagnosis, Natural History, and Treatment

Once the athlete has been removed from the playing field, the stability of the fracture and a method for repair can be determined. These steps differ, depending on the location of the fracture.

Posterior Element Fractures Fractures involving the neural arch of the second vertebra are called a "hangman's fracture." These injuries occur mechanically by cervical hyperextension while a vertical force is applied to the body. Because the vertebral canal is opened by the fracture, neurologic signs are usually not present. If there is a subluxation of the second vertebra on the third, halo immobilization is indicated because of associated disruption of the anterior and posterior longitudinal ligaments. If no subluxation is present, a brace that limits flexion may be sufficient.

A "clay shoveler's fracture" is an avulsion fracture of the spinous process that occurs when the neck is flexed and the posterior ligaments cause a distraction force that splits the spinous process vertically. This fracture occurs most commonly at C7, followed by C6 and T1. These are stable injuries without neurologic symptoms except for localized pain that may radiate to the upper shoulders. Soft collar immobilization is indicated until pain is decreased.

Unilateral or bilateral facet dislocations occur with rotation and severe flexion. Unilateral injuries are stable but may compress the nerve root at the neural foramen and may present with motor or sensory changes involving that nerve root. There is moderate anterior displacement of the vertebral body width (usually less than 50 percent) shown on a lateral x-ray. Closed reduction by cervical traction with halo immobilization is the method of treatment. Bilateral facet dislocations occur with forced flexion. The intervertebral disk, posterior longitudinal ligament, and the capsule surrounding the facet may all be involved. Neurologic deficit involving either sides or complete quadriplegia may be presenting symptoms. Lateral radiographs demonstrating more than 50 percent anterior displacement of the anteroposterior width of one vertebra on another is present. These are unstable injuries requiring posterior fusion after reduction.

Anterior Element Fractures Anterior element fractures are compression fractures caused by axial loading and flexion. They are categorized as one of four types:

1. Teardrop fracture: a chip fracture off the anterior lip of the vertebral body, breaking the cortical endplate.

2. Fracture that involves the upper half of the

vertebral body, breaking off a larger portion anteriorly.

3. Fracture of the superior and inferior vertebral endplates with the posterior cortex intact.
4. Burst-type fracture of the vertebral body, often with fracture fragments into the spinal canal.

Types 1 and 2 fractures do well with simple immobilization. Decompression and anterior fusion are indicated for types 3 and 4 fractures. Flexion and extension views as well as CT or EMG may be necessary to determine the extent of the injuries.

When to Refer

Neurologic compromise associated with a cervical fracture requires immediate neurosurgical consultation. Referral for fractures without neurologic injuries is determined by the degree of instability of the fracture. There should be no hesitancy to refer if concern arises.

Guidelines for Management

- Follow the ABCs of emergency management for these injuries with cervical spine immobilization and remove from the field of play.
- Leave the helmet on if there is any question of a cervical fracture.
- Neurologic compromise requires immediate neurosurgical consultation.
- For any unstable fracture consultation should be obtained.

Key Points

- Hyperextension, flexion, or rotational forces cause posterior element fractures.
- Axial loading and flexion cause anterior element fractures.
- Neurologic compromise may or may not be present initially with these injuries, but extreme care should be maintained to prevent it.

Cervical Disk Herniations

Presentation and Progression

Sports-related cervical disk herniations are uncommon. The nucleus pulposus may extrude through the annulus with asymmetric compressive forces.[11] The nucleus may progress into the vertebral canal and neural foramen, causing impingement on the cervical nerve root.

Pain in the neck, shoulder, or arm may be the presenting complaints of cervical disk herniations. There may be associated motor weakness or sensory changes in the segmental nerve distribution. Reflex impairment may also be present.

Diagnosis

Conservative methods are instituted in the treatment of these injuries and include rest, ice, and nonsteroidal anti-inflammatory or possibly oral corticosteroid medication. With persistent symptoms or neurologic deficits MRI is used to make the definitive diagnosis. CT scanning with EMG may be preferred by some practitioners.

Natural History

Similar to lumbar disk herniations, many cervical disk herniations resolve with time and conservative treatment.

Treatment

For persistent symptoms, epidural steroid injections may be indicated to resolve the condition. Cervical disk excision and fusion should be considered if all conservative methods fail. Return-to-play decisions are made on an individual case-by-case basis and depend on the athlete's recovery, sport position and level of competition, age, risk of future injury, and activity level.

When to Refer

MRI-documented cervical disk herniations that do not resolve with conservative care should be referred to a neurosurgeon or orthopaedic spine specialist.

Key Points

- Conservative treatment is indicated for initial symptoms.
- MRI scanning should be obtained for persistent symptoms.

- If all conservative treatment is unsuccessful, epidural steroid injections and consultant referral is indicated.
- Surgical disk excision combined with fusion may be indicated if all conservative treatment fails.
- Return to sport after surgery is determined on a case-by-case basis.

SUMMARY

Neck and cervical spine injuries have potential devastating long-term consequences. Along with cardiac events and head injuries, they are the most troubling injuries that team physicians face. Familiarity with the basics of recognition, evaluation, and treatment of these injuries is a necessary requirement for anyone involved with event coverage or sports participation that could affect the cervical spine. Injury prevention is accomplished by teaching appropriate techniques, adjusting rules, providing appropriate supervision, wearing protective equipment, and educating players, coaches, parents, and athletes, because care is necessary to lessen the potential life-threatening or life-altering consequences of these injuries. Serial neurologic evaluations are required to identify sensory or motor involvement. Appropriate use of radiographs and supplemental tests (i.e., MRI, CT, electromyelography or nerve conduction velocity, and myelography) are indicated to provide appropriate care.

In those rare instances in which further sports participation should cease based on the type of injury and the potential for paralysis, cases should be individualized. These circumstances are trying for the physician as well as the athlete. Objective evidence and comprehensive information should be presented to the athlete in this regard. Prevention of severe injury and paralysis is of extreme importance. There is no need for prompt return to play until appropriate evaluation is complete, for inadequate assessment or recovery may have lifelong consequences.

For the unfortunate athlete who suffers a disabling neck or cervical spine injury emotional, physical, and rehabilitation support should be provided. Continued athletic participation as a disabled athlete may be considered.

REFERENCES

1. Bailes JE: Spinal injuries in athletes. *In* Menezes AH, Sontagg VKH (eds): Principles of Spinal Surgery. New York, McGraw-Hill, 1996, p. 465.
2. Clarke KS: Epidemiology of athletic neck injury. Clin Sports Med 17(1): 86, 1998.
3. Gargan MF, Bannister GC: Long-term prognosis of soft-tissue injuries of the neck. J Bone Joint Surg Br 72(5):901–903, 1990.
4. Gennis P, Gallagher EJ, Giglio J, et al: The effect of soft cervical collars on persistent neck pain in patients with whiplash injury. Acad Emerg Med 3(6):568–573, 1996.
5. Sallis RE, Jones K, Knopp W: Burners: Offensive strategy for an underreported injury. Phys Sportsmed 20(11):47–55, 1992.
6. Wilberger JE: Athletic spinal cord and spine injuries. Guidelines for initial management. Clin Sports Med 17(1):111–120, 1998.
7. Wiesenfarth J, Briner W: Neck injuries. Urgent decisions and actions. Phys Sportsmed 24(1):35–41, 1996.
8. Ferriter PJ, O'Leary PF: The relationship between cervical spine injury and the upper extremity. *In* Nicholas JA, Hershman EB: The Upper Extremity in Sports Medicine. St. Louis, Mosby, 1990, p. 12.
9. Clancy WG, Brand RL, Bergfield JA: Upper trunk brachial plexus injuries in contact sports. Am J Sports Med 5(5):209–216, 1977.
10. Weinstein SM: Assessment and rehabilitation of the athlete with a "stinger." A model for the management of noncatastrophic athletic cervical spine injury. Clin Sports Med 17(1):127–135, 1998.
11. Roaf R: A study of the mechanics of spinal injuries. J Bone Joint Surg 42B:8, 1960.

Chapter 11 | Injuries to the Upper Extremity

DAVID J. GRONSKI, M.D.

The upper extremity is of pivotal importance in common sports such as baseball, football, basketball, and swimming. It is also extremely important in volleyball, lacrosse, and field events. Although each sport is unique in the demands that it places on the upper extremity and the relative frequency of various injuries, certain common injuries may occur in various sports. Any medical professional evaluating patients in a primary care setting will encounter athletes and nonathletes with upper extremity problems. These problems may result from acute trauma or overuse.

Books have been written on the complexities of diagnosis and treatment of problems related to the shoulder, elbow, hand, and wrist as single entities. Therefore, any chapter discussing injuries to the upper extremity must be abridged. This chapter attempts to cover the more common upper extremity injuries that lend themselves to evaluation and management in the primary care setting. It will highlight important epidemiologic information that may affect the differential diagnosis in the evaluation and treatment of an individual athlete involved in one activity or various sports. Pertinent history, physical examination findings, and differential diagnosis are reviewed for the most common injuries. Treatment and referral recommendations are summarized. When appropriate, return-to-play guidelines are discussed.

THE SHOULDER

The shoulder is a complex joint. In order to assess the problems most commonly affecting the shoulder, one must have a basic understanding of shoulder anatomy. The scapula, clavicle, and humerus come together to form the shoulder joint. Injuries may occur at the articulations of these bones, in the bones, or in the soft tissue around these joints.

Because of the shoulder anatomy of the acromion overlying the rotator cuff muscles and the subacromial bursa, overhead movements and activities that require arm movement away from the body can lead to problems. The subacromial tissues may be easily pinched in flexion, abduction, and internal rotation. This is a common cause of shoulder pain and will be the focus of further discussion (Fig. 11–1).

Most of the motion of the shoulder as a whole takes place at the glenohumeral joint. No other joint in the body allows the same versatility in range of motion. To allow such range of motion, a joint must sacrifice inherent stability. The bony structures of the shoulder offer very little stability, with a spherical humerus articulating with a shallow glenoid. The glenoid labrum offers some extension of the glenoid "socket" to enhance stability but is made up of flexible cartilaginous tissue. The ligaments and joint capsule of the shoulder provide some stability but, in some cases, may comprise very flexible connective tissue.

The rotator cuff muscles (the subscapularis, supraspinatus, infraspinatus, and teres minor) act as the dynamic stabilizers of the shoulder, helping to maintain integrity of the joint during extremes of motion and throughout activity in general. Weakness or fatigue of the rotator cuff muscles may allow abnormal motion of the shoulder or even varying degrees of instability. Trauma, high forces, and repetitive forces may also lead to instability.

Complete displacement of the humeral head out of the glenoid fossa is termed dislocation. In most instances, a second person is needed to "relocate" the humerus. This adjustment may be attempted on the field of play or in a medical setting. Subluxation is the term used for an episode of instability that is not severe enough to classify as a dislocation. Athletes may have vary-

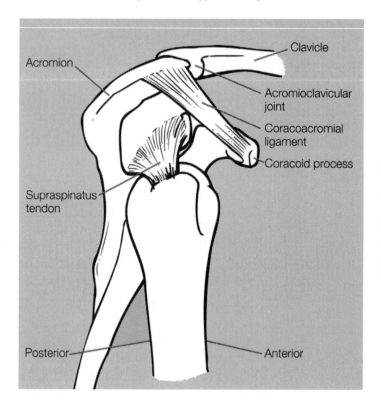

Figure 11-1. A lateral perspective of the shoulder demonstrating the coracoacromial arch. This includes the acromion, the acromioclavicular joint, the coracoid process, and the coracoacromial ligament, all of which form a roof over the supraspinatus tendon. (From Wolin PW, Tarbet JA: Rotator cuff injury: Addressing overhead overuse. Physician Sportsmed 25(6):54, 1997. Figure ©1997, Mary Albury-Noyes.)

ing degrees of pain and disability with glenohumeral instability.

Impingement Syndrome

Mechanism of Injury

Repetitive motion of the shoulder in several sports puts athletes at risk of impingement or pinching of the subacromial tissues between the acromion, coracoclavicular ligament, and the humerus. Pain often results from impingement. Fatigue of the rotator cuff muscles during activity may play a role in impingement by allowing superior displacement of the humerus. The serratus anterior, trapezius, and rhomboid muscles act as scapular rotators and stabilizers. The importance of the scapular stabilizing muscles must also be stressed. Without proper scapular rotation during flexion and abduction activities, the acromion is in a lower position, decreasing the size of the subacromial space. Electromyographic studies in swimmers have shown that fatigue of the serratus anterior may make impingement much more likely. Any sport that involves overhead use of the shoulder may be problematic. Common sports that seem to put athletes at higher risk of impingement include swimming, baseball and softball, football (throwing), tennis, and volleyball.

Hawkins and Kennedy describe a continuum of symptoms as they develop over time. Symptoms of impingement may initially include minimal pain with activity and no weakness or lack of range of motion. At this stage, patients may be pain-free if the offending activity is avoided. As time passes without adequate treatment or rehabilitation and the insult to the tissues continues, patients may report pain with activities of daily living, especially activities involving overhead movement or lifting movement away from the body. Eventually, complaints may progress to more significant pain with loss of range of motion and night pain while lying on the affected side. These symptoms may reflect both rotator cuff tendinitis and subacromial bursitis. If the disorder is left untreated and the offending activity is continued, rotator cuff tear may ultimately result as a consequence of repeated insult to the rotator cuff musculature.

A related condition that may mimic impingement syndrome is acute traumatic subacromial bursitis. This type of bursitis usually follows a single injury that drives the humerus against the acromion and causes an acute contusion to the bursa. Treatment is similar to that for impingement syndrome.

Diagnosis

The history is always crucial in making the diagnosis of impingement syndrome. A history of repetitive use or rapid increase in the intensity or frequency of use of the shoulder is almost always present. The likelihood of the diagnosis is increased if activities involve repetitive flexion and internal rotation, which increase the risk of impingement.

The examination of the shoulder can seem very complex. It can, however, be improved with a basic understanding of the anatomy, a systematic approach, and repetition. For a description of the various physical examination maneuvers cited here, see Chapter 1, on the musculoskeletal examination.

In the examination of the patient with shoulder pain, it is often wise to begin with a thorough examination of the neck. Cervical radiculopathy with referred pain to the shoulder, which lies in the C5 dermatome, is an often missed diagnosis. If shoulder pain is exacerbated by neck movement or performance of a Spurling's maneuver, cervical radiculopathy should be considered. It is also recommended that strength, sensation, and reflex testing be done in both upper extremities to look for evidence of cervical radiculopathy. If uncertainty about the source of the pain persists after a thorough examination and the practitioner is trying to differentiate between cervical radiculopathy and impingement syndrome, injection of the subacromial space of the shoulder with an anesthetic agent could be helpful. If the patient's pain is eliminated by this injection, cervical radiculopathy is highly unlikely.

Physical examination should also include a full shoulder evaluation. Range of motion (flexion, abduction, extension, internal and external rotation) should be assessed (Fig. 11–2). Loss of motion may be associated with adhesive capsulitis, subacromial bursitis, or rotator cuff tear. Acromioclavicular (AC) joint testing is done to rule out inflammation and degenerative change. "Crossover testing" may cause generalized pain in patients with impingement syndrome and is a sign of AC joint pathology only if pain localizes to the AC joint. Impingement testing in one, if not all, of the many positions described is positive. Rotator cuff strength testing may show weakness

related to inflammation or rotator cuff tear (Fig. 11–3). In addition, stability testing of the glenohumeral joint should be done to rule out instability, which may be an underlying problem contributing to impingement syndrome. Instability of the glenohumeral joint is often seen in swimmers and young females. A "clunk test," "crank test," or O'Brien's test (pp. 12–13) can be performed to help rule out possible labral tear. A "drop test" may be positive if a rotator cuff tear exists. In the author's experience, patients with rotator cuff tears may also be weak with resisted abduction of the affected shoulder.

Imaging is seldom necessary in the initial evaluation of a patient who presents with symptoms consistent with impingement syndrome. Possible exceptions include history or findings consistent with possible arthritic change (e.g., advanced age, presence of degenerative arthritis in other joints, history of remote injury including shoulder separation or dislocation) or history of recent trauma that suggests possible fracture of the clavicle, scapula, or humerus. X-rays may be indicated under these circumstances or if conservative treatment is not successful. The presence of subacromial spurring secondary to degenerative change may make conservative management less likely to be successful. Radiographs may also show evidence of calcific tendinitis in the rotator cuff tendons, which may be present after years of impingement.

Magnetic resonance (MR) imaging may be considered if initial treatment is not successful and the diagnosis is unclear. MR imaging should not be used as a substitute for a complete history and examination, however. A careful and complete history and physical examination combined with proper conservative treatment will often eliminate the need for further imaging beyond radiographs in the majority of patients. The arthrogram is an alternative to MR imaging to rule out rotator cuff tear or labral tear.

Injection may be used diagnostically to rule out a rotator cuff tear. Subacromial injection of corticosteroids is discussed under Treatment.

Differential Diagnosis

Impingement syndrome may be concurrent with or be confused with adhesive capsulitis (which is especially prominent among middle-aged women), calcific tendinitis, rotator cuff tears, cervical ra-

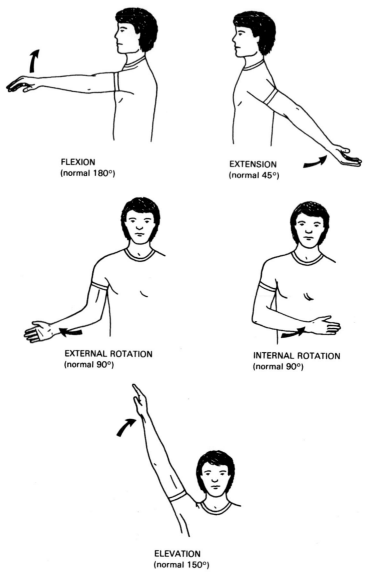

FLEXION
(normal 180°)

EXTENSION
(normal 45°)

EXTERNAL ROTATION
(normal 90°)

INTERNAL ROTATION
(normal 90°)

ELEVATION
(normal 150°)

Figure 11–2. Shoulder range of motion. (From Birnbaum, JS: The Musculoskeletal Manual, 2nd ed. Philadelphia, W. B. Saunders, 1986, p. 62.)

diculopathies, AC arthritis, acute traumatic bursitis, and shoulder instability.

Treatment

Treatment may vary based on the intensity and duration of symptoms. Initially, physical therapy designed to strengthen the rotator cuff and posterior scapular stabilizers is the cornerstone of treatment. Strengthening of the rotator cuff muscles leads to improved depression of the humeral head with use of the shoulder, functionally increasing the subacromial space and reducing the likelihood of impingement. Strengthening the muscles that

rotate and stabilize the scapula (the trapezius, serratus anterior, and rhomboid muscles) can also help to elevate the acromion with activities. This also helps to increase the subacromial space to prevent impingement.

On the basis of the severity of symptoms, one may consider adjunctive treatments. If the history and physical examination show evidence of significant subacromial bursitis or tendinitis, oral anti-inflammatory agents may be given, or even subacromial injection of corticosteroids (Fig. 11–4). These injections may be both diagnostic and therapeutic. If local anesthetic is included in the injection, range of motion and strength testing

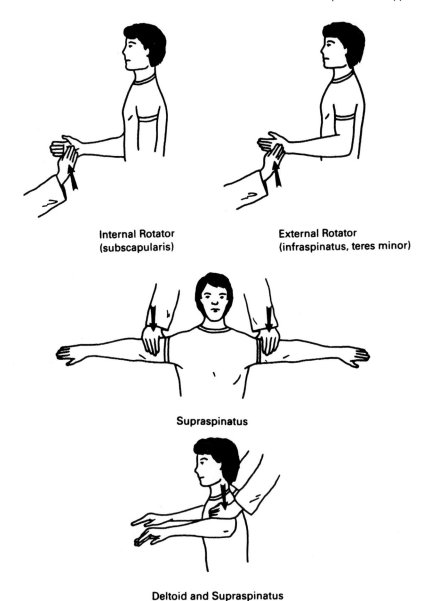

**Internal Rotator
(subscapularis)**

**External Rotator
(infraspinatus, teres minor)**

Supraspinatus

Deltoid and Supraspinatus

Figure 11–3. Shoulder signs, strength testing. (From Birnbaum JS: The Musculoskeletal Manual, 2nd ed. Philadelphia, W. B. Saunders, 1986, p. 63.)

may be repeated after the injection. If strength and range of motion improve to near normal, significant rotator cuff tear is unlikely. Modalities including icing, ultrasound, phonophoresis, and iontophoresis may be used as symptomatic treatment.

Ideally, the athlete will avoid the offending activity and begin cross training until symptoms are well controlled. Often this is either not possible or desirable for the athlete. With mild symptoms in a competitive athlete, instructions to discontinue the activity will often result in poor compliance or loss of the patient from one's care.

If symptoms are mild, a rehabilitation program may be begun, with patient follow-up within the next 3 to 4 weeks. If gradual improvement is achieved, this approach may be continued. Improvement may be slowed or prevented by continued participation in the offending activities, and the patient should be educated about this possibility. If symptoms do not improve, the athlete should be instructed to eliminate the offending activity until symptoms do improve.

Most patients will gradually respond to conservative management over 1 to 2 months. In patients who are not responding to conservative

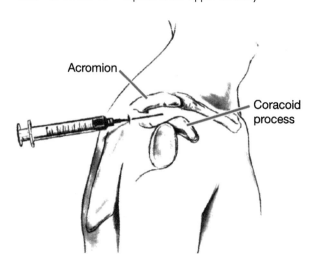

Acromion

Coracoid process

Figure 11–4. Lateral view showing the level and depth of a subacromial space injection, posterior approach. The needle is parallel to the undersurface of the acromion, directed slightly cephalad, and inserted approximately 2.5 cm. (From Bach BR Jr, Bush-Joseph C: Subacromial space injections: A tool for evaluating shoulder pain. Physician Sportsmed 20(2):93, 1992. Illustration ©1992, Pat Thomas.)

management, the possibility of rotator cuff tear, labral tear, or other injury or inflammation must be considered. The possibility of rotator cuff tear is increased in patients over the age of 40.

Surgery may be necessary to adequately evaluate and treat impingement syndrome that does not respond to conservative management. Surgical treatment usually consists of a decompression procedure.

When to Refer

Referral should be considered if there are uncertainties in the diagnosis, concerns of possible rotator cuff tear, or lack of improvement with conservative treatment.

Return to Play

The return to sports participation is based on functional ability. Athletes should have full shoulder range of motion, full rotator cuff strength, and minimal or no pain after the activity. It will always be challenging to successfully rehabilitate and treat athletes involved in high-risk activities such as swimming or pitching, especially for those who present early in the season and wish to continue the aggravating activity. With an organized rehabilitation program and patience, however, success is often possible.

Unfortunately, recurrence seems to be common. The incidence of recurrence may be decreased by a maintenance physical therapy program to be done three or four times per week during the season of any sport that involves repetitive use of the shoulder joint. One can also advo-

cate restarting the rehabilitation program 3 to 4 weeks before the season of the sport begins.

Shoulder Instability

History and Presentation

As previously outlined, the shoulder is an inherently unstable joint. A common cause of pain and disability is underlying instability. History is again pivotal in diagnosing this disorder. Patients who are experiencing dislocation or subluxation will often describe feelings of instability if allowed to characterize their symptoms. Fairly frequently, however, mild instability will present as pain and may often cause secondary impingement symptoms. In this case, the physical examination is very important in making the diagnosis. Swimmers will commonly present in this way. Other sports with a high incidence of instability include wrestling, racquet sports, volleyball, and gymnastics.

Instability may be multidirectional or isolated to one plane. Patients with multidirectional instability may have laxity at other joints as well. Isolated anterior or posterior instability may come with acute injury or follow repetitive insult.

Anterior dislocation accounts for approximately 85 to 95 percent of all shoulder dislocations. A family history of shoulder instability may be found in 25 percent of patients. Anterior instability is most likely to occur with the shoulder in the abducted and externally rotated position and the application of a posterior directed force on the more distal arm, which may partially or completely lever the humeral head out of the glenoid fossa. Football players are at risk if they attempt to make "arm tackles" with their shoulders in this position. This anterior type of injury may also occur with a backward fall on an outstretched arm.

Posterior injury may occur with a forward fall on an outstretched arm. Posterior injury may also occur with weight lifting or other activities that place the shoulder in a flexed and neutral to internally rotated position with an axial load to the upper arm. This causes posterior displacement of the humeral head with respect to the glenoid fossa. Football offensive linemen, while "pass blocking," are also at risk for posterior injury.

Physical Examination

Physical examination findings will vary based on the underlying diagnosis. With early examination after an acute dislocation or significant subluxation episode, one may find decreased range of motion and pain at rest. With acute dislocation, one study found a 100 percent incidence of hemar-

throsis, which undoubtedly contributes to these findings. In this setting the pain and limited movement due to the injury may preclude a complete examination of the shoulder. More complete examination may often be performed after a period of conservative treatment.

In the subacute setting or in a patient suffering from subluxation, examination may often be completed. Limitation in external rotation may be present with anterior instability. Impingement findings may be present, as previously discussed. Apprehension testing (described in Chapter 1) is usually helpful in diagnosing anterior instability. A "relocation test," which relieves pain brought on by apprehension testing, may help to confirm anterior instability. One may assess for posterior instability with an axial posteriorly directed load to the humerus with the shoulder in the forward flexed position. Pain during this maneuver is considered evidence of possible posterior instability (Fig. 11–5).

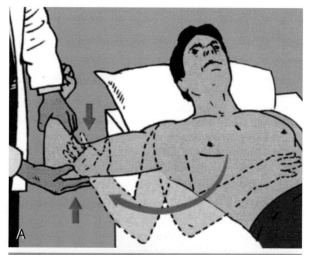
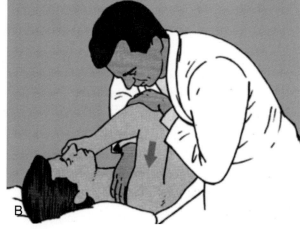

Figure 11–5. *A,* To perform the anterior apprehension test to assess shoulder instability, the examiner slowly abducts and externally rotates the supine patient's shoulder. Supporting the elbow, the examiner applies a posterior force to the forearm. The test is positive if the maneuver is painful. *B,* To perform the posterior apprehension test to assess posterior shoulder instability, the examiner flexes the patient's arm to 90 degrees, rotates the patient's shoulder medially by holding the arm, and applies a posterior force to the patient's elbow. The test is positive if this maneuver elicits apprehension. (From Greenfield G, Stanish WD: Relieving shoulder pain without surgery. Physician Sportsmed 22(4):67, 1994.)

Instability may also be demonstrated by directly testing for evidence of subluxation at the glenohumeral joint. In the patient with multidirectional instability, this testing in a relatively relaxed individual may result in pronounced findings that are evident to the patient, examiner, and any other observers.

The examiner should also include provocative testing for evidence of labral tears. Clunk testing is one such test. Rotator cuff strength testing should also be included to establish any significant weakness. One may also look for evidence of global hypermobility by searching for laxity at other joints, including evidence of significant hyperextension at the elbows and knees. Hypermobility may also be noted at the ankles or hands as well.

Imaging

In the setting of possible acute dislocation, radiographs may be helpful to confirm the diagnosis and to rule out associated fracture. X-rays may also be used to ensure proper position after reduction of the dislocation. One may also see evidence of a Hill-Sachs lesion after acute and recurrent anterior dislocation. This lesion is caused by an impression fracture of the posterolateral humeral head. Standard scapular anteroposterior and lateral views are commonly ordered. An internal rotation or Stryker view may be added to look for the Hill-Sachs lesion.

Further imaging may be considered if the patient does not respond to conservative management. The use of arthrography or MR imaging to diagnose labral tears, ligamentous injuries, or associated rotator cuff injuries may be discussed with a radiologist, sports medicine specialist, or consulting orthopaedic surgeon.

Treatment

Treatment of the acute dislocation is well described in orthopaedic and emergency medicine texts. Various maneuvers may be performed, and outlining each is beyond the scope of this chapter. One technique for reducing anterior dislocations that may be used on the playing field (and that is often used by trainers because manipulation by the treating practitioner is not necessary) is worth mentioning. With the patient in a seated position with knees and hips flexed to approximately 90 degrees, the patient interlocks the fingers of both hands and places them around the lower legs. The patient then leans back with a steady force as tolerated. This places a steady traction on the humerus and often will result in relocation, which markedly decreases the patient's pain. The effectiveness of this maneuver seems to be inversely related to the interval of time between dislocation and attempted relocation. Following successful or failed relocation the patient should be transferred to an acute care facility for radiographs and treatment with relocation if necessary. Documenting any evidence of vascular or neurologic compromise in the affected extremity before relocation attempt may be helpful with respect to further treatment and medicolegal concerns.

Treatment after the acute dislocation is somewhat controversial. Some sources advocate a period of immobilization for younger patients, with more aggressive return to range of motion for patients over 40 years of age to avoid the possibility of adhesive capsulitis. One study, however, has shown no difference in the rate of recurrence between early motion and 3 to 4 weeks of immobilization in adduction and internal rotation. There is a much higher rate of recurrence in younger patients. This rate may be as high as 100 percent in those under 10 years of age and gradually decreases to approximately 50 percent in patients who are 30 to 40 years old. One study showed that recurrence rates are higher in athletes (87 percent) than nonathletes (30 percent) over a wide variety of ages. Because of this high recurrence risk, some orthopaedic surgeons advocate a surgical repair in the acute setting, but this is controversial.

Conservative treatment may consist of short-term immobilization for comfort with early progression to range of motion exercises and gradual resumption of strengthening exercises. Attention should be directed to strengthening the rotator cuff muscles and the scapular stabilizers. Patients should be seen in follow-up to assess the level of instability and to advance their physical therapy. When patients regain full range of motion and strength, exercises may be advanced to include eccentric training, which puts the shoulder in the "at risk" position with gradually increasing load or resistance. Resistance may be obtained by using elastic bands designed for this purpose. The rate of recovery is quite variable.

When to Refer

Orthopaedic consultation should be obtained if conservative treatment is unsuccessful. In this case, one may see recurrent subluxation or dislocation or persistent pain. Stabilization procedures are often successful in this setting. Glenoid labral tear is easy to miss and may be a cause of persistent pain despite appropriate conservative management. This may often be treated successfully with arthroscopic surgery, and orthopaedic or sports medical consultation may help in discerning this diagnosis.

Return to Play

Return to play is based on the patient's functional ability. Full range of motion and strength should be attained prior to consideration. The patient should be counseled about the high rate of recurrence of subluxation and dislocation. Some sports are higher risk, and the level of risk should play a part in deciding how soon the practitioner should consider sending the athlete back to full participation. One may wish to offer orthopaedic consultation to discuss possible surgical options.

Acromioclavicular Injuries (Shoulder Separation)

Mechanism of Injury

The clavicle is attached to the scapula by both the AC and coracoclavicular ligaments. The mechanism of injury to the AC joint is usually a fall directly on "the point" of the shoulder, which causes a subluxation or dislocation of the distal clavicle. This type of fall causes downward and medial displacement of the scapula and clavicle. The clavicle then collides with the first rib, which causes the clavicle to stop while the scapular motion continues. This may cause fracture of the clavicle or injury to the ligaments of the AC joint.

Allman described a classification scheme for AC injuries. Grade 1 injuries involve sprain or tear of the AC ligament without laxity or elevation of the distal clavicle. Grade 2 injuries involve tearing of the AC ligaments along with stretch of the coracoclavicular ligaments and perhaps injury to the aponeurosis of the deltoid and trapezius muscle attachment at the distal clavicle. Elevation of the distal clavicle is minimal if present and may be seen only on stress x-rays. Grade 3 injuries involve tearing of both ligamentous restraints and aponeurosis injury. Clavicle elevation is pronounced and can usually be appreciated without stress radiographs.

Patients will usually present with pain over the AC joint and various degrees of limitation of shoulder range of motion.

Diagnosis

The diagnosis should be suspected if the appropriate history is obtained. Findings from the physical examination are also important. In grade 3 injuries asymmetry in clavicular elevation may be noted on inspection. In all grades of AC injury, the patient will have tenderness over the AC joint. Limited range of motion is often present. Secondary rotator cuff weakness may be due to pain. Crossover testing (passive adduction in a forward flexed position) is often positive for increased pain at the AC joint. The examiner should inspect and palpate the entire clavicle to rule out evidence of clavicle fracture.

Radiographs of the shoulder and clavicle are necessary to rule out clavicle fracture. Distal clavicle fracture is easily confused with AC separation. Stress views that involve weighting of the affected extremity may be done but may be of only limited clinical value.

Treatment

Treatment for grades 1 and 2 injuries is conservative and consists of use of frequent icing. A sling may be used for comfort initially. Exercises to regain range of motion are to be done as tolerated. Rotator cuff strengthening exercises may be done while healing occurs to prevent atrophy, which might result from relative disuse. It is hoped that this may prevent future impingement problems. Anti-inflammatory drugs or acetaminophen may be used for analgesia. Occasionally narcotic analgesics may be used for initial severe pain.

In grade 3 injuries, conservative treatment may be offered. Some, however, advocate surgical repair. Tenting of the skin by the distal clavicle or patient concern about the cosmetic result should prompt referral to an orthopaedic surgeon.

The usual course of recovery depends on the severity of the injury. Most patients will eventually regain full function of the shoulder. Some may have residual pain at the AC joint or may develop degenerative arthritis of the AC joint. Surgical excision of the distal clavicle is often recommended and should be curative in these circumstances.

If pain continues after conservative treatment,

one may consider injection of the AC joint as further treatment before orthopaedic referral.

When to Refer

One should refer to an orthopaedist for grade 3 injuries with tenting of the skin by the distal clavicle or a cosmetic result that is unsatisfactory for the patient. Patients who have continued pain after conservative treatment should be referred as discussed.

Return to Play

The major risk of return to play is reinjury and increased pain. In most circumstances, the patient should have full shoulder range of motion and rotator cuff strength. Padding over the AC joint with a "donut pad" may be helpful in return to contact sports. This may be placed under shoulder pads in football and hockey players. Icing may be continued or restarted for increased or recurrent pain.

THE ELBOW

The elbow is primarily a hinge joint composed of three bones. The humerus of the upper arm articulates with both the radius and ulna of the forearm (Fig. 11–6A). Flexion, extension, pronation, and supination are the primary motions of the elbow. Injuries to the elbow can be acute, chronic, or a combination of the two. The elbow is stabilized by the medial and lateral collateral ligaments and the annular ligament, which surrounds the radial head (Fig. 11–6B). Overall, the elbow is a fairly stable joint. Dislocation and frac-

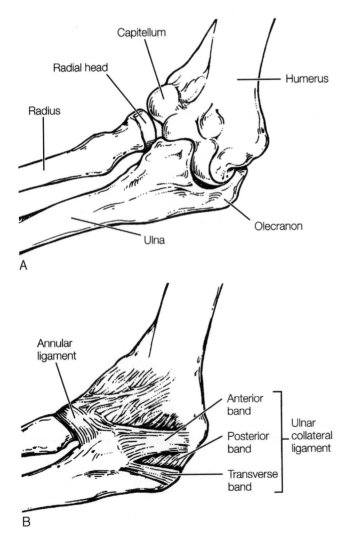

Figure 11–6. *A*, The elbow is a hinge joint consisting of articulations of the humerus, radius, and ulna. Pronation and supination of the forearm occur about the proximal radioulnar articulation. *B*, Several ligaments assist in elbow motion. The ulnar (or medial) collateral ligament consists of anterior, posterior, and transverse bands. The anterior band remains tight throughout elbow range of motion, making it the most important medial stabilizer. The radial (or lateral) collateral ligament (not shown) originates from the lateral epicondyle and inserts into the annular ligament, which is the main stabilizer of the radial head. (From Fox GM, Jebson PJL, Orwin JF: Overuse injuries of the elbow. Physician Sportsmed 23(8):58, 1995. Figures ©1995, Mary Albury-Noyes.)

ture are possible but usually require significant trauma.

Radial Head Fracture

Mechanism of Injury

The most common cause of a radial head fracture is a fall on an outstretched hand with an axial load to the forearm while the wrist is in a pronated position. Rarely, a direct blow to the radial head will cause a fracture. Any sport that puts the athlete at risk of falls can lead to radial head fractures.

Diagnosis

The patient will usually present complaining of elbow pain and may avoid extension and supination of the elbow. Physical examination should include inspection for visible swelling, which may or may not be present. Range of motion may be limited, especially with respect to extension and supination. The patient will often have tenderness over the proximal radius. The examination should also include testing for instability of the elbow to varus and valgus stress.

Radiographs will often be helpful in making the diagnosis. One should always look for evidence of a joint effusion on the lateral view. The presence of a visible posterior fat pad on this view without evidence for another fracture in the elbow should prompt very careful inspection for evidence of a radial head fracture, which will often be present. If initial x-rays do show evidence of effusion but no evidence of radial head fracture, follow-up films after initial empirical treatment will often show the fracture.

Treatment

For radial head fractures with no or minimal displacement (less than 2 mm), early mobilization within the first week is the appropriate treatment and helps to avoid loss of extension and supination range of motion. If splinting is necessary, due to pain, the patient could be splinted in a posterior splint at 90 degrees with as much supination as tolerated. This position will help to prevent further loss of range of motion caused by splinting. The splint should be removed within 3 to 5 days, and physical therapy can be initiated to attempt to restore full range of motion.

If the radial head fracture is comminuted or significantly displaced, treatment may at times be no different, but orthopaedic consultation is recommended. Management in these cases is somewhat controversial.

Usual Course and Recovery

Good recovery with a functional range of motion is the rule with appropriate treatment. Small deficits in extension and supination are possible but rarely impair function due to the range of motion in the shoulder.

When to Refer

If the fracture is comminuted or significantly displaced (more than 2 mm) or there is associated instability of the elbow, consultation with an orthopaedic surgeon is recommended. Referral should also be considered if conservative treatment does not result in functionally adequate range of motion.

Return to Play

The athlete should have regained full range of motion and strength with no tenderness over the radial head before returning to athletic activities. This rehabilitation may require at least 6 weeks.

Lateral Epicondylitis

Mechanism of Injury

The lateral epicondyle of the humerus is the origin of the common extensor muscles. Included in this group is the extensor carpi radialis brevis, which lies beneath the extensor carpi radialis longus. The origin of the extensor carpi radialis brevis is the most common site of microscopically identified degeneration associated with the pain present in lateral epicondylitis. The angiofibroblastic hyperplasia may eventually extend to involve the extensor carpi radialis longus and extensor digitorum communis (Fig. 11–7).

Although this injury is commonly called "tennis elbow," the majority of sufferers are not tennis players. This condition may occur in any athletes or nonathletic individuals who use their hands and wrists in a repetitive manner. Among tennis players who suffer from this malady, some risk factors

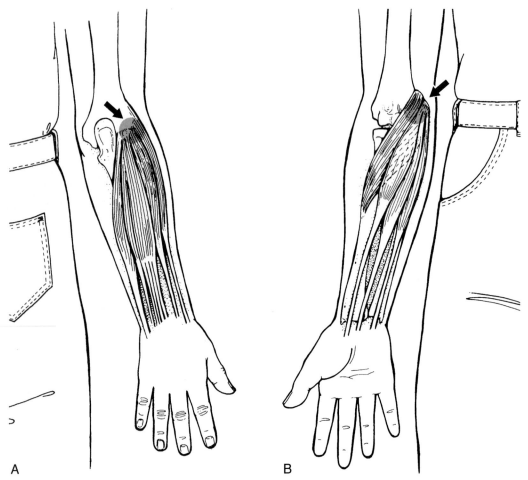

A   B

Figure 11–7. *A,* A posterior anatomic view of the elbow and forearm demonstrates the location of the affected tissues in lateral epicondylitis (tennis elbow)—insertion of the extensor tendons of the wrist on the lateral epicondyle *(arrow)*; the site to palpate for tenderness *(shaded circle)* is also shown. *B,* An anterior anatomic view of the elbow and forearm demonstrates the sources of golfer's elbow pain—the insertion of the pronator teres tendon or common flexor tendon on the medial epicondyle *(arrow)*; the site to palpate for tenderness *(shaded circle)* is also shown. (From Hannafin JA, Heinz Schelkun P: How I manage tennis and golfer's elbow. Physician Sportsmed 24(2):63, 1996. Figure ©1995, Mary Albury-Noyes.)

have been suggested but not completely proved. These risk factors include age over 40 years, use of larger rackets, tighter stringing of the racket, and increased playing time. Weakness of the rotator cuff musculature and subsequent compensation of the ipsilateral forearm musculature have been proposed as etiologic factors in lateral epicondylitis by at least one author.

Patients will often present with pain over the lateral epicondyle extending over the proximal extensor mass. Early in the course, pain may occur only during and shortly after the offending activity. Later, pain may occur with lesser provocation. Patients often complain of pain with activities of daily living including shaking hands or lifting a coffee cup or jug of milk.

Diagnosis

Often the first sign of lateral epicondylitis is a grimace on the face of the patient during a greeting handshake. A history of increased use of the hand or wrist in a sporting or work activity should also raise the possibility of lateral epicondylitis. One should ask about repetitive use of the upper extremity.

Physical examination is remarkable for full range of motion of the elbow or wrist in most cases. Tenderness is present over the lateral epicondyle and may extend to the proximal extensor musculature. Pain may be increased by gripping, resisted wrist and finger extension, and wrist supination. These maneuvers should be done with the elbow in full extension. Some examiners use pain

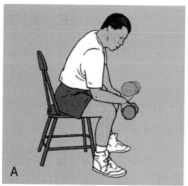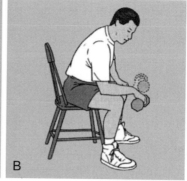

Figure 11–8. To do wrist curls, sit in a chair with the forearm resting on the thigh (or on a table). With the palm up *(A)* and holding a dumbbell, slowly bend the wrist up as high as possible and hold for 2 seconds before slowly lowering it. Repeat in a similar fashion but with the palm down *(B)*, extending the wrist upward. A more advanced technique is to do wrist curls with the upper arm held horizontal and not supported. (From Nirschl RP, Kraushaar BS: Keeping tennis elbow at arm's length: Simple, effective strengthening exercises. Physician Sportsmed 24(5):61, 1996. Figure ©1996, Terry Boles.)

upon resisted extension of the long finger to differentiate posterior interosseus nerve syndrome and radial tunnel syndrome from lateral epicondylitis. Reflex and sensory loss are not found in isolated lateral epicondylitis.

Radiographs can be used to rule out tumor in younger patients and the presence of degenerative change or bony exostoses in older individuals. Often imaging is not necessary with the initial assessment and could be reserved for cases that do not respond to conservative treatment.

Treatment

The initial treatment of lateral epicondylitis is conservative. The effectiveness of nonsurgical treatment may be as high as 82 to 93 percent. The first goal of treatment is pain relief. If possible,

the patient should curtail the offending activity. Pain may be managed with the use of frequent icing (15 to 20 minutes two or three times per day). Nonsteroidal anti-inflammatory drugs may be used. Modalities such as ultrasound, phonophoresis, and iontophoresis have been used, but well-controlled studies demonstrating their effectiveness is lacking. Bracing that places pressure over the proximal wrist extensor musculature can help to reduce stress with activity at the musculotendinous junction at the lateral epicondyle.

A home exercise program that improves the flexibility and endurance strength of the wrist and finger extensor and wrist supinator musculature is very important to prevent recurrence after pain is reduced (Figs. 11–8 and 11–9).

If pain is severe or the patient is not responding to initial conservative management, one

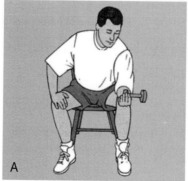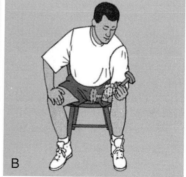

Figure 11–9. To do the forearm rotation exercise, sit with one elbow resting as in Figure 11–8 and palm facing up *(A)*. Hold a dumbbell by one end (not in the middle). Slowly rotate the forearm until the palm is facing down *(B)*. Hold for 2 seconds, then slowly return to the starting position. (From Nirschl RP, Kraushaar BS: Keeping tennis elbow at arm's length: Simple, effective strengthening exercises. Physician Sportsmed 24(5):61, 1996. Figure ©1996, Terry Boles.)

may consider corticosteroid injection as a means to decrease discomfort and decrease inflammation. Controversy does exist about the potential to weaken the muscular attachment site. Although some investigators are cautious about using one injection, others advocate a series of injections on an as-needed basis. Most arbitrarily advocate no more than three injections in any year because of these concerns.

Various steroid preparations exist and are often mixed with local anesthetic. The mixture is injected at the site of maximal tenderness, deep to the extensor carpi radialis brevis, which is anterior and distal to the lateral epicondyle. Substantial immediate reduction of the patient's pain is often seen. The possibility of hypopigmentation and subcutaneous fat atrophy should be discussed with the patient before injection. The possibility of increased pain (postinjection flare) over the 1 to 3 days after the injection in a minority of cases should also be discussed. Incidence of postinjection flare is thought to be approximately 10 percent with a corticosteroid and local anesthetic mixture and may be as high as 50 percent with corticosteroid used alone. Pain can be managed with icing and use of analgesics as necessary. Although evidence is lacking to demonstrate the effectiveness of these injections, they seem to be relatively safe and they help with short-term pain relief.

An alternative approach includes prolotherapy. These injections, which are designed to temporarily increase inflammation and promote a healing response, are somewhat controversial and not widely used, but they have been advocated as an alternative treatment. A full discussion of this technique is beyond the scope of this chapter.

Various sport modifications have been advocated. Nirschl advocates proper grip sizing of rackets for tennis players by measuring from the proximal palmar crease to the radial aspect of the ring finger to correspond with girth. He also advocates decreasing racquet string tension and the size of the racquet. Temporary or permanent use of a two-handed backhand stroke in tennis may be helpful. In golf, one may consider increasing the girth of grips and decreasing the intensity of grip as conservative measures. Use of a tennis elbow strap during activity can also be helpful.

Complete recovery may take several weeks to months. The length of recovery often depends on the patient's ability and willingness to modify or decrease the frequency of the offending activity.

Recurrence is frequent and may occur in 10 percent or more. Recurrence rate may be reduced by a continuation of the stretching and strengthening home exercise program.

When to Refer

Referral may be necessary if conservative treatment fails. Various surgical treatments are advocated for the treatment of lateral epicondylitis.

Return to Play

If pain is mild, play may often be continued during treatment. The use of a tennis elbow strap should be considered. If pain is severe, a period of avoidance or marked reduction in the offending activity may be very helpful.

Medial Epicondylitis

Mechanism of Injury

Medial epicondylitis is very similar to lateral epicondylitis except for its location and the muscles involved. The medial epicondyle is the muscular attachment site of the pronator teres, flexor carpi radialis, and palmaris longus. Inflammation may also involve the flexor carpi ulnaris and flexor digitorum superficialis. Because of the proximity of the ulnar nerve, symptoms of neuritis have been reported in up to 60 percent of cases. This condition may occur with ipsilateral lateral epicondylitis.

Although commonly called ''golfer's elbow,'' this overuse disorder may occur with any repetitive use of the flexor and pronator musculature. This might include hammering, overhead serving in tennis, or doing biceps curls in weight training. Weakness of the rotator cuff musculature and subsequent compensation of the ipsilateral forearm musculature has been proposed as an etiologic factor in medial epicondylitis by at least one author.

Patients will often present with pain that is present over the medial epicondyle and may extend over the proximal flexor mass. Early in the course, pain may occur only during and shortly after the offending activity. Later, pain may occur with lesser provocation. Patients may ultimately complain of pain with activities of daily living or at rest.

Diagnosis

One should ask about a recent history of repetitive use of the hand and wrist preceding the onset of medial elbow pain. On physical examination, patients with medial epicondylitis will invariably have tenderness near the medial epicondyle and it may extend into the proximal flexor mass. Pain may be increased with resisted wrist flexion and pronation. Range of motion should be noted. The presence of a flexion contracture may indicate more significant pathology. Ulnar nerve symptoms may be seen. Ulnar nerve subluxation should be ruled out. One may wish to test for ulnar collateral ligament laxity, which could be present in a throwing athlete. This test is done by applying a valgus stress to the elbow with the joint flexed at 20 to 30 degrees. The contralateral side may be used as a control. This diagnosis might be confused with medial epicondylitis.

Radiographic imaging is seldom necessary on initial presentation but may be used in the older patient to rule out bony spurring near the medial epicondyle or other degenerative change. In the younger patient, it may be used to rule out tumor. One might reserve imaging for patients in whom initial conservative management fails to provide relief.

Treatment

Initial treatment should include stopping or decreasing the frequency of the offending activity. A common sense approach is often helpful. One may instruct the patient to use pain as a guide to determine an acceptable activity level. Rehabilitation should concentrate on improving the flexibility and endurance strength of the wrist flexor and pronator musculature. If pain is severe, strengthening exercises may be postponed. Use of a "tennis elbow strap" placed over the proximal forearm with the pressure just distal to the medial epicondyle may be recommended. This may allow some patients to continue to participate in their sport without worsening the symptoms.

Icing may be very helpful in relieving pain and decreasing inflammation and should be recommended at least twice per day, if not more frequently. Nonsteroidal anti-inflammatory drugs may be prescribed, although their benefit has not been proved. Corticosteroid injections may also be used but are often reserved for those patients in whom initial conservative treatment fails. Evidence is lacking to demonstrate the effectiveness of these injections, but they seem to be relatively safe and may help with short-term pain relief. One should, however, discuss the risks of subcutaneous fat atrophy and overlying skin hypopigmentation as potential risks of corticosteroid injections. Most sources advocate no more than three injections in one area per year because of concern about weakening the tendinous attachments. This topic is discussed in the treatment section under lateral epicondylitis.

An alternative approach includes prolotherapy. These injections, which are designed to temporarily increase inflammation and promote a healing response, are somewhat controversial and not widely used but have been advocated as an alternative treatment. A full discussion of this technique is beyond the scope of this chapter.

An important part of treatment is ensuring that the patient is using proper technique. If the practitioner's knowledge of the sport or sports is not sufficient to assess this, a recommendation that the patient work with an instructor in the sport may be very helpful. This type of intervention may be crucial in preventing recurrence.

Usual Course and Recovery

Patients with medial epicondylitis will often improve over 4 to 12 weeks with appropriate conservative management. The speed of the recovery may depend on the ability and desire of the patient to limit the offending activity. It is helpful for patients to continue a maintenance physical therapy program if they are returning to the offending activity. This program should include both flexibility and strength exercises for the forearm musculature. Also, continuing the physical therapy into the off season and restarting the program a few weeks before the next season should decrease the recurrence rate. Convincing patients to adhere to this recommendation is challenging and not always successful.

When to Refer

Surgical consultation should be considered if conservative treatment fails. If no progress is evident after 6 months or if symptoms are increasing despite conservative management, surgery may be a good alternative. Surgical success rates are often cited to be as high as 90 to 95 percent.

Return to Play

Patients with mild medial epicondylitis may often continue the offending activity during treatment. Technique modification may help some athletes remain active with less pain. With more severe cases, the decision on resuming play should be individualized. Often a trial-and-error approach is used, with patients returning to the activity minimally at first, with self-assessment of symptoms over the next 24 to 48 hours. If symptoms are increasing within this time frame, the patient is being too aggressive in returning to play. In this case, the patient may decrease the amount of participation, or a longer course of conservative treatment should be pursued. If symptoms are not increasing, patients may slowly increase their activity level with continued self-assessment. Pain may be used as a signal of progressing too rapidly.

Little Leaguer's Elbow

Injuries to the elbow related to throwing are not limited to the younger athlete, but a discussion of little leaguer's elbow will include a brief overview of the stress applied to the elbow by the throwing motion, and these principles may be applied to the older throwing athlete and the potential injuries in these patients. Diagnosis of this disorder and appropriate management are very important because one may potentially prevent long-term damage to the elbow and a premature end to a young athlete's ability to continue throwing.

Mechanism of Injury and Presentation

In order to understand the mechanism of injury to the elbow with throwing, one must consider the anatomy of the elbow. The major motions of the elbow are flexion, extension, pronation, and supination. Ligaments on the ulnar aspect of the elbow stabilize the joint in the face of a valgus stress. The humerus articulates with both the radius and ulna. The radius articulates with the humeral capitellum, which may be injured with repetitive loading. In immature athletes the picture is further complicated by the presence of growth plates at the sites of ligamentous attachment. In these younger athletes, the epiphysis may be displaced or the physis can become inflamed by acute or repetitive traction forces.

Little leaguer's elbow is a term used to describe a constellation of symptoms and pathologic findings associated with the repetitive forces involved in throwing. This condition is usually seen in 8- to 16-year-olds. The repetitive stress may cause progressively more damage as throwing continues. Initially, a stretch injury occurs to the medial supporting structures. As the process continues, compression forces on the lateral structures may lead to cartilaginous injury, including possible osteochondritis dissecans. If treatment is not instituted, one may see flexion contracture and even osteoarthritis.

The throwing motion generates a great deal of force in the wind-up and early cocking phase. In the late cocking phase, delivery, and follow-through phase of throwing, this force is transmitted to the arm. The elbow sustains a significant valgus stress in this throwing motion. The delivery also involves active pronation of the elbow. In a well-conditioned arm, the elbow flexor and pronator musculature helps to minimize the stress through the medial (ulnar) collateral ligament and to avoid compression injury to the radial side of the elbow. Injury is usually a result of overuse, causing fatigue of these muscles and subsequent distraction forces on the ulnar side and compression forces on the radial side. As with all overuse injuries, "too much, too soon" is often the cause of throwing injuries (Fig. 11–10).

The patient will often present with pain over the medial and anterior elbow. If presentation is late, a flexion contracture may be present. Pain is exacerbated by throwing. Early in the course, pain may be present only after pitching and may resolve with short periods of rest. As the condition worsens, pain may occur with fewer pitches, and if pitching continues, the pain often begins to occur with activities of daily living and even at rest. One should elicit a history of throwing, including the number of pitches, frequency, and intensity. Some investigators suggest an association between this condition and beginning to throw curve balls before physeal closure. A change in throwing motion or improper delivery may also be an etiologic agent. Pitchers may, however, change their motion after pain occurs in an effort to protect their elbow and minimize pain.

The presence of an osteochondritis dissecans (OCD) lesion of the humeral capitellum might cause pain over the radial aspect of the joint. It might also cause mechanical symptoms of "catching" in the elbow. An OCD lesion is analogous

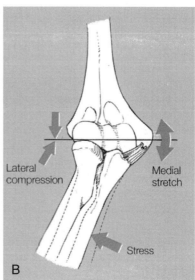

Figure 11–10. Valgus stress on the elbow created by the throwing motion *(A)* stretches the medial compartment and compresses the lateral compartment *(B)*. (From Congeni J: Treating—and preventing—Little League elbow. Physician Sportsmed 22(3):54, 1994. Figure ©1994, Tom Campbell.)

to a "pothole" in a road. This lesion extends into the underlying bony structure and may be displaced or nondisplaced. A fixed or nondisplaced lesion will often cause this symptom in the same position each time. A loose body, which might occur with a displaced OCD lesion or other cartilaginous fragmentation, might cause more unpredictable mechanical locking or catching, with subsequent swelling and restricted range of motion.

Differential diagnosis includes ulnar neuritis or ulnar nerve subluxation, stress fracture, and isolated ulnar collateral ligament sprain.

Diagnosis

One should begin the examination by inspecting the elbow for swelling, which may be present medially and anteriorly. Range of motion should be assessed. One may find evidence of flexion contracture. One may also see lack of supination range due to inflexibility and inflammation of the pronator musculature. Palpation will often elicit tenderness over the medial epicondyle and the course of the ulnar collateral ligament as well as over the anterior forearm in the area of the pronator musculature. In the setting of an OCD lesion, the examiner might elicit tenderness over the anterolateral portion of the joint. A mechanical catching may rarely be present with range of motion testing.

Stability should be assessed by applying a valgus and varus stress to the elbow joint in 20 to 30 degrees of flexion. This positioning is necessary to unlock the olecranon from the olecranon fossa and allow true assessment of the collateral ligaments. Instability with valgus stress may be present if the ulnar collateral ligament has been stretched or the medial epicondylar apophysis has been displaced. There is variability in stability in different patients, which makes comparison with the uninvolved side mandatory. Strength assessment may show weakness of elbow flexion, pronation, and wrist flexion.

Imaging

Radiographs should be done routinely to rule out apophyseal displacement or avulsion. Some displacement may be present in asymptomatic throwers. This finding makes it necessary to consider the degree of tenderness in this area and the use of comparison views of the uninvolved elbow. Radiographs may also help to identify the OCD lesion, which may be present at the humeral capitellum from repetitive compression injury. It should be noted that plain radiographs may not be sensitive enough to identify early lesions of the humeral capitellum. One should also look for evidence of degenerative change and spurring. Radiographs also allow the practitioner to rule out a bony tumor as the source of elbow pain.

Bone scan may be used to rule out stress fracture and may show evidence of traction injury at the medial epicondyle and early OCD lesions of the humeral capitellum. This may be helpful in patients with severe pain or in whom the diagnosis is uncertain. The author has rarely used a bone scan in this setting.

MR imaging may be used in the evaluation of elbow pain. Obviously, this involves considerable cost but can in the right hands be very sensitive in diagnosing these problems. If radiographs are negative and the physical examination is reassuring, MR imaging may be reserved for patients who have mechanical symptoms or whose condition does not respond to initial conservative treatment.

MR imaging should not be used to substitute for a thorough physical examination. It should also be noted that the sensitivity of MR imaging does depend on the ability and experience of the person interpreting the scan. This includes the primary physician and the radiologist. Collaboration between the examining physician and a radiologist with experience in reading such scans should be the rule in using this modality to evaluate all musculoskeletal injuries, including the elbow of a throwing athlete.

MR imaging is helpful to rule out displacement of an OCD lesion or fluid behind the fragment, which might prompt surgical consultation. It may also show evidence of bone bruise and other lesions, the significance of which is often unknown.

Treatment

Elbow pain in an adolescent thrower should always be evaluated and the diagnosis of "little leaguer's elbow" considered. Too often, pitchers continue to throw on misguided "no pain, no gain" advice or do not report their pain because of a fear that they will not be allowed to pitch. This often delays diagnosis and prolongs recovery. As in most overuse injuries, early treatment often will allow quicker return to play and lower incidence of recurrence.

If there is no instability on examination, no mechanical symptoms, and no concerning radiographic changes, conservative treatment is indicated. The first goal of therapy is to eliminate pain and inflammation. Complete rest from throwing is necessary. The amount of time may vary from 2 to 6 weeks. Ice massage can be helpful to decrease pain and inflammation. Nonsteroidal anti-inflammatory medicines are often used to reduce inflammation.

Once pain decreases, the athlete can begin stretching and strengthening exercises for the forearm musculature, including pronator strengthening. Strength and flexibility training for the shoulder, abdominal, and back musculature should also be added to form a comprehensive pitching rehabilitation program. Pitching technique should be examined by a skilled observer to look for flaws in the delivery that may be causing or contributing to the elbow pain.

Recovery and Return to Play

Once the athlete is pain-free and has improved strength and flexibility, he/she may gradually return to throwing. The resumption of throwing must be gradual. Tossing is first, with gradual progression to throwing, and then to pitching over about 2 weeks. Along the way, the progression is slowed if significant pain is encountered. Congeni has outlined a reasonable schedule for returning to pitching.

Once the athlete returns to competition, the number of pitches in each outing should be limited. About 100 pitches per outing is a reasonable number. A lesser number early in recovery may be quite reasonable. Counting pitches, rather than innings, is an important distinction because there is great variability in the number of pitches thrown by any given pitcher in one inning.

Preventing first occurrence and recurrence of this condition may be possible through proper preseason and in-season conditioning. In addition, education of the pitchers and coaches about appropriate workout schedules, limiting the number of pitches thrown, and cautioning against the introduction of breaking pitches in skeletally immature athletes are all very important. Practices should focus on quality rather than quantity.

Pitchers who experience this disorder should continue to do the rehabilitation in the off season and should be doing the rehabilitation for 4 to 6 weeks before planning to restart throwing.

When to Refer

Consultation should be obtained if the diagnosis is uncertain. If the examiner's skill does not allow assessment of stability of the elbow or if there is question of an OCD lesion and the practitioner is not comfortable with treatment, consultation is wise.

WRIST AND HAND

The anatomy of the wrist and hand is extremely complex. As noted previously, entire volumes have been written pertaining to the wrist and hand individually. Because of space limitations, this section cannot hope to address the full scope of injuries that may be seen in a primary care setting. Therefore, the focus in this discussion is on injuries that can be successfully managed by a primary care physician. The management of common hand fractures is beyond the scope of this discussion. Several helpful texts are available to guide the primary care practitioner in evaluation and management of these injuries. A few references are cited at the end of the chapter to assist the reader (Fig. 11–11).

Scaphoid Fracture

Mechanism of Injury

The scaphoid bone is the most commonly fractured carpal bone. It is seen more frequently among the young and active. The fracture usually occurs as the result of a fall on an outstretched hand or with longitudinal forces along the first metacarpal bone. Most patients will complain of wrist pain that may be somewhat diffuse. They will often have associated swelling. Many will assume that they have a "wrist sprain" and may not seek care immediately. Diagnosis may be complicated in this circumstance because of a temporary resolution of symptoms followed by aching pain and intermittent symptoms that the patient may not connect with the earlier injury. In unrecognized or inadequately treated scaphoid fractures, nonunion may result. This may be associated with chronic wrist pain, degenerative arthritis, and the need for wrist surgery.

Diagnosis

The physical examination may vary with the amount of time from the acute injury. Within a few days of the injury, inspection may reveal significant swelling and bruising. There may be marked limitation in range of motion and strength. Pain may be present with supination and pronation. Tenderness in the anatomic snuffbox, which is formed by the extensor pollicis brevis and extensor pollicis longus, is usually present. Tenderness may also be elicited with palpation of the volar aspect of the scaphoid bone. One may elicit pain in the area of the scaphoid bone with axial load of the first metacarpal through the thumb (Fig. 11–12).

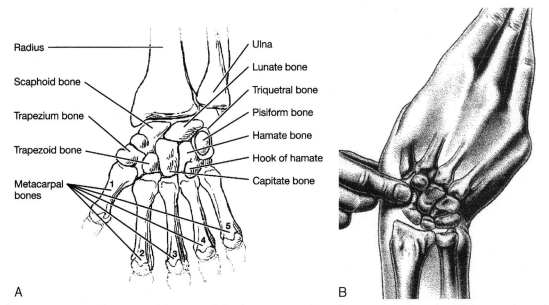

A   B

Figure 11–11. A palmar view of the wrist's skeletal anatomy (A) shows the structures to be palpated during a thorough wrist examination. A dorsal view of the wrist's surface and skeletal anatomy (B) shows that to palpate the distal pole of the scaphoid, the thumb is opposed to the little finger with the wrist in ulnar deviation. (Reprinted with permission from Whipple TL: Preoperative evaluation and imaging. *In* Arthroscopic Surgery: The Wrist. Philadelphia, J. B. Lippincott, 1992, p. 16. Figure 11–11A ©1994, Williams & Wilkins.)

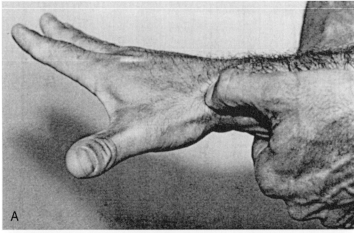

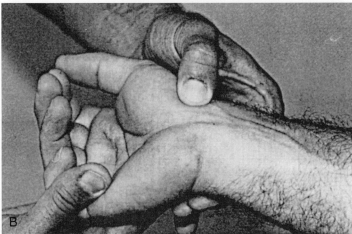

Figure 11–12. *A,* Palpating the anatomic snuffbox with the wrist in ulnar deviation. *B,* Palpating the scaphoid tubercle. (From Mirabello SC, Loeb PE, Andrews JR: The wrist: Field evaluation and treatment. Clin Sports Med 11:5, 1992.)

As time passes after the acute injury, symptoms and physical findings may decrease. Tenderness is still often present, and patients may complain of intermittent pain with activity. With scapholunate dissociation, pain may be increased over the area between these bones.

Differential diagnosis includes scapholunate or scaphotrapezoid ligament injury, scaphocapitate syndrome, perilunate fracture and dislocation, and distal radius fracture.

Imaging

Radiographs should be done if tenderness is elicited in the area of the scaphoid in the setting of acute injury, even if months have passed since the acute injury. Three views of the wrist should be obtained. A "scaphoid view," a posteroanterior film with the wrist in partial supination and ulnar deviation, may also be done to increase the sensitivity. Approximately 10 percent of scaphoid fractures may not be visible on initial x-rays. A clenched fist view may also be done to rule out scapholunate dissociation, which may be easily confused with scaphoid fractures. Up to 12 percent of scaphoid fractures have associated radial styloid, ulnar styloid, or distal radius fractures (Fig. 11–13).

If a fracture is identified, further testing is unlikely to be necessary unless CT scanning is needed to quantify displacement. If the initial x-rays are negative and snuffbox tenderness is present, the diagnosis of scaphoid fracture has not been ruled out. In this setting, one may continuously splint the patient in a thumb spica splint for 10 to 14 days.

Upon follow-up, one should repeat plain radiographs if tenderness over the scaphoid persists. Repeat radiographs are unnecessary if tenderness is no longer present after immobilization. The vast majority of unrecognized scaphoid fractures will be identified with this approach. If suspicion is still strong for scaphoid fracture, a bone scan may be used to rule out fracture. An alternative

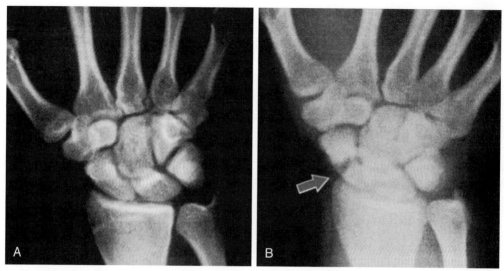

Figure 11–13. *A,* An early postinjury anteroposterior radiograph of a patient's wrist shows no evidence of scaphoid fracture. *B,* The same view of the patient's wrist seen 6 months after injury shows an obvious nonunion scaphoid fracture *(arrow).* (From Rettig AC: Wrist injuries: Avoiding diagnostic pitfalls. Physician Sportsmed 22(8):33, 1994.)

approach is to continue immobilization for an additional 2 weeks and then repeat the original assessment at follow-up.

If empirical immobilization is not an acceptable alternative, a bone scan may be done at least 2 days after the injury to definitively rule out fracture. CT or MR imaging may be used as alternatives in this setting but are more expensive unless limited scanning, priced competitively, is available.

Treatment and Consultation

Acute treatment in the setting of snuffbox tenderness without positive radiographs has been discussed. If a fracture is identified, treatment depends on location of the fracture, the presence of displacement or angulation, and time from injury to diagnosis. One must consider the blood supply of the scaphoid bone when deciding the method of treatment. Because the blood supply runs distal to proximal, more proximal fractures are prone to delayed healing or nonunion despite treatment. Fractures through the midportion or waist of the scaphoid are most common.

In a fracture without angulation or displacement, the goal of treatment is to immobilize the thumb and wrist in a thumb spica cast. The question of long arm versus short arm casting is controversial. With waist or distal fractures, short arm casting for 6 to 12 weeks should be adequate in most circumstances. Casting should be done after

acute swelling has been controlled to ensure a good fitting cast and adequate immobilization. Splinting may be required before casting to ensure immobilization while swelling is reduced. In fractures through the proximal third of the scaphoid, some sources recommend long arm thumb spica casting for 6 weeks followed by short arm thumb spica casting for 6 weeks. Because of the high risk of nonunion in this type of injury, many practitioners might wisely consider orthopedic consultation in these cases.

With displacement of greater than 1 mm or more than 20 degrees of angulation, the risk of nonunion, malunion, and avascular necrosis is quite high and should prompt referral for consideration of open reduction with internal fixation.

With delayed presentation, the risk of poor healing increases. If the fracture is stable and without displacement or angulation, one may treat as noted here, but the patient should be made aware of the increased risk of nonunion. Offering the patient orthopaedic consultation is quite reasonable in this situation. With displacement or angulation, orthopaedic consultation is indicated.

Return to Play

If the diagnosis is uncertain and splinting and reexamination are pursued, return to play should wait until the diagnosis is determined. If a fracture is identified and casting is used, the patient may be allowed to return to play in noncontact sports if the reinjury and fall risk is minimal. The return to full contact sports with a cast in place may be allowed in some areas if the cast is padded. It may be wise to obtain consultation before recommending this course because displacement of a stable fracture might occur with a fall or other injury to the fractured wrist.

If the fracture is adequately treated with casting, the return-to-play decision after the cast is removed may be individualized. Strengthening of the hand and wrist musculature should be completed before the patient returns to contact sports.

De Quervain's Tenosynovitis

Mechanism of Injury

De Quervain's tenosynovitis is an inflammatory condition involving the first dorsal compartment of the wrist. The abductor pollicis longus and extensor pollicis brevis reside in a groove of the radius and are held in place by a segment of the extensor retinaculum. Repetitive motion that involves a firm grip with ulnar deviation is cited as the most common cause of this condition. Trauma over the first dorsal compartment in the area of the retinaculum has also been cited as a potential cause of this condition.

Approximately 30 percent of the population has a septum that divides the two tendons in the first dorsal compartment. Patients with de Quervain's tenosynovitis seem to be more likely to have this variation, and it may play a role in its etiology.

Pain over the radial and dorsal aspect of the wrist is the presenting complaint. Golfers, athletes in racquet sports, and new mothers are often affected.

Diagnosis

Examination should include inspection of the wrist for swelling in the area of the first dorsal compartment just proximal to the radial styloid in the area of the extensor retinaculum. Tenderness is usually present in this same area. Provocative testing with Finkelstein's test reproduces the pain by causing maximum excursion of the two tendons involved. This test is done by having the examiner ulnarly deviate the patient's wrist while the patient flexes the thumb into the palm with the fist closed around the thumb. Pain may also be reproduced by re-

sisted thumb extension with the wrist in maximum radial deviation. Crepitus may be palpable with active use of the tendons. Triggering may also rarely be present.

Imaging is rarely necessary. Radiographs may be helpful to rule out any bony spurring in the area of the first dorsal compartment.

This condition should be distinguished from intersection syndrome and tenosynovitis of the flexor carpi radialis or of the common digital extensors. It should be noted that this condition may coexist with intersection syndrome.

Treatment and Consultation

Initial treatment is aimed at reducing inflammation. Ice massage at least two to three times per day can be quite beneficial. Relative rest is important. Protective splinting that restricts abduction and extension is often helpful. There are many "off the shelf" splints that may be used. Some even contain a gel pad that sits over the inflamed area. If these splints are not available, one may be fashioned with orthoplast or other splinting material. A hand therapist may be consulted for fabrication of less cumbersome splints if this is desired. Splinting may be used constantly for 2 to 6 weeks, depending on the rate of recovery. It may then be used only for aggravating activities as the condition improves.

Nonsteroidal anti-inflammatory drugs are often used and can minimize pain and may also reduce inflammation. Modalities such as phonophoresis and iontophoresis may also be used.

If there is no improvement with this approach or if pain is more intense at initial presentation, injection of a corticosteroid mixed with a local anesthetic may be considered. Injection into the first dorsal compartment just proximal to the radial styloid is often immediately effective in dramatically reducing pain and speeding recovery. Casting with a short arm thumb spica cast may be combined with injection if compliance with use of a removable splint is questionable. Injections may be repeated, but the success rate seems to decrease with repeat injections.

If evaluation and subsequent treatment is not begun until the condition has become chronic, conservative treatment is still indicated, but a shorter period of treatment may be considered before pursuing orthopaedic consultation.

The vast majority of patients will respond to this conservative regimen. If the condition recurs or does not resolve despite adequate conservative treatment, the practitioner can consider restricting activity to avoid abduction and extension. If this is not practical or acceptable, orthopaedic consultation for consideration of release of the first dorsal compartment should be pursued. As always, if the diagnosis is uncertain, consultation is warranted.

Return to Play

The athlete may occasionally be returned to play with appropriate splinting if this is acceptable. If not, return to play should be postponed until the pain has resolved with treatment.

Intersection Syndrome

Mechanism of Injury

Intersection syndrome, which is also known as "squeaker's wrist," is commonly seen in athletes who participate in racquet sports, weight lifting, rowing, and canoeing. It may be triggered by repetitive flexion and extension of the wrist or by local trauma. It is caused by inflammation of the peritendinous or bursal tissue that lies under the abductor pollicis longus and extensor pollicis brevis as they cross the extensor carpi radialis longus and brevis. This area is located 4 to 6 cm proximal to the radiocarpal joint. The inflammation is thought to be caused by overuse of these muscles and subsequent friction.

Pain in the area of the intersection is usually present at initial examination. Palpable and sometimes audible crepitus may be present with movement of the thumb and wrist. Pain may be increased with resisted abduction or extension of the thumb or resisted extension of the wrist.

Diagnosis and Imaging

The practitioner should inspect for swelling in the area of the intersection. Tenderness and palpable or audible crepitus may be present in this same area. One should also consider the diagnosis of de Quervain's tenosynovitis, which may be confused with or coexist with intersection syndrome. Tendinitis of the common digital extensors should also be considered.

Imaging is seldom necessary.

Treatment and Consultation

Treatment is again aimed at decreasing inflammation. Avoidance or limitation of the aggravating activity will often be helpful. Local ice massage is very effective and should be done at least two to three times per day. Splinting of the wrist in approximately 20 degrees of extension is reportedly helpful. Oral nonsteroidal anti-inflammatory drugs may also be helpful. Injection of a corticosteroid mixed with a local anesthetic in the area of bursal inflammation combined with the preceding measures may also be helpful. Modalities such as phonophoresis or iontophoresis may also be of benefit.

If conservative treatment is unsuccessful, orthopaedic consultation should be recommended.

Return to Play

This decision should be individualized, depending on the degree of discomfort and initial success of conservative treatment.

Skier's Thumb

Mechanism of Injury and Presentation

Skier's thumb, also known as gamekeeper's thumb, is an injury to the ulnar collateral ligament (UCL) of the thumb's metacarpophalangeal joint that usually occurs with forced abduction or valgus stress at this joint. This may occur with a fall on an outstretched hand (Fig. 11–14). The presence of a ski pole in the palm increases the frequency of this injury, hence the popular nickname of this disorder.

C. S. Campbell also described this injury as an occupational chronic injury among gamekeepers, hence the term gamekeeper's thumb. This injury was sustained during the practice of killing a wounded rabbit by breaking the neck of the rabbit while holding the head and neck in the potentially injured hand. This maneuver was repeated several times each day and resulted in a stretch injury to the ligament. Thus, a history of overuse with a similar mechanism of injury may be present in some patients.

Patients with an acute injury have pain and swelling that may be generalized at the thumb's metacarpophalangeal joint. Bruising is often present.

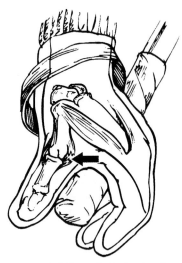

Figure 11–14. A fall in which the thumb is forcefully abducted against a ski pole may cause an injury to the ulnar collateral ligament *(arrow)*. (From Rettig AC, Wright HH: Skier's thumb. Physician Sportsmed 17(12):65, 1989. Figure ©1992, Brenda Q. Kester, Ph.D., C.M.I.)

Diagnosis

Physical examination should include inspection for the presenting signs. Palpation should elicit tenderness over the course of the UCL. If the mechanism of injury is appropriate and the physical examination suggests this injury, radiographs should be done to rule out avulsion fracture. With this injury, radiographs should be done before stress testing to eliminate the risk of displacing a formerly stable fracture. If no fracture is present, stress testing should be done to assess for the presence of the injury and to classify the degree of injury.

Along with testing for stability of the joint as a whole, one must specifically test the UCL. This is done with the joint in approximately 30 degrees of flexion to eliminate stability provided by the volar plate. One must compare the involved with the contralateral side, because there is a wide variability in baseline stability (Fig. 11–15).

Injury to the ligament is graded I through III. This classification is similar to grading systems for other ligamentous injuries. Grade I is associated with microtears in the ligament without any loss of stability. Many of these patients may not present for evaluation. Grade II is associated with a partial tear with some increased laxity but the presence of an end point. Grade III is complete disruption of the UCL. With a grade III injury there is no end point on manipulation. This is an

important distinction to make because treatment will be based on this.

With grade III injury, a Stener's lesion may be present. In this lesion, the two ends of the UCL are separated by the adductor aponeurosis (Fig. 11–16). In this case, the ligament cannot heal. This may be present in 14 to 30 percent of grade III injuries. Some authors report being able to palpate Stener's lesions in some cases. In practice, however, reliably differentiating a Stener's lesion from a grade III injury without a Stener's lesion solely on the basis of a physical examination may be very difficult. MR imaging or exploratory surgery may be necessary to reliably differentiate these two types of grade III injuries. Some sources advocate empirical conservative treatment rather than imaging with grade III injuries. This will be discussed under Treatment.

Treatment and Consultation

Grade I injuries may be treated with a removable splint to protect from further injury. These injuries usually fully resolve within a few weeks with relative rest and splinting. Icing can be helpful to minimize swelling and pain. Analgesics may be used as needed.

Grade II injuries should be treated with immobilization. Casting is helpful to ensure compliance. A removable splint is too often removed by the patient. Early removal often hampers treatment and prolongs recovery. Two to 3 weeks of casting in a short arm thumb spica cast with the thumb in a partially flexed position is recommended. If the condition improves over this period, the patient can be switched to a hand thumb spica cast or splint. Splinting during this phase may be desirable to allow range of motion and gentle strengthening. If after immobilization, significant pain without instability remains, hand therapy with possible use of modalities is a reasonable approach. If instability is still present after immobilization, orthopaedic consultation is indicated. A trial of immobilization or splinting may be helpful even if initial presentation for care is well after the acute injury.

The treatment of grade III injuries is somewhat controversial. Because MR imaging or exploratory surgery may be necessary to identify a Stener's lesion, some experts advocate one of these options in the initial evaluation of a grade III lesion. There is some concern about delaying a surgical procedure to repair a grade III lesion

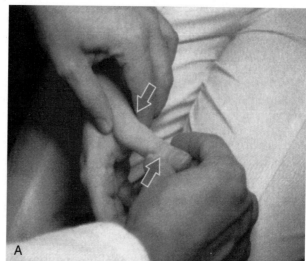

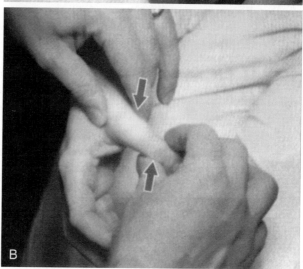

Figure 11–15. During a stress examination of the thumb, the physician stabilizes the metacarpal to prevent rotation, then applies radial stress *(arrows)* to the distal end of the phalanx. *A,* With the thumb in full extension, stability of the volar plate and accessory collateral ligaments is assessed by this technique. *B,* When the thumb is maximally flexed, the accessory stabilizers relax and allow assessment of the integrity of the ulnar collateral ligament. (From Wadsworth LT: How to manage skier's thumb. Physician Sportsmed 20(3):69, 1992.)

because it has been claimed that patients did more poorly following the delay. Some hand surgeons now think that the delay does not affect outcome. For this reason, some hand surgeons advocate an empirical trial of immobilization. If instability

persists, surgery is indicated. This has the potential of saving some patients from an unnecessary surgery or the expense of MR imaging. The drawback of this approach is that those patients with Stener's lesions will undergo immobilization without any chance for benefit. Patients should be informed of this possibility before immobilization. Because of the controversy, it seems wise to discuss the treatment plan or the possibility of consultation with an orthopaedic or hand surgeon.

Return to Play

Patients with grade I injuries may often be allowed to return to play with the aid of a splint or protective taping. Recurrent or worsened injury is possible and patients should be informed of this potential risk.

Figure 11–16. Stener's lesion. The displaced ulnar collateral ligament *(arrow)* lies superficial to the adductor aponeurosis and will not heal without surgical repair. (From Rettig AC, Wright HH: Skier's thumb. Physician Sportsmed 17(12):65, 1989. Figure ©1992, Brenda Q. Kester, Ph.D., C.M.I.)

The return-to-play decision in patients with grade II injuries with a cast in place may be feasible. Again, there is some risk of worsened or recurrent injury with the cast in place. When casting is discontinued, splinting for several weeks followed by protective taping would be wise to prevent recurrent injury. This can be discontinued when strength has returned fully and there is no pain with stress testing.

Patients with grade III injuries should be returned to play as with grade II injuries. It may be wise, however, for the patient to forego participation in contact sports until stability of the joint is achieved.

Mallet Finger

Mechanism of Injury and Presentation

The mallet finger is common among athletes participating in ball sports. This injury is characterized by loss of function of the extensor mechanism at the distal interphalangeal (DIP) joint. Thus, the DIP joint will rest in partial flexion, and the patient will be unable to fully extend the DIP joint. The mechanism of injury is usually forced passive flexion of the extended distal phalanx. This often occurs against intrinsic contraction of the extensor mechanism at the DIP joint.

Different types of injuries may lead to the mallet finger deformity. A stretch injury to the extensor tendon may occur. Complete disruption of the tendon itself may also be present. The other possible anatomic defect may be a small avulsion fracture at the extensor tendon attachment site at the dorsal aspect of the distal phalanx.

If a larger fracture fragment is seen on radiographs, the mechanism of injury may have been hyperextension combined with an axial load to the DIP joint. This combination forces the dorsal portion of the middle phalanx to act as an anvil to break off a large portion of the articular surface. This injury is more appropriately seen as a "true fracture" and may be unstable. Treatment may differ with this type of injury. An accurate history may allow the practitioner to discern the probable type of injury before radiographs are taken (Fig. 11–17).

In children, one may see a fracture or dislocation of the epiphyseal plate.

The patient will often complain of pain near the DIP joint, especially dorsally. A flexion deformity is seen at the DIP joint at rest. Swelling and pain may be seen at the proximal interphalangeal (PIP) joint as well.

Diagnosis and Imaging

The physical examination should include inspection of the entire finger, including the metacarpophalangeal (MCP), PIP, and DIP joints. Lack of complete active extension at the DIP joint is the hallmark of this injury. One may also find swelling and tenderness over the DIP joint. With this type of injury one may see evidence of hyperextension

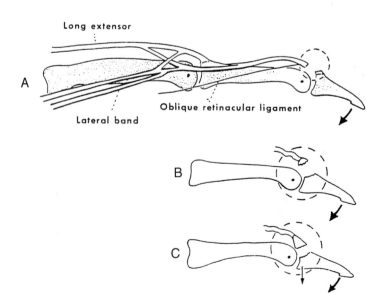

Long extensor

A

Oblique retinacular ligament

Lateral band

B

C

Figure 11–17. The mallet deformity results from a disruption of the insertion of the extensor mechanism into the base of the distal phalanx by tendon avulsion *(A)* or by fracture *(B, C)*. The extensor mechanism then slides proximally and may result in extensor imbalance at the proximal interphalangeal joint. The lesions in *A* and *B* are treated closed, but treatment of *C* requires open reduction. (From Burton RI, Eaton RG: Common hand injuries in the athlete. Orthop Clin North Am 4:809, 1973.)

deformity of the PIP joint. This deformity is due to unsuccessful attempts at extension of the DIP joint, leading to increased extension at the PIP joint, which may cause dorsal subluxation of the lateral band and possible stretch injury of the volar plate.

Plain radiographs should be done to rule out fracture throughout the involved finger. Special attention is given to the dorsal portion of the distal phalanx. A small avulsion fracture or larger "true fracture" may be seen. In the setting of a larger fracture, the collateral ligaments may be attached to the fracture fragment allowing volar displacement of the distal fragment.

Treatment

Treatment of this injury, without evidence of a larger fracture, consists of splinting the DIP joint in full extension to slight hyperextension for a period of 6 to 8 weeks. Various types of splints have been advocated. The best option is a dorsal Alumafoam splint taped in place over the middle and distal phalanx. This immobilizes only the DIP joint. Some practitioners use a "stack splint," which is acceptable but increases the chances for skin breakdown due to the potential to trap more moisture against the skin. Because of the potential for maceration, skin hygiene is very important, regardless of the type of splint chosen for treatment.

It must be emphasized to the patient that full extension must be strictly maintained during this 6- to 8-week period. This includes the periods of time when the splint is removed for skin care. During these times, the finger should be placed on a firm surface to maintain extension. If flexion occurs at the joint at any time during the splinting phase, the 6 to 8 weeks of splinting should be restarted. Ensuring compliance with this treatment regiment is challenging but very important.

Follow-up within about 2 weeks is helpful to reinforce the importance of maintaining continuous extension and to inspect for skin problems. If skin problems are identified, more frequent follow-up is recommended.

If the 6 to 8 weeks of splinting is successful in restoring the majority of extension, the patient may be weaned from splinting. Splinting during sleep over the next 2 to 3 weeks is recommended. Splinting should be continued for higher risk activities including sporting activities for an additional 6 weeks. This intermittent splinting will help to avoid reinjury.

In the setting of late presentation for care, conservative treatment several weeks after the acute injury may be successful and should be pursued.

If a larger fracture is seen on x-rays, treatment is somewhat controversial due to concerns over the potential for loss of function and degenerative change. If the fracture involves more than 25 percent of the joint surface, one may wish to splint in full extension and obtain orthopaedic consultation. If there is persistent volar displacement of the distal fragment despite splinting, orthopaedic consultation should be pursued.

When to Refer

If conservative treatment is unsuccessful, the practitioner should first explore the possibility of inadequate compliance with the splinting regimen. If a history of inappropriate splinting is obtained, a repeat attempt at conservative treatment is reasonable. If the patient has been compliant and treatment has failed, orthopaedic consultation should be sought.

With the presence of a larger fracture, one should consider consultation. With epiphyseal fracture and dislocation in a child, orthopaedic consultation is recommended.

Return to Play

With appropriate splinting, players may often return to participation in sports during treatment. Playing while wearing a splint obviously increases the risk of reinjury, and this decision should be discussed with the patient.

Boutonnière Deformity of the Finger

Mechanism of Injury and Presentation

The classic boutonnière deformity of the finger is characterized as a flexion deformity at the PIP joint combined with an extension deformity at the DIP joint. Initially the lack of extension at the PIP joint may be the only finding. This injury is caused by either a severe flexing force to the PIP joint or a direct blow to the dorsum of the PIP joint. The injury involves the rupture of the central slip of the extensor mechanism at the insertion site at the base of the middle phalanx. Rupture of the central slip allows volar migration of the lateral bands of the more distal extensor mechanism. This volar migration causes the more distal portion of the extensor mechanism to function as a PIP flexor when finger extension is attempted. Attempted extension still causes extension at the DIP joint, and this may be exaggerated, causing the boutonnière deformity. Also, the remaining central slip, no longer attached to the middle phalanx, now acts as an extensor at the metacarpophalangeal joint, causing hyperextension at the MCP joint. Reviewing the complex anatomy of the finger extensor anatomy is necessary to understand this somewhat complex relationship (Fig. 11–18).

This injury may be easily confused with a "jammed finger" and inappropriately treated. Patients with this injury will often lack the terminal 15 to 30 degrees of extension. It is easy to incorrectly dismiss this finding as secondary to swelling from the acute injury. Swelling and pain at the PIP joint will be presenting symptoms.

Diagnosis and Imaging

This diagnosis is easy to miss. When pain and tenderness exist over the dorsum of the PIP joint along with a lack of extension, the diagnosis needs to be considered. In order to differentiate this disorder from less serious injuries, it is necessary to demonstrate true lack of extension. In order to eliminate the possibility of pain causing lack of extension, a digital block can be done. If the patient, with pain eliminated, still cannot fully extend the PIP joint, boutonnière injury should be assumed and appropriate treatment given.

Radiographs should be done to rule out fracture. Avulsion fracture at the attachment site of the extensor mechanism at the proximal portion of the middle phalanx may occur but is relatively rare. In the setting of a chronic boutonnière deformity an x-ray may show calcification in the area of the volar plate of the PIP joint. This is characteristic of the pseudo-boutonnière deformity, which usually follows hyperextension injury to the PIP joint, causing rupture of the volar plate and subsequent scarring and flexion contracture. The absence of associated MCP and DIP hyperextension is helpful in differentiating these disorders.

Treatment

Treatment of a boutonnière injury consists of immobilization of the PIP joint in full extension. This may be done using Orthoplast splinting or

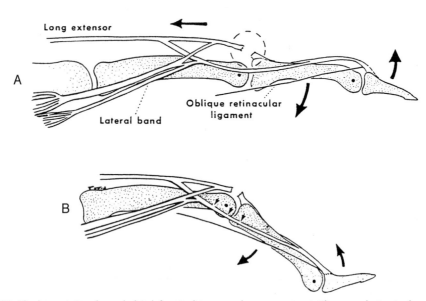

Figure 11–18. The boutonnière (buttonhole) deformity has several components. *A,* The acute lesion in the athlete involves the central slip (encircled). The proximal interphalangeal joint then drops into flexion and the extensor mechanism shifts proximally. *B,* The lateral bands then fall anterior to the axis of proximal interphalangeal joint motion *(small arrows).* If the extensor system heals in this position, the lateral bands and oblique retinacular ligaments will tether the proximal interphalangeal joint in flexion and the distal interphalangeal joint in extension. (From Burton RI, Eaton RG: Common hand injuries in the athlete. Orthop Clin North Am 4:809, 1973.)

Alumafoam splinting. With this treatment the proximal extensor mechanism has a chance to heal much as a mallet finger heals with splinting. This also helps to prevent permanent slippage of the lateral bands of the extensor mechanism in the volar direction, thus preventing the perpetuation of the boutonnière deformity. The DIP joint is allowed to have unrestricted motion, and active flexion is actually encouraged. Splinting should be recommended for 6 to 8 weeks continuously, with splinting for high-risk activities for an additional 2 to 6 weeks.

This treatment regimen is contrasted with that commonly used for "jammed" or sprained fingers. With this injury, splinting in flexion with subsequent "buddy taping" to an adjacent digit is often used. If the anatomy of the boutonnière deformity is understood, one can appreciate how this treatment actually prevents healing of the central slip and may lead to a permanent boutonnière deformity.

Correctly treated, this injury may not be associated with as much long-term deformity and disability. Unfortunately, with inappropriate treatment, permanent deformity is the norm. In the case of a more chronic presentation, one should recommend consultation with a hand therapist for a more complex treatment regimen involving dynamic splinting and exercises. Surgery for this deformity may follow failure of conservative treatment, and reported results are mixed.

When to Refer

In the setting of a large avulsion fracture of the proximal portion of the middle phalanx, orthopaedic consultation is recommended. If the practitioner is uncertain of the diagnosis, consultation is wise.

Return to Play

With appropriate splinting, most athletes may return to participation as tolerated.

SUGGESTED READINGS

Shoulder Injuries

Cox JS: The fate of the acromioclavicular joint in athletic injuries. Am J Sports Med 9(1):50–53, 1981.

Hawkins RJ, Kennedy JC: Impingement syndrome in athletes. Am J Sports Med 8(3):151–157, 1980.

Hawkins RJ, Mohtadi MG: Controversy in anterior shoulder instability. Clin Orthop 272:152–161, 1991.

Matsen FA, Harryman DT, Sidles JA: Mechanics of glenohumeral instability. Clin Sports Med 10(4):783–788, 1991.

Neer CS, Welsh RP: The shoulder in sports. Orthop Clin North Am 8(3):583–591, 1977.

Elbow Injuries

Ciccantelli P: Avoiding elbow pain (tips for young pitchers). Physician Sportsmed 22(3):65–66, 1994.

Congeni J: Treating and preventing little league elbow. Physician Sportsmed 22(3):54–64, 1994.

Davidson PA, Moseley JB, Tullos HS: Radial head fracture. Clin Orthop Related Res 297:224–230, 1993.

Nirschl RP, Kraushaar BS: Assessment and treatment guidelines for elbow injuries. Physician Sportsmed 24(5):43–60, 1996.

Nirschl RP, Kraushaar BS: Keeping tennis elbow at arm's length (simple, effective strengthening exercises). Physician Sportsmed 24(5):61–62, 1996.

Plancher KD, Halbrecht J, Lourie GM: Medial and lateral epicondylitis in the athlete. Clin Sports Med 15(2):283–305, 1996.

Wrist and Hand Injuries

Amadio PC: Scaphoid fractures. Orthop Clin North Am 23(1) January, 1992.

Burton RI, Eaton RG: Common hand injuries in the athlete. Orthop Clin North Am 4(3):809–837, 1973.

Culver JE: Injuries of the hand and wrist. Clin Sports Med 11(1) January, 1992. (The entire volume is an excellent reference.)

Landsman JC, et al: Splint immobilization of gamekeeper's thumb. Orthopedics 18(12):1161–1165, 1995.

Mastey RD, Weiss AC, Akelman E: Primary care of hand and wrist athletic injuries. Clin Sports Med 16(4):705–723, 1997.

Chapter *12* | Injuries to the Lower Extremity

JIM MACINTYRE, M.D., M.P.E., FACSM
AND STEPHEN M. SIMONS, M.D., FACSM

This chapter deals with a variety of injuries to the hip, pelvis, and lower extremity. It is not intended to be an exhaustive review of all possible injuries to these areas, but merely an overview of common and clinically important problems that might be encountered by a primary care practitioner. The chapter outlines the mechanisms of injury, pertinent history and physical findings, and appropriate use of imaging for assessment and diagnosis. The therapeutic options and usual recovery course are discussed, along with guidelines for return to practice and competition. Injuries are divided into two types: (1) acute traumatic injuries and (2) overuse injuries due to repetitive microtrauma.

ACUTE INJURIES

Acute injuries are associated with single episodes of macrotrauma to the bones or soft tissues. These injuries include ligamentous sprains, muscular strains, and bony fractures. It is important to remember that a fracture includes a soft tissue injury associated with the broken bone. The general principles of soft tissue treatment and rehabilitation will still apply once the bone has healed.

Treatment of acute injuries involves the PRICE principle: *p*rotection from further injury, *r*est, *i*ce, *c*ompression, and *e*levation (detailed in Chapter 6). The athlete's fitness should be maintained during recovery through alternative exercise that does not affect the injured area.

Quadriceps Contusions

Definition

Quadriceps contusions occur most commonly in contact sports such as soccer, football, and hockey.

A direct blow to the anterior thigh compresses muscle against the femur, usually injuring the deepest muscle. Hematoma formation and inflammation characterize the initial pathology, which may progress to be replaced by dense connective tissue.[1] The sport-related incidence of quadriceps contusions is unknown, although these contusions were responsible for 1.4 percent of injuries among military recruits.[2]

Signs and Symptoms

Athletes present with pain and swelling following direct trauma to the thigh. Grading of contusion severity is based on the range of passive knee flexion with the athlete lying prone: over 90 degrees is considered mild; 45 to 90 degrees is moderate; and less than 45 degrees is severe. Grading these injuries assists with management decisions, predicting the period of disability, and alerting the physician to possible complications.[3] Diagnostic imaging is generally not helpful initially. Consideration of other conditions including muscle rupture and acute compartment syndrome is important if the muscle girth does not stabilize in 48 hours.

Treatment

Early treatment emphasizes controlling bleeding, reducing swelling, and managing pain. The thigh should be iced frequently, and heat is avoided, as it may provoke increased bleeding. Follow the PRICE principles. The West Point study[4] showed that the use of crutches and non–weight-bearing immobilization of the thigh are much more effective than previously recommended protocols.[3] The knee is immobilized in a position of maximally

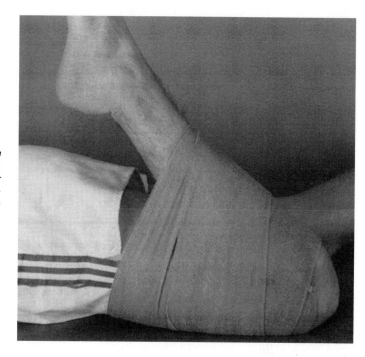

Figure 12–1. Method of maintaining knee flexion with circumferential elastic wrap. (From Garrick JG, Webb DR: Sports Injuries: Diagnosis and Management, 2nd ed. Philadelphia, W. B. Saunders, 1999, p. 255.)

tolerated flexion using double 6-inch Ace bandages for 24 to 48 hours (Fig. 12–1). This wrap provides compression, tamponades bleeding, and maintains range of motion. Early rehabilitation involves gentle passive pain-free motion emphasizing flexion as well as stationary cycling with low resistance to shorten disability time and reduce the risk of myositis ossificans.[4]

The most significant complication of quadriceps contusions is the development of myositis ossificans, which occurred in 9 percent of the cadets in the West Point study. Factors that increased the risk of developing myositis ossificans included poor initial range of motion, injury in football, treatment delay of longer than 72 hours, and ipsilateral knee effusion. Heterotopic bone can become radiographically evident in 2 to 4 weeks. Myositis ossificans is treated conservatively with pain control and range of motion exercises. Surgical intervention should be considered only after the heterotopic bone matures.[2]

Return to Activity

Disability time and return to participation in the sport following quadriceps contusions varies by injury severity. The West Point Cadet study showed average disability of 13 days for mild contusions, 19 days for moderate, and 21 days for severe contusions. Returning to activity too quickly may predispose to reinjury and increases

the risk of myositis ossificans, especially if repeat trauma occurs.

When to Refer

The primary care provider can usually manage quadriceps contusions. If pain and thigh girth progressively increase, or the patient develops paresthesias over the anterior aspect of the knee and the medial calf, referral should be made to rule out acute compartment syndrome.

Key Points

- Direct blow to the anterior thigh can lead to contusion.
- Initial management with PRICE, and immobilization in knee flexion.
- Gentle passive range of motion should begin early.
- Observe for myositis ossificans.
- Consider acute compartment syndrome if pain and quadriceps girth increase and paresthesia develops.

REFERENCES

1. Best TM: Muscle-tendon injuries in young athletes. Clin Sports Med 14(3):669–686, 1995.

2. Best TM: Soft-tissue injuries and muscle tears. Clin Sports Med 16(3):419–434, 1997.
3. Jackson DW, Feagin JA: Quadriceps contusions in young athletes. Relation of severity of injury to treatment and prognosis. J Bone Surg A 55(1):95–105, 1973.
4. Ryan JB, Wheeler JH, Hopkinson WJ, et al: Quadriceps contusions. West Point update. Am J Sports Med 19(3):299–304, 1991.

Acute Knee Ligament Injuries

The ability to diagnose and treat knee ligament injuries requires an accurate history of the mechanism of the injury as well as a careful physical examination. An understanding of the ligamentous restraints of the knee will assist in determining which structures may have been injured. Any blow to the knee will cause tension on one side of the knee and compression forces on the other. Ligaments are particularly vulnerable to the combination of rotational and tension forces. Menisci and articular cartilage are injured by compression forces combined with twisting or shearing forces. Initially patients may be unable to describe the exact mechanism of the injury; however, carefully determining the foot position (internal versus an external rotation), leg position, and the direction of the force may allow the patient to recreate the injury. Additional important factors include the sensation of a pop or snap at the time of the injury. This feature is common in anterior cruciate ligament tears, and less common in other ligamentous injuries. The patient should be questioned as to whether any movement occurred; the caregiver should attempt to differentiate whether that movement was the patella moving out of place or the whole lower leg moving upon the upper leg. This determination will assist in distinguishing ligamentous injuries from patellar dislocations. Also, if the patient was able to continue the activity after the injury, a serious ligamentous injury is less likely.

Information regarding the timing of the onset, location, and extent of swelling is crucial. Immediate tense hemarthrosis results from arterial bleeding, indicating a probable bony injury such as osteochondral fractures or patellar dislocations. Swelling that occurs over the first 6 to 12 hours after an injury is probably also bleeding, often from a tear of the anterior or posterior cruciate ligament. Swelling that accumulates over 24 to 48 hours is more commonly associated with meniscal injuries. It is important to determine the location of the swelling and differentiate local medial swelling associated with medial collateral ligament injury from intra-articular swelling from an effusion or hemarthrosis.

Other associated symptoms following the injury must also be noted. It is important to document the presence of any locking, keeping in mind that the patient's idea of "locking" may be different from the examiner's. True locking is the intermittent or continued inability to fully extend the knee, either actively or passively. True locking will often release with a click after the patient flexes and twists the knee. Other mechanical symptoms that are important include a sense of deep intra-articular catching or a sense of something loose within the knee. True locking contrasts with "pseudolocking," which is often associated with patellofemoral pain. Pseudolocking is a muscular inhibition whereby the patient is unable to actively extend the knee due to pain. This gradually resolves over a few minutes with the patient regaining full motion. The patient will usually indicate that someone else would have been able to passively extend the knee during this time.

Buckling is a sudden giving way of the knee due to pain inhibition. Buckling has many causes, and it is important to differentiate buckling from true knee instability. In true instability, the patient will feel a sense of movement of the lower leg upon the upper leg, or the patella out of the femoral sulcus. Ligamentous injury or patellar dislocation can result in feelings of instability. Ideally, a detailed history will allow the clinician to arrive at a provisional diagnosis with a high degree of certainty before examining the patient. This assessment is especially important in patients with significant guarding and pain because they may be very difficult to examine. The physical findings can then be used to confirm the diagnosis.

Key Point

A precise history of the mechanism of injury coupled with an understanding of the anatomy and biomechanics of the knee and followed by a detailed examination will allow the clinician to reach an accurate diagnosis of knee ligament injuries.

Anterior Cruciate Ligament Injury

Definition

The anterior cruciate ligament (ACL) is an intra-articular structure joining the tibia to the femur. It is the primary restraint for anterior translation of the tibia on the femur as well as for rotational movements. It is a secondary restraint for varus and valgus stress, and can be injured alone or in combination with other ligamentous structures, depending on the knee position and the magnitude and direction of the injuring force. Because of its location within the joint, the ACL will not heal on its own, and treatment may require surgical reconstruction in many athletes.

ACL injuries are common in a wide variety of contact and noncontact sports. Contact injuries usually occur from a direct blow to the knee while the foot is planted, creating a varus or valgus force on the knee, with ACL injury occurring in conjunction with other ligamentous injuries. The ACL may also be injured with hyperextension.

Most injuries to the ACL are noncontact in origin, usually due to a valgus, deceleration, or external rotation injury with attempts to cut or pivot on a planted foot. This injury has reached epidemic proportions in women's competitive basketball and soccer.[1] The exact reasons why female athletes are at particularly high risk for cruciate injuries are not clear, but a number of theories have been proposed. These theories include smaller ligament size, a narrowed intercondylar notch, inadequate strength, ligamentous hyperlaxity, defects of neuromuscular coordination, and hormonally induced laxity during certain phases of the menstrual cycle. All these theories should be considered conjecture at present, because ACL injuries appear to be multifactorial in nature.[1]

Signs and Symptoms

Knee pain, swelling, and instability are the common complaints of athletes with ACL injuries. They frequently will state that they felt a pop or snap within the knee and may report that they felt the lower leg move on the upper leg. They are usually unable to continue with the activity. Swelling is usually prominent and appears within 6 to 12 hours of injury. Immediate swelling should alert the examiner to the possibility of a bony injury, especially in the older athlete who may be at higher risk of osteoporotic fractures of the tibial plateau. ACL injuries are frequently misdiagnosed by the first examining physician. This problem could be prevented by having a high index of suspicion for ACL injury in athletes with this injury mechanism and clinical history. It is inappropriate to tell injured athletes with a large knee

effusion that they have "sprained the knee" and that they should rest and then return to sports when the swelling and pain are gone. If untreated, the swelling will decrease over the next 1 to 2 weeks and the patient may feel a false sense of security with the knee. Any attempt to return to cutting, pivoting, or deceleration sports will cause a recurrence of instability with pain and repeated hemarthrosis. Repeated giving way episodes result in further stretching of the secondary restraints, as well as injury to the menisci and articular cartilage. On a more chronic basis, the athlete will complain about symptomatic giving way of the knee with cutting and pivoting activities, often referred to as a "trick knee."

An intra-articular effusion is common following an ACL injury. Range of motion is often restricted. The Lachman test is the primary diagnostic indicator of an ACL injury, and should be compared with the uninjured knee. It consists of the loss of a firm end point to the anterior translation of the tibia on the femur at 30 degrees of flexion. Anteroposterior (AP) translation is usually increased. The more traditional drawer test of anterior and posterior translation performed with the knee at 80 to 90 degrees of flexion is less sensitive for the ACL injury and is a better position to assess the end point feel of the posterior cruciate ligament. The pivot shift maneuver recreates the anterior subluxation of the tibia on the femur and is pathognomonic for ACL injury. It is performed by placing an axial load and valgus stress on the knee and then taking the knee from an extended to a flexed position. In the fully extended position the tibia is subluxated anteriorly on the femur, and as the knee is flexed, the pull from the iliotibial band causes the tibia to reduce under the femoral condyles. The sudden shift that occurs with reduction is visible and palpable. The pivot shift is generally not performed in the acute situation because it may be extremely uncomfortable for the patient. It is more useful in the chronic situation to document rotational instability. Joint line tenderness following ACL injury may indicate a concomitant meniscal injury. This finding is a more reliable predictor of meniscal injury in the chronic situation than with an acute injury.

Adjunctive tests include the use of the KT1000 arthrometer, which gives a reliable and objective measurement of the degree of AP translation of the tibia on the femur. A side-to-side difference of greater than 4 mm is highly suggestive of ACL injury.

Imaging

Radiographs are often normal but may show avulsion of the tibial spine, especially in younger patients. Capsular avulsion fractures from the lateral tibial plateau (Segond fractures) are virtually pathognomonic of ACL injury, although their significance is unfortunately often ignored. Magnetic resonance (MR) imaging should not be routinely used to diagnose ACL injury, as a careful history and clinical examination have been shown to be equivalent or superior in diagnostic accuracy.[2, 3] MR imaging is generally not indicated if ACL reconstruction surgery has been planned based on a clinical diagnosis. The information confirmed by the study will be immediately apparent upon initial arthroscopic evaluation and does not justify the cost of the test.

Treatment

Treatment of ACL injuries can be either nonoperative or operative, with the choice depending on a number of factors, including the habitual demands on the knee, the associated damage to other structures, and the desire and willingness of the patient to undertake surgical treatment with its attendant prolonged rehabilitation.[4, 5] The activity level is the prime consideration for surgical reconstruction, which is recommended in highly active individuals who regularly participate in cutting and pivoting sports. Age was once considered to be a prime factor, but with better surgical treatment and rehabilitation, age is less of a consideration. Adolescents with open physes should be considered for reconstruction, because the long-term outlook for the knee of an ACL-deficient teenager is poor.[6, 7] Gender is considered to be a relatively unimportant factor, although women were once thought to be less likely surgical candidates. Associated injuries are a prime factor; athletes with grade 3 injuries to the collateral ligaments or posterior corners frequently require surgery.

The natural history of an untreated ACL injury is variable[8, 9] and depends to a large extent on the damage to other structures at the time of the injury. Isolated injuries are thought to have a much more benign course than those with significant associated trauma to the secondary restraints, articular cartilage, and menisci. Individuals with repeated pivoting episodes will be much more prone to meniscal and articular cartilage deterioration and progressive arthritis. Individuals who are prepared to modify their lifestyle to avoid cutting, pivoting, and jumping will generally have a better outcome than those who continue to participate in high-risk sports.[9, 10]

Reconstruction has been shown to improve stability and allow a higher activity level as well as to reduce the incidence of meniscal tears. Long-term studies have failed to show that ACL reconstruction results in a significant reduction in arthritis,[8] although the studies have some methodological problems. It should be stressed to these patients that surgical treatment does not provide a new knee and that, regardless of treatment, they will have a higher risk of problems with their knee in the future because of the trauma that occurred at the time of the injury.[5]

Surgical treatment requires the reconstruction of the ligament, as primary ACL repairs have a high rate of failure. Reconstruction is usually performed arthroscopically using either the hamstrings or the central third of the patellar tendon. Allografts and artificial ligaments such as Gore-Tex or Dacron have a limited place at present because of an unacceptably high rate of failure. ACL reconstruction is not an emergency and is best carried out after the swelling has dissipated and the knee has regained its range of motion. The decision to proceed with surgical or nonsurgical treatment is best made in conjunction with a consulting surgeon who has significant experience in dealing with this type of injury.

Nonoperative treatment is appropriate for "low-demand" patients who are prepared to modify their lifestyle to avoid cutting, pivoting, and jumping sports.[9] Early bracing can be helpful to prevent episodes of buckling and giving way that some patients experience. Local physical therapy modalities reduce swelling and regain range of motion. Strengthening is essential with specific emphasis on the hamstrings. Balance, proprioception, and functional retraining are essential prior to any return to activity. Bracing is controversial, and there is no consensus about its utility.[10–12] Individuals who do not have surgery and wish to return to sports requiring cutting, pivoting, and change of direction should probably be fitted with a functional derotational brace to minimize recurrent episodes of giving way, although it is clear that no brace can protect the knee under all circumstances.[11, 12] Return to practice and competition should be allowed when the athlete has full range of motion and good strength, and has demonstrated adequate balance and proprioception to complete a progressive functional activity test. Many individuals do quite well through a combination of appropriate rehabilitation, activity modification, and the use of functional bracing.

When to Refer

Athletes with ACL injuries should generally be referred to an orthopedic surgeon with considerable experience in their treatment. Reconstruction is a technically demanding procedure and is best left to surgeons with subspecialty training in sports medicine.

Key Points

- Have a high index of suspicion for ACL injury with a twisting injury associated with a pop, a sense of movement, early swelling, and a sense of instability.
- Examination will reveal increased AP translation with a soft anterior end point.
- Failure to diagnose an ACL injury can lead to permanent disability if the athlete is allowed to return to participation and suffers further injury.
- Treatment is individualized with the assistance of an experienced surgeon.

REFERENCES

1. Arendt E, Dick R: Knee injury patterns among men and women in intercollegiate basketball and soccer: NCAA data and review of literature. Am J Sports Med 23:694–701, 1995.
2. Rose NT, Gold SM: A comparison of accuracy between clinical examination and magnetic resonance imaging in the diagnosis of meniscal and anterior cruciate ligament tears. Arthroscopy 12:398–405, 1996.
3. Liu SH, Osti L, Henry M, et al: The diagnosis of acute complete tears of the anterior cruciate ligament: Comparison of MRI, arthrometry and clinical examination. J Bone Joint Surg B 77:586–588, 1995.
4. Johnson RJ, Beynnon BD, Nichols CE, et al: Current concepts review: The treatment of injuries to the anterior cruciate ligament. J Bone Joint Surg A 74:140–151, 1992.
5. Frank CB, Jackson DW: The science of reconstruction of the anterior cruciate ligament. J Bone Joint Surg A 79:1556–1576, 1997.
6. Lo IKY, Kirkley A, Fowler PJ, et al: The outcome of operatively treated anterior cruciate ligament disruptions in the skeletally immature child. Arthroscopy 13:627–634, 1997.
7. McCarroll JR, Shelbourne KD, Patel DV: Anterior cruciate ligament injuries in young athletes: Recommendations for treatment and rehabilitation. Sports Med 20:117–127, 1995.
8. Daniel DM, Stone ML, Dobson BE, et al: Fate of the ACL injured patient: A prospective outcome study. Am J Sports Med 22:632–644, 1994.
9. Buss DD, Min R, Skyhar M, et al: Nonoperative treatment of acute anterior cruciate ligament injuries in a selected group of patients. Am J Sports Med 23:160–165, 1995.
10. Shelton WR, Barrett GR, Dukes A: Early season anterior cruciate ligament tears: A treatment dilemma. Am J Sports Med 25:656–658, 1997.
11. Liu SH, Mirzayan R: Functional knee bracing. Clin Orthop 317:273–281, 1995.
12. Wojtys EM, Kothari SU, Huston LJ: Anterior cruciate ligament functional brace use in sports. Am J Sports Med 24:539–546, 1996.

Posterior Cruciate Ligament Injuries

Definition

The posterior cruciate ligament (PCL) is an intra-articular structure joining the tibia to the femur. It is the primary restraint for posterior translation of the tibia on the femur and provides secondary support for rotational movements in conjunction with the supports of the posterolateral corner: the lateral collateral ligament, popliteus tendon, and arcuate ligament complex.

Isolated PCL injuries result from a hyperflexion injury or a posteriorly directed force on a flexed knee. This injury can occur when athletes fall on a flexed knee while the foot is plantar flexed. The PCL is commonly injured in a motor vehicle accident when an unrestrained passenger strikes the tibial tubercle on the dashboard, driving the tibia posteriorly. The PCL can also be injured in conjunction with other ligaments during forced hyperextension or varus or valgus stress after the collateral ligaments fail.

Signs and Symptoms

When the PCL is acutely injured, a hemarthrosis usually develops within 6 to 12 hours. The patient usually complains of pain and swelling. Instability is a less common complaint unless there is concomitant injury to other ligaments. There may be associated soft tissue trauma to the anterior tibia. Athletes with a history suggestive of PCL injury should undergo a careful examination to exclude this possibility.

The hallmark of PCL injury is posterior subluxation of the tibia on the femur. The posterior drawer test is performed with the knee flexed to 90 degrees and demonstrates increased posterior translation of the tibia on the femur with a soft end point when compared with the uninjured side. Posterior sag of the tibia can be detected in several ways. With the knee flexed to 70 to 80 degrees, the examiner's thumbs are moved distally on the femoral condyles and onto the tibial condyles, which will feel less prominent than those on the uninjured side. If the hips and knees are flexed to 90 degrees with the heels supported, posterior sag of the tibia can be demonstrated by comparing the levels of the tibial tubercles.

The quadriceps active drawer test is performed with the patient lying supine with the knee flexed to 70 to 80 degrees and the foot on the examining table. The examiner stabilizes the foot on the table and asks the patient to attempt to slide the foot down the table by contracting the quadriceps. The examiner watches the position and movement of the tibia from the side as the quadriceps are contracted. If the PCL is torn, the tibia will move anteriorly with quadriceps contraction. Sensitivity may be increased by having the patient contract the hamstrings and pull the heel proximally to ensure a neutral position before the active quadriceps contraction is undertaken.

With isolated PCL injury, there is no increased lateral opening on varus stress at 30 degrees. Opening indicates that the posterior lateral corner is also injured. If both the PCL and posterior lateral corner are injured, external rotation of the tibia on the femur will be increased when examined with the knee and hips flexed to 90 degrees.

Adjunctive tests include the use of the KT1000 arthrometer, which gives a reliable and objective measurement of the degree of AP translation of the tibia on the femur. Correction factors to separate anterior from posterior translation are applied to assist in diagnosing a PCL injury.

Imaging

Plain radiographs are frequently normal. Lateral radiographs may reveal subtle posterior subluxation of the tibia on the femur or a bony avulsion fragment of the PCL origin from the posterior aspect of the tibial plateau. Merchant views in chronic cases may demonstrate patellofemoral arthrosis. MR imaging reliably demonstrates PCL injury and can also show damage to other ligamentous structures and the menisci.

Treatment

The natural history of a chronic PCL injury is not well understood and is still debated, because many

remain undiagnosed. Many athletes with isolated injury return to full activity in the short term.[1, 2] It is thought that isolated PCL injuries can do well treated nonoperatively, although many patients go on to have chronic pain, especially with activity.[3–5] Many patients develop patellofemoral pain due to increased joint reactive forces resulting from posterior sag of the tibia. Current surgical techniques are unable to restore total knee stability. Thus, surgery is indicated only in patients with a significant posterior sag (over 10 to 15 mm), those with combined ligamentous instabilities, and those patients in whom there is a large avulsion fragment that is suitable for open reduction and internal fixation.[5, 6] Nonoperative treatment is symptomatic initially, with rehabilitation emphasizing quadriceps function. Patients with chronic, symptomatic posterior instability should be considered for reconstruction if rehabilitation fails.[6]

Return to Activity

Return to participation is allowed when the patient has recovered range of motion, strength, and balance and proprioception.

When to Refer

Athletes with PCL injuries should generally be referred to an orthopedic surgeon. The decision to proceed with surgical or nonsurgical treatment is best made in conjunction with a consulting surgeon who has significant experience in treating PCL injuries. Reconstruction is a technically demanding procedure and is best left to surgeons with subspecialty training in sports medicine.

Key Points

- PCL injury results from a fall on a hyperflexed knee or a direct blow to the tibial tubercle.
- Physical findings include significant local soft tissue trauma, hemarthrosis, and increased posterior translation of the tibia on the femur associated with posterior sag.
- Treatment is generally nonoperative unless there are combined ligamentous instabilities.

REFERENCES

1. Parolie JM, Bergfeld JA: Long term results of nonoperative treatment of isolated posterior cruciate ligament injuries in the athlete. Am J Sports Med 14:35–38, 1986.
2. Fowler PJ, Messieh SS: Isolated posterior cruciate ligament injuries in athletes. Am J Sports Med 15:553–557, 1987.
3. Keller PM, Shelbourne KD, McCarroll JR, et al: Nonoperatively treated isolated posterior cruciate ligament injury. Am J Sports Med 21:132–136, 1993.
4. Dejour H, Walch G, Peyrot J, et al: The natural history of rupture of the posterior cruciate ligament. Rev Chir Orthop Reparatrice Appar Mot 2:112–120, 1988.
5. Fanelli GC, Giannotti BF, Edson CJ: Current concepts review: The posterior cruciate ligament arthroscopic evaluation and treatment. Arthroscopy 10:673–688, 1994.
6. Veltri DM, Warren RF: Isolated and combined posterior cruciate ligament injuries. J Am Acad Orthop Surg 1:67–75, 1993.

Meniscal Injuries

Definition

The menisci are semilunar wedges of fibrocartilage situated in the tibiofemoral joint. They provide joint stability, load transmission, shock absorption, joint lubrication and nutrition, and proprioception. Menisectomy leads to joint space narrowing, flattening of the articular surface, and osteophyte formation due to increased local contact pressure.

Mechanism of Injury

Menisci are injured by compressive loads, often accompanied by twisting or shearing forces. They are frequently torn in acute ACL injuries and are vulnerable in pivoting episodes in the chronic ACL-deficient knee. With age, they degenerate and become more friable and are vulnerable to injury with lesser trauma. There are a number of tear patterns, including longitudinal, radial, flap, and horizontal cleavage tears.

Signs and Symptoms

The main complaints are pain, swelling, and mechanical symptoms.[1] These symptoms may vary with time, and intervals relatively free of symptoms may occur. The pain is frequently localized on the medial or lateral joint line, and is aggravated by flexion and squatting. Swelling will usually accumulate over the 24 hours following an acute injury, with chronic injuries often associated with small effusions. Chronic lateral meniscal tears may go on to develop cysts along the joint line. Locking may occur with an acute injury. The immediate loss of extension following the injury suggests a meniscal tear, whereas effusion and muscle spasm result in the gradual loss of extension in the hours following the injury. Chronic meniscal injuries may present with repeated episodes of deep catching and locking.

Ligamentous stability should always be assessed in both acute and chronic tears. Quadriceps atrophy is common in chronic tears. The squat test is a good indicator of a meniscal tear. In a deep squat the patient will experience point pain localized to the joint line. Pain while descending or arising from the squat is more suggestive of patellofemoral problems. Pain on knee hyperflexion and localized joint line tenderness and fullness are also specific findings. McMurray's test can be a useful adjunct, but it has been shown to be relatively nonspecific.[2] It is performed with the patient supine and relaxed, with the hip flexed. To test the medial meniscus, the knee is fully flexed and externally rotated with a slight varus load applied as the knee is gradually extended. The lateral meniscus is tested with internal rotation and valgus stress. A positive test consists of pain and a palpable pop or click localized to the specific joint line. This test can be nonspecific, and can cause pain in other conditions, but an associated click improves its sensitivity.

Imaging

Plain radiographs are frequently normal in the acute injury but may show some soft tissue prominence localized to the joint line. Chronic tears can lead to degenerative changes, including joint space narrowing, spurring, subchondral cysts, and sclerosis. MRI can be useful for diagnosis, but there can be false-positive age-related changes, and occasional false-negative findings, especially with the posterior horn of the lateral meniscus. Several studies have shown no advantage of the routine use of MRI if clinical findings support the diagnosis of meniscal injury.[3, 4] Arthrograms are sensitive, but less commonly used with the wide availability of MRI.

Treatment

The initial management of meniscal tears is often conservative, including PRICE principles, nonsteroidal anti-inflammatory drugs (NSAIDs), and physical therapy.[1] The indications for surgery are chronic swelling, pain, or mechanical symptoms. Meniscal repair can be successful, especially in younger patients, or in conjunction with ACL reconstruction. If repair is not possible, partial meniscectomy is performed. Many reports indicate an increased risk of arthritis following meniscectomy with the risk thought to be increased in proportion to the amount of meniscus removed.[5, 6] Other studies, however, have demonstrated a somewhat better prognosis.[7] Newer treatments such as meniscal transplants or collagen meniscal implants are being evaluated for their potential in reducing future arthritis.

Return to Activity

Return to competition will depend on the extent of the meniscectomy and a return to full motion, strength, and completion of a functional agility program.

When to Refer

Referral is generally indicated after the failure of conservative treatment, if the knee is locked following an acute injury, or if a lateral meniscal cyst is present.

Key Points

- Meniscal injuries result from compression and shearing forces.
- Complaints are pain, swelling, mechanical symptoms, and locking.
- Physical findings include joint line pain in a deep squat, pain on hyperflexion, focal joint line tenderness and swelling, and a positive McMurray's test.
- Treatment is initially symptomatic in the absence of mechanical symptoms, with arthroscopic treatment for locking, cysts, or failed conservative therapy.

REFERENCES

1. Newman AP, Daniels AU, Burks RT: Principles and decision making in meniscal surgery. Arthroscopy 9:33–51, 1993.
2. Evans PJ, Bell GD, Frank C: Prospective evaluation of the McMurray test. Am J Sports Med 21:604–608, 1993.
3. Rose NT, Gold SM: A comparison of accuracy between clinical examination and magnetic resonance imaging in the diagnosis of meniscal and anterior cruciate ligament tears. Arthroscopy 12:398–405, 1996.
4. Miller GK: A prospective study comparing the accuracy of the clinical diagnosis of meniscus tear with magnetic resonance imaging and its effect on clinical outcome. Arthroscopy 12:406–413, 1996.
5. Rangger C, Klestil T, Gloetzer W, et al: Osteoarthritis after arthroscopic partial meniscectomy. Am J Sports Med 23:240–244, 1995.
6. Jaureguito JW, Elliot JS, Lietner J, et al: The effects of arthroscopic partial lateral meniscectomy in the otherwise normal knee: A retrospective review of functional clinical and radiographic results. Arthroscopy 11:29–36, 1995.
7. Burks RT, Metcalf MH, Metcalf RW: Fifteen year follow-up of arthroscopic partial meniscectomy. Arthroscopy 13:673–679, 1997.

Achilles Tendon Rupture

Definition

Achilles tendon rupture occurs most often in the middle-aged athlete participating in basketball, racquet sports, soccer, and other sports with explosive movement. Rupture occurs when there is rapid eccentric loading from abrupt deceleration such as landing from a rebound or changing directions. The average age of patients with rupture is 37.9 years.[1] The incidence of Achilles tendon rupture is increasing, probably due to more athletic exposure in middle-aged males. The male-to-female ratio for injury averages 5:1, probably reflecting greater participation in such sports by men.[2, 3] The left Achilles tendon is ruptured more often than the right, as right-side-dominant people will more often push off the left foot.[4] Corticosteroids either directly injected or taken orally have been implicated to predispose the Achilles tendon to rupture.[5] There is also concern that fluoroquinolones may cause collagen degradation and Achilles tendon rupture.[6]

Signs and Symptoms

The patient sustaining an Achilles tendon rupture experiences a sudden "pop" to the Achilles tendon and often describes this sensation as being struck from behind with a direct blow to the lower leg. There may be only modest pain, usually in the heel or ankle. With the onset of edema the patient is often unable to ambulate or bear weight. The diagnosis is initially missed in 25 percent of injuries,[7] often because the patient is still able to plantarflex the foot fairly forcibly by using the muscles of the posterior compartment. The patient, however, is almost always unable to do a one-legged toe raise on the affected side.

Local examination reveals a palpable defect over the tendon, although this may be difficult to detect if there is significant swelling (Fig. 12–2). The defect is usually 3 to 4 cm proximal to its insertion but may occur anywhere in the tendon, or at the muscle-tendon junction. The Thompson test is also helpful, with comparison of the injured leg to the normal, contralateral calf. The test is performed with the patient prone or kneeling on a chair. The examiner squeezes the midportion of the gastrocnemius and observes the resultant foot motion, with the normal response being plantarflexion of the foot. If the tendon is ruptured, passive plantarflexion does not occur.

Imaging

Clinical examination is usually sufficient to diagnose an acutely ruptured tendon. Subacute or chronic ruptures may be more difficult. Although MR imaging closely correlates with surgical findings, it is probably not necessary in most cases.[8, 9] Ultrasound examination of the Achilles tendon is also used to assess tendon integrity and as follow-up to surgery.[10, 11]

Treatment

Treatment of Achilles tendon rupture is somewhat controversial and must be individualized, depending on the patient's circumstances and expectations. Nonsurgical care involves immobilization wearing a non–weight-bearing cast with the foot in maximum plantarflexion for 4 weeks, intermediate plantarflexion for 4 weeks, followed by the use of a heel lift while out of the cast. For surgical treatment, a number of operative repair techniques can be used, with the subsequent rehabilitation protocol determined by the type of repair. In most cases casting is required for 4 to 6 weeks, although

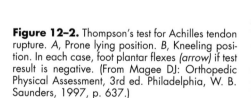

Figure 12–2. Thompson's test for Achilles tendon rupture. *A*, Prone lying position. *B*, Kneeling position. In each case, foot plantar flexes *(arrow)* if test result is negative. (From Magee DJ: Orthopedic Physical Assessment, 3rd ed. Philadelphia, W. B. Saunders, 1997, p. 637.)

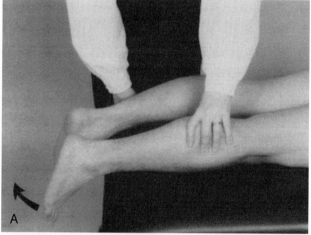

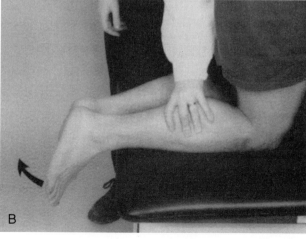

some are now allowing unprotected ambulation and a more aggressive return to activity.[12–14]

Crucial issues in the decision to proceed with surgical versus nonsurgical management include the patient's desire to return to high-level sport, potential surgical complications, and the risk of re-rupture. With conservative treatment, the tendon may heal with some elongation, leading to a loss of power for push-off and vertical jump. The advantages of nonsurgical management are lack of wound and surgical complications, less discomfort, and decreased cost, which may be a vital factor in individuals with no insurance. The disadvantages include a higher re-rupture rate and greater patient dissatisfaction because of a loss of power, strength, and endurance. The two main advantages of primary surgical repair include lower re-rupture rate and better strength and power, essential factors for athletes. Disadvantages of surgery include the costs and the possible complications, including wound problems, deep venous thrombosis, and pulmonary embolism.[12, 13]

When to Refer

Patients should be referred for consultation if there is some doubt as to the diagnosis. All athletes and most "high-demand" individuals with Achilles tendon ruptures should be referred for surgical consultation. Some fully informed patients will choose conservative management when presented with the pros and cons of both management options. Others will be unsuitable for surgical management. These groups can be managed by physicians who are comfortable and experienced in treating this problem.

Key Points

- The patient feels a sudden pop to the back of the ankle following a sudden push-off or load.
- Patients are generally unable to do a toe raise on the affected side but may have fairly good strength on resisted plantarflexion.
- Palpable defects in the tendon are common.
- The Thompson test is the principal examination procedure to diagnose acute rupture.

- Diagnostic testing with MR imaging or ultrasound may be helpful in a few cases.
- Surgical treatment is recommended for athletes to avoid loss of strength and power.

REFERENCES

1. Lo IKY, Kirkley A, Nonweiler B, Kumbhare DA: Operative versus nonoperative treatment of acute Achilles tendon ruptures: A quantitative review. Clin J Sports Med 7(3):207–211, 1997.
2. Moller A, Astrom M, Westlin NE: Increasing incidence of Achilles tendon rupture. Acta Orthop Scand 67(5):479–481, 1996.
3. Leppilahti J, Puranen J, Orava S: Incidence of Achilles tendon rupture. Acta Orthop Scand 67(3):277–279, 1996.
4. Stein SR, Luekens CA: Closed treatment of Achilles tendon ruptures. Orthop Clin North Am 7:241–246, 1976.
5. Waterston SW, Maffulli N, Ewen SWB: Subcutaneous rupture of the Achilles tendon: Basic science and some aspects of clinical practice. Br J Sports Med 31:285–298, 1997.
6. Royer RJ, Pierfitte C, Netter P: Features of tendon disorders with fluoroquinolones. Therapie 49:75–76, 1994.
7. Inglis AE, Scott WN, Sculco TP, Patterson AH: Ruptures of the tendo Achilles. J Bone Joint Surg A 58:990–993, 1976.
8. Marcus DS, Reicher MA, Kellerhouse LE: Achilles tendon injuries: The role of MR imaging. J Comput Assist Tomogr 13(3):480–486, 1989.
9. Keene JS, Lash EG, Fisher DR, DeSmet AA: Magnetic resonance imaging of Achilles tendon ruptures. Am J Sports Med 17:333–337, 1989.
10. Kalebo P, Allenmark C, Peterson L, Sward L: Diagnostic value of ultrasonography in partial ruptures of the Achilles tendon. Am J Sports Med 20(4):378–381, 1992.
11. Maffulli N, Dymond NP, Regine R: Surgical repair of ruptured Achilles tendon in sportsmen and sedentary patients: A longitudinal ultrasound assessment. Int J Sports Med 11:78–84, 1990.
12. Lo IKY, Kirkley A, Nonweiler B, Kumbhare DA: Operative vs. nonoperative treatment of acute Achilles tendon ruptures: A quantitative review. Clin J Sports Med 7(3):207–211, 1997.
13. Cetti R, Christensen SE, Ejsted R, et al: Operative versus nonoperative treatment of Achilles tendon rupture. A prospective randomized study and review of the literature. Am J Sports Med 21(6):791–799, 1993.
14. Mandelbaum BR, Myerson MS, Forster R: Achilles tendon ruptures: A new method of repair, early range of motion and functional rehabilitation. Am J Sports Med 23:392–395, 1995.

Ankle Sprains

Definition

Ankle sprains are the most common musculoskeletal injury, with thousands occurring every day.

An understanding of the anatomy of the ankle combined with a detailed history of the mechanism of injury will allow the clinician to assess and treat these injuries. The ankle joint complex is stabilized by three major ligamentous groups. The medial or deltoid ligament is a strong structure attaching the tibia to the talus and calcaneus. The lateral ligament complex comprises three ligaments—the anterior and posterior talofibular ligaments as well as the calcaneofibular ligament. The tibia and fibula are joined by the distal tibiofibular ligaments (syndesmotic ligaments). Inversion injuries usually damage the lateral structures, with the anterior talofibular ligament being most commonly injured. Eversion injures the medial deltoid ligament. Combined injuries, especially with rotation, can injure the syndesmosis along with the medial or lateral ligaments. External rotation forces can damage the syndesmosis, with possible extension of the injury proximally to tear the interosseus ligament, leading to potentially serious ankle instability. Combined plantarflexion and inversion can injure the lateral ligament complex, as well as cause damage to the midfoot ligaments. Women may be particularly vulnerable to ankle sprains because they often have tight heel cords, which maintain the foot in a plantarflexed position in which there is reduced stability of the talus within the ankle mortice. Wearing high-heeled shoes presents a similar risk.

Signs and Symptoms

Pain is the usual presenting complaint. Occasionally individuals will be unable to bear weight, which is suggestive of a fracture. The degree of swelling often does not correlate with the presence of fracture. It is important to assess the integrity of the interosseus membrane and tibiofibular ligaments. For this reason, a squeeze test is performed in which the examiner grasps the proximal tibia and compresses the tibia and fibula together, gradually moving distally toward the ankle. Pain can indicate an occult fracture of the proximal fibula, injury to the interosseus membrane, or a syndesmotic injury. Tenderness over the individual ligaments is indicative of injury to that ligament. Bony tenderness may be present even in the absence of fracture but should alert the examiner to rule out fracture. Ankle instability can be demonstrated by the anterior drawer test, in which a posteriorly directed force on the tibia allows excessive anterior movement of the talus on the

tibia, or by the demonstration of medial or lateral tilting of the talus within the mortise.

Imaging

Radiographs are frequently used in the evaluation of ankle sprains, yet most are negative for fracture. The Ottawa Ankle Rules were derived in an attempt to minimize the time and expense for treating ankle injuries in the emergency department and have been validated by several prospective studies.[1, 2] The rules state that in adults ankle radiographs are needed if the patient is unable to walk for three steps (limping is OK) after the injury and in the emergency department, *or* there is tenderness over the posterior portion of the lateral or medial malleolus. Foot radiographs are needed if the patient is unable to walk for three steps (limping is OK) after the injury and in the emergency department, *or* there is tenderness over the navicular or the base of the fifth metatarsal. A recent study has suggested that tenderness over the midportion or crest of the malleolus from the tip to 6 cm proximally is more sensitive for fracture.[3] Children or adolescents with open physes may require radiographs more frequently. Radiographic findings include fractures, widening of the ankle mortice, and avulsion fragments from the malleoli. Soft tissue swelling is common, and in children, significant swelling overlying the physis is suggestive of an epiphyseal fracture. If the squeeze test is positive over the proximal lower leg, a long ankle view or separate views of the proximal lower leg must be performed to rule out a Maisonneuve fracture (see below). Chronic syndesmotic sprains will lead to irregularity over the region of the insertion of the interosseus membrane.

Injuries that Mimic Ankle Sprain

A number of other injuries can mimic or accompany an ankle sprain. Ankle sprains that fail to resolve should be investigated to rule out other causes of persistent disability. Easily overlooked fractures include those to the medial or lateral domes of the talus, the lateral process of the talus, the os trigonum, and the anterior process of the calcaneus. Occult fractures of tarsal bones can be easily missed. If a patient has significant swelling and remains unable to bear weight after an injury despite apparently negative radiographs and symptomatic treatment for 4 to 5 days, a computed tomography (CT) scan of the ankle and midfoot is indicated.

Inversion injury can cause tearing of the syndesmosis and a diastasis of the distal tibiofibular joint. The force can be transmitted proximally, resulting in tearing of the interosseus membrane, eventually releasing through a fracture of the proximal fibula, known as a Maisonneuve fracture. Physical examination will reveal significant tenderness and swelling over the proximal fibula, as well as a positive squeeze test. Standard ankle radiographs may show widening of the mortice but will not reveal the fracture. It is important to recognize the possibility of this injury in order to perform the proper radiographs and reach the correct diagnosis.

Osteochondral injuries to the talar domes can occur as the talus inverts within the mortice. These injuries can result in persistent deep ankle pain, ankle effusions, and a catching or a loose body sensation within the ankle. Physical findings include tenderness over the talar dome. Osteochondral injuries may be detected radiographically but may require CT or MR imaging for diagnosis. Chondral injuries can be demonstrated and staged by MR imaging.

Longitudinal tears or subluxation of the peroneal tendons can cause persistent lateral pain and swelling. These will cause persistent symptoms and can cause a clicking and sense of something moving out of place on the lateral aspect of the ankle. MR imaging can demonstrate insubstance rupture or persistent tendinopathy. Resisted eversion with the examiner's fingers over the posterior aspect of the lateral malleolus can provoke and demonstrate tendon subluxation.

Subluxation of the cuboid bone may occur in association with inversion ankle sprains but can also occur with repetitive plantar-dorsiflexion in dancers. As the medial border of the cuboid subluxates in a plantar direction, the fourth metatarsal base is displaced dorsally and the metatarsal head is plantarflexed. Cuboid subluxation interferes with the function of the peroneal tendons and can lead to tendonitis. Cuboid subluxation presents with persistent lateral midfoot pain, often following a sprain that does not respond to the usual treatments. The patient often will be unable to bear weight or walk normally, frequently having difficulty rolling onto the forefoot. Physical findings include significant tenderness over the cuboid bone, reduced mobility of the cuboid when compared to the opposite foot, reduced lateral midfoot mobility on passive pronation-supination, a step-off at the base of the fourth metatarsal, and a plantarflexed fourth metatarsal head. Treatment is directed at mobilizing the rear foot and midfoot and then reducing the cuboid, using a squeeze technique as described by Marshall and Hamilton.[4]

Treatment

Treatment of ankle sprains follows the PRICE principles. Casting is no longer recommended for even the most severe ankle sprains, as protection with taping or commercially available braces is usually sufficient. Individuals who have difficulty fully bearing weight should be placed on crutches to allow partial weight bearing for a few days until it is better tolerated. Individuals who remain completely unable to bear weight after 3 or 4 days should undergo CT to rule out occult tarsal fractures. Early range of motion is important and should begin with plantarflexion and dorsiflexion and progress to making circles with the foot. Finally, more complex motions can be employed, such as writing the alphabet with the big toe. Strength training with specific emphasis on the evertors should be part of the later stage of the rehabilitation. Flexibility of the gastrocnemius and soleus is important, especially in women with shorter Achilles tendons. Retraining of balance and proprioception is very important. The simplest way to perform this is standing on one foot with the eyes closed, attempting to maintain balance. As balance improves, more complex body positions are attempted. Agility drills should be employed before the patient returns to sports participation. This should start with jogging lazy S's or figure 8's, and progress to tighter and tighter turns until full cuts and pivots are achieved. Braces should be worn during initial stages of the rehabilitation and during the return to play.

Surgery is rarely required to treat ankle sprains and is virtually never indicated for early treatment of sprains. Recurrent instability, which may require surgery, should not be confused with or equated with recurrent inversion sprains. Many individuals with incomplete rehabilitation will suffer recurrent injuries. The restoration of normal subtalar and ankle motion, lower leg strength, and balance and proprioception will often allow a return to full function without surgery. Individuals with recurrent sprains associated with radiographic evidence of increased talar tilt and anterior drawer of the tibia on the talus when compared with the contralateral ankle and in whom an adequate trial of rehabilitation fails may be surgical candidates.

Of the ankle sprain mimics, cuboid subluxation can be treated with mobilization, taping, and physical therapy. The remainder of the sprain mimics discussed here frequently require surgical treatment, and referral should be made to an orthopedist.

Return to Competition

Athletes are allowed to return to competition when they have full range of motion; can hop on tip toes; have regained 90 percent strength, balance, and proprioception; and have passed functional agility tests such cutting and moving equally well to both sides.

When to Refer

Referral is indicated if the patient has recurrent instability despite adequate rehabilitation and radiographic evidence of instability. Patients who fail to progress and are found to have ankle sprain mimics will also require referral.

Key Points

- Ankle sprains are common.
- Suspect fracture if patient unable to bear weight.
- Treatment is symptomatic with PRICE followed by restoration of range of motion, strength, balance, and proprioception.
- If the patient fails to progress as expected, have a high index of suspicion for the ankle sprain mimics, and perform repeated, detailed examination and additional investigations.

REFERENCES

1. Stiehll IG, Greenberg GH, McKnight RD, et al: Decision rules for the use of radiography in acute ankle injuries. JAMA 269:1127–1132, 1993.
2. Pigman EC, Klug RK, Sanford S, et al: Evaluation of the Ottawa clinical decision rules for the use of radiography in acute ankle and midfoot injuries in the emergency depart-

ment. An independent site assessment. Ann Emerg Med 24:41–45, 1994.
3. Leddy JJ, Smolinski RJ, Lawrence J, et al: Prospective evaluation of the Ottawa ankle rules in a university sports medicine center—With a modification to increase specificity for identifying malleolar fractures. Am J Sports Med 26:158–165, 1998.
4. Marshall P, Hamilton W: Cuboid subluxation in ballet dancers. Am J Sports Med 20:169–175, 1992.
5. Bassewitz HL, Shapiro MS: Persistent pain after ankle sprain: Targeting the causes. Physician Sportsmed 12:58–68, 1997.

Proximal Fifth Metatarsal Fractures

Definition

Proximal fifth metatarsal fractures are represented by at least three and possibly six distinct fracture types. The common fractures are the avulsion fracture of the tuberosity, the acute Jones fracture, and the proximal diaphyseal stress fracture, which can be further subdivided into three subtypes. Occurring less frequently are apophyseal distraction injuries and injuries to accessory ossicles.[1] Diagnosis and management of these fractures can be controversial. Determining the cause of the fracture, chronicity, and precise anatomic location is necessary to manage these sometimes frustrating fractures. Inappropriate diagnosis of Jones fractures has contributed to confusion regarding management.

Avulsion fracture is the most common proximal fifth metatarsal fracture and is sometimes called the tennis fracture.[2] Historically, this injury was thought to be caused by avulsion of the peroneus brevis tendon during a sudden inversion. More recently, the lateral band of the plantar aponeurosis is implicated as the structure responsible for the avulsion.[3] This fracture most commonly presents accompanying a lateral ankle sprain.

True Jones fractures are acute fractures at the metaphyseal diaphyseal junction without extension to the medial side of the metatarsal at the fourth and fifth metatarsal articulation.[4] Jones fractures are indiscriminate by age, gender, or sport.[2] The exact mechanism of injury is adduction of the fifth metatarsal, often while the foot is plantarflexed.

Diaphyseal stress fractures are typical fatigue fractures of the proximal 1.5 cm of the fifth metatarsal shaft. These are often confused with the acute Jones fractures.[2] These fractures occur as result of repetitive adduction forces such as occur in cutting or pivoting. Patients often present with an acute event that was preceded by a prodrome of chronic pain to the lateral side of the foot. The diaphyseal-metaphyseal junction is a vascular watershed zone; therefore, both acute and stress fractures in this area are prone to delayed healing or nonunion.

Signs and Symptoms

The diagnosis depends on a careful history of the mechanism of injury. A history of prodromal activity-related aching—especially with night pain—is suggestive of a chronic stress fracture that may have gone on to completion following trauma.

When acute, all these fractures present with tenderness, swelling, and ecchymoses at the base of the fifth metatarsal, and it is often difficult to differentiate them on the basis of physical examination. Weight bearing is usually possible, but painful. The exact diagnosis is based on careful examination of the radiographs to determine the anatomic site of the fracture, and the presence or absence of ongoing, antecedent stress reaction.

Imaging

Avulsion fractures have a fracture line through the tuberosity of proximal metatarsal, most commonly perpendicular to its long axis. This fracture is generally extra-articular and involves the most proximal 1 cm of the metatarsal. The jagged and irregular fracture margins and perpendicular orientation help distinguish this fracture from the apophysis in the young athlete. The physis in the skeletally immature is usually directed along the long axis of the metatarsal, helping to distinguish this growth plate from a fracture. Radiographs of the contralateral foot may help to demonstrate the physeal appearance.

The Jones fracture is best seen on an oblique radiograph. It is an acute transverse fracture, which is directed toward, but does not progress to, the medial cortex at the fourth and fifth intermetatarsal articulation.

Torg has proposed a radiographic classification system for fifth metatarsal diaphyseal stress fractures to assist prognosis and management.[5] Type I fractures display a clean fracture line without medullary sclerosis or cortical hypertrophy. There may be some periosteal reaction belying an early stress fracture. Clinically the patient lacks

antecedent pain. Type II fractures demonstrate a widened fracture line and some intramedullary sclerosis. The patient has a previous history of chronic pain or fracture. Patients presenting with pain of less than 2 weeks' duration may have normal radiographs. Type III fractures resemble fracture nonunions with a widened fracture line and extensive intramedullary sclerosis. These patients have a longstanding history of repetitive trauma to the fifth metatarsal.

Treatment

Avulsion fractures are treated by wearing of a hard-soled shoe, by walking cast immobilization, or rarely open reduction internal fixation (ORIF) if the proximal fragment involves greater than 30 percent of the articular surface and is displaced greater than 2 mm.[2] Healing usually takes place within 5 weeks.[6] Activity is advanced depending on the level of symptoms. Avulsion fractures have an excellent prognosis, and patients usually recover well enough to return to the sport within a few weeks.

Acute, nondisplaced Jones fractures should be casted and remain non–weight-bearing for 6 to 8 weeks. In one series, 72 percent of these fractures healed using a non–weight-bearing (NWB) cast for 8 weeks.[6] The high performance athlete or the informed patient who refuses conservative care may elect to proceed with early operative management.[1, 2] Acute displaced Jones fractures should be treated with early ORIF. Patients treated conservatively should have repeat radiographs at 6 to 8 weeks. If intramedullary sclerosis or lucent fracture line is present, most patients will require ORIF, but patients who are unsuitable for or who decline surgery can be treated with continued immobilization. The individual patient's desires and expectations contribute to this decision. Operative failure is rare and is usually related to inappropriate intramedullary screw size, inadequate bone graft size, incomplete reaming of medullary canal, and the patient's too-early return to vigorous activity.[7] A cautious, slow return to activity should follow rehabilitation efforts to regain ankle and foot range of motion and strength.

Proximal diaphyseal stress fractures are treated more aggressively. Type I fractures are treated much the same as acute nondisplaced Jones fractures. NWB immobilization may be quite prolonged—up to 20 weeks,[2] with active patients frequently choosing surgical treatment.

Operative intervention becomes necessary for fracture nonunion. Most authors agree that the type II diaphyseal stress fractures should be treated with bone graft or intramedullary screw fixation, especially in athletes. The sedentary, non-obese patient may elect to try prolonged cast immobilization.[1, 2] Type III fractures are officially fracture nonunions and require operative management with intramedullary screw fixation or inlay bone grafts.[5, 8]

When to Refer

Acute Jones fractures can be managed by the primary care physicians who are comfortable with supervising cast immobilization, unless the patient opts for operative treatment. Nonhealing or displaced Jones fractures and type II and type III diaphyseal stress fractures should be referred for early surgical opinion. These patients may expect to return to their sport 2 to 4 months after surgery.[9]

Key Points

- Avulsion fractures occur as a sudden inversion of the ankle. These injuries generally heal without complication when the patient wears hard-soled shoes or a cast.
- Avulsion fractures must be differentiated from the true acute Jones fracture, or diaphyseal stress fractures, which may heal poorly because of compromised blood supply.
- Nondisplaced fractures can be treated with non–weight-bearing cast immobilization for 6 to 8 weeks.
- Athletes require early surgical treatment.
- Diaphyseal stress fractures are subdivided into three types. Type I can be treated conservatively, similar to a Jones fracture, but may require surgery. Types II and III require surgical treatment.

REFERENCES

1. Quill GE: Fractures of the proximal fifth metatarsal. Orthop Clin North Am 26(2):353–361, 1995.
2. Lawrence SJ, Botte MJ: Jones fractures and related fractures of the proximal fifth metatarsal. Foot Ankle 14(6):358–365, 1993.
3. Richli WR, Rosenthal DJ: Avulsion fractures of the fifth
metatarsal: Experimental study of pathomechanics. AJR 143:185–187, 1984.
4. Stewart IM: Jones' fracture: Fracture of the base of the fifth metatarsal. Clin Orthop 16:190–198, 1960.
5. Torg JS, Balduini FC, Zelko RR, et al: Fractures of the base of the fifth metatarsal distal to the tuberosity. J Bone Joint Surg A 66:209–214, 1984.
6. Clapper MF, O'Brien TJ, Lyons PM: Fractures of the fifth metatarsal. Clin Orthop Related Res 315:238–241, 1995.
7. Glasgow MT, Naranja J, Glasgow SG, Torg JS: Analysis of failed surgical management of fractures of the base of the fifth metatarsal distal to the tuberosity: The Jones fracture. Foot Ankle Int 17(8):449–457, 1996.
8. DeLee JC: Fractures and dislocations of the foot. In Mann RA (ed): Surgery of the Foot. St. Louis, C. V. Mosby, 1986.
9. Rettig AC, Shelbourne KD, Wilckens J: The surgical treatment of symptomatic nonunions of the proximal (metaphyseal) fifth metatarsal in athletes. Am J Sports Med 20(1):50–54, 1992.

Turf Toe

Definition

Turf Toe is a potentially debilitating injury to the first metatarsal phalangeal (MTP) joint. First described in 1976, this injury is most commonly suffered by football players playing on artificial surfaces.[1] Traumatic dorsiflexion of the MTP causes a stretch injury to the plantar joint capsule. The sprain usually occurs at the capsular attachment to the proximal metatarsal, as this is weaker than the phalangeal attachment.[2] There may be a concomitant compression injury to the articular cartilage surfaces on the dorsum of the joint.

Artificial surfaces are harder and have a higher coefficient of friction than natural surfaces. These factors allow for greater forces transmitted to the MTP joint when the foot is forcibly dorsiflexed against a fixed toe. The shoes used on artificial surfaces are usually less rigid than those used for natural surfaces, which contributes to the deforming forces at the MTP. Players wearing stiffer shoes are less likely to have a turf toe injury.[3] Athletes with hyperpronation and pes planus may be predisposed to turf toe through increased valgus stress on the medial side of the joint.[4]

Signs and Symptoms

The athlete complains of pain in the first MTP, usually following a single traumatic episode. The degree of symptoms is determined by the extent of the injury. Pain, swelling, ecchymoses, and restriction of motion are all present to varying degrees. Careful physical examination should be performed to ensure that the sesamoid bones are not the site of injury.

Management and return to play depend on the sprain severity. A grading system proposed by Clanton and Ford can assist with assessment and prognosis for return to participation.[2] Grade 1 injuries have minimal swelling, medial tenderness, and minimal joint motion restriction. Athletic participation is usually possible. Grade 2 injuries have more diffuse and intense tenderness, moderate swelling, ecchymoses, and mild to moderate motion restriction. Return to play takes 1 to 2 weeks as pain subsides and motion is restored. Grade 3 injuries have severe pain and tenderness encompassing the joint, and significant swelling and ecchymoses. Range of motion is severely restricted, and weight bearing is difficult. Return to sport may take 3 to 6 weeks.

Imaging

Diagnostic imaging is usually not necessary. Radiographs are usually normal with the exception of occasional small periarticular flecks of bone, which probably represent small joint margin avulsions. Severe or chronic cases may require careful determination of the tissue injured to rule out sesamoid or metatarsal and phalangeal fractures. Bipartite sesamoids are not uncommon, and comparison radiographs of the contralateral foot or a bone scan can be helpful in differentiating this from an acute sesamoid fracture. This assessment can be done best using MR imaging.[5]

Treatment

Treatment of turf toe initially utilizes PRICE principles. All too often this injury is dismissed by the coach and athlete as a minor problem, only to recur, requiring further convalescence after returning to play too quickly. Early range of motion activity is important to minimize the time to return to sport. Rest from further stress to the joint is crucial to speed the recovery. Nonsurgical treatment for turf toe requires reducing the stress on the MTP. Early on, this can be accomplished through taping. Increased support to the MTP joint can also be accomplished by using a stiffer athletic shoe, inserting an insole with a rigid stainless steel forefoot, or using a custom-molded orthotic with a Morton's extension.[2]

Return to Sport

There is a variable time frame for return to participation, with average times ranging from 1 to 6 weeks, as described earlier. Athletes should have minimal pain and be able to push off the affected side without difficulty, using appropriate taping or shoe modifications.

When to Refer

Surgical management of an MTP capsular sprain is rarely indicated. Sesamoid injury can have a clinical presentation similar to that of a turf toe. A bipartite sesamoid can separate at the cartilage interface, creating a recalcitrant turf toe syndrome that may be best managed surgically.[6] Referral should be made if the injury fails to respond to conservative treatment within the expected time frame.

Key Points

- Turf toe occurs more commonly on artificial playing surfaces and in players using more flexible athletic shoes.
- Athletes with a flexible flat foot are at greater risk for turf toe.
- Early identification and treatment of turf toe is mandatory to reduce time loss from sport.
- PRICE principles and joint range of motion exercises are crucial to return to play.
- Restricting the first MTP dorsiflexion with taping, stiff shoes, inserts with stainless steel forefoot, and custom orthotics with a Morton's extension aid the athlete's return to play.

REFERENCES

1. Bowers KD Jr, Martin RB: Turf-toe: A surface related football injury. Med Sci Sports 8(2):81–83, 1976.
2. Clanton TO, Ford JJ: Turf toe injury. Clin Sports Med 13(4):731–741, 1994.
3. Clanton TO, Butler JE, Eggert A: Injuries to the metatarsophalangeal joints in athletes. Foot Ankle 7:162–176, 1986.
4. Rodeo SA, O'Brien S, Warren RF, et al: Turf-toe: An analysis of metatarsophalangeal joint sprains in professional football players. Am J Sports Med 18(3):280–285, 1990.
5. Tewes DP, Fischer DA, Fritts HM, Guanche CA: MRI findings of acute turf toe. A case report and review of anatomy. Clin Orthop 304:200–203, 1994.

6. Rodeo SA, Warren RF, O'Brien SJ, et al: Diastasis of bipartite sesamoids of the first metatarsophalangeal joint. Foot Ankle 14(8):425–434, 1993.

OVERUSE INJURIES

In contrast to traumatic injuries, overuse injuries result from repetitive microtrauma to bony, ligamentous, or musculotendinous structures. They generally arise from the inability of the body to absorb the forces generated by the repeated cyclic loading of the musculoskeletal structures. Although it might seem that these injuries occur randomly, it is possible to identify numerous factors involved in their development. Factors extrinsic to the athlete include the biomechanical demands of the activity, training methods, training shoes, and training surfaces. Intrinsic factors related to the athletes themselves include primary intrinsic factors such as overall fitness, strength and flexibility, biomechanics and alignment, and individual variations in bony and ligamentous structures. Secondary or acquired intrinsic factors also play a significant role, including previous injuries that have been incompletely rehabilitated and which have led to imbalances, functional asymmetries, and gait abnormalities.

Extrinsic Factors

One of the most frequent causes of overuse injuries is inappropriate training methods, which usually take the form of doing too much activity too soon. Training errors include excessive duration or intensity of training, failure to allow adaptation to new training levels, and failure to allow for individual differences in adaptation and performance.

The training surface may predispose to injuries. Excessively hard surfaces such as concrete can lead to increased shock transmission to the legs. Running on a steeply cambered road may cause asymmetric stresses on the pelvis and lower leg. The leg on the uphill side will tend to pronate and externally rotate in order to shorten the leg and level the pelvis, applying increased forces to the medial musculoligamentous structures. The foot of the downhill leg will tend to supinate, leading to increased tension on the lateral structures, and possible injuries.

The characteristics of the dance floor are important in dance injuries. Most professional companies have specially designed and suspended floors that allow for good shock absorption with jumping and landing. Injuries can occur when dancers are on location and train on excessively hard surfaces, or in young dancers rehearsing or performing in small studios with poorly constructed floors.

Many individuals suffer running-related injuries because of the use of inappropriate footwear. Footwear design is generally a compromise between motion-control features and shock absorption. Increases in one will often lead to decreases in the other. Problems arise when individuals buy footwear that is not appropriate for their type of individual biomechanics, foot type, or activity.

Intrinsic Factors

Intrinsic factors play a crucial role in the etiology of overuse injuries. The primary factors are those related to the individual athlete's physical characteristics. Secondary or acquired intrinsic factors are those that result from postural and movement dysfunctions arising from previous incompletely rehabilitated injuries.

Primary Intrinsic Factors

Inadequate Strength and Flexibility The muscles are the shock absorbers for the joints. They are required to absorb the forces involved with the repeated impacts and movements associated with repetitive activities. If there is inadequate strength or endurance of the muscular structures, fatigue will result and overload can occur to the muscles, ligaments, tendons, or bones. Inadequate flexibility can cause relative tissue tightness, leading to the improper mechanics or imbalances of the forces acting on the joints. Imbalances in the muscle strength between agonist and antagonist groups may lead to acute muscle tears and injuries. Athletes with excessive joint laxity may be predisposed to injury unless muscular support and balance are optimized.

Hormonal and Nutritional Status Highly trained female athletes are at significant risk for the development of the Female Athlete Triad of disordered eating, amenorrhea, and osteoporosis. Lower circulating estrogen levels can lead to an increased risk of stress fractures. Nutritional deficiencies can lead to loss of muscle mass and early muscle fatigue, predisposing to overuse injuries. There is a significant relationship between dance injuries and both body mass index and menstrual function.[1]

Biomechanics and Alignment It has long been thought that intrinsic factors are important in the genesis of overuse injuries in running. Many investigators have studied injured runners and made pronouncements as to why these injuries have occurred, including theories that biomechanical factors, such as excess pronation and abnormalities of lower leg and knee alignment, lead to injury. Unfortunately, most of these conclusions were obtained by examining injured runners only, and well-controlled studies have been unable to confirm that these factors are important in running injuries.[2, 3]

Secondary (Acquired) Intrinsic Factors

Acquired factors for overuse injuries are the result of mechanical movement dysfunctions, usually resulting from previous injuries. Repetitive movements in running and dance require the action of muscular forces on a series of rigid limb segments joined by mobile linkages, commonly referred to as the kinetic chain. Optimal performance requires that all segments of the kinetic chain be appropriately positioned to support the body's weight and allow for movement. Anything that interferes with normal joint mobility or stability will necessitate compensatory postural and movement changes, which can lead to increased stresses on other sites in the kinetic chain. Once the capacity of the chain to compensate is exceeded, tissue breakdown and injury will occur. This failure may be at the site of the abnormal mobility; however, the overt injury can also occur at a site distant from the dysfunction. One could simplistically compare this to "culprit" and "victim" in the injury. The presenting injury may merely be the victim, which has suffered an injury as a result of an inability to compensate for a dysfunction at a distant site in the chain (the culprit). When an athlete presents with an injury, it is easy to assume that the injury has occurred in isolation, but it is essential to consider that the injury may be secondary to an underlying dysfunction.[4, 5]

Kinetic chain dysfunction has been described in overuse injuries in the general population[6] and in runners.[5] Individuals with plantar fasciitis have been shown to have reduced static and dynamic range of motion and reduced lower leg strength in addition to the symptomatic plantar fasciitis.[7] No joint mobility testing was performed in this study; however, it quite possibly would have been abnormal. It would be logical to predict that these dysfunctions, if left untreated, could cause gait alterations and predispose to other injuries at other sites in the chain.

Kinetic chain dysfunction has been implicated in overuse dance injuries.[4, 8] In a retrospective study, 11 of 16 (69 percent) injured dancers were found to have kinetic chain dysfunctions, including 9 of 12 with overuse injuries and 2 of 4 with acute injuries.[4] Evaluation of a similar group of uninjured dancers revealed that only 44 percent of 108 uninjured dancers had dysfunctions.[9] Of the 9 dancers with overuse injuries to the lower leg and foot, 8 had abnormal functional foot movements and 7 of these 8 reported a history of previous injury to the same region.[4] Another study found a significant correlation between previous injury and a new injury in a prospective study of dancers.[8] Those dancers with previous injuries had significantly less ankle and foot mobility than uninjured dancers.

It would appear that previous ankle sprains are significantly related to new overuse injuries. In addition to the studies in dancers, a prospective study of army recruits found that previous injury, specifically sprained ankles, was a significant risk factor for new injuries.[10] This finding can be explained by a loss of normal subtalar motion and function, with resultant increased stress on the muscle tendon units attempting to stabilize the foot and ankle. Impaired balance and proprioception can follow ankle sprains and have been shown to persist for several weeks despite active rehabilitation.[11] Following ankle sprains, it is important to strengthen the peroneal muscles, because failure to do so could lead to repeated injuries. Because the subtalar joint acts as a rotational transducer between the ankle and the lower leg and knee, persistent abnormal pronation or supination can result in increased compensatory stresses on the proximal chain.

Physicians and therapists have traditionally focused solely on the injury site when dealing with overuse injuries, yet it is important to recognize that any injury may be a manifestation of a local or distant dysfunction in the kinetic chain. For this reason, the entire kinetic chain must be screened to rule out any primary or underlying injury. This process is especially important in individuals who have had recurrent injuries to the same site or limb, because there may be an underlying dysfunction that places increased stress on elements of that limb, resulting in serial episodes of tissue breakdown and injury.

Treatment of Overuse Injuries

Treatment for overuse injuries depends on four steps. Unfortunately, many athletes are treated only until their symptoms are resolved, and then are sent back to physical activities without being completely rehabilitated. All four steps in rehabilitation and treatment are important, and failure to deal with any one of the factors can lead to repeated injuries.

1. Relief of Symptoms Relief of acute-injury symptoms depends on use of ice, massage, anti-inflammatory medications, and physical therapy. Modified rest is prescribed in which the offending activity is slowed or stopped and other activities are substituted that can still provide an aerobic workout without stressing the injured part.

2. Rehabilitation of Muscle Function Rehabilitation is the most important step of treatment, yet it is often neglected. Muscle strength and the balance between muscle groups must be restored. These exercises can consist of general nonspecific exercises later progressing to more functional, sports-specific exercises. Flexibility should also be addressed, with a full functional joint range of motion being reestablished prior to return to activities.

3. Correct Underlying Factors Any factor that has been identified as the cause of the injury should be corrected. These steps might include modifications in training schedules, the use of specific strengthening or flexibility exercises, the choice of appropriate footwear or equipment, or possibly a supportive orthotic, gait retraining, or the proper alignment and adjustment of equipment to that individual's biomechanics. Contributing imbalances and kinetic chain dysfunctions should also be addressed and rehabilitated appropriately. It is important to treat joint mobility and strength deficiencies proximal and distal to the joint in question to ensure the proper function of all segments required in the activity. Braces may be important to allow an earlier return to activities or to help alleviate the symptoms in ongoing activities.

4. Reintroduction of Activities Activities must be restarted gradually, with training reintroduced at a lower level to allow a progressive buildup of frequency, intensity, and duration. Repeat injuries often occur if training is reintroduced too quickly. Training should be done on a hard/easy basis with at least one rest day per week. Balance and proprioception retraining is very important, especially in the treatment of ankle and foot injuries and in knee injuries. It is also important for the athlete to work on agility drills before returning to activities that require any cutting, pivoting, or change in direction.

Key Points

- Overuse injuries are not random occurrences and usually have an identifiable cause.
- Extrinsic factors such as training errors, training surface, and footwear are important.
- Primary intrinsic factors include strength, flexibility, and hormonal and nutritional status.
- Secondary intrinsic factors are crucial, specifically incomplete rehabilitation of previous injuries, especially ankle sprains.
- Identification of the underlying cause of the injury will allow the rehabilitation program to be tailored to correct the underlying problem, rather than using a cookbook approach.
- Treatment includes relief of symptoms, restoration of strength and flexibility, and functional return to activity, but also must include correction of the underlying factors.

REFERENCES

1. Benson JE, Geiger CJ, Eiserman PA, Wardlaw GM: Relationship between nutrient intake, body mass index, menstrual function and ballet injury. J Am Dietetic Assoc 89(1):58–63, 1989.
2. Reid DC: The myth, mystic, and frustration of anterior knee pain. Clin J Sport Med 3(3):139–143, 1993.
3. Wen DY, Puffer JC, Schmalzried TP: Lower extremity alignment and risk of overuse injuries in runners. Med Sci Sport Exerc 29(10):1291–1298, 1997.
4. Macintyre JG: Kinetic chain dysfunction in ballet injuries. Med Prob Perf Art 99(2):39–42, 1994.
5. Macintyre JG, Lloyd-Smith DR: Intrinsic factors in over-

use running injuries. In Renstrom P (ed): International Olympic Committee Encyclopedia Series. 4. Sports Injuries: Basic Principles of Prevention and Care. Oxford, Blackwell Scientific Publications, 1994.

6. Kibler WB, Chandler TJ, Stracener ES: Musculoskeletal adaptations and injuries due to overtraining. In Holloszy JO (ed): Exercise and Sports Science Reviews, Baltimore, Williams & Wilkins, 1992.

7. Kibler WB, Goldberg C, Chandler J: Functional biomechanical deficits in running athletes with plantar fasciitis. Am J Sports Med 19(1):66–71, 1991.

8. Weisler ER, Hunter DM, Martin DF, et al: Ankle flexibility and injury patterns in dancers. Am J Sports Med 24(6):754–757, 1996.

9. Macintyre JG: Unpublished data, 1995.

10. Jones BH, Cowan DN, Tomlinson JP, et al: Epidemiology of injuries associated with physical training among young men in the army. Med Sci Sports Exerc 25(2):197–203, 1993.

11. Leanderson J, Eriksson E, Nillson C, Wyckman A: Proprioception in classical ballet dancers: A prospective study of the influence of an ankle sprain on proprioception in the ankle joint. Am J Sports Med 24(3):370–374, 1996.

Lower Back Pain

Definition

Lower back pain is a common phenomenon in the North American population that affects almost everyone to some degree at some stage in life. Management is often frustrating and depends on an accurate diagnosis and treatment that is specific to that diagnosis. Fortunately, most back pain is self-limiting, and even in the absence of an accurate diagnosis, excellent treatment results are frequently obtained with conservative management.

The cause of lower back pain is multifactorial in nature. The pain can arise from any of the structures in the back, including the muscles, ligaments, facet joints, intervertebral disk, or sacroiliac joints. Acute back strain can involve any of these structures and usually is initiated by one acute episode of lifting or twisting. Falls can also cause acute pain. Chronic overuse syndromes can also occur with the back and are predisposed by poor posture, including increased lumbar lordosis, tightness of the hamstrings and iliopsoas, and lack of strength of the abdominal and paraspinal musculature. Two of the most common causes of lower back pain in athletes are spondylolysis and pelvic instability/sacroiliac joint dysfunction (SIJD).

Spondylolysis

Definition

Spondylolysis is a stress fracture of the pars interarticularis, and is thought to arise from repetitive extension and flexion of the spine. Both the pathology and the clinical presentation of spondylolysis are variable. Many cases are asymptomatic, with 6 percent of the population having radiographic evidence of a pars defect, although there are higher rates in adolescent athletes, especially gymnasts, dancers, and divers. The specific pathologic picture extends over a continuum and may range from an asymptomatic painless fibrous defect discovered on an x-ray to a stress fracture with disabling pain. It is thus important to correlate the clinical findings with any imaging studies.

Signs and Symptoms

Spondylolysis usually presents with activity-related lower back pain, usually exacerbated by extension or twisting, which load the posterior elements of the spine. It is often unilateral and can be relieved by rest, although night pain may occur in acute cases.

Adolescents with spondylolysis will usually demonstrate defective posture with lumbar hyperlordosis, poor abdominal tone, tight hip flexors, and weak hamstrings. Unilateral extension frequently reproduces the back pain. This is tested by having the athlete stand on one leg while bringing the contralateral knee up to the chest, and then extending the back, which stresses the pars on the side of the standing leg. There is occasional unilateral tenderness over the posterior elements on the involved side.

Imaging

Radiographs will frequently show the characteristic "scottie dog" lesion on the oblique view, but the clinical significance must be interpreted with caution because of the high prevalence of asymptomatic lesions. The technetium radionuclide bone scan is the diagnostic test of choice, and improved diagnostic accuracy can be gained through the use of single photon emission computed tomography (SPECT), which can accurately localize the lesion to the pars. A positive x-ray with a negative bone scan should prompt the clinician to search for another cause of the patient's back pain, including sacroiliac joint dysfunction, which is common in this group of athletes.

Some athletes will suffer anterior slippage of a vertebra on the one below through bilateral spondylolytic pars defects, which is termed spondylolisthesis. It is graded on the degree of radiographic slippage.

Treatment

The treatment of spondylolysis is controversial, and depends on the stage of the defect. Early stress fractures with positive bone scans and negative radiographs have the best chance of healing. Well-established fractures with sclerotic margins have little healing potential. There is general agreement that the pain-producing activities should be stopped. Some clinicians recommend cessation of all activities, but it seems more reasonable, and equally effective, to maintain activities that can be performed on a pain-free basis. Early fractures can heal with soft bracing, but well-established fractures are unlikely to show radiographic healing (normalization of x-rays so the defect is no longer detectable).[1] Rigid Boston bracing for 6 to 12 months resulted in radiographic healing in only 12 of 67 patients, mostly in those patients with recent onset of symptoms. Despite the lack of radiographic healing, bracing provided symptomatic improvement in the majority of patients.[2] Long-term studies have shown that patients with spondylolysis and spondylolisthesis can perform at high levels of athletics without symptoms.[3, 4] These findings would suggest that activity modification and possibly soft bracing for symptomatic relief should be the treatment of choice. Early lesions with negative radiographs and positive bone scans should possibly be treated with more rigid activity restrictions.

Other rehabilitation should be undertaken while the patient is in the restricted activity phase. Lumbar stabilization exercises have been shown to have beneficial results, although the study has some methodologic shortcomings.[5] The athlete should work at stretching the hip flexors and hamstrings and should correct lumbopelvic mechanics and hyperlordosis.

Return to Activity

Athletes should be allowed a gradual return to activity when they are asymptomatic and have completed a posture and stabilization program. They should be allowed to gradually progress in their level of activity so long as it can be accomplished without provoking an increase in pain.

When to Refer

Patients with spondylolysis usually can be managed by the primary care practitioner. They should be referred to a specialist if there is some question as to the diagnosis, higher grade spondylolisthesis, or neurologic compromise.

Key Points

- Spondylolysis is a common condition, especially in athletes in sports requiring repetitive extension loading of the spine.
- In many cases patients are asymptomatic, and the presence of a radiographic defect does not indicate that the spondylolysis is the cause of the pain, unless a bone scan is positive.
- Most patients will do well with activity modification and with strengthening, stabilization, and flexibility exercises.
- Symptomatic bracing may be useful in some patients, but there is no clear advantage to the use of prolonged rigid immobilization.

REFERENCES

1. Morita T, Ikata T, Katoh S, Miyake R: Lumbar spondylolysis in children and adolescents. J Bone Joint Surg B 77:620–625, 1995.
2. Steiner ME, Micheli L: Treatment of symptomatic spondylolysis and spondylolisthesis with the modified Boston brace. Spine 10:937–943, 1985.
3. Seitsalo S, Antila H, Karrinaho H, et al: Spondylolysis in ballet dancers. J Dance Med Sci 1:51–54, 1997.
4. Muschik M, Hahnel H, Robinson PN, et al: Competitive sports and the progression of spondylolysis and spondylolisthesis. J Paediat Orthop 16:364–369, 1996.
5. O'Sullivan P, Phyty GD, Twomey LT, et al: Evaluation of specific stabilizing exercise in the treatment of chronic low back pain with radiographic evidence of spondylolysis or spondylolisthesis. Spine 22:2959–2967, 1997.

Pelvic Instability: Sacroiliac Joint Dysfunction

Definition

Sacroiliac joint dysfunction (SIJD) is a common, frequently overlooked, and almost universally controversial condition. The pelvic ring is composed of the innominate bones, which meet at the symphysis anteriorly and articulate with the sacrum posteriorly at the sacroiliac joints. Conventional medical wisdom frequently maintains that the SI joint is immobile, despite numerous studies that have demonstrated that movement does indeed occur.[1] Movement is increased during pregnancy when production of the hormone relaxin is increased, leading to ligamentous laxity. Excessive mobility can lead to instability and lumbopelvic pain. The pain can be variously attributed to mechanical stresses on ligamentous structures, facet joints, disks, and muscles. The significant role of the SI joint in chronic back pain has been well documented in a pain ablation injection study.[2]

The most common dysfunctions occur with rotational subluxation of the innominate bones, leading to an asymmetry in the pelvic ring structure. Some patients will show an upslip pattern in which the innominate bone is subluxated superiorly. Once the subluxation has been corrected, these patients may demonstrate an underlying hypermobile SI that allows the subluxation and then locking into a position at the extremes of motion. Tightness of the hip capsule will limit its movement, thus transferring increased stress to the SI joints, leading to dysfunction.

Signs and Symptoms

Sacroiliac dysfunction and pelvic instability can present with pain in either an acute or chronic manner, with the clinical presentation determined by the actual site and type of dysfunction. In athletic individuals, there may be a history of trauma, often a fall onto the buttocks, or an axial load onto one leg, such as can occur with stepping unexpectedly off a curb or into a hole in the ground. Overstriding during downhill running or performing kicks or vigorous hip flexion or extension movements in martial arts or dance may also lead to SIJD. It is not uncommon to see SI dysfunction following motor vehicle accidents in which patients have braced their legs against the brake pedal or floor in anticipation of impact. In pregnancy, back pain from SIJD may have gradual onset with activities of daily living or acute onset with a twisting motion. Some women suffer significant pain and disability that, if untreated, can leave them bedridden for the duration of their pregnancy.

The pain is often localized to the SI joint itself but may also be found in the buttocks, pubic symphysis, lower abdomen, or lateral thigh. Occasionally there is pain referred to the posterior thigh and lower leg and foot. This can mimic pain of a protruded intervertebral disk, which creates a common source of confusion, as many individuals interpret leg pain as originating only from disks. SIJD pain differs in that there are no associated neurologic findings such as weakness, restricted straight leg raising, pain on forced knee-chest flexion, or reflex changes. Additionally, SI joint pain is often discontinuous within the leg, with discrete areas of pain over the buttock, posterior thigh, posterior calf, and rarely the plantar surface of the foot. The pain is patchy and does not radiate in a continuous band-like manner. Pressure over the SI joint can also reproduce leg symptoms in some individuals. Movement is painful, with extension often more painful than flexion. Prolonged sitting can cause pain in the lower back and buttocks.

Patients will occasionally complain of increased pain with coughing or sneezing. This is often thought to indicate disk pathology; however, pelvic instability due to an SI joint dysfunction can also cause pain with this maneuver. A good way of distinguishing them is to have the patient cough while the pelvis is being stabilized by a compressive force across the iliac crests to support the SI joint. If this abolishes the cough-induced pain, it suggests that the pain may be due to an SI dysfunction.

Patients with SI dysfunction will often present with a secondary injury arising from gait alterations but will admit to underlying activity-related back pain. Patients may also complain that they feel as if they are out of alignment and that their gait is abnormal, but many will not volunteer this sensation unless specifically questioned.

Dysfunction of the SI joint leads to compensatory changes at other sites in the axial skeleton, including sacral torsion, rotation of the lumbar vertebrae, and frequently secondary rotations of thoracic and even cervical vertebrae. These changes can produce pain at sites distant from the SI joint, as well as in the characteristic findings of flexible dual scoliosis, and rotations of the upper thorax and shoulder girdle. If the SI joint remains unstable and malaligned, it will do little good to try to correct more proximal problems in the upper back or neck until the SI is treated.

The most common finding on physical examination is that of tenderness over the SI joint, which can be assessed by applying direct pressure while the patient is lying prone. There is often local tenderness over the region of the posterior superior iliac spine. Examination is also directed at the identification of functional asymmetries of the pelvic girdle and SI joint. These are manifested by asymmetric positioning of the levels of the anterior and posterior superior iliac spines in the frontal plane. In addition to rotation of the innominates, the sacrum may tilt to one side, resulting in a sacral torsion.

Additional clues are leg lengths that are asymmetric and change when the patient goes from a supine position to a long sitting position in which the patient sits upright on the examination table with the hips flexed to 90 degrees and the knees extended. An asymmetric range of hip motion is also suggestive of an SI dysfunction. Usually one hip will have a predominant range of external rotation and the other a predominant range of internal rotation. Hamstring flexibility is affected by SIJD, with the hamstring on the side of the anterior rotation having a reduced flexibility relative to the other. Although these findings are not diagnostic, they are certainly suggestive of this problem. More detailed tests are well described by Lee[1] and Woerman.[3]

Imaging

Imaging of lower back pain is controversial. The diagnosis of SIJD must be made on a clinical basis, using history and detailed physical examination, with imaging studies of little use in its management. In the patient with acute, nontraumatic lower back pain without neurologic signs, or symptoms suggestive of systemic problems such as infection or neoplasm, it is generally recommended that plain x-rays be performed only after the failure to respond to 6 weeks of conservative treatment. With current cost consciousness, this would appear to be a good policy, although it may be difficult to convince patients to wait.

There is a high prevalence of radiographic abnormalities in the asymptomatic population, with MRI demonstrating disk disease in up to 35 percent of subjects between 20 and 39 years of age, and in 13 of 14 subjects over 60 years old.[4] Thus, it is very difficult to assess the results of an imaging study, especially when the radiographic findings do not correlate with the clinical picture.

As a general rule of thumb, imaging should be reserved for cases in which it will change the immediate management of the patient. If a disk herniation is suspected but nonoperative treatment is planned, it is unnecessary to perform an MRI unless the patient has signs and symptoms that might suggest the need for surgery if the pathology is confirmed by the MRI.

It must be kept in mind that SIJD is a diagnosis of exclusion and that the presence of neurologic signs or symptoms should make SIJD a secondary diagnosis. Because the signs and symptoms of disk herniation may evolve and progress over time, careful, serial neurologic examination should be performed at each patient assessment.

Treatment

It is important to emphasize to these patients that there is no magic treatment for back pain, and that the responsibility for treating back pain lies with them. All treatments ultimately require the patient's active participation and cooperation and the adherence to a regular program of maintenance exercises. The patient who is unwilling to accept responsibility for the pain and unwilling to do these exercises should be told to learn to live with the pain.

The treatment of almost all lumbosacral problems is directed toward relief of symptoms, followed by restoration of strength and flexibility. It was once thought that bed rest for 1 to 2 weeks was a good treatment of a lumbosacral strain. However, this is no longer thought to be the case, and patients who maintain their mobility within the limits of their pain tolerance have the most rapid recovery time. Acetaminophen and NSAIDs are used for symptomatic relief. Narcotics can be used for short time periods but may be inappropriate for longer periods of time due to the potential for habituation in cases in which there is no "quick fix" to the problem. Ice massage over the lumbosacral region is often effective. Physical therapy is occasionally helpful, although the use of modalities alone for symptomatic relief for any longer than a few days should be discouraged. Mobilization has shown to be effective in some cases. Strengthening and pelvic stabilization drills are essential. Muscle tone must be improved in the abdominals and paraspinals. It is crucial to restore flexibility of the hamstrings, quadriceps, hip flexors, and hip capsule.

Specific treatment of SIJD and pelvic instability consists of correcting the underlying dynamics and positional defects of the pelvis. The scope of this chapter does not allow a full discussion of this, but good reference texts are available.[1, 3] SI support belts place a compressive force around the pelvis and stabilize the SI joint and are useful in treating pelvic instability, especially during pregnancy. Lumbar stabilizing drills and Kegel exercises should also be recommended.

Return to Activity

The pain from SI dysfunction is often not disabling. As long as there is no evidence of diskogenic pain, neurologic compromise, or lumbar stress fracture, participation may be allowed to continue, within the limitations of pain.

When to Refer

If there is a suspicion of an SI dysfunction on clinical examination, the patient should be referred to an allopathic or osteopathic physician, or a physical therapist with specific training in manual therapy. These practitioners can recommend and perform specific stretching exercises to return the pelvis to its normal alignment.

Key Points

- Lumbosacral pain is a common problem and its effective management requires patient participation.
- Sacroiliac joint dysfunction is a common cause of lower back pain, but it must be a diagnosis of exclusion. Patients must have no evidence of infection, tumor, or systemic process and a normal neurologic examination.
- The hallmark of physical examination is asymmetry of pelvic landmarks, hip range of motion, and hamstring flexibility, and changing leg lengths.
- Treatment requires referral to an experienced practitioner for correction of the dysfunction.

REFERENCES

1. Lee D: The Pelvic Girdle: An Approach to the Examination and Treatment of the Lumbo-Pelvic-Hip Region. New York, Churchill Livingstone, 1989.
2. Schwarzer AC, Aprill CN, Bogduk N: The sacroiliac joint in chronic low back pain. Spine 20:31–37, 1995.
3. Woerman AJ: Evaluation and treatment of the lumbar-pelvic-hip complex. In Donatelli R, Wooden MJ (eds): Orthopedic Physical Therapy. New York, Churchill Livingstone, 1989.
4. Boden SD, Davis DO, Dina TS, et al: Abnormal magnetic resonance scans of the lumbar spine in asymptomatic subjects. J Bone Joint Surg A 72:403–408, 1990.

Groin Pain

Groin pain in athletes encompasses a variety of problems involving any of the structures in the lower abdomen, inguinal region, upper adductor muscles, symphysis pubis, or scrotum. A detailed history and physical examination will assist the clinician in arriving at an appropriate diagnosis. Sports hernia is covered in Chapter 15.

Osteitis Pubis

Definition

Osteitis pubis is an inflammatory, overuse disorder of the symphysis pubis that occurs in running, ice hockey, wrestling, rugby, tennis, football, soccer, and basketball.[1] Several mechanical factors are thought to contribute to increased stress at the symphysis. If hip rotation or extension is limited due to inherent structural tightness or capsular tightness after an injury, more force is transmitted to the symphysis.[2] Other factors include instability of the sacroiliac joint, adductor muscle strains, and excessive pelvic up and down motion or sway.

Signs and Symptoms (Table 12–1)

Athletes present with insidious onset of pain in the groin aggravated by kicking, running, or pivoting. Sit-ups may also cause more pain. Examination shows tenderness directly over the symphysis, adductor muscle tightness, and pain with resisted adductor activity. Patients with osteitis pubis should always have specific examination to exclude underlying SI joint dysfunction and hip capsular tightness. Rarely, the symphysis can become infected, so the patient should be questioned re-

Table 12–1
Presenting Complaints and Physical Findings of 12 Athletes With Osteitis Pubis

Symptoms (Findings)	No. of Athletes	Percentage
Acute onset	2	17
Gradual onset	10	83
Groin pain	9	75
Adductor pain		
Unilateral	11	92
Bilateral	1	8
Lower abdominal pain	2	17
Hip pain	3	25
Scrotal/peroneal pain	1	8
Tenderness at symphysis	12	100
Pain with hip flexion	5	42
Decreased hip abduction	12	100
Resistive pain		
Abductors	8	67
Rectus abdominis	4	33

Source: Holt MA, Keene JS, Graf BK, et al: Treatment of osteitis pubis in athletes. Results of corticosteroid injections. Am J Sports Med 23:601–606, 1995.

garding the presence of systemic signs such as fevers, chills, and night sweats.

Imaging

Diagnostic tests include plain radiographs, technetium-99 bone scan, or MR imaging.[3] An x-ray may show erosion, sclerosis, and widening of the margins to the symphysis. "Flamingo views" are radiographs taken while the patient is standing first on one leg and then while standing on the other leg. Joint movement greater than 2 mm suggests pelvic instability, although this is not specific for osteitis pubis.[2] A bone scan will show increased activity, although it will not differentiate between osteitis pubis and infection.

Treatment

Rest, anti-inflammatory medicines, and adductor stretching are used to manage this problem. Corticosteroid injections directly into the symphysis pubis may decrease the time to pain-free recovery and return to play[1] (Figs. 12–3 and 12–4). Strengthening of the hip abductor and adductor musculature should be undertaken using high repetitions and low resistance (3 sets of 30 to 40 repetitions). This maintains symmetric forces on the pubis, thereby preventing shearing of the sym-

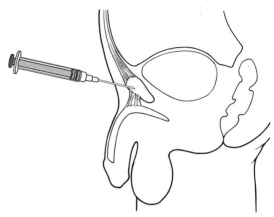

Figure 12–3. Needle placement in the anteroposterior plane. (From Holt MA, Keene JS, Graf BK, et al: Treatment of osteitis pubis in athletes. Results of corticosteroid injections. Am J Sports Med 23:602, 1995.)

physis and helping to maintain the alignment of the SI joints. Underlying factors such as SI joint dysfunctions and hip capsular tightness are corrected. A physical therapist experienced in manual therapy will be invaluable in providing treatment for this difficult problem.

Return to Competition

Osteitis pubis can be prolonged and debilitating to athletes in a competitive season, with one study showing that the average time to full athletic recovery was 9.6 months.[4] The athlete should be pain-free and have completed a functional agility

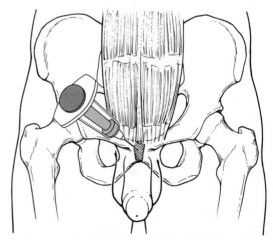

Figure 12–4. Needle placement in the sagittal plane. (From Holt MA, Keene JS, Graf BK, et al: Treatment of osteitis pubis in athletes. Results of corticosteroid injections. Am J Sports Med 23:602, 1995.)

program prior to return to sports. Kicking athletes should progress through a graded kicking program, starting with small numbers of short kicks, and progressively increasing the distance and force during successive practices, so long as the athlete remains pain-free.

Key Points

- Osteitis pubis presents with midline groin pain of insidious onset, with pain worsened by kicking, pivoting, or running.
- SI joint dysfunctions and hip capsular tightness are common predisposing factors.
- X-ray changes show marginal erosions. Flamingo views may show pelvic movement. Bone scan is typically active in the symphysis.
- Treatment includes rest, NSAIDs, correction of underlying factors, restoration of strength and flexibility, and possible corticosteroid injection into the symphysis.

REFERENCES

1. Holt MA, Keene JS, Graf BK, et al: Treatment of osteitis pubis in athletes. Results of corticosteroid injections. Am J Sports Med 23(5):601–606, 1995.
2. Williams JG: Limitation of hip joint movement as a factor in traumatic osteitis pubis. Br J Sports Med 12:129–133, 1978.
3. Fricker PA: Management of groin pain in athletes. Br J Sports Med 31:97–101, 1997.
4. Fricker PA, Taunton JE, Ammann W: Osteitis pubis in athletes: Infection, inflammation, or injury? Sports Med 12:266–279, 1991.

Stress Fractures

Definition

Stress fractures represent the end point of a continuum of bony stress reactions to repetitive loading. When a mechanical load is applied to a bone, remodeling accelerates to maintain skeletal integrity. Early in this process, osteoblastic activity to lay down new bone generally lags behind osteoclastic resorption, resulting in a net loss of bone and the development of microfractures. In most instances, the bone is able to adapt to the new level of stress. However, when loading is increased too rapidly, the imbalance can be of sufficient magnitude to lead to a clinically significant weakening of the bone.[1, 2]

The etiology of stress fractures is multifactorial. The primary factors are similar to those of all overuse injuries as previously described. Women seem to have a greater predisposition to stress fractures than men.[3, 4] Numerous reasons have been postulated, including differences in bone mass, lower ratio of muscle to body mass, lower levels of musculoskeletal strength and cardiovascular fitness, and hormonal and endocrine factors. Although none of these theories has been properly validated in a prospective study, there is consensus that a significant relationship exists between stress fractures, reproductive hormone levels, and bone mass. There is significant concern that women suffering from the Female Athlete Triad are at a greater risk for stress fractures during their athletic career, and that they will have significant risk for premature osteoporotic fractures later in life.

Stress fractures account for up to 10 percent of all sports injuries, and represent a higher proportion of running injuries. They can occur in some areas of the spine, as well as in almost every bone of the appendicular skeleton. The most common site is the tibia, followed by the tarsals, metatarsals, and femur.[1] Stress fractures of the shaft and neck of the femur, the proximal tibia, the base of the fifth metatarsal, and the tarsal navicular are considered to be at high risk for complications if they are not diagnosed and treated with appropriate rest and rehabilitation.

Signs and Symptoms

Stress fractures usually present with pain, initially following activity, and with worsening, the pain may progress to be present during and after the activity, and finally being present with the activities of daily living. Night pain is a common feature, which should alert the clinician to the possibility of a stress fracture. The pain is often poorly localized and may be easy to dismiss due to the lack of physical findings. It is essential for the clinician to have a high index of suspicion in order not to miss these fractures.

Imaging

Radiographic findings often lag several weeks behind the clinical picture and are frequently negative in the early symptomatic stages. It is therefore essential to understand that a negative x-ray does not rule out a stress fracture. Technetium radionuclide bone scans are quite sensitive to stress fractures, and can be positive as soon as 3 days after the onset of the injury. They represent the most cost-effective means to diagnose stress fractures. MR imaging is also very sensitive but is more expensive. In individuals symptomatic for a high-risk fracture, activity should be curtailed until a bone scan or MR imaging has been performed to confirm or rule out fracture.

Treatment

It is important that the patient understand the significance of the injury and its potential complications, in order to have compliance with treatment, because athletes who exercise with sufficient intensity to suffer a stress fracture are often reluctant to stop their activity. Stress fractures are treated with modified rest. Ambulation is permitted for the activities of daily living, but all other weight-bearing activities and skeletal loading must cease until symptoms have abated. Alternative forms of nonimpact activity are substituted. Cycling and swimming are recommended, and runners can run in the deep end of a pool. Aerobic dancers can still participate in the warmup, strengthening, and stretching segments of the workout but should ride a stationary cycle or rest during the hopping and bouncing portions of the workout. During the period of relative rest, underlying factors are corrected, and strength training is undertaken.

Return to Activity

Once the athlete has been pain free in normal daily activities for 14 days, he/she is allowed to gradually reintroduce weight-bearing activities, so long as this can be done on a pain-free basis.

Key Points

- Stress fractures are a common athletic injury.
- Clinical features include activity-related pain that might be poorly localized, night pain, and focal bony tenderness and swelling.
- Diagnosis depends on bone scans, CT,

or MR imaging with plain radiographs frequently normal, especially early.
- Treatment requires modified rest, symptomatic relief, correction of underlying factors, strengthening, and flexibility, with a gradual return to activity depending on symptoms.

REFERENCES

1. Matheson GO, Clement DB, McKenzie DC, et al: Stress fractures in athletes: A study of 320 cases. Am J Sports Med 15:46–58, 1987.
2. Matheson GO, Clement DB, McKenzie DC, et al: Scintigraphic uptake of ^{99m}Tc at nonpainful sites in athletes with stress fractures: The concept of bone strain. Sports Med 4:65–75, 1987.
3. Bennell KL, Malcolm SA, Thomas SA, et al: Risk factors for stress fractures in track and field athletes. Am J Sports Med 24:810–818, 1996.
4. Brukner P, Bennell KL: Stress fractures in female athletes: Diagnosis, management and rehabilitation. Sports Med 24:419–429, 1997.

Medial Tibial Stress Syndrome

Definition

Medial tibial stress syndrome (MTSS) is most often used synonymously with "shin splints," a common descriptive term for leg pain of musculotendinous origin. MTSS is common and may account for up to 18 percent of overuse syndromes, most commonly among athletes involved in running sports.[1] As with many syndromes, the precise source of the pain may be elusive with muscle, connective tissue, or periosteum variously implicated. It is now thought that MTSS represents one end of a continuum of bony stress injury, with a focal stress fracture representing the other.[2, 3]

Biomechanical factors were once thought to predispose to developing MTSS. Structural alignments including passive subtalar joint mobility, greater Achilles tendon angle, excess pronation, forefoot and rearfoot varus, and increased Q angle have been postulated to predispose to MTSS,[4–6] but well-controlled studies that carefully evaluated both injured and uninjured athletes cast some doubt on this hypothesis.[7]

Signs and Symptoms

Patients present with lower leg pain, which becomes progressive with continued activity. Pain initially begins preexercise, progressing to pain during and after exercise. If the activity continues, the pain will eventually become present during activities of daily living. If the athlete continues the offending activity, the injury may progress from a diffuse periostitis to a focal tibial stress fracture. Pain with daily activities helps to distinguish MTSS from chronic exertional compartment syndromes. Pain experienced more posteriorly in the calf may result from chronic exertional compartment syndrome of the deep posterior compartment, or popliteal artery entrapment syndrome.

Physical examination shows diffuse tenderness along the posterior medial aspect of the proximal metaphysis and diaphysis of the tibia, which may be exquisite.[8] Swelling or other objective physical findings are usually absent. Discrete, localized tenderness suggests focal stress fracture. Provocative tests of alternating active plantarflexion and dorsiflexion will be positive in compartment syndromes. Similarly, progressive pain with prolonged active plantarflexion or passive dorsiflexion suggests popliteal artery entrapment.

Imaging

Diagnostic imaging is able to differentiate MTSS from focal stress fracture. MTSS is usually a clinical diagnosis, but it is occasionally necessary to have a definitive diagnosis. The expense of the study must be balanced by the potential of a positive or negative test to change the immediate management of the patient. Plain radiography is generally not useful to diagnose MTSS, but it can confirm a focal stress fracture. Bone scans have been used to distinguish MTSS from stress fracture. MTSS is suggested by a diffuse, linear radioisotope uptake in the cortex, present only in the delayed static phase of the scan. Stress fractures show more focal uptake, as well as increased activity during the angiogram and blood pool phases.[2, 9] MR imaging has proved useful in differentiating MTSS from focal stress fractures. A grading system utilizing fat suppression, T2 and T1 imaging provides diagnostic and prognostic information superior to scintigraphy.[10] This grading system correlates well with a previously described scintigraphic scale and can assist in the clinical management of the highly performing athlete.[2, 11]

Treatment

Rest is the primary treatment modality for MTSS. Avoidance of the precipitating weight-bearing ac-

tivities while cross training in the pool is followed by use of the stationary bicycle, cross-country ski machine, or stair climber. Strengthening of the lower leg musculature is essential. Restoration of normal foot mobility is important. Progressive weight-bearing exercises are added as symptomatic recovery occurs. NSAIDs and local physical therapy modalities such as ultrasound may help provide symptomatic improvement. Orthotic devices to normalize foot position may be helpful.[5]

Surgical management of MTSS is controversial and seldom indicated. Posterior compartment fasciotomy and periosteal stripping procedures have produced mixed results, with little certainty that surgically treated patients can expect pain relief or return to a previous level of athletic activity.[12] If the patient fails to recover as expected, other diagnostic possibilities should be excluded before any consideration is given to surgery.

Return to Practice and Competition

The athlete can expect to return to a gradual training regimen as symptoms subside. The scintigraphic and MR imaging classification systems have been used to predict typical recovery times as 2 to 3 weeks in mild cases and up to 16 weeks for severe cases. Considering the high risk of recurrence, caution is necessary in outlining a progressive rehabilitation and training regimen. The athlete must restart activity using an alternating hard-easy program with gradual progression of frequency, duration, and intensity. Recurrence of symptoms should cause the athlete to reduce the activity level.

When to Refer

Referral for surgical opinion should occur in cases of uncertain diagnosis, or for patients in whom conservative treatment plans have failed, including adequate rest. Patients with other causes of lower leg pain, including exercise-induced chronic compartment syndrome and popliteal artery entrapment, should be referred to an appropriate surgeon. Consultation for biomechanical evaluation and orthotics should be considered if the practitioner does not offer such expertise.

Key Points

- Medial tibial stress syndrome is one of the most common athletic injuries.
- MTSS probably results from a diffuse periostitis and should be distinguished from focal tibial stress fractures, chronic compartment syndromes, and other vascular problems.
- Physical findings include diffuse tenderness along the length of the distal medial tibial border.
- Plain radiography is helpful if positive for focal stress fracture but is insensitive at distinguishing MTSS from early stress fracture.
- Triple phase bone scans or MR imaging can be helpful to clarify the diagnosis and provide prognostic clues to recovery.
- Rest from athletic activity remains the hallmark of treatment. Return to play should be gradual and very carefully directed to avoid symptom recurrence.

REFERENCES

1. Orava S, Puranen J: Athlete's leg pain. Br J Sports Med 13:92–97, 1979.
2. Batt ME, Ugalde V, Anderson MV, et al: A prospective controlled study of diagnostic imaging for acute shin splints. Med Sci Sport Exerc 30:1564–1571, 1998.
3. Matheson GO, Clement DB, McKenzie DC, et al: Stress fractures in athletes: A study of 320 cases. Am J Sports Med 15:46–58, 1987.
4. Vitasalo JT, Kvist M: Some biomechanical aspects of the foot and ankle in athletes with and without shin splints. Am J Sports Med 11:125–130, 1983.
5. Sommer HM, Vallentyne SW: Effect of foot posture on the incidence of medial tibial stress syndrome. Med Sci Sports Exerc 27:800–804, 1995.
6. Cowan DN, Jones BH, Frykman PN, et al: Lower limb morphology and risk of overuse injury among male infantry trainees. Med Sci Sports Exerc 28:945–952, 1996.
7. Ilahi OA, Kohl HW: Critical review: Lower extremity morphology and alignment and risk of overuse injury. Clin J Sport Med 8(1):38–42, 1998.
8. Beck BR, Osternig LR: Medial tibial stress syndrome. J Bone Joint Surg A 76:1057–1061, 1994.
9. Matin P: Basic principles of nuclear medicine techniques for detection and evaluation of trauma and sports medicine injuries. Semin Nucl Med 18(2):90–112, 1988.
10. Arendt EA, Griffiths HJ: The use of MR imaging in the assessment and clinical management of stress reactions of bone in high-performance athletes. Clin Sports Med 16(2):291–306, 1997.
11. Fredrickson M, Bergman G, Hoffman KL, Dillingham MS: Tibial stress reaction in runners: Correlation of clinical symptoms and scintigraphy with a new magnetic resonance imaging grading system. Am J Sports Med 23(4):472–481, 1995.
12. Abramowitz AJ, Schepsis A, McArthur C: The medial tibial syndrome: The role of surgery. Orthop Rev 23(11):875–881, 1994.

HIGH-RISK STRESS FRACTURES

Femoral Stress Fractures

Definition

Femoral stress fractures are relatively uncommon, accounting for less than 10 percent of stress fractures in a large series.[1] They can occur in the shaft or less commonly the neck of the femur. Femoral neck fractures are further subdivided, depending on the location and extent, into the superior, or tension side, and the inferior or compression side, and complete undisplaced transverse fractures. Femoral stress fractures can go on to completion with devastating consequences, including displacement and avascular necrosis of the femoral head. It is thought that tension side fractures of the femoral neck are at highest risk of progressing to completion. Unfortunately, some femoral stress fractures present acutely with displacement because the athlete or physician has ignored the warning signs of persistent and increasing pain. Physicians must maintain a high index of suspicion for stress fracture in any athlete with unexplained activity-related hip, groin, or thigh pain.

Signs and Symptoms

Femoral stress fractures may produce dull aching in the anterior or lateral hip with pain radiating down the leg. There is usually no point tenderness, due to the overlying musculature, although this can occasionally be found in shaft fractures in thin women. Gentle hopping on the affected leg will reproduce the hip pain, although this must be performed with caution in individuals who are acutely symptomatic. Femoral neck fractures can occasionally present with decreased hip flexion and internal rotation. The femoral fulcrum test may be a useful adjunct to diagnosis.[2] With the athlete sitting on the edge of the table, the examiner places an arm under the patient's thigh. The examiner's other hand places a downward force over the patient's knee, flexing the femur over the fulcrum created by the arm. The fulcrum (arm) can be moved proximally, with increased pain occurring when it is exactly below the site of the fracture.

Imaging

The results of imaging will depend on the stage of the fracture and duration of symptoms. Early fractures will have normal radiographs, and usually positive bone scans, although SPECT scanning may be necessary to demonstrate very early fractures. MR imaging is also sensitive and can demonstrate early stress fractures. As the fracture progresses, endosteal or periosteal reaction may appear on plain radiographs. Later, overt fracture lines may be apparent on either the tension or compression side, and may progress to a complete, nondisplaced fracture. Finally, stress fractures may present with a complete, displaced fracture of the femoral neck.[3, 4]

Treatment

The management of femoral stress fractures is controversial. Treatment options have included complete bed rest,[5] crutches and avoidance of weight bearing, or modified rest with avoidance of offending activities.[1] Bone scan positive, x-ray negative fractures can be treated with activity modification to eliminate impact activity, but allow pain-free activities of daily living. X-ray positive compression or tension side fractures can be treated similarly but these patients may require crutches until they are symptom-free in daily activity. Tension side fractures should probably be treated more conservatively, although some studies have shown no displacement of either type with this treatment.[4] It is essential that the patient understand the significance and potential complications of the injury and adhere to the activity restriction.

Surgical fixation of femoral neck stress fractures has been used in cases of both displaced and nondisplaced fractures.[3–5] Displaced fractures have a high risk of avascular necrosis and nonunion.[3, 4, 6] Clearly, diagnosis of femoral stress fractures is essential before the fracture completes or displaces.

Return to Competition

As already described, patients are allowed to resume a graded return to activity when they have been pain-free in normal weight-bearing activities

for 14 days. They may then begin a progressive walk-run program. This program breaks the activity period into 5-minute units, with 4 to 6 units (20 to 30 minutes) a common starting point. To start, the athlete walks for 4 minutes, then runs for 1 minute (W4–R1) during each of the 5-minute periods, and repeats this pattern for the allotted time. As the condition improves, the walking is gradually decreased, and the running increased (W3–R2, W2–R3, W1–R4, and finally R5, a return to full running), so long as this can be accomplished without pain.

When to Refer

Patients with x-ray positive fractures and any degree of displacement should be referred immediately. Other fractures can be managed by the primary care physician who has the requisite experience and confidence.

Key Points

- The physician must have a high index of suspicion for femoral neck stress fracture in any patient with unexplained activity-related groin or hip pain.
- Impact activity must be stopped until stress fracture has been ruled out.
- Radiographs are negative early, but a bone scan or MR imaging will be positive.
- Treatment is based on the fracture classification, depending on the bone scan and radiographic findings.
- Most stress fractures can be treated with activity modification, although some require surgical treatment.

REFERENCES

1. Matheson GO, Clement DB, McKenzie DC, et al: Stress fractures in athletes: A study of 320 cases. Am J Sports Med 15:46–58, 1987.
2. Johnson AW, Weiss CB, Wheeler DL: Stress fractures of the femoral shaft in athletes: More common than expected: A new clinical test. Am J Sports Med 22:248–256, 1994.
3. Johansson C, Ekenman I, Tornkrist H, et al: Stress fractures of the femoral neck in athletes: The consequence of a delay in diagnosis. Am J Sports Med 18:524–528, 1990.
4. Fullerton LR, Snowdy HA: Femoral neck stress fractures. Am J Sports Med 16:365–377, 1988.

5. Volpin G, Hoerer D, Groisman G, et al: Stress fractures of the femoral neck following strenuous activity. J Orthop Trauma 4:394–398, 1990.

6. Visuri T, Vara A, Meurman KOM: Displaced stress fractures of the femoral neck in young male adults: A report of twelve operative cases. J Trauma 28:1562–1569, 1988.

Focal Tibial Stress Fractures

Definition

Tibial stress injury presents as a continuum ranging from diffuse tibial periostitis (see previous discussion of MTSS) to focal tibial fractures associated with radiolucent defects on plain radiographs. MTSS presents with generalized anterior tibial pain. If impact activity is continued, progressive injury may result in a focal stress fracture of the posterior medial tibial border, most commonly at the junction of the proximal two-thirds and the distal one-third of the tibia. Fractures in this region are on the compression side of the tibia and usually behave relatively benignly without frequent or significant complications. They contrast with focal stress fractures of the anterior cortex of the midshaft of the tibia, which occur on the tension side of the bone. These anterior fractures have a high rate of delayed healing and nonunion and can progress to complete displaced fractures[1–4] and thus must be treated with caution. Repetitive push-off and landing has been proposed as a potential etiologic factor in the development of anterior stress fractures.[5]

Signs and Symptoms

Activity-related anterior tibial pain is the usual presentation. There is progressive pain with continued activity, and night pain may develop. The pain initially may be diffuse, but it will localize with continued activity. Physical examination reveals focal areas of tenderness over the anterior tibia, associated with local thickening and periosteal reaction. Hop test is positive. Lower leg musculature will often be weak.

Imaging

Radiographs reveal diffuse cortical thickening and periosteal elevation. Single or multiple transverse radiolucent lines extend about half way through the anterior cortex. In late cases, CT scanning may reveal sclerosis of the fracture edges suggestive of nonunion.

Treatment

Because of the potential for significant complications, it is essential to prevent the progression of MTSS to focal stress fractures. Patients with activity-related anterior tibial pain must reduce the level of impact activity until they are asymptomatic. Specifics of early treatment were previously outlined under stress fractures and MTSS.

Once an athlete has developed a radiolucent line on x-ray, it is essential to discontinue activity (especially collision, jumping, and cutting sports) in order to prevent the fracture from progressing to completion.[1, 3] Various conservative treatments have been proposed, including electromagnetic bone growth stimulators.[4] Surgery is often necessary and usually consists of curetting or drilling out the fracture and area of fibrous nonunion followed by bone grafting. Other authors have recommended intramedullary rodding,[6] but this should probably be reserved for failures of drilling and grafting. ORIF will be required for displaced fractures.

When to Refer

Most athletes with radiographic stress fractures of the anterior tibial cortex should be referred for a surgical opinion. Even if it is successful, nonsurgical treatment will be prolonged.

Key Points

- Focal stress fractures of the anterior tibial cortex associated with a radiolucent line on plain radiographs are prone to complications of delayed or nonunion, and progression to complete fracture.
- Prevention and activity restriction are the best early treatment to avoid progression to a focal fracture.
- Established fractures with a radiolucent line should be treated initially with rest and immobilization but will often require drilling and bone grafting.

REFERENCES

1. Beals RK, Cook RD: Stress fractures of the anterior tibial diaphysis. Orthopedics 14:869–875, 1991.

2. Orava S, Karpakka J, Hulkbo A, et al: Diagnosis and

treatment of stress fractures located at the midtibial shaft in athletes. Int J Sports Med 12:419–422, 1991.

3. Green N, Rogers R, Lipscomb B: Nonunions of stress fractures of the tibia. Am J Sports Med 13:171–176, 1985.
4. Rettig AC, Shelbourne KD, McCarroll JR, et al: The natural history and treatment of delayed union stress fractures of the anterior cortex of the tibia. Am J Sports Med 16:250–255, 1988.
5. Ekenman I, Tsai-Fetlander L, Westblad P, et al: A study of intrinsic factors in patients with stress fractures of the tibia. Foot Ankle Int 17:477–482, 1996.
6. Chang PS, Harris RM: Intramedullary nailing for chronic tibial stress fractures. Am J Sports Med 24:688–692, 1996.

Tarsal Navicular Stress Fractures

Definition

Tarsal navicular stress fractures are relatively uncommon in sports and rare in nonathletes. Tarsal navicular stress fractures account for up to 28.6 percent of all stress fractures in athletes,[1] and up to 35.2 percent of stress fractures in track athletes. They are common in running sports, particularly middle distance running, sprints, and hurdles,[2] but are also found in soccer, basketball, and racquet sports. Neither cavus nor planus foot structure has been shown to predispose to this injury; however, limitation of ankle and subtalar joint dorsiflexion has been implicated.[3] Diagnosis of a tarsal navicular stress fracture is often delayed many months.[3, 4] Therefore, a high index of suspicion for tarsal navicular stress fracture is necessary when treating any athlete with unexplained midfoot pain.

Signs and Symptoms

Patients present with the insidious onset of dorsomedial foot pain. The pain is worse with activity and becomes better with rest. Night pain may be present. Rarely, a history of inversion or trauma will be present. The pain may be poorly localized and radiate along the medial longitudinal arch, first or second metatarsal ray, or the dorsum of the midfoot. Some patients experience pain in the anterior ankle.

The hallmark finding on physical examination is tenderness to palpation over the dorsum of the navicular. The N spot, described by Brukner and Khan,[1, 2, 4] is located at the dorsalmost point of the navicular, slightly distal to the talonavicular joint and adjacent to the tibialis anterior tendon. Torg reported tenderness at this location in 17 of 21 patients with these fractures.[3] One-legged hopping may reproduce the pain.[5] In early cases, the patient usually demonstrates normal strength, symmetric range of motion, and absence of swelling. As pain progresses, there will be loss of strength and mobility.

Imaging

Tarsal navicular stress fractures are usually not well visualized on plain radiography, although close scrutiny of plain films may demonstrate sclerosis at the proximal articular border of the navicular.[6] Although radionuclide bone scans are very sensitive, they cannot differentiate between a bony stress reaction and a true stress fracture with cortical defect. The presence of a cortical defect is an important consideration for treatment, so a follow-up CT scan is necessary in cases with a positive bone scan. For this reason, proceeding with a CT scan as the initial diagnostic study may be more cost effective. All fractures occur in the middle third of the proximal aspect of the tarsal navicular. They usually occur as straight or curvilinear fractures in the sagittal plane. The majority of these fractures are incomplete, partial fractures extending from the dorsal cortex. A small percentage will completely transect the navicular, extending to the plantar cortex.[7] MR imaging does not provide substantive additional information to assist in managing these fractures but may be useful if the diagnosis is in question, as it may reveal other causes of midfoot pain.

Treatment

Most sports-related stress fractures are successfully treated by restricting impact and weight-bearing activity. This approach may work for a navicular stress injury shown on bone scan with no cortical defect seen on CT scan. Navicular stress fractures with a cortical defect rarely heal with this limited approach to treatment. Six to 8 weeks in an NWB cast has been shown to heal 86 percent of these fractures.[3, 4] Following cast immobilization, extensive rehabilitation to restore normal mobility of the ankle, subtalar, and midfoot joints will be required. Restoration of lower leg strength is essential.

Surgical treatment with screw fixation, bone grafting, or both is considered for initial treatment of complete or displaced fractures and as secondary treatment for failed nonsurgical treatment.

Return to Activity

NWB cast treatment usually allows athletes' return to play in an average time of 5.6 months following diagnosis. Aggressive efforts at joint mobilization, ankle flexibility, muscle strengthening, and gradual return to activity is implemented following cast removal. The progression of activity is determined by clinical examination and the patient's ability to run on a pain-free basis. The patient may experience periarticular soreness with return to activity; however, the absence of tenderness at the N spot is a sensitive test for clinical recovery. Repeat bone scan or CT is not helpful to gauge healing, as the radiographic abnormality may persist indefinitely despite clinical recovery.[2, 4]

When to Refer

Incomplete tarsal navicular stress fractures may be managed following protocols as stated in the treatment section. Displaced fractures and fractures that fail conservative treatment should be referred for surgical or prolonged nonsurgical management.

Key Points

- Tarsal navicular stress fractures present with poorly localized activity-related midfoot pain.
- A high index of suspicion is necessary for this diagnosis.
- CT scanning should be done early in suspected cases, as plain radiographs are frequently negative.
- Treatment of stress fractures associated with a cortical defect is prolonged NWB casting. Displaced fractures require open reduction and internal fixation.
- Functional rehabilitation and a gradual return to activity are required.

REFERENCES

1. Brukner P, Bradshaw C, Khan KM, et al: Stress fractures: A review of 180 cases. Clin J Sports Med 6(2):85–89, 1996.

2. Khan KM, Brukner PD, Kearney C, et al: Tarsal navicular stress fractures in athletes. Sports Med 17(1):65–76, 1994.
3. Torg JS, Pavlov H, Cooley LH, et al: Stress fractures of the tarsal navicular: A retrospective review of twenty-one cases. J Bone Joint Surg (A) 64(5):700–712, 1982.
4. Khan KM, Fuller PJ, Brukner PD, et al: Outcome of conservative and surgical management of navicular stress fracture in athletes. Am J Sports Med 20(6):657–666, 1992.
5. Fitch KD, Blackwell JD, Gilmour WN: Operation for nonunion of navicular stress fracture of the tarsal navicular. J Bone Joint Surg B 71:105–110, 1989.
6. Pavlov H, Torg JS, Freiberger RH: Tarsal navicular stress fractures: Radiographic evaluation. Radiology 148:641–645, 1983.
7. Kiss ZS, Khan KM, Fuller PJ: Stress fractures of the tarsal navicular bone: CT findings in 55 cases. AJR 160:111–115, 1993.

PATELLOFEMORAL PAIN

Definition

Patellofemoral pain (PFP) represents a spectrum of disorders of the patellofemoral (PF) joint, resulting in activity-related anterior knee pain. The exact source of the pain is unknown, although it is variously postulated to come from the subchondral bone, patellar retinaculum, and the synovium around the knee joint.[1] Other structures that are occasionally implicated are the patellar tendon origin, peripatellar plicas, and occasionally arthrosis of the PF joint.

There are numerous reported causes for PF pain, including bony problems such as dysplastic femoral condyles, and abnormalities of patellar size, shape, and height. It is thought that the underlying cause is poor patellar tracking with lateral tracking of the patella, leading to abnormal distribution of the PF joint reactive forces. Soft tissue causes would include generalized ligamentous laxity with poor patellar tracking, reduced patellar mobility with tethering of the lateral facet leading to lateral patellar compression syndrome, tightness of the hamstrings leading to increased PF joint reactive forces, and deficiency of the vastus medialis, leading to lateralization of the tracking. Biomechanical and alignment factors have been implicated in the genesis of PFP; however, this cause has not been supported by research.[2] Other factors include excess pronation, leading to obligatory internal torsion of the tibia on the femur and lateral tracking of the patella. Restrictions of hip, SI joint, or foot mobility frequently lead to patellar tracking abnormalities, reinforcing the notion that it is important to examine the entire kinetic chain in patients with overuse injuries.[3]

Signs and Symptoms

Activity-related anterior knee pain is the characteristic complaint. It is frequently worse with walking up stairs and is commonly associated with "theater knees," in which the patient's knees stiffen and become painful after being maintained in a flexed position for a prolonged period of time. Swelling is not uncommon; however, if swelling is severe or prolonged, consideration should be given to other intra-articular disorders. Pain is generally activity-related and subsides with rest. With continued activities, the pain may become constant and plague the athlete even during activities of daily living.

Patients with PFP often have pain with squatting. The pain generally is worse during the movement phase, and not in a deep squat. Pain localized to the joint line in a full deep squat is suggestive of meniscal injury. Local examination will generally demonstrate tenderness over the medial or lateral patellar retinaculum and patellar facets. Patellar mobility and tilting should be assessed. Mobility may be increased with excessive lateral or medial glide and patellar instability, or may be decreased, with significant tethering of the patella. Patellar tilt in the femoral sulcus should be assessed. An inability to tilt the lateral border of the patella above the horizontal plane of the condyles is a contributory factor to PF pain.[1] Patients with lateral subluxation and dislocation of the patella will also have a positive apprehension sign, in which the patient has a marked reaction to sudden attempts to subluxate the patella laterally.

Some physicians rely on the PF compression test, in which the patella is compressed into the sulcus while the quads are actively contracted, resulting in pain provocation. This test should be avoided because it will lead to pain in a high proportion of normal individuals and can cause significant pain in susceptible patients.

Retropatellar crepitus is common and may range from fine to rather coarse, which is palpable as well as audible. Patients with patellar tendinitis will have point tenderness at the origin of the patellar tendon from the lower pole of the patella. The patellofemoral joint can often refer pain to the medial joint line, especially the anterior third.

A biomechanical assessment is essential to identify factors underlying the PF pain. This is accomplished observing patellar tracking while the patient performs closed chain flexion of the knee. The patient stands with the feet 6 to 8 inches apart and then dorsiflexes at the ankle while flexing the knee. Normally, the center of the patella will track over the second metatarsal. In individuals with ideal alignment, the midpoint of the patella tracks approximately over the web space between the first and second toes in this position. If excessive pronation is present, then the midpoint of the patella often lies medial to the great toe. This results in increased lateral patellar tracking forces, which can lead to symptomatic PF problems. Both knees should track symmetrically. Unilateral abnormal tracking should alert the examiner to the possibility of a kinetic chain dysfunction, with abnormal mobility of the foot, hip, or SI joint on the affected side.

Imaging

Radiographs usually do not demonstrate any acute bony pathology. The Merchant view may show variations of PF anatomy such as lateral tracking and tilting of the patella, patellar subluxation, and a shallow femoral sulcus. PF arthrosis may be present, especially involving the lateral compartment. In cases of frank dislocation there will occasionally be osteochondral fragments in the lateral gutter or defects from the lateral condyle or the medial patellar facet. In adolescents, it is always important to carefully examine the radiographs for evidence of osteochondritis dissecans, which can present in a similar manner.

Treatment

In general, treatment for PF pain follows the same principles outlined previously for all overuse injuries. Extrinsic factors, such as training errors and footwear, should be addressed and corrected. Intrinsic factors such as muscle imbalances, inflexibility, and strength deficiencies should all be identified and remedied. When the symptoms are bilateral and the patellar tracking is abnormal but symmetric, custom orthotic foot beds may help correct excess pronation, normalize tracking, and alleviate the problem. Although not the definitive treatment, these devices certainly can play a role in part of a total management plan for this problem.

Kinetic-chain dysfunctions resulting in abnormal and asymmetric patellar tracking should be identified and treated. Restricted subtalar or talocrural joint motion should be restored. Tight hip capsules should be stretched and released. SI joint alignment and mobility should be normalized.

Stretching is used to improve the flexibility of the quadriceps and hamstrings. It is also important to stretch the iliotibial band, which sends insertions to the lateral retinaculum and may contribute to lateral tracking of the patella. The Achilles and heel cords should be stretched, as tightness decreases ankle dorsiflexion, resulting in increased pronation and PF joint reactive forces.

Strengthening is generally done using a graduated program of eccentric quadriceps strengthening drills in the form of a mini-squat. The patient stands with the feet approximately 8 inches apart and gradually slowly does a squat. This initially is done to a very minimal flexion angle of the knee. As the patient's tolerance to the activity progresses, the angle of the squat can be deepened and the velocity increased. Two cautions must be exercised. First, it should be stressed to the patient that the midpoint of the patella should be centered over the second toe throughout the entire squat. Second, the squats should be done without pain both during and after the exercise. If the exercises cause pain, then the patient should reduce the speed in the angle of the drop.

Patellar stabilizing sleeves work well in cases in which the individual has a hypermobile patella, especially if he/she has had problems with subluxations and/or dislocations. Individuals with lateral tracking and a very tight lateral retinaculum and decreased medial glide generally do not benefit from the sleeves and may in fact have their symptoms provoked. McConnell taping is useful in some patients. This uses a firm adhesive taping procedure to attempt to normalize the patellar position within the sulcus and allow for improved patellar tracking. Taping and bracing are not treatments in and of themselves, but they are only adjuncts to allow the patient pain-free mobility to improve the level of symptomatology while the rest of the treatment is undertaken.

When to Refer

The vast majority of patients with PFP respond to conservative treatment. Patients with abnormal patellar tracking, especially negative patellar tilt and restricted patellar mobility, may be candidates for lateral release if prolonged conservative treatment has failed.[1, 4] Patients with mechanical symptoms following trauma might likewise benefit from arthroscopic evaluation.

Key Points

- Patellofemoral pain is the most common overuse knee injury in runners.
- Patients complain of diffuse anterior and peripatellar pain, worse with activity.
- Treatment consists of normalization of patellar tracking, and the correction of kinetic chain dysfunctions, strength and flexibility.
- Surgery is rarely indicated.

REFERENCES

1. Fulkerson JP, Kalenak A, Rosenberg TD, et al: Patellofemoral pain. Chicago, AAOS Instructional Course Lectures, 1992, pp. 57–70.
2. Reid DC: The myth, mystic, and frustration of anterior knee pain. Clin J Sports Med 3(3):139–143, 1993.
3. Macintyre JG, Lloyd-Smith DR: Intrinsic factors in overuse running injuries. In Renstrom P (ed): International Olympic Committee Encyclopedia Series. 4. Sports Injuries: Basic Principles of Prevention and Care. Oxford, Blackwell Scientific Publications, 1994.
4. Kolowich PA, Paulos LE, Rosenberg TD, et al: Lateral release of the patella: Indications and contraindications. Am J Sports Med 18:359–365, 1990.

ILIOTIBIAL BAND FRICTION SYNDROME

Definition

The iliotibial band friction syndrome (ITBFS) is a common cause of lateral knee pain, especially in runners.[1, 2] This overuse syndrome is caused by friction between the posterior edge of the iliotibial band as it passes over the underlying lateral femoral condyle. The friction occurs maximally when the knee is flexed about 20 degrees in early stance phase of gait. Predisposing factors include tightness of the ITB, weakness of the hip abductors that allows tilting of the pelvis to the contralateral side, and SI joint dysfunction. Running on a steeply cambered road surface may increase the tension in the ITB, especially if the patient always runs on the same side of the road relative to traffic. ITBFS can be difficult to treat, with frequent recurrences as the athlete returns to running, if the underlying factors are left uncorrected.

Signs and Symptoms

Athletes present with lateral knee pain following a change in training, terrain, and footwear. The pain is in the vicinity of the lateral femoral condyle. Downhill running and hiking frequently provoke the symptoms of ITBFS.[3] Cross training on bicycle, stairmaster, or nonimpact type activity often does not cause pain. ITBFS is one of the few conditions that will stop runners in their tracks. Victims will often be able to continue walking or running so long as they maintain the affected leg in full extension.

Physical examination reveals significant tenderness over the lateral femoral condyle with crepitus and pain as the leg is passively flexed and extended. Less commonly, there will be tenderness over the distal IT band and Gerdy's tubercle. Maximal tenderness usually occurs when the knee is flexed to about 30 degrees. Ober's test for tightness of the IT band is helpful. This is accomplished with the patient sidelying with the affected side up. The examiner flexes the knee and then first abducts then extends the hip, and then lets the hip drop back into adduction in order to place the IT band under tension. A useful modification of this test can be performed by flexing and extending the knee in this position while pressing over the lateral femoral condyle. This position will usually reproduce the athlete's symptoms and is more sensitive than simple palpation over the condyle. Hip abductor musculature strength is almost universally reduced. SI joint dysfunction is frequently present.

Imaging

Plain radiographs are usually normal. MR imaging may assist the clinical diagnosis if there is any suggestion of an intra-articular process causing lateral knee pain.[4-6]

Treatment

Initial treatment for ITBFS consists of the PRICE principles. Stretching of the IT band can be accomplished by lateral trunk bending while standing. It is essential to correct SI joint dysfunction and restore adequate strength of the hip abductors. Transverse friction massage, NSAIDs, and occasionally corticosteroid injections can be used.[7] Biomechanical factors may be addressed with orthotics. Training errors should be corrected, including avoiding banked surfaces, alternating the direction of running on a track or cambered streets, and attention to shoe choice and wear. ITBFS is notorious for recurring in patients who return to running too soon, so it is essential to

gradually increase training stress and avoid sudden increases in training volume. Although surgery is rarely indicated, resection of a portion of the IT band can be quite successful in recalcitrant cases.[8]

Return to Activity

Most athletes respond to the preceding measures and return to training in a few days to weeks. Surgical referral is indicated when the symptoms do not respond to all conservative efforts, including substantial rest, and the patient still is unable to train for the sport activity adequately. Mild symptoms should not preclude an athlete from participating in important competition.

Key Points

- Iliotibial band friction syndrome occurs most often in runners.
- ITBFS is characterized by lateral knee pain, which is worse with downhill running or descending stairs.
- Maximum tenderness is over the lateral femoral condyle at 30 degrees of knee flexion.
- Treatment involves PRICE principles, NSAIDs, lateral stretching, hip abductor strengthening, correction of SI joint dysfunction, and occasionally corticosteroid injections.
- Biomechanical factors and training methodology must be reviewed and corrected.

REFERENCES

1. Linenger JM, West LA: Epidemiology of soft-tissue/musculoskeletal injury among U.S. Marine recruits undergoing basic training. Milit Med 157(9):491–493, 1992.
2. Jordaan G, Schwellnus MP: The incidence of overuse injuries in military recruits during basic military training. Milit Med 159(6):421–426, 1994.
3. Orchard JW, Fricker PA, Abud AT, Mason BR: Biomechanics of iliotibial band friction syndrome in runners. Am J Sports Med 24(3):375–379, 1996.
4. Ekman EF, Pope T, Martin DF, Curl WW: Magnetic resonance imaging of iliotibial band syndrome. Am J Sports Med 22(6):851–854, 1994.
5. Murphy BJ, Hechtman KS, Uribe JW, et al: Iliotibial band friction syndrome: MR imaging findings. Radiology 185(2):569–571, 1992.
6. Nishimura G, Yamato M, Tamai K, et al: MR findings in iliotibial band syndrome. Skeletal Radiol 26(9):533–537, 1997.

7. Schwellnus MP, Theunissen L, Noakes TD, Reinach SG: Anti-inflammatory and combined anti-inflammatory/analgesic medication in the early management of iliotibial band friction syndrome. A clinical trial. S Afr Med J 79(10):602–606, 1991.

8. Martens M, Libbrect P, Burssens A: Surgical treatment of the iliotibial band friction syndrome. Am J Sports Med 17:651–654, 1989.

TARSAL TUNNEL SYNDROME

Definition

Tarsal tunnel syndrome is a collection of symptoms in the foot and ankle analogous to carpal tunnel syndrome at the wrist. Although it is rare compared to carpal tunnel syndrome, it is the most common nerve entrapment syndrome in the foot. This symptom complex is characterized by predominantly sensory and sometimes motor symptoms to the plantar aspect of the foot, heel, and medial ankle due to compression of the tibial nerve or its branches as it courses through the tarsal tunnel on the medial side of the ankle.[1]

The fibro-osseous tarsal tunnel is bordered primarily by osseous structures of the foot, with the flexor retinaculum forming the roof. Static compression of the tibial nerve at the tunnel can be caused by any space-occupying mass intrinsic or extrinsic to the tunnel. Tumors, ganglion cysts, tenosynovitis, fractures, varicosities, and accessory or anomalous muscles and bone account for many of the anatomically identifiable causes of tarsal tunnel syndrome. Dynamic compression, unrelated to an anatomic lesion, can be due to biomechanical factors such as excessive pronation. Muscle engorgement with exercise can also transiently compress the tibial nerve. Medical causes of neuropathy such as diabetes, alcoholism, and hypothyroidism must also be considered.[2–4]

Signs and Symptoms

Patients present with a variety of sensory complaints. They may experience burning, numbness, tingling, parasthesias, or pain on the medial ankle or plantar heel and foot. The neurologic symptoms often radiate to the toes or proximally to the ankle and lower leg. Brief, intense, and sharp pain often begins with exercise and then resolves with cessation of activity. These symptoms may progressively worsen until they are present constantly with weight bearing, eventually leading to night pain. The patient may notice local swelling at the medial ankle.[2]

Pain may be reproduced by careful palpation along the entire course of the tibial nerve and its branches from a point proximal to the medial malleolus, across the retinaculum, and into the plantar aspect of the forefoot. Tinel's sign is elicited by tapping over the nerve as it courses through the tunnel. Symptoms may be exaggerated by forcing the foot into a dorsiflexed and valgus position. Atrophy of the intrinsic musculature of the foot can be a subtle but late finding.[5] Local nerve examination is accompanied by a complete neurologic examination of the lower extremities including the low back to rule out a proximal cause for the patient's symptoms.

Diagnosis

Diagnostic evaluation of the suspected tarsal tunnel syndrome requires consideration of the wide differential diagnosis. Laboratory tests to rule out rheumatologic diseases and other medical causes for peripheral neuropathy should be considered in light of the clinical findings. Electrodiagnostic studies can aid the clinical diagnosis. Motor and sensory function should be evaluated on the symptomatic side and compared to the contralateral nerve. When both sides are abnormal, comparison to accepted norms is necessary. Sensory deficits are more common than motor deficits.[5] Although a positive test can confirm the diagnosis, a negative test does not preclude tarsal tunnel syndrome.[6]

Imaging

Diagnostic imaging is necessary to rule out anatomic factors resulting in nerve compression. Radiographs can reveal degenerative changes, old fractures, bone spicules, and accessory ossicles.[5] MR imaging may demonstrate soft-tissue lesions such as neurilemomas, ganglion cysts, lipomas, post-traumatic fibrosis, or neuromas.[6]

Treatment

The treatment of tarsal tunnel syndrome depends on the underlying cause of the nerve compression and dysfunction. Many cases without clear anatomic nerve compression are due to mechanical compression and tensioning of the nerve by abnormal foot biomechanics and excess pronation. Conservative measures include NSAIDs, activity modification, and occasional local corticosteroid injections. Careful attention to the runner's biomechanics, including shoe modifications and orthoses is necessary for nonsurgical management success.[5] Surgical decompression with retinaculum release and nerve dissection is most successful when a space-occupying lesion is identified.[7, 8]

When to Refer

Patients with tarsal tunnel syndrome should be referred for a surgical opinion after the failure of an adequate trial of conservative measures.

Return to Activity

Return to practice and competition with nonsurgical management is based on symptom control and the identification and correction of any underlying factors. Gradual resumption of training is necessary.

Key Points

- Tarsal tunnel syndrome results in activity-related sensory and motor symptoms to the plantar aspect of the foot.
- Examination findings are consistent with nerve entrapment in the tarsal tunnel.
- Investigations may reveal underlying medical causes, anatomic nerve compression, and abnormal nerve conduction findings.
- Conservative care is directed at symptom relief and attention to abnormal biomechanics.
- Surgical management is used for cases recalcitrant to conservative efforts.

REFERENCES

1. Beskin J: Nerve entrapment syndromes of the foot and ankle. J Am Acad Orthop Surg 5:261–269, 1997.
2. Schon LC: Nerve entrapment, neuropathy, and nerve dysfunction in athletes. Orthop Clin North Am 25(1):47–59, 1994.
3. Sammarco GJ, Conti SF: Tarsal tunnel syndrome caused by an anomalous muscle. J Bone Joint Surg A 76(9):1308–1314, 1994.
4. Sammarco GJ, Chalk DE, Feibel JH: Tarsal tunnel syndrome and additional nerve lesions in the same limb. Foot Ankle 14(2):71–77, 1993.
5. Jackson DL, Haglund B: Tarsal tunnel syndrome in athletes: Case reports and literature review. Am J Sports Med 19(1):61–65, 1991.
6. Finkel JE: Tarsal tunnel syndrome. MRI Clin North Am 2(1):67–78, 1994.
7. Pfeiffer WH, Cracchiolo A: Clinical results after tarsal

tunnel decompression. J Bone Joint Surg A 76(8):1222–1230, 1994.
8. Stull PA, Hunter RE: Posterior tibial nerve entrapment at the ankle. Oper Tech Sports Med 4(1):54–60, 1996.

PLANTAR FASCIITIS

Definition

Plantar fasciitis is a very common overuse syndrome in running athletes. The plantar fascia originates on the plantar aspect of the calcaneus, runs anteriorly along the arch, and inserts on the base of the proximal phalanges. An understanding of the biomechanical forces applied to the plantar fascia may help identify predisposing conditions for plantar fasciitis.[1] At heel-off, dorsiflexion of the toes causes the plantar fascia to tighten, thereby raising the longitudinal arch, inverting the hindfoot, and externally rotating the leg, the so-called "windlass effect." This movement assists the foot in converting from the pronated, shock-absorbing position to the supinated position, which provides a rigid lever for the push-off phase of gait.[2] Although both the excessively mobile hyperpronated foot and the rigid cavus foot have been associated with increased risk of plantar fasciitis, runners' injuries are multifactorial, and it is often impossible to precisely identify cause-and-effect relationships.[3] Nerve entrapments, rheumatic disorders, and gout may predispose to or mimic the symptoms of plantar fasciitis, and should be considered in recalcitrant cases.

Signs and Symptoms

The main complaint is pain at the plantar aspect of the medial heel. The pain is worse with activity and particularly noticeable with the first few steps in the morning, with the initial minutes of running, after exercise, and after any period of inactivity and immobility. The pain of plantar fasciitis is often described as a "burning or aching" character that sometimes precludes sports or impairs activities of daily living.

Examination includes palpation of the plantar fascia followed by a general examination of foot structure and function. Maximum tenderness usually occurs at the origin of the plantar fascia from the medial calcaneal tuberosity. The examiner should also palpate along the course of the plantar fascia and longitudinal arch for other tender sites or nodules. Palpation of the plantar fascia while the toes are dorsiflexed may be more sensitive to reproduce symptoms. Tinel's sign over the tarsal tunnel may elicit paresthesias if the medial calcaneal nerve is entrapped.

The biomechanical examination attempts to identify the excessively mobile hyperpronated foot or the high arched pes cavus foot. The supple foot applies excessive traction forces to the plantar fascia, while the high arched foot dissipates shock poorly. Individuals with plantar fasciitis have been shown to have reduced static and dynamic range of motion and reduced lower leg strength in addition to the symptomatic plantar fasciitis.[4] Examination should therefore include an assessment of the mobility of the ankle, subtalar, and midfoot joints, with comparison to the uninjured side.

Imaging

Imaging studies are usually not required for a clinical diagnosis. If initial conservative treatment measures are not successful, roentgenograms will provide information about the bony structures of the foot. A calcaneal heel spur is often seen on lateral views of the foot. The significance of a heel spur is controversial, but most authorities agree that the bony spur is unlikely to be the source of the heel pain.[5] Many individuals with pain have no spurs, while others with spurs have no pain. Ultrasonography demonstrates thickened and hypoechoic fascia in those suffering plantar fasciitis when compared to control subjects.[6, 7] MRI may be useful for delineating a precise tissue diagnosis, although this usually has limited clinical value for management.[8, 9]

Treatment

The treatment of plantar fasciitis begins with the PRICE principles, along with the use of heel cups to improve intrinsic heel pad cushioning, simple arch supports, and supportive shoes (Fig. 12–5). Mobility must be restored to the ankle and subtalar and midfoot joints, and this alone may provide significant relief for many patients.[10] Strengthening of the intrinsic foot and lower leg musculature is recommended. A program of eccentric strengthening of the gastrocnemius-soleus complex is useful, as it also reintroduces eccentric tensioning to the plantar fascia.

If these measures fail, then custom orthotics, a short leg walking cast, corticosteroid injections, and night splints can be helpful.[11–14] Iontophoresis of dexamethasone may be helpful to the athlete needing to return to training promptly but has not

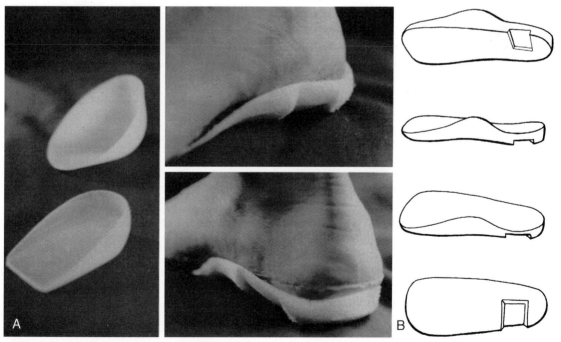

Figure 12–5. *A,* Over-the-counter heel cups designed to compress the fat pad and cushion the heel. *B,* Custom orthoses used for treatment of subcalcaneal pain syndrome. These may be made of many types of material. Consistent features are support of the arch, presence of cushioning material, recess for area of pain beneath the heel, and slight medial elevation. (From DeLee JC, Drez D Jr: Orthopaedic Sports Medicine: Principles and Practice, Vol. 3. Philadelphia, W. B. Saunders, 1994, p. 1826.)

demonstrated any discernible benefit compared with placebo at 1 month.[15] Corticosteroid injections are controversial because of concerns of fat pad necrosis and plantar fascia rupture.[16]

When to Refer

Surgical management for chronic plantar fasciitis should be reserved for the relatively few patients failing to respond to prolonged conservative measures.[17] Many cases of recalcitrant heel pain may be relieved surgically through plantar fascia release and spur removal, if the proper diagnosis is made and the most appropriate procedure performed.[18] Endoscopic plantar fascial release has been popularized but remains controversial.[17, 19] It is important to exclude proximal nerve entrapment producing heel pain and stress fractures of the calcaneus prior to surgery. Surgical complications include persistent numbness and neuroma or painful neural stump. A long-term concern for plantar fascia release is the effects on biomechanics. Cadaver surgeries and biomechanical modeling have demonstrated decreased arch stability and reduced foot stiffness, which may lead to future midfoot problems in those patients undergoing surgical release.[20-22]

Key Points

- Plantar fasciitis is characterized by inferior heel pain, which is worse in the morning, after inactivity, or upon initiating exercise.
- Maximum tenderness is at the origin of the plantar fascia on the calcaneus.
- Imaging studies are generally not required for diagnosis.
- Conservative therapy consists of PRICE principles; mobilization of talocrural, subtalar, and midfoot joints; strengthening; wearing heel cups, arch supports, custom orthotics, short leg walking cast, or night splints; and corticosteroid injections. These measures are successful in most cases.
- Surgical management is reserved for only the most recalcitrant cases.

REFERENCES

1. Chandler TJ, Kibler WB: A biomechanical approach to the prevention, treatment and rehabilitation of plantar fasciitis. Sports Med 15(5):344–352, 1993.
2. Kwong PK, Kay D, Voner RT, White MW: Plantar fasciitis: Mechanics and pathomechanics of treatment. Clin Sports Med 7(1):119–126, 1988.
3. Warren BL, Jones CJ: Predicting plantar fasciitis in runners. Med Sci Sports Exerc 19(1):71–73, 1987.
4. Kibler WB, Goldberg C, Chandler J: Functional biomechanical deficits in running athletes with plantar fasciitis. Am J Sports Med 19(1):66–71, 1991.
5. Bordelon RL: Heel pain. In DeLee JC, Drez D (eds): Orthopaedic Sports Medicine. Philadelphia, W.B. Saunders, 1994, pp. 1806–1830.
6. Wall JR, Harkness MA, Crawford A: Ultrasound diagnosis of plantar fasciitis. Foot Ankle 14(8):465–470, 1993.
7. Cardinal E, Chem RK, Beauregard CG, Pelletier M: Plantar fasciitis: Sonographic evaluation. Radiology 201(1):257–259, 1996.
8. Kier R: Magnetic resonance imaging of plantar fasciitis and other causes of heel pain. MRI Clin North Am 2(1):97–107, 1994.
9. Roger B, Grenier P: MRI of plantar fasciitis. Eur Radiol 7(9):1430–1435, 1997.
10. Macintyre JG, Palmer T: Treatment outcomes for plantar fasciitis. Unpublished data, 1999.
11. Gill LH, Kebzak GM: Outcome of nonsurgical treatment for plantar fasciitis. Foot Ankle Int 17(9):527–532, 1996.
12. Batt ME, Tanji JL, Skattum N: Plantar fasciitis: A prospective randomized clinical trial of the tension night splint. Clin J Sport Med 6(3):158–162, 1996.
13. Mizel MS, Marymount JV, Trepman E: Treatment of plantar fasciitis with a night splint and shoe modification consisting of a steel shank and anterior rocker bottom. Foot Ankle Int 17(12):732–735, 1996.
14. Powell M, Post WR, Keener J, Wearden S: Effective treatment of chronic plantar fasciitis with dorsiflexion night splints: A crossover prospective randomized outcome study. Foot Ankle Int 19(1):10–8, 1998.
15. Gudeman SD, Eisele SA, Heidt RS, et al: Treatment of plantar fasciitis by iontophoresis of 0.4% dexamethasone. A randomized double blind, placebo controlled study. Am J Sports Med 25(3):312–316, 1997.
16. Sellman JR: Plantar fascia rupture associated with corticosteroid injection. Foot Ankle Int 15(7):376–381, 1994.
17. Baxter DE: The heel in sport. Clin Sports Med 13(4):683–693, 1994.
18. Sammarco GJ, Helfrey RB: Surgical treatment of recalcitrant plantar fasciitis. Foot Ankle Int 17(9):520–526, 1996.
19. Kinley S, Frascone S, Calderone D, et al: Endoscopic plantar fasciotomy versus traditional heel spur surgery: A prospective study. J Foot Ankle Surg 32(6):595–603, 1993.
20. Thordarson DB, Kumar PJ, Hedman TP, et al: Effect of partial versus complete plantar fasciotomy on the windlass mechanism. Foot Ankle Int 18(1):16–20, 1997.
21. Kitaoka HB, Luo ZP, An KN: Effect of plantar fasciotomy on stability of arch of foot. Clin Orthop 344:307–312, 1997.
22. Arangio GA, Chen C, Kim W: Effect of cutting the plantar fascia on mechanical properties of the foot. Clin Orthop 339:227–231, 1997.

Chapter 13 | Back Injuries

CRAIG C. YOUNG, M.D.

The lower back is a common site of injury in athletes and nonathletes alike, with 5 to 35 percent of the population being injured each year and 60 to 90 percent being injured during their lifetime.[1-6] In 1990, lower back pain was the fifth most common reason for visiting a physician's office, accounting for almost 15 million office visits, over half of which were at a primary care physician's office.[7] Primary care physicians should be able to identify and treat most causes of lower back pain with a careful history and physical examination.

HISTORY TAKING GUIDELINES

The initial history should identify the onset, location, duration, and character of pain, as well as any aggravating or relieving factors, and treatments tried. Factors that must be considered when evaluating acute low back pain include the mechanism of and the forces involved in the injury. In the younger athlete, acute low back pain is frequently related to a traumatic event, which causes a contusion, muscle strain, or ligamentous sprain. In the older athlete, much lower forces caused by a simple overrotation of the trunk, such as occur with a golf stroke or backhanded swing in tennis, may be sufficient to cause a painful injury. Herniated disks are much more common in this older patient group.

Common locations for pain include the midline, paraspinal muscles, buttocks, and legs. Patterns of radiation and referral should be noted not only for pain but also for tingling and numbness. Radicular symptoms occur in specific dermatomal patterns with associated motor weakness and reflex and sensory changes. Pain radiating into the lower leg or foot suggests nerve root impingement.

Mechanical pain is aggravated by activity and relieved with rest, and tends to get progressively worse over the course of the day. People with mechanical pain often will favor certain positions.

Standing aggravates extension-related pain, whereas sitting aggravates flexion-related pain. Nonmechanical pain is independent of activity and often worse at night. Nonmechanical pain may be caused by tumor or infection and warrants a more aggressive investigation into its cause. Patients suffering from pain referred from vascular or visceral sources frequently shift positions in an attempt to relieve the pain.

A complete review of systems may identify potential intrinsic and extrinsic risk factors (Table 13–1) or raise the suspicion of nonmusculoskeletal causes of back pain (Table 13–2). Weight loss, night pain, and constitutional signs and symptoms may be associated with tumors or systemic disease. Alteration of bowel and bladder control may be related to cauda equina syndrome.

LOWER BACK STRAINS AND SPRAINS

Muscle strains and ligament sprains are very common and account for approximately one quarter of

---

Table 13–1
Potential Intrinsic and Extrinsic Risk Factors for Back Pain

Intrinsic Factors

Abnormal back curvature
    Excessive lumbar lordosis
    Scoliosis
Bony pathology
    Degenerative disk disease
    Leg length inequality
    Scheuermann's disease
    Spondylolysis
Hyper- or hypomobility
Muscle imbalance
Obesity
Older age
Poor conditioning

Extrinsic Factors

Improper equipment
Poor technique
Repetitive motions
Training errors

Table 13–2
Nonmusculoskeletal Causes of Back Pain

Referred pain from other organ systems	
Aortic dissection	Neoplasm
Abdominal aortic aneurysm	Intraspinal tumors
Cardiac disease	Metastatic tumors
Myocardial infarction	Primary bone tumors
Gastrointestinal disorders	Neurologic diseases
Pancreatitis	Demyelinating diseases
Pancreatic cancer	Neuropathies
Peptic ulcer disease	Transverse myelitis
Ruptured abdominal viscus	Pulmonary diseases
Gynecologic disorders	Pneumonia
Ectopic pregnancy	Spontaneous pneumothorax
Hematocolpos	Urologic disorders
Pelvic inflammatory disease	Prostatitis
Tumors	Urinary disorders
Hip pathology	Nephrolithiasis
Infections	Pyelonephritis
Diskitis	Ureteral colic
Epidural abscess	Vascular disorders
Osteomyelitis	**Other nonmusculoskeletal causes**
Metabolic diseases	Abusive relationship
Gout	Compensable injury
Hyperparathyroidism	Conversion disorder
Osteoporosis	Depression
Paget's disease	Disability seeking
	Drug seeking
	Psychiatric disorder
	Somatoform disorder

all physician visits for lower back pain.[8] Sports that involve extensive or repetitive twisting motions (e.g., baseball, golf, gymnastics), repetitive extension and flexion motions (e.g., football, swimming), weight-lifting activity (e.g., ballet, pairs figure skating), or maintenance of a flexed position for extended periods (e.g., bicycling, downhill racing) place an athlete at risk for muscle strains and ligament sprains. The most common location for a muscle strain in the lower back is in the distal tendons of the paraspinal muscles in the lower lumbosacral and iliac crest areas. Common locations for ligament sprains in the lower back include the supraspinous, interspinous, and iliolumbar ligaments. Localized tissue damage results in bleeding and causes muscle spasm, swelling, and tenderness in the region of the injury.

History

The history is usually of sudden onset of pain after an incident that often has involved sudden motion and poor body mechanics. Occasionally,

muscle strains in athletes will result from overuse and present with a more gradual onset of pain. In either case, pain is usually aggravated by specific motions and activities. The pain may radiate into the buttock or upper posterior thigh, but it rarely radiates below the knee.

Physical Examination

Muscle spasms, limited range of motion, and a functional scoliosis are frequently found on examination. Usually the diagnosis is clinically apparent and no imaging is needed on initial evaluation. Plain radiographs should be considered if the mechanism of injury suggests possible fracture or if the injury is not responding to appropriate treatment.

Treatment

The treatment of acute muscle spasms is controversial. Most athletic trainers prefer ice and stretching, but a sizable group prefer heat and stretching. Ice causes local vasoconstriction, which results in minimizing the aggravation of inflammatory mediators at the injury site. Heat causes local vasodilatation, which results in increased blood flow and increased plasticity and flexibility of the tissue. However, the effects of heat and ice have not been well studied in the treatment of muscle spasms.

Acute lower back strains and sprains are treated with modified activity, avoiding aggravating motions. Nonsteroidal anti-inflammatory drugs (NSAIDs) may be used in more severe cases. Bed rest has not been shown to be very effective at treating back pain and should be limited to less than 2 days, if used at all, because immobility leads to rapid cardiovascular deconditioning.[9] Muscle relaxants should also be avoided in most cases. They are occasionally useful for individuals who are having difficulty sleeping, but side effects such as sedation, dizziness, and nausea frequently preclude their use. In some cases of chronic strains, the use of modalities such as ultrasound and transcutaneous electric nerve stimulation (TENS) may prove to be beneficial. The usual course and recovery time from an acute muscle strain is days to weeks; nearly all will heal within 2 months.[2, 6, 10, 11]

Long-term management and prevention include a strengthening, stretching, and posture program that emphasizes abdominal strengthening, proper posture, and hamstring flexibility. Athletes should make sure that they are adequately warmed up prior to activities, because basic science studies have shown that connective tissue has greater plasticity at higher temperatures and is able to withstand greater forces before sustaining damage.

Referral

Referral to a musculoskeletal specialist should be considered if the problem does not respond to appropriate treatment and in chronic recurrent cases, especially in the adolescent athlete, who is rarely seen in the physician's office for lower back strain.[8, 12] Referral to a physical therapist or an athletic trainer to provide proper instruction should be strongly considered if the physician is not comfortable in instructing the athlete in a rehabilitation program. Most teams at the college level and many teams at the high school level have their own athletic trainers.

Return to Practice and Competition

The athlete should start cross training as soon as possible to maintain cardiovascular conditioning and may return to activities as pain tolerance permits. Functional drills should be used to test an athlete's ability to return to activity.

Key Points

- Lower back strains and sprains usually resolve within 2 months.
- Muscle strains are relatively rare in the pediatric age group.
- Limit bed rest to 2 days.
- Emphasis should be placed on preseason conditioning and pregame warmup to prevent lower back strains and sprains.

SCIATICA

Sciatica is radicular pain that radiates down the leg in a dermatomal pattern owing to nerve root irritation. The most frequently involved nerves are the L5 and S1 nerve roots. Because sciatica is relatively rare in young athletes, other causes such as ring apophysitis should be considered.[8, 12, 13]

Disk herniation and bony hypertrophy are the most common causes of sciatica in athletes between 40 and 65 years of age. For athletes over 65 years old, degenerative osteophytes are the most common cause of sciatica.[14] Other causes to consider include spinal stenosis, lumbar facet syndrome, and tumors.

History

Patients with sciatica often complain of pain that is aggravated by coughing, deep breathing, laughing, and straining with bowel movements. Up to 10 percent of patients with L5 or S1 nerve irritation experience only leg pain with no back pain.[15] Cauda equina syndrome is caused by a large central disk herniation compressing the cauda equina. This rare condition is a surgical emergency, which requires decompression of the nerve to prevent permanent loss of function. Cauda equina syndrome should be suspected in the presence of (1) saddle anesthesia, which is the reduction of sensation over the buttocks, upper posterior thighs, and perineum; (2) urinary retention; or (3) back pain that is more prominent than radicular symptoms. Other signs and symptoms associated with cauda equina syndrome include bilateral leg weakness, bilateral leg pain, loss of bowel or bladder control, and impotence.

Physical Examination

Nerve root tension signs, which include the straight leg test, crossed straight leg test, and prone knee bending test, are useful in reproducing sciatic pain. The *straight leg test* is performed with the pelvis in a stable fixed position and the knees extended (Fig. 13–1). The straight leg test is positive if raising the leg between 35 and 70 degrees of hip flexion reproduces radicular symptoms. Dural motion occurs between 35 and 70 degrees; above 70 degrees the sciatic nerve is completely stretched.[16] Pain at less than 35 degrees is frequently caused by hamstring and other soft-tissue tightness, whereas pain at greater than 70 degrees is from the lumbar or sacroiliac joints. The sensitivity of the straight leg test for detection of nerve root compression is 80 percent, but specificity is only 40 percent.[17] When a positive straight leg test is caused by nerve root irritation, the location of the lesion is most likely at the L5, S1, or S2 level.[16] To further confirm a sciatic source of pain, have the patient lower the leg from the

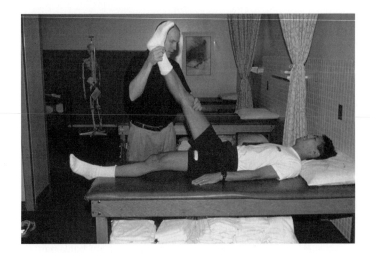

Figure 13–1. Straight leg test.

height at which the straight leg raise sign was positive until the symptoms resolve, then dorsiflex the foot, which should reproduce the radicular symptoms.

The *crossed straight leg* or well straight leg test is a more specific (75 versus 40 percent for the straight leg test) but less sensitive (25 versus 80 percent) measure of sciatic irritability.[17] A positive crossed straight leg test frequently indicates a large disk protrusion, usually medial to the nerve root.[16] The patient is placed in the same position as described for the straight leg test. The test is positive when raising the asymptomatic leg reproduces radicular symptoms in the symptomatic leg. The *prone knee bending test* or femoral stretch test is most useful for evaluations of a higher nerve root irritation (L2 to L4), the femoral nerve, or vascular claudication. The patient lies prone with the hip in neutral position while the examiner

places the knee in maximum flexion (Fig. 13–2). A positive test reproduces the radicular pain. Absence of peripheral pulses in this position suggests vascular claudication.

The *L4 nerve root* innervates the dermatome that includes the medial ankle and anterior shin (Fig. 13–3). The patellar reflex is predominately an L4 function (Table 13–3). L4 motor function is tested by resisting ankle dorsiflexion and inversion. The *L5 nerve root* is associated with a dermatome that includes the lateral calf and the first dorsal web space (Fig. 13–3). The L5 nerve root has no easily reproducible reflex in most patients; however, a medial hamstring reflex or a peroneal reflex has been found by some clinicians to be useful. L5 motor function is tested by resisting great toe extension (Table 13–3). The *S1 nerve root* is associated with a dermatome that includes the lateral foot (Fig. 13–3). The Achilles tendon

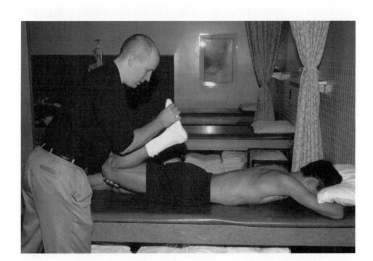

Figure 13–2. Prone knee bending test.

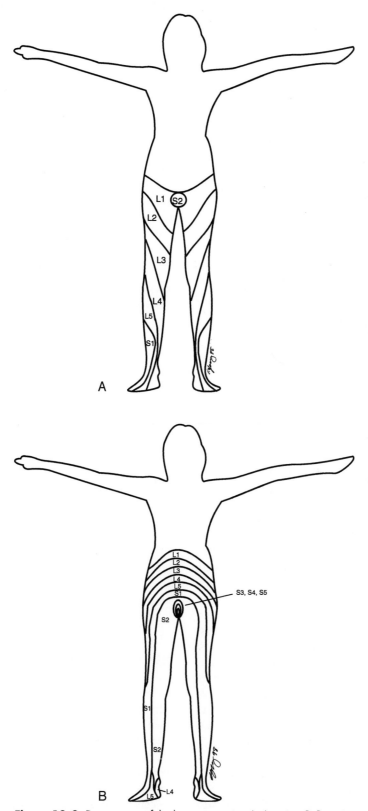

Figure 13–3. Dermatomes of the lower extremity. *A,* Anterior. *B,* Posterior.

Table 13–3
Neurologic Examination of the Lower Extremities

Root	Reflex	Muscles	Sensation
L4	Patellar	Tibialis anterior	Medial ankle and medial leg
L5	None*	Extensor hallucis longus	First dorsal web space and lateral leg
S1	Achilles	Peroneus longus and brevis	Lateral foot

*A medial hamstring reflex or a peroneal reflex has been found useful by some clinicians.

reflex is predominately an S1 function. S1 motor function is tested by resisted plantar flexion and eversion of the foot (Table 13–3).

Imaging

Usually the diagnosis is clinically apparent and imaging is rarely needed on initial evaluation. Plain radiographs should be considered if the mechanism of injury suggests a possible fracture or if the injury is not responding to appropriate treatment. Plain radiographs may be useful for evaluating fracture, infection, tumor, or impinging osteophytes. Bone scans provide relatively non-specific information, but they may be useful for evaluating metastatic disease, osteomyelitis, and reflex sympathetic dystrophy. Other special tests are indicated only if the results will change patient management; the decision to obtain additional testing is often best left to musculoskeletal specialists.

Treatment

Treatment of sciatica depends on the cause. Most cases will respond to conservative treatment with relative rest, NSAIDs, and physical therapy. A few days of bed rest may prove helpful, but longer periods should be avoided because of adverse effects on the athlete's cardiovascular fitness, strength, flexibility, and athletic skills.[2, 17–19] Most causes of sciatica, in the absence of cauda equina syndrome, resolve spontaneously. Almost half of the patients will recover in a month.[6] Conservative treatment for up to 3 months can be used to treat individuals with stable neurologic symptoms without adversely affecting the outcome.[20]

Referral

Patients in whom cauda equina syndrome is suspected should be referred for an emergency surgical consultation. Patients with worsening neuro-logic symptoms despite treatment should be referred for further evaluation. Patients with stable neurologic symptoms usually respond quite well to conservative management and need referral only after a prolonged course of conservative treatment with unsatisfactory results.

Return to Practice and Competition

The athlete should start cross training as soon as possible to maintain cardiovascular conditioning and may return to activities as pain permits.

Key Points

- Sciatica usually resolves within 3 months.
- Patients with stable neurologic symptoms usually respond to conservative management.
- Limit bed rest to 2 days.
- Patients with saddle anesthesia, bilateral leg weakness and pain, loss of bowel or bladder control, urinary retention, and impotence may have cauda equina syndrome and should be referred for an emergency surgical consultation.

HERNIATED DISK

A herniated disk occurs when the central semigelatinous nucleus pulposus extends through a weakened section of the outer fibrous annulus fibrosis. The 30- to 50-year-old athlete is most likely to suffer a herniated disk because of the combination at this age of a relatively large nucleus pulposis and a relatively weak annulus fibrosis. Over 90 percent of all disk herniations are in a posterolateral direction in either the L4 or L5 disk, which usually causes compression of the L5 and S1 nerve roots, respectively.[21, 22] Activities that repetitively load the back as well as a genetic predisposition place an athlete at increased risk for degenerative disk disease.[23–26]

History

The pain related to a herniated disk usually occurs in the absence of a specific traumatic event. Patients with herniated disks usually describe 24 to 48 hours of localized lower back pain followed by the onset of radicular pain.[27] Most patients will complain of radicular pain aggravated by sitting and relieved by lying down. The radicular patterns are described in the earlier section on sciatica. A careful review of systems should include questions about saddle anesthesia, bilateral leg weakness and pain, loss of bowel or bladder control, urinary retention, and impotence, which are all signs and symptoms associated with cauda equina syndrome.

Physical Examination

Athletes with a herniated disk will often develop a listing posture to alleviate nerve root irritation. The athlete will lean away from the side of more common posterolateral disk herniation or toward the side of the rarer medial disk herniation. This listing posture also causes an asymmetry in forward flexion and in lateral bend range of motion. Usually, radicular signs and positive nerve root tension signs are found as described in the sciatica section and in Table 13–3.

Imaging

Imaging is rarely needed on initial evaluation. Plain radiographs will not show the herniated disk and should be considered only if the diagnosis is not clear or if the injury is not responding to appropriate treatment. Occasionally, computed tomography (CT) or magnetic resonance (MR) imaging is useful in evaluating patients who are not responding to treatment, but in most cases these tests are more cost effective when ordered by specialists who may consider ordering them to appraise a person's surgical options.

Treatment

Most patients with herniated disks will eventually respond to conservative management.[20, 28] Conservative management usually starts with NSAIDs or analgesics and may include a few days of bed rest. As previously noted, prolonged bed rest should be avoided. Traction has been shown to provide relief in some cases. Posture and sports maneuvers should be analyzed for flaws, and corrections should be made if necessary. A strengthening and stretching program of the back, abdomen, and extremities should be prescribed. Running may often be continued because the lumbar spine receives less than 5 percent of ground reaction forces during this activity. Drills specific to the patient's sport, if they do not aggravate the back, should be continued as well. The usual time for resolution depends on the location and size of the herniation and may range from 6 to 24 weeks or longer.

Referral

Five to 10 percent of patients with a herniated disk may eventually require surgery.[20, 28] Although studies have found that the outcomes of surgical and conservative management are similar, surgical treatment appears to offer a more rapid resolution of symptoms.[20, 28–31] Because many athletes have a limited sporting career, they may choose the higher-risk, more invasive surgical treatment in order to speed recovery.

Return to Practice and Competition

Athletes should have near-normal strength and range of motion and be able to pass sport-specific functional drills prior to return to full sporting activity.

Key Points

- Patients with stable neurologic symptoms usually respond to conservative management.
- Limit bed rest to 2 days.
- Patients with saddle anesthesia, bilateral leg weakness and pain, loss of bowel or bladder control, urinary retention, and impotence may have cauda equina syndrome and should be referred for an emergency surgical consultation.

FACET SYNDROME

Facet syndrome is recurrent irritation of the facet joint with associated synovitis. The joint irritation results from bony hypertrophy, osteophytes, and the loss of disk space associated with degenerative disk disease. Irritation may also be caused by repetitive extension and rotation.

History

A typical patient with facet syndrome is an older athlete who complains of intermittent episodes of midline lower back pain. Occasionally the pain is referred to the buttock and the posterior thigh. The patient may have a history of twisting the spine or lifting in rotation followed by acute onset of pain.

Physical Examination

On examination patients exhibit findings similar to those of herniated disks, although frequently with more diffuse lower back pain. The pain is often aggravated by extension or rotation of the spine. Motion is limited and painful toward the involved side.

Imaging

Plain radiographs are useful for evaluation of bony changes, including the bony hypertrophy, osteophytes, and the loss of disk space associated with degenerative disk disease. CT scans may show bony impingement.

Treatment

Acute pain is usually controlled with NSAIDs and rest. In recalcitrant cases, referral for a facet injection with cortisone may be useful.[12, 32] Other potential treatments include traction, mobilization, and manipulation.[33] Sporting techniques should be analyzed for flaws, and corrections should be made if necessary. Athletes with facet syndrome should learn to recognize the early signs of pain associated with facet syndrome and start early prophylactic treatment with NSAIDs and activity modification.[33]

Referral

Referral to a specialist should be considered in recurrent or recalcitrant cases.

Return to Practice and Competition

The athlete should start cross training as soon as possible to maintain cardiovascular conditioning and may return to activities as pain permits.

Key Points

- Sporting techniques should be analyzed for flaws, and corrections should be made if necessary.
- Athletes should learn to recognize the early signs and start early prophylactic treatment with NSAIDs and activity modification.

SPONDYLOLYSIS AND SPONDYLOLISTHESIS

A spondylolysis is a stress fracture that results in a defect in the pars interarticularis. Forty to 50 percent of lower back pain in young athletes is caused by a spondylolitic lesion.[8, 34, 35] Athletes in sports that expose them to repetitive extension and flexion (e.g., gymnastics, ballet, rowing, and diving) or to repetitive hyperextension of the back (e.g., football) are at increased risk. Other risk factors include genetic predisposition and developmental defects.[12, 36, 37] The most frequent location of spondylolysis is at the L4 or L5 level.[37]

A spondylolisthesis is a bilateral pars interarticularis defect that results in forward displacement of the superior vertebral body in relation to the inferior vertebral body. Spondylolisthesis is graded by percentage of slippage: grade I represents 0 to 25 percent slippage; grade II represents 25 to 50 percent slippage; grade III represents 50 to 75 percent slippage; grade IV represents 75 to 100 percent slippage.

In general, female athletes have lower bone mass than males; therefore, women are at higher risk for stress fractures. The review of systems for female athletes should include questions about their menstrual history. Important information to investigate includes date of menarche and history of periods of amenorrhea or oligomenorrhea. Both amenorrhea and oligomenorrhea have been associated with an increased risk of stress fractures. Other questions should investigate calcium intake.

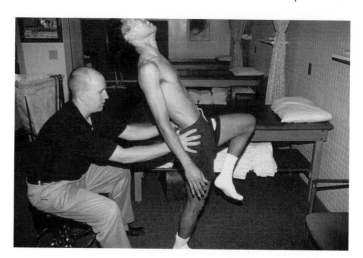

Figure 13–4. One-legged hyperextension test.

History

Rarely is an acute injury associated with a spondylolitic lesion; instead, there is a gradual worsening of pain with continued activity. Spondylolitic pain is primarily aggravated by hyperextension activity.

Physical Examination

The athlete often has an area of point tenderness over the spine. The pain is reproduced by back extension. This pain is worsened with hyperextension while standing on the ipsilateral leg (one-legged hyperextension test, Fig. 13–4). The athlete may also have pain with flexion and rotation away from the side of the lesion and lateral bending toward the side of the lesion. A step-off may be palpated over the spine in athletes with spondylolisthesis. With either type of lesion, athletes may have hamstring tightness or spasm secondary to a postural reflex.[36, 37]

Imaging

Oblique lumbar films may reveal the classic "Scottie dog" deformity, which consists of a decapitation of the Scottie dog at the neck (Fig. 13–5). Although this classic finding may not be visible on plain radiographs until 3 to 6 weeks after the onset of back pain, a three-phase bone scan will be positive within 24 hours 95 percent of the time and should be considered if the clinical index of suspicion is high.[11, 27, 37]

Spondylolisthesis is usually visible on a lateral lumbar radiograph. An inverted "Napoleon's hat" sign may be visible on the anteroposterior (AP) radiograph.

Treatment

The key to treating spondylolysis is modification of activity. Some physicians use a rigid lumbosacral brace to treat athletes with hot bone scans.[27, 37–39] The athlete is allowed to resume sporting activity while wearing the brace when the athlete becomes asymptomatic, usually approximately 3 weeks after starting treatment. Use of the brace is continued until there is radiologic evidence of healing or the bone scan becomes cold. Bracing does not appear to improve the treatment outcome in patient with bone scans that are initially negative.[33, 37] Patients should also be

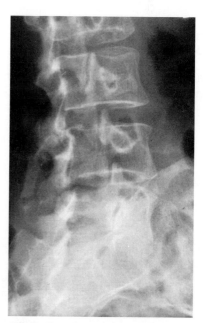

Figure 13–5. The "Scottie dog" deformity associated with spondylolisthesis.

placed in a physical therapy program that emphasizes strengthening the abdomen and the back and stretching the lower extremities. The posture and sporting techniques of the athlete should be analyzed and corrected if necessary.

For patients with an inactive spondylolysis or with a spondylolisthesis, treatment consists of activity modification and a physical therapy program as just described. The posture and sporting techniques of the athlete should be analyzed and corrected if necessary. For athletes with grade I spondylolisthesis, there is no evidence that participation in contact sports is related to progression of slippage.[27, 37] Athletes with grade II or higher spondylolisthesis should be counseled about the risk of increased slippage with continued activity; however, they should not be unilaterally excluded from sports. Athletes with grade II or higher spondylolisthesis who choose to continue participation in high-risk activities should be followed with annual radiographs until they reach skeletal maturity. Both spondylolysis and spondylolisthesis usually become stable after skeletal maturity is reached.[37]

Referral

Referral to a musculoskeletal specialist should be strongly considered with athletes who want to remain active during treatment.

Return to Practice and Competition

Sporting activity is allowed while wearing the brace when the athlete becomes asymptomatic, usually approximately 3 weeks after initiating treatment.

Key Points

- Obtain oblique lumbar spine films if spondylolysis is suspected. Consider bone scans if plain films are negative but spondylolysis is highly suspected.
- Both spondylolysis and spondylolisthesis usually become stable after skeletal maturity is reached.

- Athletes with grade II or higher spondylolisthesis who choose to continue participation in high-risk activities should be followed with annual radiographs until skeletal maturity is reached.

SCOLIOSIS

Scoliosis is lateral curvature of the spine greater than 10 degrees. Scoliosis is found in up to 5 percent of the population, and is seen more frequently in females with late menarche (i.e., gymnasts and ballet dancers).[40–42] The cause is idiopathic in 80 percent of the cases.[40] However, there is a strong genetic predisposition, with a positive family history in 70 percent of the cases.[40] Because most cases of scoliosis are asymptomatic, the deformity is usually first detected in young adolescents on routine preseason screening.

Physical Examination

Shoulder asymmetry is often the first noted sign of scoliosis. A rib hump can be accentuated by having the athlete lean forward. In some cases the lateral curvature of the spine can be seen in the standing athlete.

Imaging

If an inclinometer placed at the apex of the curve with the athlete bending forward measures 5 degrees or less, radiographs are probably not needed. The Cobb method of curve measurement is usually performed on a standing posteroanterior (PA) spine radiograph.

Treatment

A skeletally immature athlete with mild scoliosis is followed clinically every 4 to 6 months until skeletal maturity is reached or the curve reaches 25 degrees. Scoliosis is usually treated with bracing once the curve reaches 25 degrees or if it is progressing rapidly. Surgical stabilization is usually considered when the curve reaches 40 degrees.

Usual Course

Most cases of scoliosis are mild, have minimal progression, and do not require any treatment other than clinical follow-up.

Referral

Patients with scoliosis that is moderate (greater than 25 degrees), rapidly progressing (greater than 10 degrees per year), or severe (greater than 40 degrees) should be referred to a pediatric orthopedic surgeon.

Clearance

Patients with mild scoliosis are not restricted from sports. Patients who are braced may participate in sports while wearing their brace. Patients who have had a spinal fusion should be counseled against participating in collision sports, contact sports, gymnastics, and diving.[43] Patients with a short spinal fusion may in some cases be allowed to participate in light contact sports at the discretion of the spine surgeon.

Key Points

- In general, patients with mild scoliosis are allowed to participate in unrestricted activity.
- Follow patients with scoliosis closely with sequential curve measurements, and refer to a specialist if necessary.

ANKYLOSING SPONDYLITIS

Ankylosing spondylitis is a seronegative spondyloarthropathy that affects both the peripheral and axial skeleton.

History

The most common presentation is in young men in their late teens who complain of gradually worsening morning stiffness and of lower back pain. The pain is initially concentrated in the thoracolumbar area, but gradually spreads throughout the spine. The pain is aggravated by sudden motions and only partly relieved by rest.

Physical Examination

Decreased chest expansion and decreased spinal flexibility are seen on examination. A Schober test can be used to measure decreased spinal flexibility (Fig. 13–6). A mark is placed over the spine at the level of the posterior superior iliac spine. A second mark is placed 10 cm above this level and a third mark is placed 5 cm below the first mark. The distance between these marks is measured as the patient attempts to touch his/her toes. The distance between the end marks will be at least 20 cm in persons with normal flexibility.[10]

Imaging and Laboratory Tests

Initially, plain radiographs will appear normal, but with time the vertebral bodies become squared. Eventually, widespread development of syndesmosphytes along the lateral and anterior surfaces of the intervertebral disks completes the characteristic appearance of "bamboo spine." Finally, the sacroiliac joints narrow and fuse. A bone scan is usually positive at the sacroiliac joints. Most individuals who develop ankylosing spondylitis are HLA-B27 antigen positive.

Treatment

Treatment includes postural and breathing exercises and avoidance of painful activities. Treatment of exacerbations is with NSAIDs.

Clearance for Return to Play

Patients with mild ankylosing spondylitis usually have no restrictions placed on sports activities. However as ankylosing spondylitis becomes more advanced, the spine becomes more rigid and osteoporotic and may be at increased risk for fractures.[44, 45] Thus, individuals with advanced ankylosing spondylitis should avoid participation in collision sports and other high-impact loading sports (e.g., vaulting, high jumping).

SCHEUERMANN'S DISEASE

Kyphosis or roundback deformity is a compensatory posture seen in children who have inflexibility of the back muscles and tight hamstrings. In most cases the deformity is only postural and transient. However, some patients develop anterior

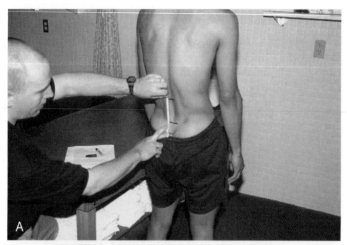

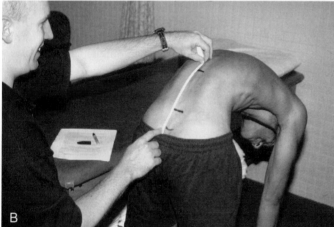

Figure 13–6. The Schober test.

wedging of the vertebral bodies. Scheuermann's disease is the development of three or more consecutive vertebrae with anterior wedging of greater than 5 degrees. The disease is usually diagnosed in adolescents and has a genetic predisposition.

History

Usually the patient presents with the development of a painless kyphotic deformity in the absence of any traumatic injury.

Physical Examination

The patient with Scheuermann's disease will have kyphosis of the thoracic spine and lordosis of the lumbar spine when examined in the standing position. The patient usually also has tight hip flexors and hamstring.

Imaging

In addition to the anterior wedging, irregular vertebral end plates, Schmorl's nodes and narrowed disk spaces are seen on the AP radiograph.

Treatment

Initial treatment consists of flexibility exercises that emphasize stretching of the back and hamstrings and of abdominal strengthening exercises. When kyphosis reaches 50 degrees or is progressive, strong consideration should be given to back bracing. Progression of kyphosis beyond 70 degrees usually is treated surgically. After at least 1 year after operation for a spinal fusion for

Scheuermann's disease, patients may return to light noncontact activities.[43] Patients who are treated nonoperatively have no restrictions once they have completed their treatment program and are asymptomatic.

Referral

Patients with progressing kyphosis or with kyphosis greater than 50 degrees should be referred to a musculoskeletal specialist.

VERTEBRAL APOPHYSITIS

Vertebral apophysitis or ring apophysitis is similar to Scheuermann's disease except for a lack of the kyphotic deformity. The disease occurs almost exclusively in adolescents. Radiographic findings are similar to those of Scheuermann's disease, except for the absence of anterior wedging on the radiographs of patients with vertebral apophysitis. Treatment is similar to that for Scheuermann's disease.

OSTEOPOROSIS

Osteoporosis is the end stage of loss of bone density. Osteoporosis has been related to over a million fractures each year in the United States at the cost of nearly 4 billion dollars.[44] Weight-bearing exercise plays a major role in prevention of osteoporosis. Recent studies have linked both amenorrhea and oligomenorrhea to lower bone density, which places the athlete at increased risk for developing both stress fractures and osteoporosis. Female athletes have a higher incidence of amenorrhea and oligomenorrhea than nonathletes.[45–50]

Important aspects of prevention of osteoporosis include regular weight-bearing exercise, adequate intake of calcium, and avoidance of irregular menses. Irregular menses may be avoided by adequate calorie intake, decreasing activity level, or hormonal replacement. Some athletes participate in sports that provide high levels of cardiovascular exercise but minimal weight-bearing exercise (e.g., swimming and crew). The current daily recommendation of calcium is at least 1500 mg for amenorrheic women and 1200 mg for women with regular periods. In addition, at least 5 to 10 mg of vitamin D should be included in the daily diet.

Key Points

- Both amenorrhea and oligomenorrhea are related to increased risk of stress fractures and osteoporosis.
- Adequate calcium and vitamin D intake are needed to ensure good bone health.

CHRONIC LOW BACK PAIN

Low back pain that persists longer than 3 months in spite of treatment can be considered chronic. Although 2 to 10 percent of patients with low back pain will have chronic low back pain, this condition is relatively rare in athletes.[2, 6, 51, 52] In these patients, the history and physical examination should be carefully repeated and alternative diagnoses should be considered. Secondary gain issues such as disability, lawsuits, and drug addiction need to be explored.

Narcotics should be avoided in these patients because their use tends to lead to an addiction in a patient who still has inadequate pain control. These patients often benefit from a multidisciplinary approach, which combines the skills and knowledge of primary care physicians, orthopaedic surgeons, physical therapists, occupational therapists, athletic trainers, nurses, physiatrists, psychologists, psychiatrists, and social workers. The program should include pain management, physical and occupational therapy, biofeedback, and counseling. In addition, many of these patients will seek relief from alternative treatment modalities, such as acupuncture and chiropractic manipulation.

REFERRED PAIN

Although most low back pain is musculoskeletal in origin, physicians must be careful not to miss back pain caused by other sources. Pain can be referred to the back from many diseases in different structures (see Table 13–2), including gastrointestinal disorders, genitourinary disorders, gynecologic disorders, hip pathology, obstetric disorders, pelvic pathology, pulmonary disease, and secondary gain (e.g., malingering, seeking compensation) issues. A thorough discussion of all these sources is beyond the scope of this chapter.

Piriformis Syndrome

Piriformis syndrome is caused by irritation or impingement of the sciatic nerve by the piriformis muscle. Patients will complain of deep pain in the lower back or in the posterior hip. This pain often radiates down the leg. On examination the patients have sciatic notch tenderness and pain to resisted hip external rotation and to passive internal hip stretching. Piriformis syndrome is treated by activity modification, NSAIDs, and physical therapy.

Sacroiliac Dysfunction

Pain from the sacroiliac joint often presents as unilateral low back pain. On physical examination the athlete often has tenderness over the sacroiliac joint, posterior superior iliac spine, or buttock region. The patient may have pain when flexing the hip such as when bringing the knee to the chest. Various pelvic stress tests have been described to reproduce this pain.[53]

Neoplasm

The most common spinal tumor is metastatic carcinoma, usually from cancer of the breast, lung, prostate, gastrointestinal, or genitourinary systems. The most common primary tumor is multiple myeloma. The pain is typically insidious in onset, located in the midline, and aggravated by activity. Night pain, unrelieved by sleep or lying down, is found in almost 90 percent of back pain caused by neoplasm. Plain radiographs may be normal, especially early in the course of the disease. Bone scans can be useful in confirming clinical suspicion of neoplasm. CT scan and myelograms are useful in the evaluation of neurogenic tumors.

Infection

The most common source of spinal osteomyelitis is from hematologic spread from a respiratory tract infection in the younger patient and from a urinary tract infection or procedure in an older patient. The presence of a fever should raise suspicions about infection. The pain associated with osteomyelitis is usually well localized and is aggravated by motion, which results in limitation of motion and paraspinal muscle spasm. Early radiographs are usually normal. Bone scans are useful in confirming clinical suspicion and in localizing the infection. A gallium- or indium-labeled white blood cell scan is very specific in confirming infection. MR imaging is also used by some physicians to confirm osteomyelitis.

SUMMARY

Most causes of back pain in athletes are relatively benign and will heal with time. Proper diagnosis and treatment will help speed the athlete's recovery. A careful review should be done for potentially serious underlying causes of back pain. Red flags to increase clinical suspicion include (1) pain that lasts longer than 12 weeks, (2) new pain in patients under the age of 20 years and over the age of 50, (3) history of major trauma, (4) history of cancer, (5) systemic signs, (6) constitutional signs, (7) atypical pain, and (8) severe or rapidly progressive neurologic deficit.

ACKNOWLEDGMENTS

I would like to thank Sharon L. Busey, M.D., and Chris McLauglin for their assistance with editing and Chris Geiser, P.T., A.T.,C., and Michael Ribar, A.T.,C., for their help with the photographs.

REFERENCES

1. Hainline B: Low back injury. Clin Sports Med 14:241–265, 1995.
2. Gillete RD: A practical approach to the patient with back pain. Am Fam Physician 53:670–676, 1996.
3. Ferguson RJ, McMaster JH, Stanitski CL: Low back pain in college football lineman. Am J Sports Med 2:63–69, 1974.
4. Pope MH, Novotny JE: Spinal biomechanics. J Biomech Engineering 115:569–574, 1993.
5. Papageorgiou AC, Croft PR, Ferry S, et al: Estimating the prevalence of low back pain in the general population: Evidence from the South Manchester back pain survey. Spine 20:1889–1894, 1995.
6. Wheeler AH: Diagnosis and management of low back pain and sciatica. Am Fam Physician 52:1333–1341, 1995.

7. Hart LG, Deyo RA, Cherkin DC: Physician office visits for low back pain: Frequency, clinical evaluation and treatment patterns from a U.S. national survey. Spine 20:11–19, 1995.

8. Micheli LJ, Wood R: Back pain in young athletes. Arch Pediatr Adolesc Med 149:15–18, 1995.

9. Waddell G, Feder G, Lewis M: Systematic reviews of bed rest and advice to stay active for acute low back pain. Br J Gen Pract 47:647–652, 1997.

10. Wilhite J, Huurman WW: Thoracic and lumbosacral spine. *In* Mellion (ed): The Team Physician's Handbook. Philadelphia, Hanley & Belfus, 1990, pp. 374–400.

11. Micheli LJ: Spine and chest wall. *In* Johnson RJ, Lombardo J (eds): Current Review of Sports Medicine. Philadelphia, Current Medicine, 1994, pp. 1–16.

12. Gerbino PGI, Micheli LJ: Back injuries in the young athlete. Clin Sports Med 14:571–590, 1995.

13. Kujala UM, Taimela S, Erkintalo M, et al: Low-back pain in adolescent athletes. Med Sci Sports Exerc 28:165–170, 1996.

14. Oegema TTJ: Biochemistry of intervertebral disc. Clin Sports Med 12:419–439, 1993.

15. Friis M, Gulliksen GC, Rasmussen P, et al: Pain and spinal root compression. Acta Neurochir 39:241–249, 1977.

16. Scham SM, Taylor TKF: Tension signs in lumbar disc prolapse. Clin Orthop Relat Res 75:195, 1971.

17. Boyd RJ: Evaluation of back pain. *In* Goroll A, May L Jr, Mulley AG Jr (eds): Primary Care Medicine: Office Evaluation and Management of the Adult Patient, 3rd ed. Philadelphia, J.B. Lippincott, 1995, pp. 742–751.

18. Deyo RA, Diehl AK, Rosenthal M: How many days of bed rest for acute low back pain? N Engl J Med 315:1064, 1986.

19. Deyo R: Conservative therapy for low back pain. Distinguishing useful from useless therapy. JAMA 250:1057–1062, 1983.

20. Weber H: Lumbar disc herniation. A controlled, prospective study with ten years observation. Spine 8:131–140, 1983.

21. Frymoyer JW: Back pain and sciatica. N Engl J Med 318:291–300, 1988.

22. Deyo RA, Loeser J, Bigos SJ: Herniated lumbar intervertebral disc. Ann Intern Med 112:1990, 1990.

23. Battié MC, Videman T, Gibbons LE, et al: Determinants of lumbar disc degeneration: A study relating lifetime exposures and magnetic resonance imaging findings in identical twins. Spine 20:2601–2612, 1995.

24. Frymoyer JW, Pope MH, Clements JH, et al: Risk factors in low-back pain. J Bone Joint Surg A 65:213–218, 1983.

25. Haher TR, O'Brien M, Kauffman C, Liao KC: Biomechanics of the spine in sports. Clin Sports Med 12:449–464, 1993.

26. Videman T, Sams S, Battié MC, et al: The long-term effects of physical loading and exercise lifestyles on back-related symptoms, disability, and spinal pathology among men. Spine 20:699–709, 1995.

27. Eismont FJ, Kitchel SH: Thoracolumbar spine. *In* DeLee JC, Drez D Jr (eds): Orthopaedic Sports Medicine: Principles and Practice. Philadelphia, W.B. Saunders, 1994, pp. 1018–1062.

28. Bush K, Cowan N, Katz DE, Gisher P: The natural history of sciatica associated with disc pathology. Spine 17:1205–1212, 1992.

29. Saal JA, Saal JS: Nonoperative treatment of herniated lumbar intervertebral disc with radiculopathy. An outcome study. Spine 14:431–437, 1989.

30. Hoffman RM, Wheeler KJ, Deyo RA: Surgery for herniated lumbar discs: A literature synthesis. J Gen Intern Med 8:487, 1993.

31. Hall S, Bartleson JD, Onofrio BM, et al: Lumbar spinal stenosis: Clinical features, diagnostic procedure, and results of surgical treatment in 68 patients. Ann Intern Med 103:271, 1985.

32. Helbig T, Lee CK: The lumbar facet syndrome. Spine 13:61–64, 1988.

33. Reid DC: Injuries and conditions of the neck and spine. *In* Sports Injury Assessment and Rehabilitation. New York, Churchill Livingstone, 1992, pp. 784–837.

34. Hardcastle RH: Repair of spondylolysis in young fast bowlers. J Bone Joint Surg Br 75:398–402, 1993.

35. Jackson DW: Low back pain in young athletes: Evaluation of stress reaction and discogenic problems. Am J Sports Med 7:364, 1979.

36. Stinson JT: Spondylolysis and spondylolisthesis in the athlete. Clin Sports Med 12:517–528, 1993.

37. Mandelbaum BR, Gross ML: Spondylolysis and spondylolisthesis. *In* Reider B (ed): Sports Medicine in the School-Aged Athlete. Philadelphia, W.B. Saunders, 1996, pp. 144–156.

38. Steiner ME, Micheli LJ: Treatment of symptomatic spondylolysis and spondylolisthesis with the modified Boston brace. Spine 10:937–943, 1985.

39. Micheli LJ, Hall JE, Miller ME: Use of a modified Boston brace for back injuries in athletes. Am J Sports Med 8:351–356, 1980.

40. Sponseller P: Bone, joint and muscle problems. *In* Oski F, DeAngelis C, Feigin R, et al (eds): Principles and Practice of Pediatrics, 2nd ed. Philadelphia, J.B. Lippincott, 1994, pp. 1016–1048.

41. Nattiv A, Stryer B, Mandelbaum B: Gymnastics. *In* Agostini R (ed): Medical and Orthopedic Issues of Active and Athletic Women. Philadelphia, Hanley & Belfus, 1994, pp. 378–387.

42. Hamilton W: Ballet. *In* Reider B (ed): Sports Medicine: The School Age Athlete, 2nd ed. Philadelphia, W.B. Saunders, 1996, pp. 543–581.

43. Yancey RA, Micheli LJ: Thoracolumbar spine injuries in pediatric sports. *In* Staniski CL, DeLee JC, Drez D Jr (eds): Pediatric and Adolescent Sports Medicine. Philadelphia, W.B. Saunders, 1994, pp. 162–174.

44. Hunter T, Dubo H: Spinal complications of ankylosing spondylitis. Ann Intern Med 88:546–549, 1978.

45. Murray G, Persellin R: Cervical fracture complicating ankylosing spondylitis. A report of eight cases and review of the literature. Am J Med 70:1033–1041, 1981.

46. National Institutes of Health: Consensus Development Conference on Osteoporosis. Pub. No. 421–132:46. Washington, DC, U.S. Government Printing Office, 1984.

47. Cann CE, Martin MC, Genant HK, Jaffe RB: Decreased spine mineral content in amenorrheic women. JAMA 251:656–659, 1984.

48. Myburgh KH, Bachrach LK, Lewis B, et al: Low bone mineral density at axial and appendicular sites in amenorrheic athletes. Med Sci Sports Exerc 25:1197–1202, 1993.

49. Drinkwater BL, Nilson K, Chestnut CHI, et al: Bone mineral content of amenorrheic and eumenorrheic athletes. N Engl J Med 311:277–281, 1984.

50. Alekal L, Clasey J, Fehling P, et al: Contributions of exercise, body composition and age to bone mineral density in premenopausal women. Med Sci Sports Exerc 27:1477–1485, 1995.

51. Micklesfield L, Lambert E, Fataar A, et al: Bone mineral density in mature, premenopausal ultramarathon runners. Med Sci Sports Exerc 27:688–696, 1995.

52. Snow-Harter C: Athletic amenorrhea and bone health. *In* Agostini R (ed): Medical and Orthopedic Issues of Active and Athletic Women. Philadelphia, Hanley & Belfus, 1994, pp. 164–168.

53. Klenerman L, Slade PD, Stanley M, et al: The prediction of chronicity in patients with an acute attack of low back pain in a general practice setting. Spine 20:478–484, 1995.

54. Hackley DR, Wiesel SW: The lumbar spine in the aging athlete. Clin Sports Med 12:465–485, 1993.
55. Magee D: Pelvis. *In* Orthopedic Physical Assessment, 3rd ed. Philadelphia, W.B. Saunders, 1997, pp. 434–459.

SUGGESTED READINGS

Gerbino PGI, Micheli LJ: Back injuries in the young athlete. Clin Sports Med 14:571–590, 1995.

Hoppenfeld S: Physical Examination of the Spine and Extremities. Norwalk, CT, Appleton, 1976.
Lachacz JG: Management and rehabilitation of athletic lumbar spine injuries. *In* Canavan PK (ed): Rehabilitation in Sports Medicine. Stamford, CT, Appleton & Lange, 1998, pp. 139–172.
Magee D: Orthopedic Physical Assessment, 3rd ed. Philadelphia, W. B. Saunders, 1997.
Stinson JT, Wiesel SW (eds): Spine Problems in the Athlete. Clin Sports Med 12(3), 1993.

ROB JOHNSON, M.D.

The spectrum of injuries or special medical problems of the chest is broad. The incidence of these injuries is, however, low. Generally, these injuries occur to athletes involved in collision or contact sports or sports in which a projectile is either thrown or struck. Injury may occur to soft tissues of the chest wall, the bones that protect the thorax, or the contents of the thorax. Barotrauma associated with scuba diving is discussed in texts on diving medicine.

CHEST WALL CONTUSION

Mechanism of Injury and Presentation

Injury to the chest wall is usually caused by a direct blow, delivered by an opponent, a projectile thrown or batted by another player (ball, hockey puck), or another piece of equipment used in a particular sport (bat, hockey stick, lacrosse racquet). The athlete presents complaining of acute onset of pain related to a specific traumatic incident. Frequently, the athlete complains of increased pain with deep breathing (especially during activity) and with coughing or wheezing. Upper extremity activity may also aggravate the pain.

Diagnosis

The diagnosis is made by clinical findings. The injured athlete may have a contusion at the site of injury and will have localized tenderness to palpation in an area of the thorax, but seldom point tenderness. Breath sounds will be symmetric, and there will be no signs of other injury such as rib fracture, and the like. There are no other tests to perform unless a rib fracture or other thoracic injury is suspected.

Treatment

Treatment is conservative, using cryotherapy during the acute phase of symptoms and analgesics for comfort.

Course and Recovery

The prognosis is good for complete recovery from this injury. Painful symptoms may, however, persist, making training and competition difficult for days to weeks.

When to Refer

Consultation is rarely necessary.

Return to Practice and Competition

The athlete may return to training and competition when symptoms permit. The clinician may offer significant latitude in return-to-play decisions because sequelae are rare.

Key Points

- Usual mechanism of injury is a direct blow.
- Treatment is symptomatic.
- Return to play is allowed as soon as symptoms permit. Sequelae are rare.

RIB FRACTURES

Mechanism of Injury and Presentation

Rib fractures increase in frequency as the elasticity of the chest wall decreases. Consequently, children experience fewer rib fractures than adults. In fact, if a child has a rib fracture, one should investigate carefully for associated injury because the force to create this fracture is significantly greater than the force necessary to fracture the adult rib. The usual mechanism of injury is a direct anterior-posterior force occurring in collision or contact sports. Deceleration forces have also been implicated. The fifth to ninth ribs are most commonly fractured at the posterior angle of the ribs, typically the weakest structural site. The floating ribs are less commonly fractured because they are not as rigidly fixed as ribs 5 to 9. The first four ribs are more protected than their lower counterparts and are also fractured less frequently. If any of the first four ribs are fractured, a careful examination is necessary to eliminate the possibility of vascular or pulmonary injury.

Nondisplaced fractures are much more common than displaced fractures. A displaced fracture can cause a pneumothorax and/or hemothorax.

The athlete with rib fracture presents with a history of acute trauma followed by point tenderness at the fracture site and pain exacerbated by deep or forced inspiration and expiration. If there is associated vascular or pulmonary injury, respiratory symptoms may be more acute and severe.

Diagnosis

Physical examination is positive for point tenderness to palpation at the fracture site. Anterior-posterior compression of the chest wall usually refers pain to the fracture site. If the rib fracture is uncomplicated, breath sounds will be symmetric.

The chest x-ray is the diagnostic test of choice when confirmation of the fracture is necessary. For those patients whose condition is stable without respiratory compromise, some clinicians do not perform the chest x-ray because the treatment plan is unaffected by the x-ray results.

Treatment

Treatment of rib fractures involves rigorous analgesia with local application of ice to relieve symptoms. Fractures complicated by pneumothorax, hemothorax, or damage of liver, spleen, or major vessels may require hospitalization and appropriate consultation.

Usual Course and Recovery

Acute symptoms may persist for 2 or more weeks. Recovery in uncomplicated rib fractures is usually uneventful.

When to Refer

Consultation should be obtained for displaced rib fractures that cause injuries to underlying lung, spleen, liver, or vascular structures.

Return to Practice and Competition

The time of return to play is as variable as the healing rate of fractures. When the fracture is no longer tender to palpation and the athlete has no respiratory symptoms, it is permissible to return to training. With successful participation in practice situations, the athlete may return to competition. Protection such as a rib belt or flak jacket is helpful as recovery continues during the athlete's participation in sport.

Key Points

- Direct blows to the chest commonly cause nondisplaced rib fractures.
- Ribs 5 to 9 are most commonly involved.
- Displaced rib fractures may cause vascular, pulmonary, or abdominal injury, and must be considered when evaluating the athlete with rib fracture.
- Elasticity of the chest wall in children results in fewer rib fractures in this age group.
- Return to play is indicated when the athlete is minimally symptomatic. Chest wall protection is necessary in collision or contact sports.

STRESS FRACTURE OF THE RIBS

Mechanism of Injury and Presentation

As with stress fractures at other sites, rib stress fractures have been reported in sports requiring repetitive upper extremity activity. Cases of rib stress fractures have been reported in rowing, golf, weight lifting, volleyball, gymnastics, rugby, tennis, baseball, surfing, and judo. The first rib is most commonly involved at the site of the groove for the subclavian artery, which is the thinnest portion of the rib. Repetitive contractions of the serratus anterior have been implicated. Typically, the athlete with a stress fracture of the rib complains of posterolateral chest pain, which is progressive and worsens with a specific offending activity of the sport of participation.

Diagnosis

The physical examination may yield little in the way of positive findings. Consequently, the clinician must have a high level of suspicion and obtain a chest x-ray to investigate the possibility. A negative chest x-ray mandates a bone scan for accurate diagnosis.

Treatment

Treatment involves pain control, stopping the offending sports activity, and strengthening the periscapular muscles and scapular stabilizers.

Usual Course and Recovery

Symptoms remit when the offending activity is discontinued. As with other stress fractures, the recovery period has a broad range of 2 to 12 weeks.

When to Refer

Consultation is rarely necessary.

Return to Practice and Competition

When the athlete is asymptomatic and has no pain while performing the sport or activity that caused the stress fracture, he or she may gradually return to training and competition.

Key Points

- Stress fractures of the ribs occur in sports that involve repetitive activity of the upper extremities.
- Cessation of the offending activity is the key to treatment.
- Recovery to the asymptomatic state signals the time to begin a progressive training program and return to competition.

FRACTURES OF THE STERNUM

Mechanism of Injury and Presentation

Fractures of the sternum are rare. To fracture the sternum, a violent direct blow or severe decelera-

tion force is necessary. The athlete presents with a history of violent trauma involving the anterior chest and complains of anterior chest pain. Violent trauma to the sternum may cause cardiac contusions or aortic rupture.

Diagnosis

On physical examination, there is tenderness to palpation at the site of fracture; occasionally, a step-off can be palpated. Radiographs of the chest, especially a lateral view, can confirm the diagnosis. If x-rays are not adequate, CT tomography can be helpful.

Treatment

Symptomatic treatment using analgesics and local therapy is indicated.

Usual Course and Recovery

Time course is variable. Complications are uncommon.

When to Refer

Consultation is seldom necessary.

Return to Practice and Competition

The athlete may return to practice as symptoms permit.

Key Points

- Sternal fractures are rare.
- Treatment is symptomatic.
- Rarely, sternal trauma may be associated with cardiac contusion or aortic rupture.

STERNOCLAVICULAR SUBLUXATION AND DISLOCATION

Mechanism of Injury and Presentation

Thirty-one per cent of all reported dislocations of the sternoclavicular (SC) joint occur in sports. Posterior dislocations result from either direct or indirect forces. A direct blow to the anterior clavicle causes posterior dislocations. An indirect force applied to the posterolateral shoulder compresses it and rolls it forward, resulting in a posterior dislocation. Anterior dislocations are caused by indirect forces as the anterolateral shoulder is compressed and rocked backward. Anterior dislocations are far more common than posterior dislocations (a ratio of 20 to 1). The athlete presents with pain at the site of injury. If the dislocation is posterior, the athlete may have symptoms of dyspnea, stridor, coughing, or dysphonia.

Diagnosis

The physical examination reveals asymmetry of the sternoclavicular joints with either prominence of the injured side (anterior subluxation or dislocation) or uninjured side (posterior subluxation or dislocation). Upper extremity motion exacerbates the pain at the SC joint. X-rays may yield the diagnosis but are difficult to interpret. CT with tomograms can be more helpful.

Treatment

Subluxations, either anterior or posterior, can be treated symptomatically. This may require brief use of a sling for comfort, analgesics, and local cryotherapy. Anterior dislocations are managed with closed reduction followed by a figure-eight splint or sling and analgesics. Posterior dislocations may be associated with injury to underlying pulmonary or vascular structures. Consequently, closed reduction may have to be performed emergently. Postreduction treatment includes a longer period of figure-eight immobilization, perhaps as long as 3 to 4 weeks.

Usual Course and Recovery

Subluxations of the SC joint heal by fibrosis and scarring. Pain usually subsides after 3 to 4 weeks. Those with dislocations usually become symptom-free after 4 to 6 weeks. Rehabilitation under a physical therapist's supervision follows this period of immobilization.

When to Refer

Unless the clinician is comfortable with the reduction of SC dislocations, consultation should be obtained to perform the procedure. If underlying vascular or pulmonary structures are injured, a thoracic surgeon may need to be involved.

Return to Practice and Competition

If the athlete is symptom-free after an appropriate period of immobilization, a gradual return to conditioning and practicing the skills of the sport. Following success at practice, the athlete may return to competition. Return to collision and contact sports may be delayed compared to noncontact sports.

Key Points

- Anterior subluxations and dislocations are more common than posterior subluxations and dislocations.
- Posterior dislocations may be associated with vascular and pulmonary injury.
- Subluxations usually do not need to be reduced.
- Dislocations are usually reduced by closed techniques.

COSTOCHONDRAL SEPARATION

Mechanism of Injury and Presentation

A sharp, direct blow to the chest may cause separation of the costochondral joint. Athletes with this problem experience intense pain initially, followed by a stabbing pain at the injury site. This pain seems to be caused by the overriding of bone and cartilage. Some athletes report "clicking" within the first week of injury. This sensation subsides later in the course.

Diagnosis

The diagnosis is usually made by the examination. A deformity due to rib displacement may be present. There is tenderness to palpation at the site of injury. A chest x-ray may or may not assist in confirming the diagnosis.

Treatment

Treatment is symptomatic with ice, analgesics, and symptom-limited activity restrictions. Injecting a local anesthetic into the costochondral space may help alleviate symptoms. If symptoms create chronic problems, the overriding cartilage may be excised.

Usual Course and Recovery

Most costochondral separations resolve without complication. Most patients become stable in about 2 weeks.

When to Refer

If the overriding cartilage continues to cause pain, consultation should be obtained to consider excision of the overriding segment.

Return to Practice and Competition

The athlete may return to practice and competition when symptoms permit.

Key Points

- Costochondral separation is a rare, painful condition caused by a sharp blow to the anterior chest.
- Treatment is usually supportive. Surgery is available for the chronically painful problem.

PULMONARY CONTUSION

Mechanism of Injury and Presentation

Blunt trauma to the chest wall, abrupt deceleration of the lung within the chest cavity, or a displaced rib fracture can result in a pulmonary contusion. This trauma results in hemorrhage and edema of the lung parenchyma. Mild and moderate injuries result in local pain at the site of injury and little or no respiratory difficulty. Athletes with severe pulmonary contusions present with hemoptysis, copious secretions, and respiratory difficulty.

Diagnosis

The physical examination of someone with mild injury may be completely normal. Those with more significant injury will be in respiratory distress and have rales with auscultation. The radiographic appearance of pulmonary contusions has been graded to highlight severity and define prognosis.

> Grade I: Up to 18 percent opacification of lung (most common sport-related level of injury)
> Grade II: 18 to 28 percent opacification
> Grade III: Over 28 percent opacification

Treatment

Treatment of a pulmonary contusion hinges largely on the x-ray grading of the injury. Grade I injuries are treated with rest and observation. Grade II contusions require hospitalization, and respiratory support may be necessary. Similarly, grade III lesions require hospitalization and ventilatory support if symptoms warrant.

Usual Course and Recovery

Those with grade I injuries by x-ray recover within days. Grades II and III injuries have a variable course.

When to Refer

Consultation should be sought for grades II and III injuries.

Return to Practice and Competition

Grade I injuries may return as symptoms permit. If hemoptysis occurs with this injury, that symptom should resolve before return to play. Some experts suggest waiting 10 days before return to collision sports. For those with grades II and III contusions, it is recommended to avoid collision sports for the remainder of the season. For subsequent seasons, the experts also recommend a follow-up computed tomography (CT) of the chest before return to collision sports.

Key Points

- Most pulmonary contusions occurring in sports are mild (grade I).
- Hemoptysis is uncommon in mild contusions.
- More serious pulmonary contusions may cause an athlete to miss the remainder of the season to ensure recovery.
- Grades II and III contusions (radiographic grading) should be observed in a hospital setting.

SPONTANEOUS PNEUMOTHORAX

Mechanism of Injury and Presentation

Spontaneous pneumothorax occurs in athletes when a congenital bleb on the surface of the visceral pleura ruptures. The typical pneumothorax most often affects males (male-female ratio of 4:1) ages 20 to 40 years and can be associated with connective tissue disease, interstitial lung disease, or obstructive lung disease. It can manifest in the athlete during activity or at rest. Presenting complaints include acute onset of pleuritic chest pain, cough, and shortness of breath. A pneumothorax of significant size can cause respiratory distress.

Diagnosis

Tachypnea, tachycardia with a shift of the apical pulse toward the side of the pneumothorax, diminished breath sounds, and hyperresonance to percussion of the chest wall on the affected side may be present. Subcutaneous emphysema is a sign that air has dissected into the mediastinum. The ECG may show an axis shift. The chest x-ray confirms the diagnosis and can allow the clinician to estimate the severity of collapse.

Treatment

A pneumothorax that is estimated at less than 15 to 20 percent can be treated by observation. Anything larger should be treated with chest tube drainage. Ventilatory support may be necessary for larger pneumothoraces. For the 50 percent who experience recurrences, each succeeding pneumothorax further increases the chances of recurrence. The athlete with recurrent pneumothorax can be treated surgically with pleurodesis.

Usual Course and Recovery

The small pneumothorax treated with observation demonstrates absorption of residual air in the chest cavity of 1.25 percent per day. This can be expedited up to three times faster by administering elevated O_2 concentrations. The athlete treated with a chest tube must demonstrate sustained lung expansion with the chest tube clamped before the therapy can be discontinued.

When to Refer

Surgical consultation may be necessary for the larger pneumothorax if chest tube drainage is indicated or for treatment of recurrences.

Return to Practice and Competition

The athlete may resume training and competition when the pneumothorax has resolved and respiratory status has returned to normal.

Key Points

- Spontaneous pneumothorax commonly affects males 20 to 40 years of age.
- Up to 20 percent pneumothorax can be treated conservatively.
- Over 20 percent pneumothorax will need a chest tube for reexpansion.
- The recurrence rate is 50 percent and increases in frequency with successive pneumothoraces.

TRAUMATIC PNEUMOTHORAX

Mechanism of Injury and Presentation

Traumatic pneumothorax may result from a blunt blow to the chest while the glottis is closed or from a displaced rib fracture that lacerates the lung. The resultant injury can be either a simple or tension pneumothorax. Simple pneumothorax causes dyspnea and chest pain. In rare situations, the athlete may be asymptomatic. The athlete with tension pneumothorax will have chest pain, but will present with acute respiratory distress, restlessness, and cyanosis.

The tension pneumothorax is caused by a tangential tear of the parenchyma that results in a flap-valve (one-way valve) phenomenon that permits air to enter the pleural space during respiration, thereby increasing intrapleural pressure. Increasing pressure reduces lung expansion and leads to decreased oxygenation and rapidly progressive respiratory compromise.

Diagnosis

The examination results in an athlete with simple pneumothorax are similar to those of spontaneous pneumothorax. The athlete with tension pneumothorax will present in acute respiratory distress with hypotension, tachypnea, tachycardia, hyperresonance to percussion, and absent breath sounds over the involved lung and apical pulse displaced away from the involved side. Tracheal deviation is also away from the side of involvement. The chest x-ray confirms the diagnosis, but may unnecessarily delay proper intervention; a tension pneumothorax may need emergent treatment.

Treatment

Simple pneumothorax can be treated as outlined for the spontaneous pneumothorax. Tension pneumothorax requires urgent insertion of a 14- to 18-gauge needle in the second intercostal space at the midclavicular line. With a rush of air, respiratory effort eases. A chest tube should be inserted as in other larger pneumothoraces. Similar guidelines for chest tube removal can be applied to this situation.

Usual Course and Recovery

The same guidelines apply to these injuries as for spontaneous pneumothorax.

When to Refer

Consultation would be appropriate for respiratory distress and ventilatory support or for chest tube management.

Return to Practice and Competition

In addition to applying return-to-play decisions as used for a spontaneous pneumothorax, there are often associated injuries that may dictate the athlete's return.

Key Points

- Chest trauma may cause either a simple or tension pneumothorax.
- A tension pneumothorax needs immediate treatment to relieve acute respiratory compromise.
- Treatment and return-to-play decisions are otherwise similar to those outlined for a spontaneous pneumothorax.

HEMOTHORAX

Mechanism of Injury and Presentation

When a rib fracture tears the pleural space or lacerates an intercostal artery, the bleeding that occurs may produce a hemothorax. Up to 400 ml of blood may fill the pleural space without producing symptoms. Larger volumes may be symptomatic. The injured athlete may complain of lightheadedness, chest pain, and dyspnea. If the bleeding fails to tamponade, the symptoms may progress to syncope and respiratory failure.

Diagnosis

The physical examination will show signs of both hypovolemia and respiratory distress. The chest x-ray confirms the diagnosis.

Treatment

Appropriate treatment involves surgical intervention (chest tube or thoracotomy) and ventilatory support.

Usual Course and Recovery

With surgical treatment, symptom recovery is prompt. Underlying chest trauma must also be treated. The length of recovery is dictated by symptom resolution and athlete recovery.

When to Refer

Consultation with a thoracic surgeon should be done as soon as the diagnosis is made.

Return to Practice and Competition

Hemothorax in an athlete is a season-ending injury. The athlete must undergo a thorough evaluation for the next sports season prior to return.

Key Points

- Hemothorax occurs in combination with other chest trauma.
- The athlete presents with symptoms of respiratory distress and hypovolemia.
- Treatment is surgical.

PULMONARY EMBOLUS

Mechanism of Injury and Presentation

Immobilization following lower extremity injury, prolonged travel, and, in women, oral contraceptive use, all increase the risk of pulmonary embolism (PE). The source of most clots is the deep venous system of the lower extremity. Ten percent of these patients die within 1 hour of the embolus. The correct diagnosis is made in only 30 percent of those experiencing the problem. But, when properly diagnosed and treated, the survival rate is 92 percent. Almost one third of those whose condition is undiagnosed eventually die of recurrent PE. The athlete presents with acute onset of pleuritic chest pain, cough, and dyspnea with no history of trauma.

Diagnosis

Physical examination reveals fever, tachypnea, inspiratory crackles, and possibly a pleural rub. Chest x-ray followed by ventilation/perfusion scan are the tests of choice.

Treatment

Heparin therapy followed by coumadin is the recommended treatment. Thrombolytic therapy has not resulted in improved outcomes.

Usual Course and Therapy

When properly diagnosed, therapy is usually successful. Oral anticoagulant therapy should be continued up to 6 months.

When to Refer

If the condition is uncomplicated, consultation is unnecessary.

Return to Practice and Competition

Collision and contact sports are to be avoided for the athlete on anticoagulant therapy. Upon completion of anticoagulant therapy, all sports may be resumed.

Key Points

- Pulmonary embolism can occur in special situations in athletes.
- Proper diagnosis demands a high index of suspicion.
- Anticoagulant therapy is the appropriate therapy.
- The athlete must avoid collision and contact sports while on anticoagulants.

MYOCARDIAL CONTUSION

Mechanism of Injury and Presentation

Myocardial contusions are a result of direct blows to the chest or a result of rapid deceleration causing the heart to strike the sternum. This injury is seen in collision sports or sports involving high speeds or falls (cycling, skiing, rock climbing, and sky diving). The symptoms of injury to the chest wall are likely to overshadow any cardiac symptoms. Thus, the clinician must have a high level of suspicion to pursue the diagnosis.

Diagnosis

An abnormal electrocardiogram (ECG) and altered cardiac enzymes may confirm the diagnosis. The initial ECG is probably a better prognostic indicator than cardiac enzymes.

Treatment

If the diagnosis is made, at least 24 hours of monitoring is appropriate. Most arrhythmias or dysrhythmias occur during the first 24 hours after injury.

Usual Course and Recovery

If symptoms remit and no rhythm disturbances occur within 24 hours, complications are unlikely and the athlete can be discharged from the hospital.

Return to Play

If no cardiac abnormalities occur, the athlete may return to practice and competition when he or she is asymptomatic.

Key Points

- The diagnosis will be missed if one fails to have a high clinical suspicion after blunt chest trauma or deceleration injury.
- The ECG is the best prognostic indicator.
- If no dysrhythmias occur in the first 24 hours, the athlete may return to play when asymptomatic.

COMMOTIO CORDIS

Definition

Blunt, nonpenetrating trauma, usually from a thrown or batted projectile (ball or puck), can trigger ventricular dysrhythmia leading to cardiac arrest. This is a rare problem, reported to occur primarily in children. Collapse and death occur almost instantaneously with the chest trauma. Sports implicated in commotio cordis are, in descending order of frequency, baseball, hockey, softball, karate, and lacrosse.

Key Points

- Commotio cordis, caused by nonpenetrating trauma to the chest wall, is a problem usually occurring in children.
- Death is instantaneous and results from ventricular dysrhythmia.

TRAUMATIC AORTIC RUPTURE

Mechanism of Injury and Presentation

This serious injury occurs in athletes who are traveling at high speeds (alpine skiing, water skiing, sky diving) and suddenly decelerate when striking immovable objects. The fixed descending aorta tears away from the mobile aortic arch. Almost 90 percent die at impact. The remaining victims survive long enough to reach an emergency hospital.

Diagnosis

A high index of suspicion is the key to diagnosis. A chest x-ray may show widening of the mediasti-num, tracheal deviation to the right, left-sided pleural effusion, and an obscure aortic knob. Other helpful imaging studies may be angiography or contrast CT of the chest.

Treatment

Immediate surgery is required.

Usual Course and Recovery

Prognosis for this injury is poor.

When to Refer

Emergency consultation with thoracic or vascular surgeon is crucial.

Return to Practice and Competition

After recovery, collision and contact sports are contraindicated.

Key Points

- The combination of high-speed sports and collision with immovable objects can cause this dangerous injury.
- Slightly more than 10 percent survive long enough to get to the operating room.

SUGGESTED READINGS

Adelman DC, Spector SL: Acute respiratory emergencies in emergency treatment of the injured athlete. Clin Sports Med 8(1):71–79, 1989.

Amara L: Thoracoabdominal injuries in the athlete. Clin Sports Med 16(4):739–753, 1997.

Baker CL, Flandry F, Henderson JM: The Hughston Clinic Sports Medicine Field Manual. Baltimore, Williams & Wilkins, 1996, pp. 43–50.

Fragoso CV, Systrom DM: The Respiratory System. *In* Strauss RH (ed): Sports Medicine. Philadelphia, W.B. Saunders, 1991, pp. 141–145.

McKeag DB, Hough DO (eds): Primary Care Sports Medicine. Dubuque, Brown and Benchmark, 1993, pp. 343–347.

Miles JW, Barrett GR: Rib fractures in athletes. Sports Med 12(1):66–69, 1991.

Chapter 15 | Gastrointestinal Problems and Abdominal Trauma

JEFF RADAKOVICH, M.D.

Primary care physicians frequently find themselves practicing sports medicine by either actively covering sporting events, serving as team physicians, or treating athletes in their ambulatory practices. Although athletes may have special needs and concerns, they also can be affected by the same injuries and conditions that nonathletes are. These conditions can include gastrointestinal (GI) problems. A survey of collegiate swimmers found that 48 percent were affected by GI symptoms over an 8-week training period.[1] Also, 50 percent of triathletes have been found to have GI symptoms at some point in training, and 10 percent had symptoms frequently enough to take medications on a regular basis.[2] In an endurance competition (swimming, biking, canoeing, running), 81 percent of respondents had GI symptoms during the competition.[3]

In addition to the medical concerns of the gastrointestinal system, traumatic injury to the abdomen can occur during sports or exercise. Abdominal trauma would be expected with contact sports such as football, wrestling, hockey, and soccer. But it also may be seen in high-speed noncontact events such as water skiing, horseback riding, cycling, and alpine skiing. A physician serving as medical consultant for a game or event should be prepared to deal with such an occurrence. Ten percent of all abdominal injuries are attributable to sports-related trauma.[4] Of all sports-related admissions to a pediatric emergency department over 2 years, 7 percent were due to abdominal trauma.[5] The physician should also be prepared to see these injuries in the office, as some patients may delay seeking medical care. In a series of ski-related splenic injuries, 50 percent of the injured subjects were able to continue skiing and had a delayed presentation for evaluation.[6]

Therefore, whether directly involved with athletics or not, primary care physicians should be competent at recognizing and providing initial management for abdominal injury.

PHYSIOLOGIC EFFECTS OF EXERCISE ON THE GASTROINTESTINAL TRACT

Understanding how exercise affects the physiology of the GI tract can help with understanding why some symptoms occur, and subsequently can help the physician formulate a rational plan for treatment. The majority of research in this area has been done in endurance athletes such as runners, triathletes, and cyclists because of the large number of participants in these sports and because of the ease of controlling experimental conditions in an exercise laboratory. It is assumed that similar results occur in other forms of exercise.

Increasing levels of exercise cause decreases in renal and splanchnic blood flow and changes in intestinal permeability.[7, 8] Numerous studies show that higher levels of exertion correlate with increased symptoms such as nausea, vomiting, cramping, and diarrhea.[9, 10] One study showed that 80 percent of runners who were 4 percent dehydrated had lower tract GI symptoms.[11] Another study showed that flow to the superior mesenteric artery (SMA) was not decreased in asymptomatic runners but was in symptomatic runners.[8] Splanchnic and renal flow is reduced less from the resting state during acute exercise in individuals who have had endurance training.[12] A liquid meal has been shown to diminish the effect of decreased SMA flow in low-intensity exercise.[8] It is unclear exactly how decreased blood flow causes symptoms, but several possibilities exist. Intestinal permeability may increase as blood flow decreases and may allow bile, pancreatic juices, or bacteria to cross into the circulation with subsequent response of chemotactic factors resulting in inflammation, which could be a source of cramps or diarrhea.[7] After endurance running, increases in endotoxemia have been shown to correlate with GI symptoms.[8] If blood flow or energy is not adequate to transport glucose out of the lumen of the small intestine, the bacteria of the colon may act on the carbohydrate, resulting in bloating or flatulence.[8] Also, the presence of carbohydrate may osmotically draw fluid to the intestinal lumen, leading to a bloated feeling.[8] Mechanical influences such as compression of the colon by the psoas muscle and the movement of the cecum during activity are unproved factors implicated in lower GI symptoms. The relationship of symptoms to GI hormones such as motilin, somatostatin, glucagon, pancreatic polypeptide, secretin, vasoactive intestinal polypeptide, and peptide histidine isoleucine has been investigated.[8] Currently, it is unclear if the changes in hormone levels are a cause or result of the changes in intestinal blood flow.

With respect to the esophagus, several changes can occur with exercise. With exercise the lower esophageal sphincter tone may decrease. This decrease in tone may result in increased reflux.[10] Esophageal pH meters have confirmed changes in pH associated with symptoms, including belching.[13]

Gastric emptying can be affected by many factors. Cool liquid is emptied most rapidly.[13] Carbohydrate concentrations higher than 10 percent decrease the rate of gastric emptying.[13] Liquids are emptied faster than solids, and higher gastric volumes stimulate higher emptying rates.[10] Exercise up to 75 percent of maximal exertion increases gastric emptying rate; exertion greater than 75 percent of maximum decreases emptying rate.[13] Also, the greater the volume of fluid in the stomach, the greater the rate of emptying from it.[10]

The effect of exercise on transit time in the small and large intestine is controversial. The presence of diarrhea with exertion would suggest increased transit time. However, studies are conflicting, with some showing decreased transit time (increased rate)[13] and others not showing changes in transit time.[14]

Upper Gastrointestinal Problems with Exercise

Presentation

Athletes can present with numerous symptoms attributable to the upper GI tract. These symptoms include heartburn, nausea, vomiting, epigastric pain, chest pain, and loss of appetite. These symptoms occur in about 10 percent of runners and occur more often in women than men, and in younger runners more than older ones.[13]

Many runners will have had these symptoms throughout their athletic careers, and they believe that such symptoms are "normal." Therefore, they may be self-medicating to control these symptoms. Those who present for evaluation may be concerned with how their symptoms have affected their performance or that a more serious medical problem may exist. Indeed, because athletes are not exempt from having other medical problems, a thorough history should be obtained not only for previous GI problems but also for diabetes, coronary artery disease, and asthma. If exertional chest symptoms occur, a cardiac history that includes cardiac risk factors should be obtained. A thorough history of the frequency, volume, and intensity of exercise should be obtained, trying to correlate inciting factors with the symptoms. It has been shown that experienced runners tend to have fewer GI symptoms. The timing of eating and drinking and the choice of foods and liquids are also crucial. A history of dehydration or heat-related illness is relevant because both are correlated with exertional GI symptoms.

Diagnosis

As for any patient presenting with GI symptoms, the physical examination should include blood pressure, weight, resting pulse, abdominal examination, and rectal examination to include testing for occult fecal blood. If the history warrants, a cardiac and pulmonary assessment may be necessary, especially in the athlete over 40 years old.

Laboratory and ancillary testing should be guided by history, physical examination, and the clinician's index of suspicion for underlying disease. Ultrasonography of the biliary system may be needed to rule out cholelithiasis. If peptic ulcer disease is suspected, endoscopy, contrast radiography, or *Helicobacter pylori* testing may be appropriate. If the presenting symptoms are compatible with cardiac disease, an electrocardiogram (ECG), stress testing, or imaging may be necessary.

Treatment

Most often, clinical suspicion will suggest an etiology and lead to suggestions for therapy. Inadequate fluid intake is not uncommon. Pre-exercise loading with 500 to 800 ml of fluid 20 to 30 minutes before activity and drinking 200 to 500 ml every 15 to 20 minutes during exercise should be encouraged. Athletes should be warned that thirst is an insensitive indicator of dehydration and that performance can be affected before they perceive thirst. The fluid should be cold and contain no more than 10 percent carbohydrate in order to avoid delayed gastric emptying, which can lead to cramping or feeling bloated. A beverage of 6 percent carbohydrate may help delay muscle glycogen depletion for exercise lasting more than 1 hour. For bouts of exercise less than 1 hour, water should be adequate. Avoiding caffeine because of its diuretic and laxative effects is necessary. Alcohol may also contribute to dehydration by its diuretic effect. Pre-exercise meals should contain around 500 kcal, should be consumed 2 to 3 hours before activity, and should be low in fat and fiber content. Each athlete is an individual and will respond differently to changes in fluid and food intake. The athlete should be aware of the need to experiment to see which regimen is best tolerated. Certainly, making changes in eating and drinking patterns should be done with adequate amount of time before a competition to assess its benefits.

The use of H_2 blockers has shown some success for those with reflux and upper GI disease and is generally well tolerated.[15] Ranitidine, 300 mg taken 1 hour before running, produced a decrease in reflux and duration of reflux symptoms.[16] Cimetidine, 800 mg taken 1 hour before an ultramarathon, ameliorated nausea and vomiting.[17] In some situations, temporarily lessening the volume or intensity of training can be helpful until the symptoms are controlled. Then, a gradual increase to previous level of activity may be better tolerated.[10]

In general, adequate hydration and altering the timing, amount, and type of food and liquid intake are often helpful for athletes with upper GI symptoms. Remembering that athletes can have common conditions such as peptic ulcer disease or gastroesophageal reflux is important so that these problems can be evaluated and treated properly.

When to Refer

Consultation for upper endoscopy should be considered for patients who have significant anemias associated with upper GI symptoms. Referral should be considered also for those who do not respond to empiric treatment or for whom a specific diagnosis cannot be ascertained despite initial workup and treatment.

Return to Practice and Competition

Those athletes who have mild symptoms without any evidence of severe underlying disease may not have to stop exercising. An example would be a case of mild reflux that promptly responds to treatment. If symptoms are severe, the athlete needs to stop exercising until a diagnosis is made and appropriate therapy started. A gradual, monitored return to activity can progress after correction of any training errors and addressing of issues related to fluid and food intake.

Key Points

- Avoid dehydration by drinking fluids 20 to 30 minutes before and every 15 to 20 minutes during exercise.
- Use cold fluids with less than 10 percent carbohydrate to avoid delayed gastric emptying.
- Avoid the use of caffeine and alcohol because of their diuretic effects, which can lead to dehydration.
- Pre-exercise meals should be consumed 2 to 3 hours before exercise and should be low in fat and fiber content.
- For reflux symptoms or belching, H_2 blockers can reduce symptoms if taken 1 hour before exercise.
- Decreasing activity to control exercise-induced symptoms may be necessary, followed by a more gradual return to full activity once symptoms are controlled.

Lower Gastrointestinal Problems with Exercise

Presentation

To affirm that lower GI problems are common in athletes one need only observe the rush to the woods or toilets at a distance running event. In one endurance event 61 percent of athletes had lower GI symptoms.[3] Runners needed to interrupt runs for bowel movements 16 percent of the time in one survey, which also showed that fecal urgency was the most common GI complaint by runners.[9]

Exercise-induced lower GI symptoms can include lower abdominal cramping, fecal urgency, increased number of bowel movements during exercise, diarrhea, or even hematochezia. These symptoms, like upper GI symptoms, correlate with level of intensity of exercise.[10]

Diagnosis and History

The history should include exercise intensity, volume, frequency, and conditions under which the patient exercises. Hyperthermia, like dehydration, can decrease splanchnic blood flow.[8] Also, the timing, quality, and volume of fluid and food intake should be detailed. Because exercise may be exacerbating an underlying condition, obtaining a nonexertional GI history is important. Younger patients may have symptoms suggestive of inflammatory bowel disease or irritable bowel syndrome. Older patients may have symptoms that warrant consideration of colon cancer, intestinal claudication, or biliary disease. The differential diagnosis for nonexertional diarrhea could include food poisoning, laxative abuse, diet desserts containing sorbitol, lactose intolerance, food allergies, exercise-induced anaphylaxis, fecal impaction, thyroid disease, pancreatic disease, antibiotic-related diarrhea, or even *Clostridium difficile*–induced pseudomembranous colitis. Also, a travel history should be obtained because the athlete may have traveled to a region in which infectious diarrhea or parasitic infections are common. Make note of family members or team members with similar symptoms, suggesting infectious causes.

Physical Examination

The physical examination should include abdominal and rectal examinations to include testing for occult fecal blood. Laboratory testing should be directed by the history and physical examination findings. If diarrhea is prominent, test the stool for leukocytes or parasites such as *Giardia lamblia* or perform cultures for bacterial pathogens. Complete blood cell count and thyroid studies may be helpful. Examination of the colon by colonoscopy, sigmoidoscopy, or barium enema may be needed if the history and physical examination are suspicious for underlying pathology, especially in athletes over 40 years old or those who have strong family histories for colon disease.

Treatment

Initial measures for treating lower GI symptoms should include ensuring adequate hydration. Pre-exercise meals should be low in residue, fat, and protein and should be eaten several hours before a workout in order to avoid the gastrocolic reflex during exercise. Because caffeine can act as a laxative, decreasing or eliminating it may be helpful. A trial of a lactose-free diet or lactase enzyme pills (purchased over the counter) may be considered.[13] Decreasing intensity and volume of exercise with a gradual return may be helpful. Some runners believe that GI symptoms lessen with conditioning.[9] Manipulation of the diet and fluid intake should be done prior to competition as a trial of its efficacy.

Despite the preceding measures, symptoms may persist in some athletes, and pharmacologic treatment may be considered. For diarrhea, loperamide has a low side effect profile, is usually effective, and may be used prophylactically, one to two tablets before exercise. Anticholinergics such as atropine, dicyclomine hydrochloride, and hycosamine may cause decreased sweating, which predisposes the athlete to heat injury.[13] Centrally acting agents such as chlordiazepoxide, phenobarbital, and diphenoxylate hydrochloride suppress the central nervous system and involve the risk of athletic performance below expectations.

Lower GI symptoms are common in athletes, especially endurance athletes. The evaluation should focus on common causes for exercise-induced symptoms; the examiner should not forget that common conditions present in the athlete can be manifested by the stress of exercise, as they are in nonathletes.

When to Refer

Occasionally an athlete may continue to have symptoms despite undergoing evaluation, treatment, and changes in training and food/fluid intake. Referral should be considered if there is suspicion of inflammatory bowel disease (IBD), intestinal claudication, or unwanted weight loss associated with the athlete's symptoms despite initial treatment, or if the patient has not responded to reasonable treatment as outlined.

Return to Practice and Competition

As with upper GI symptoms, the athlete may continue to participate if the symptoms are mild and are responding to treatment. For those with severe symptoms, a temporary cessation or decrease in activity may be needed. Then, a gradual, monitored return to activity as tolerated can be allowed once a definitive diagnosis is made, the symptoms improve as the underlying problem is being treated, and training errors and dietary problems are corrected.

Key Points

- Avoid dehydration by drinking fluids 20 to 30 minutes before and every 15 to 20 minutes during exercise.
- Pre-exercise meals should be consumed 2 to 3 hours before exercise and should be low in fat, fiber, and protein.
- Avoid caffeine because of its laxative effect.
- Try establishing a routine of having bowel movements prior to exercise.
- Avoid caffeine and alcohol, which have diuretic effects that could lead to dehydration.
- Try a lactose-free diet or lactase tablets if lactose intolerance is suspected.
- Loperamide 2 mg, one to two capsules prior to exercise, may prevent loose stools.
- Decreasing activity to control exercise-induced symptoms may be necessary, followed by a more gradual return to full activity once symptoms are controlled.

GASTROINTESTINAL BLEEDING IN ATHLETES

Presentation

Gastrointestinal blood loss in athletes may be considered in two forms: occult bleeding, which is very common, and hematochezia or hematemesis, both of which are uncommon. A survey of marathoners found 21 percent converted from heme-negative stool before a race to heme-positive stool after a race.[18] There was no correlation between being heme-positive and having GI symptoms; 27 percent of triathletes studied had heme-positive stool after a competition.[19] Another study found marathon runners to have a 2 percent prerace rate of heme-positive stool and 22 percent postrace rate. Quantitating loss in high-intensity training for runners showed an increase in daily fecal blood loss from 1.5 ml of blood loss per day while not running to 6.6 ml of blood loss per day during intensive training.[20] Also, 1.2 to 8.4 percent of cyclists have heme-positive stool after exercise.[21]

Gut ischemia is believed to be a cause for GI blood loss. In one study, 85 percent of ultramarathon runners showed heme-positive stool after racing after being prerace negative.[22] In the heme-positive group there were reports of nausea, vomiting, and diarrhea as well.[22] Colonoscopy studies done after exercise have shown areas consistent with ischemia that have resolved quickly with reperfusion.[10] Ischemic lesions in the upper GI tract have been demonstrated to be similar to those in the colon that resolved quickly with reperfusion after exercise cessation.[23]

Hematochezia is uncommon, with less than 2 percent of runners reporting gross blood in the stool after hard runs.[9] However, patients may consider rectal bleeding to be normal after a strenuous workout and may not report it. One study indicated only 25 percent of runners with gross bleeding sought medical care.[18] Therefore, it is imperative that primary care physicians ask their athletes about rectal bleeding during preseason screening or on routine examinations. Reports of death and serious hemorrhage are rare. Most sources of GI hemorrhage are in the stomach.[15]

Diagnosis and History

Most athletes, of course, will not present for occult bleeding; therefore, most patients will present for gross bleeding. It is important to determine the timing of the bleeding. Was it during the activity or during a bowel movement? Was it associated with pain? Is there a history of non–exercise-related bleeding due to hemorrhoids, anal fissures, or inflammatory bowel disease? Is there a family history of colon cancer or inflammatory bowel disease? Medication lists should be evaluated, especially for nonsteroidal anti-inflammatory drugs.

Physical Examination

GI bleeding should never be presumed to be due to exercise unless the history, physical examination, and appropriate testing show no cause or underlying GI problem. The physical examination should include checking the abdomen and rectum for masses, hemorrhoids, and fissures, and fecal occult blood. Complete blood cell count should be performed, and if anemia is present, serum iron, ferritin, and iron-binding capacity should be checked. Evaluation of the colon by endoscopy or barium enema should be considered in anyone over 40 years old or younger when risk factors or history suggests colon cancer or inflammatory bowel disease as possible causes.

Treatment

If underlying causes other than exercise are found, they should be treated as they would be in nonathletes. The initial treatment for exercise-associated GI bleeding is hydration to reduce the level of ischemia, which in turn may reduce GI blood loss. Cimetidine used before exercise has been shown to reduce occult GI blood loss.[17] However, occult blood loss has not been proved to be harmful to the nonanemic athlete, so its regular use in asymptomatic athletes without anemia may be unnecessary. Those with gastritis may benefit from an H_2 blocker.

Because athletes may have the same diseases as nonathletes, rectal bleeding should be evaluated and not simply assumed to be due to exertion. During preseason screening or physicals, the athlete should be asked about rectal bleeding because few will seek medical advice about it. This also provides an excellent opportunity to discuss adequate hydration practices, which could ameliorate or eliminate any GI symptoms.

When to Refer

Colonoscopy is indicated for any athlete over 40 years old who has frank rectal bleeding to exclude colorectal cancer as a cause. Younger athletes may need to have colon examinations when bleeding is associated with significant anemia, or the personal or family history suggests IBD as a cause.

Return to Practice and Competition

GI bleeding may not be, in itself, a contraindication to exercise. However, if exercise causes the condition to worsen, rest should be advised until the underlying problem is controlled and treatment instituted. Athletes should be warned that anemia-related fatigue may limit their abilities until the anemia is corrected. Activities may need to be adjusted as tolerated until then.

Key Points

- Never assume gastrointestinal bleeding is due only to exercise. Whether bleeding is occult or gross, investigation for the cause is necessary, as it would be in nonathletes.
- If no cause is found for occult bleeding and the athlete is not anemic and not symptomatic, no treatment is necessary.
- If the athlete has anemia attributable to gastritis, or has upper GI symptoms, then using H_2 blockers may be reasonable.
- Always encourage aggressive hydration to avoid gut ischemia, which may contribute to GI blood loss.
- Ask athletes about GI bleeding, as they rarely will seek medical help regarding this problem.

ABDOMINAL TRAUMA

As previously stated, abdominal trauma is not uncommon in athletics. Although penetrating trauma can occur in sports, blunt trauma is more common. Primary care physicians must be prepared to deal with the initial evaluation, stabilization, and diagnostic evaluation of such types of trauma.

Diagnosis

The initial evaluation for abdominal injury in the athlete is no different from that in the nonathlete. In the unusual event of loss of consciousness, one should assume that a neck injury is present and proceed with ABCs of trauma: first, establish an airway; second, begin breathing by use of pocket valve mask. Initiate chest compressions to restore circulation. Evaluate for disability or neurologic injury using the Glasgow Coma Scale. Exposure is then important for a thorough examination. Jerseys and equipment may need to be cut away.

History and Physical Examination

In most instances the patient will be conscious and somewhat cooperative for an initial on-field examination. A history should detail the mechanism of trauma, whether the pain is diffuse or localized, and if the symptoms are immediate or delayed. The examination should document vital signs, both supine and standing if possible; any ecchymoses, abrasions, bowel sounds, and localized or diffuse tenderness; and any signs of peritoneal irritation. When possible, rectal examination including testing for occult fecal blood, should be performed.

Return to Practice and Competition

Deciding whether an athlete can return to play that day can be difficult. Although intra-abdominal injury may cause diffuse pain, the pain may start out localized before becoming more generalized. Pain from abdominal wall injuries will remain isolated. Isometric contractions (tightening without movement) of the abdominal wall may reproduce localized abdominal wall pain but not for internal organ damage. Isometric contraction may aggravate pain if peritoneal irritation has occurred owing to internal organ damage, but the pain is usually more diffuse. Serial examinations should be performed before allowing return to activity. If vital signs remain stable, if bowel sounds are present, and if any tenderness is localized to the abdominal wall, the athlete may return to competition if he/she feels capable.

When to Refer

When the initial examination demonstrates lack of bowel sounds, mild tachycardia, tenderness to palpation over an internal organ, or signs of peritoneal irritation, transport to the emergency department is mandatory. The threshold of the decision to transport should be low because the initial examination can fail to pick up serious injury, and rapid worsening in the field can occur with no adequate resuscitation resources available.

In the emergency department, vital signs and physical examination should be repeated. If peritoneal signs are present, general surgical consultation is necessary and laparotomy may be necessary quickly. If peritoneal signs are equivocal, further workup may be needed. Diagnostic peritoneal lavage (DPL) is 95 percent sensitive, 98 percent specific for intraperitoneal injury, less so for retroperitoneal injury. In experienced hands DPL can be done quickly and may help expedite making a decision about laparotomy. CT scanning with intravenous and oral contrast media may be used and has an advantage over DPL in evaluation of retroperitoneal structures such as the kidneys and duodenum.

Laboratory examinations should include complete blood cell count, amylase, urinalysis, and radiographs of the abdomen and upright chest to exclude free air under the diaphragm. Liver function testing may be done if the right upper quadrant or epigastric area is involved.

SPECIFIC INJURIES TO THE GASTROINTESTINAL TRACT

Hollow Organs

Injuries, especially rupture, to hollow organs are uncommon in sports.[24] Jejunal rupture[25] and intramural hematomas of the duodenum[26] have been reported. Traumatic rupture of the stomach is rare, even in motor vehicle accidents.[27]

Mechanism of Injury and Presentation

The injury will be, of course, high energy and can result from bowel being crushed against the spine, a sudden increase in luminal pressure, or tearing at the junction of mobile and fixed segments of intestine, such as the ligament of Treitz.[27]

Diagnosis

The patient will nearly always have diffuse abdominal pain and possibly nausea or vomiting.[28] Any blood in the nasogastric aspirate must raise suspicion for ruptured viscus.[27] The examination will reveal diffuse tenderness with peritoneal signs. Radiographs may show free air under the diaphragm, retroperitoneal air if the duodenum is ruptured, or obliteration of the psoas shadow.[27] DPL may show interluminal contents, bilirubin, amylase, or bacteria on Gram stain.[26] If amylase is elevated in the peritoneal lavage, duodenal rupture should be suspected.[27] If duodenal injury is suspected, CT with oral and intravenous contrast material can be helpful.

When to Refer

Most patients with a ruptured viscus will not need extensive imaging. Their initial presentation with peritoneal signs will most often require prompt surgical referral for laparotomy. The abdominal contents can then be evaluated under direct visualization, and repairs to injured organs can be made.

Return to Practice and Competition

Because these injuries are uncommon, no guidelines exist for return to play. As after any abdominal surgery, early activity is encouraged. Theoretically, in an uncomplicated recovery, the patient should be able to return to full activity once the abdominal wall incision has healed completely, usually in 12 weeks.

Splenic Injury

The spleen is the most commonly injured solid abdominal organ and is frequently associated with left-sided rib fractures.[27] In a series of snowboarding injuries, 7 of 12 abdominal injuries involved the spleen.[29]

Mechanism of Injury

There is a strong association with mononucleosis infection, resulting in either spontaneous or traumatic rupture during the first 21 days of the illness.[30] Injuries to the spleen usually result from a blow to the left upper quadrant, left ribs, left flank, or a sudden deceleration in which the hilum is torn.[31]

Diagnosis

Pain initially may be limited to the left upper quadrant or radiate to the left shoulder (Kehr's sign). It then can progress to diffuse abdominal pain if bleeding occurs outside the capsule. The spectrum of presentations ranges from little pain to hypovolemic shock.[13] If the patient's symptoms are not initially severe, the patient may delay

seeking medical care. One report showed that 50 percent of low-speed skiing injuries that resulted in splenic laceration had delayed presentations for medical care.[6]

Physical Examination

The initial examination may show little pain initially or mild rib pain. Follow-up examinations may then show more intense pain that becomes more diffuse or signs of peritoneal irritation. In splenic injuries with significant bleeding, tachycardia, hypotension, sweating, and thirst may be seen.

Initial laboratory tests should include a minimum of complete blood cell count and amylase levels to evaluate for concomitant pancreatic injury. CT scan of the abdomen is excellent in defining splenic injury. Ultrasound can also be used but gives less information about potential damage to other organs.

Treatment

Initial treatment includes intravenous access and fluid resuscitation if hypotension is present. Serial examinations and serial hemoglobin are necessary. Bed rest is the usual course until the patient's condition has proved to be stable. Because of the importance of the spleen as an immune system organ, efforts should be made to treat the patient without splenectomy. Ninety percent of pediatric splenic ruptures are treated conservatively.[27]

When to Refer

The indications for splenectomy include hilar vascular injury, massive subcapsular hematoma, extensive fragmentation, total avulsion, and continued bleeding after attempted splenic repair.[27]

Return to Practice and Competition

Recommendations for return to play after splenic injury are somewhat empiric. If the injury is managed conservatively, return to contact sports should be delayed until the spleen has normalized on computed tomography (CT) imaging, and the athlete should return no sooner than 4 months.[32] After splenectomy, no vigorous activity for 6 to 8 weeks and no contact for 3 months should be recommended.[32] For the athlete with mononucleosis and splenomegaly, returning to activity may begin slowly 3 weeks after the onset of symptoms. If the athlete wants to return to contact or collision sports and is feeling well at 3 weeks, imaging of the spleen by ultrasound or CT should first be performed to confirm a return to normal spleen size. If the spleen is enlarged, repeat imaging studies every 10 to 14 days may be required until the spleen has normalized.

Splenic injury can be very dramatic in its presentation or very subtle on initial examination. A high index of suspicion must be kept for injuries that may result in splenic injury. Conservative treatment is appropriate in most cases. The return to athletics after splenic injury must be individualized, depending on the severity of the injury and its treatment.

Injury to the Liver

The liver is the second most commonly injured solid organ in the abdomen.[27] With better imaging techniques, clinicians are realizing that these injuries are more common than previously suspected. Nevertheless, it is not a common problem in sports.

Mechanism of Injury

The athlete will have received a blow to the right upper quadrant, right lower ribs, back, or side, or have had a collision resulting in sudden deceleration.[32] The patient may complain of right upper quadrant, shoulder, or diffuse abdominal pain. The physical examination reveals right upper quadrant pain or diffuse pain that may have signs of peritoneal irritation. When liver injury is suspected, serial abdominal examinations, hemoglobin levels, and liver function tests should be performed. CT scan of the abdomen can accurately diagnose liver injury and other associated injuries.

Treatment

If the patient is hemodynamically stable, bed rest with serial abdominal examinations is all that is required. If the patient remains stable, the CT can be repeated in 5 to 7 days. If the hemoglobin continues to fall or the patient is hemodynamically unstable, then CT is often needed sooner, and laparotomy may be required.[27]

When to Refer

Even if conservative management is expected, consultation with a surgeon is warranted in case of unexpected rebleeding that may require prompt laparotomy.

Return to Practice and Competition

Because there is little experience with traumatic injury to the liver in athletics, return to play recommendations are somewhat conservative. Return to full activity should be delayed until the liver appears normal by imaging.[31] Gradual return to lighter activity is probably acceptable prior to full return.

For the athlete with atraumatic hepatitis, splenomegaly, and elevated liver function tests, avoiding contact and collision sports would make sense. There are no formal recommendations or data to give guidance for this issue. However, it would seem that the athlete should wait until splenomegaly and liver function tests have returned to normal before engaging in contact and collision sports or other strenuous activity.

Pancreatic Injury

The pancreas is infrequently injured in sports.[24] When pancreatic injury occurs, the complications can be life-threatening. In children, trauma is the most common cause of pancreatitis, and 10 percent of blunt abdominal trauma in children can result in pancreatitis.[33]

Mechanism of Injury

In children pancreatic injury may be associated with handlebar trauma.[34] Blunt trauma by a helmet or from martial arts kicks has also been described.[24]

Diagnosis

Pain may be severe and often starts in the midabdomen to the epigastric area and subsequently may become more diffuse. The abdominal examination may show diminished or absent bowel sounds. Tenderness may be localized in the epigastric, midabdominal area, then becomes more generalized with associated peritoneal irritation.

The amylase level often is elevated. However, in one report of pancreatic trauma cases, serum elevations in amylase occurred in only 61 percent of the cases.[27] CT scanning can show evidence of laceration of the pancreas or mass effect with diffuse inflammation. Because of the potential complications of pancreatitis, complete blood cell count, arterial blood gas measurements, chest x-ray, and assessment of calcium and other electrolytes should be made.

Treatment

The treatment for pancreatic injury depends on the extent of the injury. The pancreas that is divided or lacerated may be best treated with distal pancreatectomy.[24] Reports of percutaneous drainage for pseudocysts even with ductal disruption have been published.[35] Stable patients may be treated conservatively with intravenous hydration, gut rest, and monitoring.

When to Refer

Surgical consultation is indicated for all but the most stable patients with pancreatic injury, especially if there is a suspicion of ductal disruption or if any complications of pancreatitis occur.

Return to Practice and Competition

There are no established guidelines for returning to activity after pancreatic injury. It would seem that light activity could be allowed as tolerated when the athlete feels able. Once the athlete tolerates a normal diet, noncontact activity can be advanced as tolerated. Before the athlete returns to contact/collision sports, the pancreas should appear normal on CT imaging.

It should be remembered that the symptoms immediately after blunt abdominal trauma may be minimal. The athlete should be warned about the symptoms of pancreatitis and given indications to return for evaluation. If there is any suspicion of pancreatic injury, a workup should be encouraged before an athlete is sent home.

Abdominal Wall Injuries

Mechanism of Injury

Injuries to the abdomen may be limited to the abdominal wall and may occur from a direct blow to the abdomen. Contusions are the most common type of abdominal wall injury. However, rectus sheath hematomas can result from an injury to the epigastric artery or vein.[32] The patient will complain of pain and tenderness to the touch and with movement.

Diagnosis

The examiner should look for ecchymosis, localized swelling, the presence of bowel sounds, tenderness, and rebound tenderness. Although pain may start out isolated, generally in intra-abdominal organ injury pain will be generalized and diffuse. Often isometric contraction will cause isolated, well-localized pain for abdominal wall injuries. Internal organ injury may produce pain with abdominal wall contraction, but this is usually accompanied by peritoneal signs and more generalized tenderness on examination.

It should be remembered that abdominal wall injuries do not rule out the possibility of underlying intra-abdominal injury. If any concern is present regarding intra-abdominal injury, imaging should be done.

Treatment

Ice and analgesics are all that are necessary to treat contusions. The athlete can return to play as symptoms allow. Hematomas can be observed unless the hematoma is expanding, in which case surgical ligation or aspiration may hasten the recovery to within 1 to 2 weeks.[32]

When to Refer

Surgical consultation should be requested whenever there is a concern for intra-abdominal organ injury, especially when bowel sounds are absent, peritoneal signs are present, or there is concern that a rectus hematoma is expanding and may need ligation.

Return to Practice and Competition

Athletes with abdominal wall contusions can return to unrestricted activity as soon as their symptoms allow. Those with rectus hematomas requiring aspiration and ligation may also return when symptoms allow, but this may take as long as 2 weeks.[32]

SUMMARY

As primary care physicians encourage more patients to exercise to maintain health and fitness, they should be prepared to manage the potential problems that may accompany exercise, such as GI symptoms. In addition, for those patients who are exercising, primary care physicians should ask about GI symptoms related to exercise, as the patient may be reluctant to volunteer the information or may believe that these symptoms are normal. When these symptoms do occur, it cannot be assumed that they are related to exercise. A thorough history and physical examination should be performed. Laboratory studies and other appropriate tests should be ordered, depending on the patient's risks for any underlying disorders.

In addition, primary care physicians should be prepared to begin a diagnostic workup and initial resuscitation efforts for patients who may present with abdominal trauma. Even for physicians who do not attend sporting events, a working knowledge of managing abdominal trauma is necessary to treat those patients whose presentations are delayed.

REFERENCES

1. Strauss RH, Lanese RR, Leizman DJ: Illness and absence among wrestlers, swimmers, and gymnasts at a large university. Am J Sports Med 16(6):653–655, 1988.
2. Worme JD, Doubt TJ, Singh A, et al: Dietary patterns, gastrointestinal complaints, and nutrition knowledge of recreational triathletes. Am J Clin Nutr 51:690–697, 1990.
3. Worobetz LJ, Gerrard DF: Gastrointestinal symptoms during exercise in Enduro athletes: prevalence and speculations on the aetiology. NZ Med J 98:644–646, 1985.
4. Diamond DL: Sports-related abdominal trauma. Clinics Sports Med 8(1):91–99, 1989.
5. Davis JM, Kuppermann N, Fleisher G: Serious sports injuries requiring hospitalization seen in a pediatric emergency department. Am J Dis Child 147:1001–1004, 1993.
6. Sartorelli KH, Pilcher DB, Rogers FB: Patterns of splenic injuries seen in skiers. Injury 26(1):43–46, 1995.
7. Pals KL, Chang R, Ryan AJ, et al: Effect of running intensity on intestinal permeability. J Appl Physiol 82(2):571–576, 1997.
8. Peters HPF, Akkermans LMA, Bol E, et al: Gastrointestinal symptoms during exercise; The effect of fluid supplementation. Sports Med 20(2):65–76, 1995.
9. Keefe EB, Lowe DK, Goss JR, et al: Gastrointestinal symptoms of marathon runners. West J Med 141:481–484, 1984.
10. Green GA: Exercise-induced gastrointestinal symptoms. Physician Sportsmed 21(10):60–70, 1993.
11. Rehrer NJ, Janssen ME, Brouns F, et al: Fluid intake and gastrointestinal problems in runners competing in a 25-km race and a marathon. Int J Sports Med 10:S22–25, 1989.
12. McAllister RM: Adaptations in control of blood flow with training: Splanchnic and renal blood flows. Med Sci Sports Exerc 30(3):375–381, 1998.
13. Green GA: Gastrointestinal disorders in the athlete. Clin Sports Med 11(2):453–470, 1992.
14. Kayaleh RA, Seshkinpour H, Avinashi A, et al: Effect of exercise on mouth-to-cecum transit in trained athletes: A case against the role of runners' abdominal bouncing. J Sports Med Physical Fitness 36(4):271–274, 1996.
15. Moses FM: The effect of exercise on the gastrointestinal tract. Sports Med 9(3):159–172, 1990.
16. Shawdon A: Gastro-oesophageal reflux and exercise. Sports Med 20(2):109–116, 1996.
17. Baska RA, Moses FM, Graeber G, et al: Gastrointestinal bleeding during an ultramarathon. Dig Dis Sci 35(2):276–279, 1990.
18. McCabe ME, Peura DA, Kadakia SC, et al: Gastrointestinal blood loss associated with running a marathon. Dig Dis Sci 31(11):1229–1232, 1986.
19. Worme JD, Doubt TJ, Singh A, et al: Dietary patterns, gastrointestinal complaints, and nutrition knowledge of recreational triathletes. Am J Clin Nutr 51:690–697, 1990.
20. Nachtigall D, Nielsen P, Fischer R, et al: Iron deficiency in distance runners: A reinvestigation using ^{59}Fe-labelling and non-invasive liver iron quantification. Int J Sports Med 17:473–479, 1996.
21. Wilhite J, Mellion MB: Occult gastrointestinal bleeding in endurance cyclists. Physician Sports Med 18(8):75–78, 1990.
22. Baska RS, Moses FM, Deuster PA: Cimetidine reduces running-associated gastrointestinal bleeding. Dig Dis Sci 35(8):956–960, 1990.
23. Gaudin C, Zerath E, Guezennec CY: Gastric lesions secondary to long-distance running. Dig Dis Sci 35(10):1239–1243, 1990.
24. Diamond DL: Sports-related abdominal trauma. Clinics Sports Med 8(1):91–99, 1989.
25. Murphy CP, Drez D Jr: Jejunal rupture in a football player. Am J Sports Med 15(2):184–185, 1987.
26. Henderson JM, Puffer JC: Abdominal pain in a football player. Phys Sportsmed 17(8):47–52, 1989.
27. Jurkovich GJ, Carrico CJ: Trauma: Management of the acutely injured patient. In Sabiston DC (ed): Textbook of Surgery, 15th ed. Philadelphia, W.B. Saunders, 1997, pp. 296–327.
28. Shorter NA, Jensen PE, Harmon BJ, et al: Skiing injuries in children and adolescents. J Trauma 40(6):997–1001, 1996.
29. Prall JA, Winston KR, Brennan R: Severe snowboarding injuries. Injury 25(8):539–542, 1995.
30. Maki DG, Reich RM: Infectious mononucleosis in the athlete: Diagnosis, complications, and management. Am J Sports Med 10(3):162–173, 1982.
31. Perez VM, McDonald AD, Ghani A, et al: Handlebar hernia: A rare traumatic abdominal wall hernia. Trauma 40(3):568, 1996.
32. Amaral JF: Thoracoabdominal injuries in the athlete. Clin Sports Med 16(4):739–753, 1997.
33. Arkovitz MS, Garcia VF: Spontaneous recanalization of the pancreatic duct: Case report and review. J Trauma 40(6):1014–1015, 1996.
34. Takishima T, Sugimoto K, Asari Y, et al: Characteristics of pancreatic injury in children: A comparison with such injury in adults. J Pediatric Surg 31(7):896–900, 1996.
35. Ohno Y, Ohgami H, Nagasaki A, et al: Complete disruption of the main pancreatic duct: A case successfully managed by percutaneous drainage. J Pediatric Surg 30(12):1741–1742, 1995.

Chapter **16** | Genitourinary Problems

PATRICK MORRIS, M.D.

Genitourinary problems encountered by sports medicine practitioners vary from renal trauma that is evaluated on the field to exercise-related hematuria and proteinuria that are clinical issues. Acute injuries to the male genitalia are also discussed here, as are preparticipation considerations regarding the athlete with only one kidney or with a single testicle or ovary.

RENAL TRAUMA

History and Diagnosis

Sports-related renal trauma is not uncommon, although the exact incidence is unknown. Blunt renal trauma can be categorized into four groups: (1) contusions, (2) minor lacerations, (3) major lacerations (deep cortical and calyceal lacerations), and (4) vascular pedicle injuries. Fortunately, the majority of renal injuries that occur during sports participation are contusions and minor lacerations that respond well to conservative management, with no long-term sequelae.

The athlete with blunt renal trauma most often presents with abdominal or flank pain and hematuria. A mild amount of tenderness at the injury site is to be expected, but significant pain, with or without marked tenderness, should raise suspicion of injury to the underlying viscera. Intra-abdominal bleeding should always be considered in the initial evaluation, with appropriate monitoring of the ABCs—*a*irway, *b*reathing, and *c*irculation.

The need for imaging studies following blunt renal trauma is controversial. Definite indications include gross hematuria, microscopic hematuria with signs or symptoms of shock, a falling hematocrit, and a retroperitoneal mass. Athletes whose symptoms do not rapidly improve should also undergo imaging. Computed tomography (CT scanning) is the diagnostic method of choice for most initial evaluations; it offers detailed viewing of kidney anatomy and the chance to evaluate

other intra-abdominal injury. An intravenous pyelogram (IVP) is reasonable if associated abdominal trauma is unlikely. Either extrarenal or intrarenal extravasation of dye may indicate injury, with both occurring in the case of renal fracture. IVP is often inadequate to diagnose vascular injury, and selective renal arteriography may be necessary.

Management of microscopic hematuria in otherwise stable athletes following renal trauma is challenging because the degree of hematuria may not correlate with the degree of injury. Vascular pedicle injuries may not involve any hematuria. The vast majority of athletes with isolated microscopic hematuria, however, have at most a renal contusion, and further studies can be avoided in those with a benign examination and improving clinical course. Clinical concerns such as a history of a high-force injury, overlying rib fractures, or concomitant abdominal injuries demand further imaging studies and consultation.

Treatment and Return to Play

The initial management of renal contusions or minor lacerations includes bed rest, hydration, and analgesics. Use of nonsteroidal anti-inflammatory drugs (NSAIDs) risks adverse renal side effects; other analgesic choices are more prudent. An athlete with a renal contusion whose microscopic hematuria rapidly clears and whose blood pressure and physical examination are normal can return to contact play. However, with more severe renal injuries athletes are often told to avoid strenuous activity for 2 to 3 weeks, as rebleeding may occur during this time, and to avoid contact play for 6 weeks. It is reasonable to repeat a CT scan or IVP before 6 weeks to have radiographic resolution assist in making the return-to-play decision. Protective padding should be properly fitted and worn on resuming contact or collision sports.

HEMATURIA

History and Diagnosis

Exercise-related hematuria is common in athletes who participate in both contact and noncontact sports, with the greatest incidence occurring among distance swimmers and runners. The hematuria can come from mechanical trauma, such as renal vein kinking or bladder contusion, or from pre-existing pathologies, nephrolithiasis, urinary tract infections, or medication use. The commonly accepted upper limit of the normal laboratory value is 3 red blood cells per high-power field, with a higher count considered evidence of micro-hematuria.

The physician should begin investigating hematuria in the athlete by securing detailed information about the type, duration, frequency, and intensity of workouts to see if a discernible pattern of exercise and hematuria exists. A routine review of medical systems may suggest appropriate diagnostics (e.g., urinary cultures for urinary tract infection or urethritis, or IVP for nephrolithiasis) and past medical history, family history, and medication lists can also provide clues that would point away from the assumption that exercise is the causative factor.

In the clinical examination one should be alert for hypertension, irregular heart rhythm, heart murmur, abdominal mass, petechiae, and peripheral edema. Lesions of the prostate, genitalia, and urethral opening should be considered. Skin angiomas found on an athlete with hearing loss may signal Alport's syndrome. Laboratory findings of oliguria, proteinuria, or red blood cell casts may also help to define important rheumatologic, infectious, and cardiovascular causes of hematuria.

If exercise-related hematuria still seems likely, the next step is to repeat a urinalysis in 24 to 48 hours, after an exercise-free period. No further work-up for a single episode of exercise-related hematuria is necessary after a normal repeat urinalysis. Periodic screening of urine (not preceded by exercise) is a reasonable precaution, however, especially if gross hematuria was the initial presentation. Any persistent hematuria requires further evaluation; sports hematuria should not be assumed. Serum kidney function tests, further urine studies, diagnostic imaging and consultation may be necessary to rule out extrinsic or intrinsic kidney, collecting system, or bladder disease.

Recurrent episodes of microhematuria with exercise, if they are episodes that clear in 24 to 48 hours, also have a benign prognosis, and an in-depth evaluation is not necessary in most cases. Although management of recurrent gross hematuria is controversial, pursuit of further diagnoses is advisable, especially for the older athlete.

Other conditions can mimic hematuria. Myoglobinuria and hemoglobinuria (e.g., the "foot-strike hemolysis" of endurance runners) may present with discolored urine and a dipstick urinalysis "positive" for blood. In urinary microscopic examination, however, the intact red blood cells of hematuria are absent. Certain medicines, various foods (e.g., beets, fava beans, rhubarb), natural laxatives (cascara, senna) and vegetable dyes (e.g., V-8 juice) also discolor urine.

Treatment and Return to Play

Exercise-induced microscopic hematuria is not a contraindication to athletic activity if there is no suspicion that another pathologic process is responsible. If there is gross hematuria, it is reasonable to disallow strenuous activity until clinical examination and repeat urinalysis are reassuring.

Upon return to sports activities, the athlete should maintain adequate hydration and can try not to void just before running; an empty bladder may contribute to bladder trauma. Bicycle seat hematuria is best prevented by seat adjustments, like use of a padded seat with enough width and forward tilt to ease pressure on the perineum.

PROTEINURIA

History and Diagnosis

Postexercise proteinuria is also common in both contact and noncontact sports, and the degree of proteinuria is directly related to the intensity of exercise involved. Normal protein excretion is 30 to 45 mg/day, while exertional proteinuria ranges from 100 to 300 mg/day, usually noted as 2+ to 3+ by dipstick evaluation. The proteinuria appears within 30 minutes of exercise and clears in 24 to 48 hours.

A thorough medical and family history, and repeat urinalysis after a 24- to 48-hour exercise-free interval, are the mainstays of initial evaluation. If these findings are normal, no further workup is needed. However, if the amount of proteinuria on initial presentation is 4+ or greater (over 1000 mg/dl), an additional 24-hour quantitative urinalysis is reasonable. Remember that pathologic proteinuria can be worsened by exercise. If the repeat urinalysis is abnormal, further evaluation may include serum kidney function tests, fasting blood glucose levels, complete blood cell count, urinary protein electrophoresis, imaging studies, and renal consultation.

Treatment and Return to Play

No activity restriction is recommended for those with exercise-induced proteinuria. There is no evidence that these athletes are at risk for chronic renal disease. However, a yearly evaluation of blood pressure and urinalysis has been recommended. This seems reasonable for those who present with postexercise proteinuria of 2+ (100 to 300 mg/day) or greater.

ACUTE RENAL FAILURE

Acute renal failure is an uncommon, but documented, risk of strenuous exercise. The risk is increased with prolonged exercise in the heat, especially in those who are less fit and poorly acclimated. Therefore, prevention includes adequate training, acclimatization to heat, awareness of heat stress symptoms, and adequate hydration before, during, and immediately following strenuous exercise.

MALE GENITAL TRAUMA

Testicular trauma presents with appropriate injury history and with scrotal pain and tenderness but also may involve referred pain around the groin and flank discomfort. Nausea is common, and vomiting may also occur. Palpating a painful scrotal mass in this setting may indicate testicular contusion or rupture, strangulated hernia, epididymitis, or testicular torsion.

Testicular contusion, which is the most common diagnosis, may involve minimal symptoms with brief resolution, or significant swelling and ecchymoses requiring scrotal elevation and bed rest. Initial treatment with ice impedes swelling, and in significant injuries ice application is imper-

ative for pain control. Returning to play depends on pain tolerance and on the functional ability of the athlete to meet his sport's demands. Wearing an athletic supporter can help control pain, and if recurrent trauma is possible, protection with an athletic cup is recommended.

Ruptures of the testicle or epididymis should be in the differential diagnosis of any scrotal trauma. These athletes often have persistent pain appearing out of proportion to the injury, or have progressive pain despite rest. Physical examination may reveal an expanding scrotal mass that cannot be transilluminated, or an epididymis that cannot be separated from the testicle. Ultrasound imaging may be problematic due to false-negative findings and should not delay expedient referral for urologic consultation and treatment.

Testicular cord torsion is not thought to be a direct result of sport involvement, but an athlete may be at risk if a high attachment of the tunica vaginalis on the spermatic cord allows abnormal mobility of the testis during vigorous activity. The young athlete presents with acute, excruciating testicular pain. Examination findings may include a high-riding testicle, obliteration of the space between the epididymis and the cord, an abnormal epididymal position, or induration of the overlying scrotal skin. Radionuclide scanning can accurately distinguish torsion from epididymitis, but immediate surgical consultation is required, and should not be delayed.

Finally, prolonged cycling may lead to paresthesia and numbness of the perineum, scrotum, and penis, due to compression of the genitofemoral nerve or pudendal nerve between the symphysis pubis and bicycle seat. Transient urinary retention and decreased force of voiding have also been reported. These problems are self-limited and resolve with relative rest, alteration in bicycle seat position, or change in seat style. Unless symptoms persist or progress, it is not necessary to discontinue biking.

PREPARTICIPATION CONSIDERATIONS

Allowing an athlete to participate in contact sports, or even limited contact sports, with a single kidney is controversial. Published reviews of all causes of renal trauma requiring hospitalization implicated sports in 4 to 28 percent of injuries, although the actual loss of a kidney due to a sports accident rarely occurs. Considering that the incidence of a solitary kidney (congenital or acquired) has been estimated at 1 in every 1100 to 1800 persons, and even as high as 1 in 500 persons, it is remarkable that so few catastrophic injuries related to sports are noted. The finding of a single normal kidney demands a thorough discussion with the athlete, and often the athlete's family, making sure that they have a full understanding of the risks and benefits of athletic participation before a decision allowing participation in contact or limited contact sports can be made. A single abnormal kidney (dysfunctional, deformed, or displaced) benefits from renal consultation for individualized decision making, and may warrant restriction to noncontact sports. Appropriate protective padding is recommended for both practice and games, although the type of padding is controversial, and proof of efficacy is lacking.

The athlete with a single testicle (the other testicle either absent or undescended) or single ovary usually is not restricted from contact or collision sports. A similar discussion of risks prior to participation is necessary, and a protective athletic cup is recommended for male athletes.

SUGGESTED READINGS

Anderson CR: Solitary kidneys and sports participation. Arch Fam Med 4:885–888, 1995.

Cianflocco AJ: Renal complications of exercise. Clin Sports Med 11(2):437–451, 1992.

Eichner ER: Hematuria: A diagnostic challenge. Physician Sportsmed 18(11):55–63, 1990.

Goldszer R, Siegel A: Renal abnormalities during exercise. *In* Strauss R (ed): Sports Medicine, 2nd ed. Philadelphia, W.B. Saunders, 1991, pp. 156–166.

Mee S, McAninch J: Indications for radiographic assessment in suspected renal trauma. Urol Clin North Am 16(2):187–192, 1989.

York, JP: The male genitourinary system. *In* Strauss R (ed): Sports Medicine, 2nd ed. Philadelphia, W.B. Saunders, 1991, pp. 515–528.

Chapter 17 | Special Issues of Young and Adolescent Athletes

MICHELE LaBOTZ, M.D.
BRYAN W. SMITH, M.D., Ph.D.

Although young athletes have many of the same sports-related problems as adults, their changing physiology predisposes them to some unique injuries as well. This chapter focuses on these unique aspects of sports injury in immature athletes by initially addressing some general physiologic principles and then looking at specific injury patterns that are frequently encountered in children and adolescents.

GENERAL PRINCIPLES

Growth (Physeal) Plates

Children's bones and cartilage are fundamentally different from those of adults. Bony growth requires open epiphyseal plates and apophyses (sites of musculotendinous attachment to bone). These cartilage plates are often the weak link in the kinetic chain; therefore, they are particularly vulnerable to injury. The classic example of a growth plate injury is the ankle inversion that usually leads to ligamentous injury in the adult but often results in a distal fibular growth plate injury in the child. The index of suspicion for bone injury in the child increases with any injury that involves areas near the ends of long bones. The presence of bony tenderness, even with normal x-rays, requires conservative treatment of a suspected growth plate injury.

The Salter-Harris fracture classifications are widely published and are significant to the primary care provider in that Salter-Harris I and V fractures are frequently not noticed on routine radiographs. The dividing cells that provide linear growth are located on the epiphyseal side of the growth plate. Therefore, Salter-Harris fractures III through V, or any fracture that disrupts the blood supply to these cells, have a relatively higher risk for growth disruption at a particular site. It is also important to note that some sites of physeal injury have much higher rates of growth disruption than do others. The distal femur and distal tibia are two commonly injured sites that need careful management and close follow-up to minimize this risk.

Apophyseal Plates

Apophyses are similar to epiphyseal plates because the growth cartilage at these sites is a weak link and therefore more susceptible to both acute and chronic injuries. Bones grow faster than the musculotendinous units. This discrepancy is thought to predispose the rapidly growing athletes to both acute and chronic injuries of the apophyseal plate. A force that causes muscle strain in adults may cause an avulsion injury in the adolescent athlete. Although most nondisplaced avulsions respond well to immobilization, displaced avulsions may require open reduction. Traction apophysitis results from the microtrauma of repetitive pulling of the tendon attachment, which is believed to cause microfractures at the apophyseal plate. Radiographs of apophyseal plates are often neither sensitive nor specific for diagnosing traction apophysitis.

SHOULDER INJURIES

Instability and Impingement

History and Mechanism of Injury

With the exception of acute trauma, instability is the primary cause of shoulder complaints in young athletes.[1] Children's ligaments are inherently more lax than those of adults. In the shoulder, this results in a physiologic multidirectional instability that may lead to development of a secondary impingement syndrome. This type of instability is very different from that seen in patients who have recurrent subluxations or dislocations after an initial traumatic event. In activities that place repetitive stress on the glenohumeral joint, a strong rotator cuff is required to stabilize the humeral head, and strong scapulothoracic muscles are needed to stabilize the glenoid platform. As the rotator cuff fatigues, the humeral head tends to migrate upward, which can lead to impingement of the tendons passing beneath the acromial arch. This is especially common in activities with repeated overhead motion. Rotator cuff tears are rare in young athletes.

Presentation

Atraumatic subluxations may present painlessly either voluntarily or during glenohumeral activity. Impingement presents more insidiously with vague pain over the anterior and superior aspects of the shoulder. This pain initially occurs only with activity, but it may become constant. Night pain may be reported. Range of motion—especially elevation and internal rotation—may be limited.

Diagnosis

The physical examination should focus on findings of instability. Increased glide of the humeral head in an anteroposterior direction and positive apprehension and sulcus signs suggest multidirectional instability. Rotator cuff and range of motion testing should be performed, although classic impingement signs may not be present in young athletes, as most impingement is a secondary phenomenon. Painful popping or other mechanical symptoms on range of motion testing may indicate a tear of the glenoid labrum or bony damage to the humeral head.

Imaging Studies

These studies should include internal and external rotation anteroposterior (AP) views of the glenohumeral joint, along with axillary, lateral (or scapular Y), and outlet views. In true atraumatic instability, and in most cases of impingement, these radiographs will all be normal. With instability or mechanical symptoms on examination, a Stryker notch view can be obtained to visualize lesions of the posterolateral humeral head, which can occur in anterior dislocations (Hill-Sachs lesions). The axillary view can provide visualization of fractures of the glenoid rim (Bankart lesions), but the sensitivity is low. The outlet view can demonstrate a curved acromion that can be a source of bony impingement.

Treatment

Patients with instability or impingement should be started on a vigorous rotator cuff strengthening and scapular stabilizing program. During rehabilitation, athletes need to avoid glenohumeral movements and positions that elicit feelings of instability. This usually limits abduction to activities below shoulder level and requires avoidance of excess external rotation. Most will significantly improve with conservative therapy.

When to Refer

For patients with impingement symptoms, if symptoms persist after 3 months of compliance with a rehabilitation program, orthopaedic referral may be necessary to exclude rare causes of impingement. Patients with recurrent traumatic or painful shoulder dislocation, or who have abnormalities of the humeral head or glenoid rim, need orthopaedic referral. Some orthopaedists will wait up to a year after initiation of a rehabilitation program in atraumatic dislocations before instituting operative management.

Recovery and Return to Play

Rotator cuff therapy should gradually reduce symptom frequency and severity in these patients. When patients are asymptomatic at rest they may begin a gradual return to play. Athletes may return to play after achieving full, pain-free range of motion and strength adequate for the activity. Rotator cuff rehabilitation needs to be continued during functional progression to full play and may need to be continued while the immature athlete is training or competing at an intense level.

Key Points

- Impingement in young athletes is usually secondary to multidirectional instability.
- Instability requires a rotator cuff rehabilitation program.
- Locking, grinding, painful popping, or radiologic evidence of glenohumeral bony injury needs orthopaedic referral.

Little League Shoulder

Mechanism of Injury and Presentation

This injury usually presents as pain in the dominant arm of a pitcher. It is an overuse syndrome of the proximal humeral growth plate. Osteochondrosis and articular cartilage changes are rare.

Diagnosis and Imaging Studies

Shoulder examination may reveal tenderness over the humeral head but is generally nonspecific. Shoulder radiographs reveal widening of the proximal humeral physeal plate relative to the uninvolved side.

Treatment

Treatment consists of 4 to 6 weeks of rest from pitching. Complete healing without sequelae should dictate the athlete's return to throwing.

Key Points

- This injury is readily treated with 4 to 6 weeks of rest.
- Radiographs are necessary to rule out other causes of proximal humeral bone pain.

ELBOW INJURIES

Elbows seem to be particularly vulnerable to injury in the young athlete. The valgus orientation of the elbow combined with the repetitive nature of throwing and racquet sports generate increased stress across the growth plates there. "Little League elbow" is frequently a catch-all term for medial elbow complaints, but it is important to realize that throwing injuries can affect the lateral and posterior aspects of the elbow as well. The same holds true for racquet sports and for activities such as gymnastics, in which the elbow becomes a weight-bearing joint.

Injuries to the Medial Elbow

Mechanism of Injury

The repetitive stress to the medial elbow as seen in throwing or racquet sports can result in microtrauma to the medial epicondylar apophysis. If not addressed promptly, this stress can lead to avulsion of the medial epicondyle. Numerous complications can occur, including acute and chronic fracturing of the medial epicondyle (the most common fracture in young throwing athletes) and premature closure of the growth plate. Ligamentous and ulnar nerve injuries are unusual in this age group.

Presentation

Decreased performance is often the first indicator of injury, which frequently leads to increased training and further overuse. Pain is present during and after activity and is usually localized to the medial elbow. However, lateral or posterior complaints can reflect related problems. Throwers may pinpoint a particular time in the throwing phase that exacerbates their symptoms. Medial stress is maximal during the late cocking and early acceleration phase of throwing.

Diagnosis

Physical examination often reveals a flexion contracture and tenderness over the medial epicondyle. Swelling is common but may be subtle, particularly in chronic injuries. Resisted wrist flexion and pronation is usually painful and may be restricted. It is important to do a full elbow and distal neurovascular examination. Ulnar nerve function is tested by assessing sensation of the fourth and fifth fingers and by resisted abduction of the fifth finger.

Imaging Studies

Optimally, anteroposterior, lateral, and internal and external oblique radiographs of the involved elbow are necessary. Comparison films of the un-involved side often reveal subtle growth plate injuries in the injured elbow that might otherwise go undetected (Fig. 17–1). Findings that can be seen include fragmentation, beaking, or spurring of the medial epicondyle to complete closure of the physis.

Treatment and Return to Play

The mainstay of treatment is rest and symptomatic treatment with ice and nonsteroidal anti-inflammatory drugs (NSAIDs). Four to 6 weeks are usually required for complete symptom resolution, followed by a rehabilitation program, which begins with range of motion activities followed by strengthening exercises. A progressive throwing program can usually commence once adequate strength is achieved. If pain resumes at any point during the rehabilitation process, throwing is discontinued until the athlete is asymptomatic at rest. Splinting may be required in recalcitrant cases or if compliance cannot be assured.

When to Refer

Avulsions or other bony abnormalities (spurring, premature growth plate closure) that interfere with elbow or ulnar nerve function should be referred to an orthopaedist. Displaced avulsions require surgical referral.

Key Points

- Little League elbow is not benign and requires intervention.

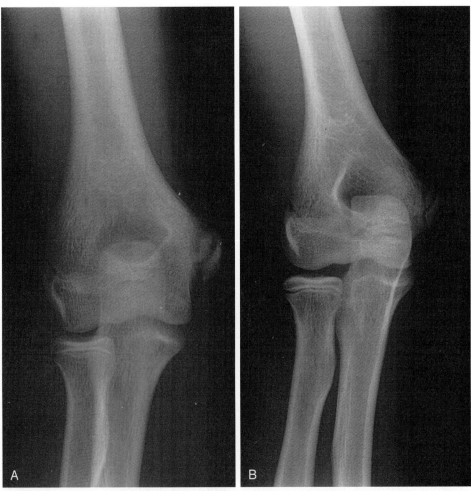

Figure 17–1. *A*, Widened medial epicondylar apophysis in a 14-year-old pitcher. *B*, Normal contralateral side for comparison.

- Adequate rest is essential; it is often several weeks until throwing can resume.
- Recurrence of symptoms requires complete rest for the remainder of the season.
- Evaluation of ulnar nerve function is important.

Injuries of the Lateral Elbow

Mechanism of Injury

Many lateral elbow complaints in children and adolescents are due to chronic compression injuries of the radial head and capitellum, which are variations of Little League elbow. The repetitive compression of throwing can result in osteochondritis dissecans (OCD) of the capitellum or the radial head. Early adolescent pitchers and gymnasts are most susceptible to injury. For gymnasts, vaulting and floor exercises seem to be the activities that most often cause this problem. Chronic lateral elbow pain in younger athletes (7 to 12 years old) is most often due to Panner's disease, which is an osteochondrosis of the capitellum. Panner's disease is considered a self-limited condition of necrosis of the capitellum with continued normal growth and subsequent recalcification. OCD, in contrast, can result in deformity and loose body formation.

Presentation

As in medial injuries, the first manifestations may be decreased performance and flexion contracture. Diffuse or lateral elbow pain is often relieved with rest. In patients with unstable fragments, locking or catching of the elbow may occur.

Diagnosis

Examination often reveals flexion contracture, diffuse pain, and swelling. Mechanical symptoms such as locking or grinding may also be present. A full elbow examination may reveal concurrent medial or posterior injury.

Imaging

Plain radiographs (Fig. 17–2) may reveal cystic and sclerotic changes of the capitellum, radial head flattening and deformity, and occasionally loose bodies. Comparison views of the uninvolved side are often helpful for evaluation. Special studies such as computed tomography (CT), arthrography, or magnetic resonance (MR) imaging may be necessary to fully assess the damage.

Treatment and Return to Play

Subchondral damage with intact articular cartilage usually responds well to relative rest and a strict avoidance of any throwing or impact-loading activities. Splinting or casting may be necessary for compliance. After symptoms resolve, range of motion and strengthening exercises can be instituted with radiographic evidence of healing expected in 6 to 12 weeks. This is followed by a slow functional progression, which may take 6 to 12 months. Lesions with large or unstable fragments will need surgical referral to either pin or removal of the involved area. Panner's disease is treated symptomatically with rest. Splinting is sometimes required, and radiographic follow-up after symptom resolution is recommended.

Key Points

- Early adolescent pitchers and gymnasts can develop OCD of the capitellum or radial head.
- Mechanical symptoms such as locking and catching are often present in OCD.
- Panner's disease in young children requires symptomatic therapy and is usually without sequelae.

WRIST INJURIES

Most wrist injuries result from a fall onto an outstretched hand with serious ligamentous injury being rare in the immature athlete. Fractures and growth plate injuries are usually seen in the distal radius and ulna. Most are treated with cast immobilization depending on the type and extent of the fracture. The scaphoid is the most common carpal bone fractured. If initial radiographs are negative, the athlete should be placed in a thumb spica cast if clinical suspicion warrants. Repeat radiographs should be obtained in 2 weeks or bone scanning performed to confirm the diagnosis.

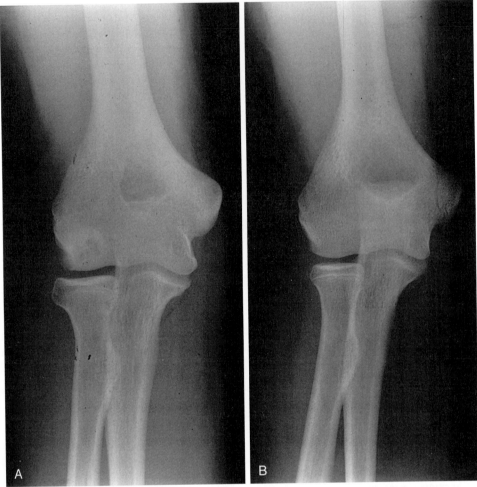

Figure 17-2. Osteochondritis dissecans of the capitellum and radial head hypertrophy in a 15-year-old pitcher. *A,* Premature medial epicondylar apophyseal closure is seen. *B,* Normal contralateral side for comparison.

Distal Radial Physeal Stress Reaction

Mechanism of Injury

This injury occurs from repeated axial loads to the hyperextended wrist. The resultant microtrauma alters the ossification and growth processes. It has been primarily reported in young (12 to 14 years old) female gymnasts who practice in excess of 35 hours per week.[2] Floor exercise and vaulting usually provoke the most symptoms.

Presentation

Symptoms are bilateral in about one third of the cases. Pain is typically elicited over the distal radial physis when the wrist is placed into forced hyperextension and axially loaded. Swelling may or may not be appreciated.

Diagnosis and Imaging Studies

The diagnosis depends on the symptoms elicited and the presence of radiographic findings. Gabel has proposed three stages of stress reaction.[2]

Stage I: Preradiographic
Stage II: Radial physeal radiographic changes
Stage III: Stage II changes with secondary positive ulnar variance

Several radiographic changes of the distal radius can be found on the AP and lateral views and include indistinct margins; a widened, beaked, or cystic appearance; and irregularity of the physis. Late radiographic findings include positive ulnar variance with shortening of the radius due to distal radial growth arrest. Comparison views may be helpful in unilateral cases.

Treatment and Return to Play

With the stage I injuries, the athlete should be restricted from activities that axially load the joint. By 2 to 4 weeks, symptoms have usually resolved and following a normal examination, the athlete may resume full activity. Any resumption of pain would necessitate further activity restriction.

Stage II injuries require similar treatment as stage I. Athletes and parents need to be informed that resolution of the symptoms usually requires longer activity restriction (up to 3 months), and the prognosis for recovery without permanent sequelae is less certain. Splinting or casting will increase compliance and may hasten resolution. Imaging plays little role in the return-to-play decision.

The likelihood of developing a stage III injury seems to be proportional to the length of time spent competing in gymnastics. These individuals may also develop ulnar pain secondary to ulnar impaction or injury to the triangular fibrocartilage complex. These athletes may be at increased risk for degenerative arthritis.

When to Refer

Proper diagnosis of this condition and recognition of complications is important in deciding whether conservative care or orthopaedic referral is indicated. Recognizing the length of time for recovery and the possibility of a less than optimal outcome, the practitioner's comfort level in managing stages II and III stress reactions dictates whether orthopaedic referral is indicated.

Key Points

- Distal radial physeal stress reaction is seen primarily in young competitive gymnasts.
- Rest from axial loading can relieve symptoms and reduce the chance for complications.
- Disregard for the symptoms can result in premature closure of the distal radial growth plate.

HAND INJURIES

Hand injuries are very common at all levels of sport. Improper treatment can result in loss of motion and decreased use. The practitioner needs to have a solid knowledge of the anatomy and function of the fingers and the hand.

Gamekeeper's Thumb

Mechanism of Injury

The mechanism of injury is a fall on an outstretched hand with the thumb abducted and a force directed radially. In the adult, this results in a sprain of the ulnar collateral ligament. In the immature athlete, a Salter-Harris type II or III fracture is more likely.

Presentation

This hand injury is common in skiing and football. The athlete presents with swelling and ecchymoses about the thumb. There is loss of range of motion. Pain may be nondistinct but is usually greatest at the ulnar side of the metacarpophalangeal joint.

Diagnosis

A radiograph should be obtained prior to stressing the joint to avoid displacing a probable fracture. If there is no evidence of fracture, the ulnar collateral ligament must be stressed by applying radial deviation in full extension and at 30 degrees of flexion. Comparison to the noninjured thumb is useful. Determination of a firm end point while stressing the ligament confirms the integrity of the ligament.

Imaging Studies

AP, lateral, and oblique views of the thumb are obtained. Any irregularity of the joint surface, rotation or displacement of 2 mm or more requires reduction.[3]

Treatment

Nondisplaced growth plate fractures as well as incomplete sprains of the ulnar collateral ligament can be treated with short arm thumb spica casting for 4 weeks. Mild sprains with no evidence of instability may only need 1 to 2 weeks of splinting. Following casting, the athlete should be placed in a rehabilitation program to regain range of motion and strength of the thumb.

Return to Play

The athlete can be allowed to participate in sports while casted. The cast can be molded to fit a ski pole grip. Following cast removal, the return of full function and strength dictates return to play.

When to Refer

Any displaced or malaligned growth plate fracture or a ligamentous injury in which the examiner cannot determine a firm end point when stressing needs orthopaedic evaluation for possible surgical intervention.

Key Points

- Gamekeeper's thumb is usually a growth plate fracture in the immature athlete.
- Do not stress the thumb until radiographs are obtained.
- Any destabilizing injury requires orthopaedic referral.

LOWER BACK PAIN AND INJURY

The natural history of lower back pain in children is very different from that in adults, and the diagnosis of mechanical lower back pain in immature athletes is one of exclusion. Back pain lasting longer than 3 weeks requires a careful evaluation to rule out significant injury or other pathologic process. Degenerative disk disease is much less common than in adults, although disk herniations can occur. During phases of rapid growth, the vertebral column exerts tension on the lumbodorsal fascia and frequently causes lower back pain. Stretching often provides rapid relief.

Spondylolysis and Spondylolisthesis

Mechanism of Injury

Spondylolysis is a stress fracture of the pars interarticularis resulting from recurrent microtrauma with repetitive back hyperextension. This most often occurs at the L5 level. With disruption of both pars in a given segment, spondylolisthesis results when one vertebral segment slips on the next.

Presentation

Spondylolysis is frequently seen in sports that promote hyperextension of the lumbar spine such as gymnastics, diving, and dancing. However, athletes in other sports such as volleyball and football can develop spondylolysis. Athletes usually present with progressive lower back pain that is worsened with back extension and twisting. Rest often provides relief. Radicular symptoms may occur, especially with spondylolisthesis. Both conditions are often associated with the beginning of the adolescent growth spurt. There may be a genetic predisposition, and many patients with spondylolysis are also found to have spina bifida occulta.

Diagnosis

Tenderness and muscle spasms may be present in the paraspinous region. Hamstrings are often relatively tight. Resisted back extension and hyperextension while standing on one leg will frequently reproduce the pain. Neurologic examination is frequently normal, but the L5 nerve root should be specifically assessed (dorsiflexion of the great toe and foot) for dysfunction.

Imaging Studies

Plain radiographs should include standing AP, lateral, and bilateral oblique films of the lumbar spine. On oblique films, the spinous processes resemble Scottie dogs and pars defects present as radiolucent "collars" about their necks. As with all stress fractures, routine x-rays are not sensitive for spondylolysis early in the course of the disease, and bone scanning has traditionally been indicated for athletes with persistent symptoms. However, one recent study showed bone scans to have a 15 percent false-positive rate when compared with axial and angled CT scans in the same subjects.[4]

Spondylolisthesis is readily visualized on standing lateral radiographs and is graded by the percentage of slip of one vertebra on its adjacent vertebra. Slippage up to 25 percent is considered grade I, 25 to 50 percent is grade II, 50 to 75 percent is grade III, and 75 to 100 percent is grade IV.

Treatment and Return to Play

Spondylolysis was previously believed to be primarily a congenital or developmental defect with little chance for repair. However, with current recognition of most cases as a stress fracture with potential for further injury, treatment is analogous to treatment for stress fractures in other parts of the skeleton. Asymptomatic patients do not require treatment. Symptomatic patients are treated with rest and immobilization. However, the intensity of the treatment regimen varies widely. Some regimens begin with a rigid antilordotic brace, which is initially worn 23 hours a day, and weaned as tolerated. This may take up to 6 months. A less restrictive program that has reported good results has been use of a nonrigid brace, avoidance of hyperextension activities, and cross training in nonextension activities (e.g., bicycling).[4] Persistent pain after 4 weeks leads to use of a rigid brace; otherwise, at 6 to 8 weeks patients began a slow progressive rehabilitation back to full activity. When athletes were pain-free at rest, with hyperextension, and with activity, they were allowed to return to competitive sports.

Treatment of spondylolisthesis depends on the amount of slippage. Any patient with over a 30 percent slip should be referred to an orthopaedist, regardless of symptoms. Symptomatic patients with less than 30 percent slip should be managed similarly to those patients with spondylolysis. Repeat radiographs should be obtained for any change in symptoms, and any progressive slip should be referred to an orthopaedist.

Usual Course and Recovery

The course is highly dependent on patient compliance with rest and bracing. Although growing athletes are particularly at risk for increased slippage, minor degrees of spondylolisthesis rarely progress to becoming symptomatic even with continuation of competitive sports.[5]

When to Refer

Referral depends on the clinician's comfort and familiarity with bracing techniques and ability to provide frequent follow-up. Compliant patients whose symptoms do not show continued improvement over the course of treatment or who are unable to wean themselves from the brace without recurrence of symptoms should be reevaluated for

other problems, and referral for surgical management should be considered.

Key Points

- Pain occurs with hyperextension.
- Back pain is frequently seen at the start of a growth spurt.
- Stress fracture often requires prolonged therapy.

HIP AND PELVIS INJURIES

Hip or groin complaints in the adolescent are frequently apophyseal injuries. The anterior superior iliac spine (origin of the sartorius) and the ischium (origin of the hamstrings) are the most frequent sites of these injuries. However, any child with hip pain, especially with limitation of internal rotation, needs AP and frog leg radiographs of the hips to rule out Legg-Calvé-Perthes disease in the young child and slipped capital femoral epiphysis in the preadolescent.

KNEE INJURIES

Although acute ligamentous and meniscal injuries are less common in immature athletes than in adults, young athletes who acutely injure the knee and have a resultant hemarthosis have a strong likelihood of ligamentous or meniscal injury. However, the practitioner must consider a physeal injury in a youngster in what would be considered an uncomplicated ligament sprain in an adult. Suspected cases warrant stress radiographs. Physeal injuries of the distal femur or tibia are uncommon but are notorious for growth disruption; these patients should have orthopaedic referral.

Most chronic knee complaints involve the extensor mechanism. In young athletes this includes apophysitis of the patellar tendon in addition to the patellofemoral disorders and patellar tendinitis that are seen frequently in adults.

Osgood-Schlatter Disease and Sinding-Larsen-Johansson Disease

Mechanism of Injury

Osgood-Schlatter disease (OSD) is an apophysitis at the distal insertion of the patellar tendon onto the tibial tubercle. Sinding-Larsen-Johansson disease (SLJ) is an apophysitis at the proximal end of the patellar tendon at the distal pole of the patella. A similar condition also occurs where the quadriceps tendon inserts onto the proximal pole of the patella. These conditions all are caused by traction on the continuous tendon that connects the quadriceps to the tibial tubercle. These conditions usually occur in early adolescent males. Up to one third of cases are bilateral. The role of pre-existing Osgood-Schlatter disease as a risk factor for tibial tuberosity avulsion is unknown.

Presentation

These conditions typically present with chronic pain during activities in which the quadriceps is working eccentrically, especially during jumping and running. Avulsions of the tibial tuberosity are rare but can be seen in adolescent males who are involved in jumping activities. They present with pain, swelling, and inability to bear weight.

Diagnosis

With OSD there is tenderness at and possible swelling and prominence of the tibial tubercle, although SLJ is typically tender at the inferior pole of the patella. The patellar tendon may be tender in either condition.

Imaging Studies

Although the diagnosis is clinical, radiographs may be helpful in ruling out other pathologic conditions. X-rays may reveal fragmentation at the tibial tubercle or the presence of a discrete ossicle in OSD (Fig. 17–3). However, these findings are frequently seen in asymptomatic athletes as well. In SLJ x-rays are often normal but fragmentation at the inferior border of the patella may be seen.

Treatment

Ice massage and relative rest can be helpful to relieve acute symptoms. NSAIDs can be used acutely for symptom relief but not for a premature return to activity. Stretching of the quadriceps, hamstring, and iliotibial band help maintain flexibility throughout the adolescent growth spurt. Activity can be titrated to the athlete's tolerance.

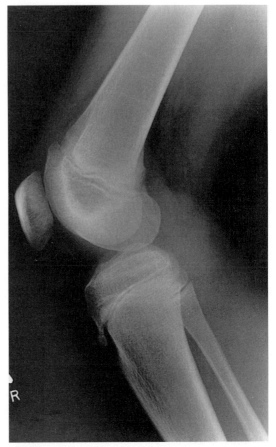

Figure 17–3. Lateral knee radiograph in a 13-year-old soccer player with Osgood-Schlatter disease.

Usual Course and Recovery

There is usually a 12- to 18-month period of waxing and waning symptoms until apophyseal closure. Increased activity brings about increased symptoms, and patients can adjust their activities accordingly. Prominence of the tibial tuberosity may be permanent. It is unclear if these conditions predispose to future patellar tendinitis.

When to Refer

If conservative management has failed, painful ossicles may require surgical excision.

Return to Play

Athletes may return to play as symptoms permit. However, the athlete might not tolerate kneeling, squatting, or jumping activities.

Key Points

- OSD and SLJ are self-limited conditions, frequently seen in adolescent males.
- Activity can be self-monitored.

Osteochondritis Dissecans

Mechanism of Injury and Presentation

Osteochondritis dissecans (OCD) is a rare lesion of the articular surface and subchondral surface that is primarily seen in the adolescent male. Its etiology is unknown, but many hypotheses center on acute or chronic disruption of the blood supply to subchondral bone. This disruption may lead to bony necrosis and subsequent fracturing and displacement of the bone and cartilage into the joint space. OCD is most frequently seen in the medial femoral condyle. The early stages may present with vague joint pain and intermittent swelling associated with activity, whereas later lesions may present with mechanical symptoms, such as joint locking or catching.

Diagnosis

The knee should be palpated in flexion to assess for intercondylar pain. Wilson's test may be positive with lesions that are located on the lateral aspect of the medial femoral condyle. In this test the patient is seated at the edge of the examining table and medially rotates the tibia. The patient then actively extends the knee. Pain at about 30 degrees may be indicative of an OCD lesion. The test is considered positive if knee extension with a laterally rotated tibia is subsequently pain-free. Patients may also have swelling and mechanical signs (locking, grinding) if there is a loose fragment.

Imaging Studies

On plain radiographs, tunnel views with the knee in flexion allows visualization of the condylar surfaces. OCD lesions may appear as a surface irregularity or a loose body on x-ray. MR imaging is sometimes required to visualize the lesion and also helps the surgeon assess stage of healing and viability of any fragments. One study recently proposed MR imaging staging of OCD lesions whereby intact cartilage, contrast enhancement of the lesion, and absent "cystic defects" indicated lesions that could be managed conservatively.[6] Lesions with cartilage defects, fragments surrounded by fluid, and detached fragments were thought to require surgical intervention.

OCD lesions are occasionally seen as incidental findings in asymptomatic patients. These patients do not require any further intervention other than observation.

Treatment

The outcome is much better if lesions are healed before physeal closure, and this should be the goal of treatment. About half of compliant patients with open growth plates heal within 10 to 18 months after starting conservative therapy.[7] Immobilization and non–weight-bearing are initiated until patients are pain-free with activities of daily living. Previous guidelines advocated prolonged periods of immobilization to assist nonoperative healing. However, it is now believed that joint motion is important in maintaining healthy articular cartilage; early, active, non–weight-bearing rehabilitation for 6 to 8 weeks is now recommended as long as patients are asymptomatic.

Usual Course and Recovery

Bone age is the primary determinant of OCD prognosis.[7] Younger patients (under 11 years for girls, and under 13 years for boys) have an excellent prognosis and usually regain normal function. Athletes older than 20 have a much higher incidence of loss of function and development of degenerative arthritis.

When to Refer

Patients who are nearing physeal closure should be referred early. Younger patients who have persistent symptoms with conservative therapy and those with fragments that have become unstable or show sclerosis on follow-up radiographs should also be referred.

Return to Play

This decision depends on the resolution of symptoms and radiographic evidence of healing.

Key Points

- OCD often presents with vague symptoms of insidious onset.
- Treatment and prognosis depend on age and stability of the OCD lesion.

ANKLE AND FOOT PAIN

Acute injuries of the ankle and foot in children require careful evaluation for bone injury. Ligamentous injury is often the exception rather than the rule, and radiographs are required when bony tenderness is elicited. Standing and comparison radiographs of the uninvolved side may help detect subtle widening or irregularity of an injured growth plate.

Several developmental abnormalities may present as acute or chronic foot pain. Tarsal coalition, an autosomal dominant trait, may present as the fibrous union ossifies during early adolescence with symptoms referable to the subtalar joint. Plain radiographs (including oblique views) may reveal the abnormality; however, CT scans are often required. Accessory ossicles are common and may be a source of pain but are also frequently incidental findings during evaluation and should not be confused with a fracture. The most common sites of these ossicles are at the base of the fifth metatarsal and posterior to the talus. If conservative therapy fails to relieve ossicle symptoms, surgical excision may be required. Freiberg's disease is an infarction of the metatarsal head and is usually seen in young adolescent females, and Kohler's disease is an irregular ossification of the navicular usually seen in young (2 to 9 years old) children. Both are treated with casting or orthotics to relieve symptoms. Kohler's disease resolves without sequelae. In Freiberg's disease the metatarsal head reossifies in 2 to 3 years, but removal of loose bodies may be required.

Ankle Sprains and Fractures

Mechanism of Injury

The ankle is the most frequently injured joint in all athletes. Injuries in children can be different from those in adults owing to the presence of open growth plates in the distal tibia and fibula. A typical history involves an inversion ("rolled my ankle over") type of injury involving the lateral ankle about 85 percent of the time. Distinct medial ankle injuries should be considered fractures until proved otherwise. Distal tibial growth plate disruptions are particularly prone to premature closure, making appropriate management crucial.

Presentation

Athletes usually present acutely with ankle pain, swelling, and inability to bear weight. Later in the time course, there are usually ecchymoses with severe sprains and growth plate injuries.

Diagnosis

The distal tibia and fibula should be palpated for bony tenderness, especially over the growth plates. Sprains will present with inframalleolar tenderness. In inversion injuries, the fifth metatarsal should be palpated to assess for an avulsion fracture at the insertion of the peroneus brevis tendon or a possible Jones fracture (fractures of the proximal third of the diaphysis).

Imaging Studies

AP, lateral, and mortise views of the ankle may reveal bone or soft tissue findings consistent with a fracture. However, x-rays are frequently normal in Salter-Harris I and V physeal injuries. In any child with open growth plates, swelling and tenderness at the physis are sufficient to make the diagnosis. It is important to obtain foot radiographs in cases of fifth metatarsal tenderness (Fig. 17–4).

Treatment

Initial treatment consists of air-splinting the Salter-Harris I fibular fracture or severe sprain in neutral position, compression wrapping, elevation, ice, and adequate analgesia. Most patients will require crutches for a short period of time. Casting is reserved for situations in which compliance is in question, and the cast should be applied after initial swelling has resolved. Three to 6 weeks of immobilization is frequently required in appropriately immobilized fractures.

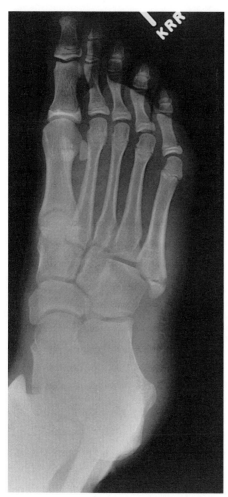

Figure 17–4. Fifth metatarsal avulsion fracture in a 12-year-old soccer player who presented with a history of a twisted ankle.

Usual Course and Recovery

As soon as possible, a functional rehabilitation program is begun. This ideally includes strengthening, range of motion, and proprioception components. These children need to be followed to ensure that normal growth continues in the affected bone. Any arrest in growth, which may occur up to 2 years after initial injury, needs to be seen by an orthopaedist for evaluation and possible surgical intervention.

When to Refer

Because of the risk for growth disruption, all Salter-Harris II to V fractures, tibial fractures, and any fracture of uncertain alignment should be referred to an orthopaedist.

Return to Play

The athlete may return to play when the ankle has been fully rehabilitated, with strength and range of motion comparable to that of the uninvolved ankle. The athlete should not exhibit any altered mechanics (e.g., a limp) that may predispose to further injury.

Key Points

- Bony tenderness on physical examination is a key diagnostic finding.
- Adequate immobilization is needed for growth plate injuries.
- Long-term follow-up is needed to ensure continued growth in affected physis.

Sever's Disease

Mechanism of Injury

Sever's disease is a traction apophysitis of the insertion of the Achilles tendon onto the calcaneus. It is common among 9- to 12-year-old athletes who are involved in repetitive impact activity, especially with poorly cushioned footwear, as seen in soccer cleats, or playing on hard surfaces. Biomechanical abnormalities that alter the pull of the Achilles tendon on the calcaneus can also contribute to symptom development.

Presentation

Athletes present with heel pain, which is exacerbated by impact activity. They may also complain of morning pain, which subsides during the day.

Diagnosis

Examination may reveal pain with side-to-side compression of the calcaneus or tenderness at the Achilles tendon insertion, but may be completely normal. There is often decreased flexibility of the gastrocnemius-soleus complex. The ankle examination is completely normal.

Imaging Studies

Radiographs are not routinely recommended, as the appearance of the calcaneal apophysis does not correlate with clinical symptoms. Irregularities and increased density of the calcaneal apophysis are frequently seen in asymptomatic patients.

Treatment

Treatment revolves around decreasing the chronic traction stress on the apophysis. Stretching of the plantarflexors and strengthening of the dorsiflexors is frequently helpful. Heel lifts or orthotics may also relieve some of the stress. A period of relative rest, ice, and NSAID treatment may be necessary for pain relief, and in severe cases casting may enforce rest. Do not consider injection of this site.

Usual Course and Recovery

Sever's disease is a self-limited condition that resolves with fusion of the calcaneal apophysis.

When to Refer

Sever's disease can routinely be managed by the primary care provider.

Return to Play

The athlete may return to play as symptoms allow. Patients need to be aware of the waxing and waning nature of their symptoms, and their willingness to "play with pain" will help determine their level of activity.

Key Points

- Heel pain and tenderness may be present without other significant findings.
- The disease is self-limited.
- Pain is the guideline for return to play.

REFERENCES

1. Ireland ML, Hutchinson MR: Upper extremity injuries in young athletes. Clin Sports Med 14:533–569, 1995.
2. Gabel GT: Gymnastic wrist injuries. Clin Sports Med 17:611–621, 1998.
3. Markiewitz AD, Andrish JT: Hand and wrist injuries in the preadolescent and adolescent athlete. Clin Sports Med 11:203–225, 1992.
4. Congeni J, McCulloch J, Swanson K: Lumbar spondylolysis. A study of natural progression in athletes. Am J Sports Med 25:248–253, 1997.
5. Muschik M, Hahnel H, Robinson PN, et al: Competitive sports and the progression of spondylolisthesis. J Pediat Orthoped 16:364–369, 1996.
6. Bohndorf K: Osteochondritis (osteochondrosis) dissecans: A review and new MRI classification. Europ Radiol 8:103–112, 1998.
7. Obedian RS, Grelsamer RP: Osteochondritis dissecans of the distal femur and patella. Clin Sports Med 16:157–174, 1997.

SUGGESTED READINGS

Nicholas JA, Hershman EB (eds): The Lower Extremity and Spine in Sports Medicine, 2nd ed. St. Louis, Mosby, 1995.
Nicholas JA, Hershman EB (eds): The Upper Extremity in Sports Medicine, 2nd ed. St. Louis, Mosby, 1995.
Stanitski CL, DeLee JC, Drez D Jr (eds): Pediatric and Adolescent Sports Medicine. Philadelphia, W.B. Saunders, 1994.

Chapter 18 | Special Issues of the Female Athlete

CONSTANCE M. LEBRUN, M.D.C.M., M.P.E., C.C.F.P.

The past several decades have seen a virtual "explosion" in the women's fitness industry, with increasing numbers of young girls and women participating in both recreational and competitive sports. This chapter briefly covers the history of sports for women, the health benefits for women of all ages, and special medical considerations unique to the female athlete. Common musculoskeletal injuries are also discussed. It is hoped that this information will be of assistance to the busy primary care practitioner managing the exercising female. Counseling and treating physically active women should be a rewarding part of medical practice.

HISTORY OF WOMEN IN SPORTS

Women did not always enjoy the relatively easy access to sport and recreation that is taken so much for granted today. For example, in the days of the ancient Greeks and Romans, merely watching Olympic events was punishable by being hurled off a cliff. Compare and contrast this with the current level of Olympic participation by women and the increasing presence of women in professional and male-dominated sports such as basketball and hockey.

Historically, there was a cultural belief that women should be feminine and inconspicuous, and that they might somehow damage their reproductive organs if they exercised too vigorously. The latter opinion was frequently supported by the medical thinking of the day. Fortunately, increased knowledge about the effects of training and competition has put some of these myths to rest. Changes in acceptable leisure and exercise clothing, such as the advent of bloomers for riding on bicycles, also literally paved the way for easier participation in sports.

This revolution came about slowly at first, beginning with women winning the right to vote, and landmark decisions, such as the Charter of Rights in Canada and the passage of Title IX of the Educational Assistance Act in the United States in 1972. Title IX decreed that all institutions receiving federal money were obligated to offer equal opportunities to both sexes (including equality of participation opportunities, scholarship dollars, and other athletic program benefits) in proportion to the numbers of women and men enrolled. This was indeed radical for the times, and although this ruling was popular among the female athletic population, it engendered some ill feelings, especially on the part of those males in traditional sports, such as football, who felt threatened and extremely protective of their level of funding. In the 1980s there was somewhat of a backlash against this edict, and the issue was taken to the Supreme Court. In 1984 athletic programs were deemed to be exempt from Title IX because they did not receive federal funding directly.

Fortunately, those in power in sport have continued to strive for greater opportunity and improved training for female athletes, coaches, and administrators, and the momentum continues in a positive direction. There remains, however, a great deal of work yet to be done at many levels. There is still a significant difference in media coverage of men's and women's sports, and even the language used to describe characteristics of female athletes can frequently be sexist and pejorative. Other barriers to exercise for women include lack of child care, as well as the demands of domestic duties, and double and triple workdays. The threat of sexual harassment or attack can cause women to alter their leisure and workout habits in order to protect their personal safety.

Professional inequity in management, coaching, officiating, and other administrative levels also needs to be addressed by the offering of more incentives and opportunities for women to pursue these professions. For example, in 1987 the Canadian Association for the Advancement of Women in Sport established the National Coaching School for Women. In addition to sport-specific coaching techniques, female coaches are educated about other important issues such as sexual harassment in sports, homophobia, and the like. Positive role models will encourage other women to follow in their footsteps.

The advocacy of large professional groups such as the American College of Sports Medicine is also crucial. In 1982, an opinion statement was issued by this group, supporting full participation of women in distance events.[1] Some believe that this was directly responsible for inclusion of the women's marathon in the 1984 Olympics in Los Angeles, whereas previously women had been limited to competing in events of 800 m or less.

Other organizations such as the Women's Sport Foundation, the Melpomene Institute, and more recently WomenSport International have continued to lobby for positive change for women and girls in sports and physical activity at all levels of involvement, as well as increased research into specific issues affecting female athletes. With the current surge of interest in the Internet as a means of effective communication and advertising, it is easy to find information about these specific groups, as well as others with similar goals. In 1994 the first International Conference on Women and Sport (Women, Sport and the Challenge of Change) was held in Brighton, England. This resulted in the Brighton Declaration on Women and Sport, the development of an International Strategy for Women in Sport, and the establishment of an International Working Group of Women and Sport. We can hope that the next millennium will continue to usher in additional advances for women in sport and recreation.

HEALTH BENEFITS OF EXERCISE FOR WOMEN

Women of all ages derive the same health benefits from regular physical activity as do their male counterparts: greater cardiorespiratory fitness, lower blood pressure, decreased percentage of body fat, and increased lean body mass. The implications for positive self-esteem, improved socialization skills, and enhanced self-confidence are also evident. Adolescents who are physically active have a substantial reduction in risk-taking health behaviors such as smoking, alcohol and drug abuse, and unprotected irresponsible sexual activity resulting in teenage pregnancy and sexually transmitted diseases. There is good epidemiologic evidence of increased longevity, lower incidence of cardiovascular disease (including atherosclerosis, dyslipidemia, and hypertension), non–insulin-dependent diabetes, and possibly some cancers. Weight-bearing activities, particularly when begun at an early age, are important for maximizing and maintaining bone mineral density.[2] In general, active women seem to suffer less from premenstrual syndrome and dysmenorrhea, the various discomforts associated with pregnancy (lower back pain, weight gain), and postmenopausal symptoms such as vasomotor instability and mood swings.

Physical activity is an important modifiable risk factor for coronary artery disease. Recent recommendations from the American College of Sports Medicine[3] on the amount and frequency of activity needed for a health-protective effect are not overly demanding and can be easily incorporated into a regular program. Daily quality physical activity in school programs and the development of community fitness and recreation programs should introduce girls to physical activity at an early age and promote lifelong interest and involvement.

PHYSIOLOGIC DIFFERENCES BETWEEN MALE AND FEMALE ATHLETES

In the past, much emphasis has been placed on the "unsuitability" of the female frame for vigorous exercise. Primarily due to the differential effects of the male and female sex hormones after puberty, there are substantial physical and physiologic differences between athletic men and women. Testosterone promotes growth of bone and lean muscle mass, and estrogen promotes breast development and increased fat distribution on the thighs and hips. Estrogen may have a protective effect on muscle membranes and an antioxidant activity that may diminish exercise-induced muscle damage. Specific glycogen-sparing effects of estrogen and progesterone may aid women in longer distance endurance events by preferentially shifting metabolism more toward fat as a substrate, rather than carbohydrate. Although it is true that, compared with male athletes, females have a lower aerobic capacity, lower hemoglobin, and less muscular strength (particularly in the upper body), several factors must be kept in mind. First, female athletes have their own specific needs for activity and do not need to compete with the males. Many of the so-called "differences" can be lessened if corrected for percentage of lean body mass, rather than just for weight. In addition, increasing opportunities for women in sport, leading to more athletic exposure at an earlier age, should help to bridge the gap.

The response to exercise training in both sexes is basically the same, including a decrease in resting heart rate and blood pressure and decreased body fat. The magnitude of change depends on the initial fitness level, as well as the specific training program. The fact that women have smaller hearts and lesser stroke volumes means that women may demonstrate a higher heart rate at the same percentage of maximal aerobic capacity. In practical terms, this has an important implication for the heart rate method of prescribing exercise, especially during more strenuous activities. It may be necessary to prescribe a sustained intensity level of 75 to 80 percent of maximal heart rate to achieve the desired training effect. Alternatively, the rating of perceived exertion (RPE) scale may be used to determine exercise intensity. Appropriate strength training for women will not result in the same muscle hypertrophy as in men, due to much lower levels of testosterone, but overall strength and conditioning can be improved, with the additional benefit of promotion of higher bone density.

Thermoregulation may be one of the important differences between male and female athletes. Women may be disadvantaged in conditions of extreme heat and humidity in the same way as children, due to a larger surface area to body mass ratio and a smaller sweat rate. In addition, in women in the reproductive age group, the thermogenic effect of progesterone during pregnancy or in the luteal phase of the cycle (increase of 0.3 to 0.4° C) may theoretically interfere with temperature regulation during prolonged exercise in conditions of high ambient heat and humidity.

Gender and regional differences in body composition also result from the actions of the sex hormones. Women have increased subcutaneous fat, particularly in the hips and thighs (gynecoidal fat pattern), while men (and postmenopausal women) are more prone to the androidal fat pattern, with fat accumulation in the abdominal area. The "pear" body type, with a waist-to-hip circumference ratio of less than 1, is thought to be associated with a lower prevalence of cardiovascular disease, hypertension, dyslipidemia, and diabetes than the "apple" silhouette, a waist-to-hip circumference ratio of greater than 1. Nevertheless, many successful female athletes have thin, narrow "boyish" hips and wide shoulders.

There are currently no completely accurate methods of determining body composition. The use of skinfold measurements is limited by the reproducibility of the instrument and technique of the measurer, as well as by the formulae used. Even the "gold standard" of underwater weighing has an estimated error range of 2 to 4 percent. Perhaps a more important consideration in the female athlete with premature osteoporosis due to menstrual abnormalities is the tendency of this method to "overestimate" percentage body fat, unless a suitable correction factor is used in the equation to compensate for the decreased bone density. In general, sport-specific "recommendations" for optimal body composition are determined by measuring the top athletes in the given sport and are not based on any scientific evidence of significant improvement in performance. There is an inherent danger of precipitating disordered eating patterns in susceptible individuals when too much emphasis is placed on body composition. It is far more effective to emphasize proper nutrition and training methods, as well as the development of lean body mass.

There are frequently biomechanical differences between men and women, but again, caution must be used in their interpretation. Women are commonly thought to have a wider, more shallow pelvis and a greater Q angle (angle between the femur and tibia) than men, as well as a higher incidence of the so-called "miserable malalignment" syndrome (increased femoral anteversion, tibial torsion, and excess pronation). These features may predispose to overuse injuries. However, most athletic injuries are more sport-specific than gender-specific, and it is not possible to generalize to such a degree. There is as much variation between body types and the shape of the pelvis among men or women as there is between them. Specifically, no biomechanical factor should discourage or preclude a healthy girl or woman from becoming physically active.

MUSCULOSKELETAL INJURIES IN FEMALE ATHLETES

There are some sports, such as rhythmic gymnastics and synchronized swimming, that are practiced exclusively by young women and girls. Other sports, such as football and boxing, still remain largely a male bastion. The lines are becoming more blurred in activities such as ice hockey, rugby, wrestling, and weight lifting. Women's ice hockey was introduced into the Winter Olympics for the first time in Nagano in 1998, and women's participation in the other sports is becoming more common at the high school, collegiate, national, and professional levels.

Sport injury data also reflect the absolute numbers of each gender taking part. Soccer, for example, is the most widely played game in the world, with scores of female athletes embracing it enthusiastically. Women's rugby is currently the fastest growing sport in North America. Gymnastics and figure skating, on the other hand, have many more female than male participants.

Lower Extremity Injuries

The feet and ankles take a beating in most sports, with the common ankle inversion sprain being the most frequent injury. Proper management includes early referral to physical therapy, and protection with tape or an ankle brace for return to sport. The chief cause of a repeat injury is inadequate rehabilitation, especially in terms of proprioceptive retraining. An injury to the high lateral ankle may actually be a fracture or stress fracture of the fibula. Stress fractures are also common in the metatarsal and tarsal bones, as well as in the tibia and femur in runners, military recruits, and dancers. There may be associated problems with disordered eating and menstrual irregularity, including amenorrhea. Stress fractures of the navicular bone, the upper anterior tibial cortex, or the shaft and neck of the femur must be diagnosed and managed appropriately to avoid progression to a complete fracture. Bony impingement at the anterior tibiotalar joint, or posteriorly due to an os trigonum, can occur as a result of excess axial loading and extremes of dorsiflexion and plantarflexion of the ankle. Bunions and hallux valgus deformities of the feet are more common in women than in men, largely due to the design of footwear.

Female athletes seem to have a greater propensity toward anterior knee problems such as patellofemoral pain syndrome. Although biomechanics and joint laxity are frequently implicated as causative factors, inadequate development of the musculature about the knee, especially the vastus medialis obliquus muscle, is also likely a factor. In a survey carried out by the National Collegiate Athletic Association,[4] women were found to have a higher incidence of tears of the anterior cruciate ligament in both basketball and soccer than did male participants. The debate continues as to whether intrinsic factors (such as size of the ligament and the notch it has to pass through) or extrinsic variables (body movement, muscular strength and coordination, and skill level) play a greater role. Extrinsic factors, of course, can be improved upon by specific training programs.

Back Injuries

Women also seem to have a slightly higher incidence of scoliosis, frequently in association with menstrual dysfunction. Spondylolysis or stress fractures of the pars interarticularis of the lumbar vertebrae are commonly seen in female gymnasts, figure skaters, divers, and dancers who perform repetitive hyperextension maneuvers. In males these injuries are not as prevalent, but they can be seen in athletes such as football linemen and pole vaulters.

Upper Extremity Injuries

A combination of increased ligamentous laxity and less upper body strength can lead to shoulder injuries such as impingement syndrome (or swimmer's shoulder) and multidirectional instability, but these injuries are treated the same in male and female athletes. About the elbow, boys will more commonly develop Little League elbow from baseball, and young female gymnasts with an increased carrying angle of the elbow and repetitive loading through the joint may present with osteochondritis dissecans and/or loose bodies in the joint. A common injury in young female gymnasts (frequently misdiagnosed as a wrist sprain) is a stress injury to the distal radial epiphysis. If this is not picked up early, there can be permanent damage to the growth plate, and subsequent overgrowth of the ulna in relation to the radius.

Head and Neck Injuries

As women increase their participation in contact sports, it is inevitable that a corresponding increase will occur in cervical spine and head injuries. Some experts believe that women, with weaker neck stabilizing muscles and a relative lack of experience in hitting or tackling, may have proportionately more injuries than men who have grown up learning the proper techniques to protect themselves. Specific criteria to determine return to play after a concussion are quite controversial and are not based on any valid scientific studies. Under these circumstances, however, it is usually better to err on the conservative side of management for both sexes.

Gender-Specific Injuries and Conditions

Female athletes can suffer from a variety of breast disorders including direct trauma, discomfort during sports activity due to large breasts, and nipple irritation from the friction of overlying clothing. Fibrocystic changes, breast lumps, and galactorrhea may be detected by regular breast self-examination and should be further investigated and treated as appropriate. For the most part the other problems can be managed with a properly fitting and supportive sports bra, although protective chest plates may be required for certain sports such as softball, hockey, and other contact sports. Fortunately, a number of companies now make such women's sports equipment.

The female reproductive organs are generally better protected from trauma than are those of males. Pain in the pelvis and groin area may be due to a sporting injury such as a femoral neck or pelvic stress fracture, but it is also important to exclude gynecologic problems. Specific menstrual dysfunction and contraception will be discussed in further detail later.

In older women, stress incontinence and other pelvic floor problems such as uterine prolapse may occur secondary to childbirth and aging of the tissues. These disorders may be embarrassing for women to discuss and should therefore be specifically inquired about, as they may frequently limit

or completely inhibit exercise participation. Conservative treatment can include Kegel exercises or biofeedback techniques and use of machines to retrain pelvic floor muscles, as well as the use of pessaries, but surgical referral may ultimately be necessary.

THE YOUNG DEVELOPING FEMALE ATHLETE

Puberty and adolescence is a time of rapid growth and physiologic change for both sexes. In most young girls, peak height velocity is reached between the ages of 10.5 and 13 years, with menarche occurring approximately 1 year later. Although growth slows after this, it continues until skeletal maturity is reached by about the age of 18 or 19 in girls. This is a crucial time for young women—their social skills are being formed, and their bodies are developing and changing. Sport can offer an outlet for them, but can also be risky in terms of injuries. Tight muscles in relation to rapidly growing bones can lead to an increased incidence of injuries to the epiphyses (or growth plates) as well as the apophyses (or attachment of tendons to bone).

Development of the reproductive organs follows a sequence of thelarche (development of pubic hair) and menarche or onset of menstruation. Clinically, the use of Tanner stages during this time may be helpful to separate prepubescent from postpubescent athletes for purposes of contact and collision sports. The average age of menarche in the United States is 12.8 years, but there is a wide range of "normal." In general, a girl should be investigated for primary amenorrhea if she has not begun to menstruate by the age of 16, or has not developed secondary sexual characteristics by the age of 14.

Currently it is debated whether vigorous athletic training prior to puberty can delay menses and adversely affect final adult height.[5] Some experts think that late-maturing girls are selectively channeled into sports, because their physique offers them a competitive advantage, while the early maturers are socialized away from them. Nevertheless, there appears to be a threshold of approximately 12 to 14 hours per week of vigorous training, the exceeding of which may cause problems. It is a well-known phenomenon that young girls participating in gymnastics or dance who have to stop training because of an injury frequently undergo a growth spurt and onset of menstruation.

ATHLETICS AND THE MENSTRUAL CYCLE

During the first several years after menarche, menstrual cycles may be irregular before they settle into the adult ovulatory pattern. There is a well-defined cascade of hormonal and physiological events that characterize an ovulatory menstrual cycle.

Events of the Menstrual Cycle

Menses (the days of menstrual bleeding) usually lasts 5 to 6 days. The endometrium or lining of the uterus is being shed. Menstrual cramps or dysmenorrhea during this time may disrupt athletic performance, and can usually be managed with antiprostaglandin medications.

The follicular or proliferative phase includes the following:

- The hypothalamus secretes gonadotropin-releasing hormone (GnRH).
- GnRH stimulates the pituitary gland to release follicle-stimulating hormone (FSH) and luteinizing hormone (LH). FSH promotes growth of the ovarian follicle(s) and synthesis of estrogen from androgen precursors, and LH stimulates androgen production from the ovary.
- One or more of the developing follicles in the ovary is stimulated to grow and become dominant.
- Average length is 14 days, but this phase is subject to variation.

Approaching ovulation, there is a sudden increase in LH and FSH secretion owing to the positive feedback of increasing estrogen levels. These hormones trigger ovulation, with subsequent formation of the corpus luteum.

The luteal phase or proliferative stage includes the following:

- Corpus luteum secretes estrogen and progesterone, which stabilize the endometrial lining and prepare it for implantation of the fertilized ovum.
- This stage generally lasts from 10 to 14 days. A luteal phase less than 10 days is termed a shortened luteal phase and may be the first sign of menstrual dysfunction.
- High levels of estrogen and progesterone can cause symptoms such as breast tenderness, fluid retention, food cravings, and mood swings. In moderation, these symptoms are known as molimina and indicate normal functioning of the hypothalamic-pituitary-ovarian axis. In excess, they can become troublesome as premenstrual syndrome (PMS).

If fertilization does not occur, gradual decline in estrogen and progesterone levels triggers desquamation of the endometrium as menstrual flow.

Definitions[6]

1. Eumenorrhea: Ovulatory menstrual cycles at intervals of 20 to 38 days.

2. Oligomenorrhea: Menstrual cycles at intervals greater than 39 to 90 days.

3. Amenorrhea

- Primary amenorrhea: No menstrual cycles by the age of 16 or no development of secondary sexual characteristics (i.e., breasts or pubic hair) by the age of 14.
- Secondary amenorrhea: No menstrual cycles for more than 6 months or less than three cycles in a year following menarche and the establishment of regular menstrual cycles.

MENSTRUAL DYSFUNCTION

Menstrual dysfunction generally follows a continuum, but there is no evidence to indicate the rate of progression from one stage to another:

1. Ovulatory menstrual cycles.

2. Shortened luteal phase.

3. Anovulatory menstrual cycles: "Regular" menstrual bleeding occurs, but ovulation does not take place and hormonal levels remain low throughout the cycle. Clues include irregular bleeding not preceded by any ovulatory symptoms. In practice, a good clinical question is, "Can you tell by how you are feeling if your period is coming?"

4. Hypoestrogenic amenorrhea.

Athletic Amenorrhea

The diagnosis of athletic amenorrhea is one of exclusion. It is thought to be a form of hypothalamic amenorrhea. In athletes, the incidence is 10 to 44 percent (compared with approximately 5 percent in the general population).

The mechanism of athletic amenorrhea is thought to be multifactorial.[7]

1. Training regimen—abrupt onset of intense exercise.

2. Reproductive maturity—onset of training after menses are well established is less likely to precipitate menstrual dysfunction, suggesting that maturation of the hypothalamic-pituitary-ovarian axis is critical.

3. Changes in body weight and composition: It was previously thought that a critical level of body fat was necessary for initiation and maintenance of menstrual cycles, but currently it is believed that each individual may have a specific threshold.

4. Dietary changes—it is more common in vegetarians.

5. Emotional and psychological stress may be factors.

6. Sport specificity? Higher incidence in runners than swimmers or cyclists.

There are two main pathophysiologic hypotheses:

1. Inhibition of hypothalamic generation of GnRH pulses and LH release is caused by adrenal axis activation and catecholamine release during exercise.

2. Concept of "energy drain" (whether by inadequate calorie intake, or excessive exercise or energy expenditure) causes a negative energy balance. Amenorrhea is an adaptive response to this, as there are not enough calories to adequately support the reproductive process.

Health consequences of amenorrhea are related mainly to the hypoestrogenic state:

1. Premature loss of bone density (similar to postmenopausal woman).[8]

2. Higher incidence of stress fractures and other musculoskeletal injuries.

3. Possibility of increased cardiovascular disease due to loss of protective effect of estrogen on blood lipids.

4. Alterations in hormone-related cancers; i.e., chronic anovulation and unopposed estrogen secretion promote endometrial proliferation, increasing the risk of hyperplasia and adenocarcinoma of the uterus.

Diagnosis and History Taking

1. Reproductive history—age of menarche, length and frequency of menstrual periods, date of last menstrual period, number of periods in past year, pregnancies, miscarriages, contraceptive use, presence or absence of moliminal symptoms, irregular heavy bleeding.

2. Family history of late menarche or menstrual disorders.

3. Physical activity—age of onset of training, duration, type, frequency and intensity of exercise, recent changes in exercise patterns.

4. Weight—"ideal," highest, lowest, recent changes.

5. Nutrition—calorie intake (note calcium and iron intake), vegetarianism, disordered eating patterns.

6. Social—pressures at school, work, sports, support systems, self-esteem, and coping mechanisms.

7. Medications—including past history of hormones and oral contraceptives.

8. Review of systems—headache, galactorrhea, visual changes, and alteration in sense of smell.

9. Estrogen deficiency—vaginal atrophy, dyspareunia, vasomotor instability.

10. Androgen excess—acne, oily skin and hair, hirsutism.

11. Symptoms of thyroid deficiency or excess—heat/cold intolerance, dry hair and skin, weight gain or loss.

Physical Examination

1. General—height, weight, BMI (body composition).

2. Indicators of chromosomal abnormalities—short stature, webbed neck, increased carrying angle of elbow (Turner's syndrome).

3. Head and neck—fundi (papilledema), visual fields, thyroid (size, nodules).

4. Breasts—development (Tanner staging), presence of galactorrhea.

5. Pelvic examination—presence of normal reproductive organs, polycystic ovaries, clitoromegaly, vaginal dryness or atrophy.

6. Hirsutism, acne, and male pattern alopecia suggest high androgen levels.

Imaging Studies (if clinically indicated)

1. Computed tomography (CT) of skull and sella turcica to rule out pituitary adenoma.

2. Pelvic ultrasound to rule out polycystic ovarian syndrome.

Laboratory and Clinical Tests

Progesterone challenge: 5 to 10 mg of medroxyprogesterone acetate (Provera) for 5 days should precipitate withdrawal bleeding. If not, this test may be repeated following "priming" of the endometrium with 0.625 mg of estradiol for 16 days. Other investigations will depend on findings from the history and physical examination and may include the following:

1. Pregnancy test

2. Thyroid function tests, prolactin

3. Gonadotropins

4. Karyotype

5. Estrogen and progesterone

6. Testosterone and dehydroepiandrosterone sulfate (DHEAS)

Treatment Considerations

1. Treat associated diseases (i.e., hypothyroidism)

2. Improvement in diet and nutrition

3. Slight reduction in training schedule (5 to 10 percent) and/or intensity

4. Slight increase in weight (5 lb)

5. Reduction in other stresses (social, psychological)

6. Hormone replacement (cyclic estrogen and progesterone or oral contraceptives) if no response after 3 to 6 months

7. Clomiphene if desiring pregnancy

8. Adequate calcium intake—1500 mg of elemental calcium per day

9. Regular weight-bearing exercise

Usual Course and Recovery

Many athletes will regain normal menses with these measures, including restoration of normal fertility. Hormonal protection may be necessary to protect bone density. There is evidence, however, that they may not completely regain their previous bone density; hence, the need for early diagnosis and therapy.

THE FEMALE ATHLETE TRIAD

In some athletes, menstrual dysfunction coexists on a background of disordered eating patterns. The hypoestrogenic state and lack of adequate calcium can, in combination, compromise bone density. The female athlete triad refers to the combination of disordered eating, amenorrhea, and osteoporosis.[6] Athletes who are diagnosed with one entity of the triad are at risk and should be screened for the others. In practice, this means when a female athlete presents with a stress fracture, the treating physician should automatically ask about menstrual and dietary history. These screening questions are also appropriate to include in the preparticipation physical examination.[8]

Disordered Eating

Disordered eating occurs along a continuum, ranging from preoccupation with body size shape and composition, all the way to the frank eating disorders of anorexia nervosa and bulimia nervosa (as described in the DSM-IV manual of the American Psychological Association[9]). The diagnostic criteria for these disorders are listed in Table 18–1. Some authors believe that disordered eating in athletes should be classified as a separate entity (Table 18–2).[10] At any stage, however, there can be significant health implications.

Mechanisms of Disordered Eating[10]

Eating disorders can be precipitated in susceptible individuals by inadvertent comments from parents, coaches, and judges. No sport participants are

Table 18–1
Diagnostic Criteria for Eating Disorders

Anorexia Nervosa

1. Refusal to maintain body weight at or above a minimally normal weight for age and height (e.g., weight loss leading to maintenance of body weight less than 85% of that expected; or failure to make expected weight gain during period of growth, leading to body weight less than 85% of that expected).
2. Intense fear of gaining weight or becoming fat, even though underweight.
3. Disturbance in the way in which one's body weight or shape is experienced, undue influence of body weight or shape on self-evaluation, or denial of the seriousness of the current low body weight.
4. In postmenarchal females, amenorrhea, i.e., the absence of at least three consecutive menstrual cycles.

Specify type:
Restricting type: During the episode of anorexia nervosa, the person does not regularly engage in binge eating or purging behavior (i.e., self-induced vomiting or the misuse of laxatives or diuretics).
Binge eating/purging type: During this episode of anorexia nervosa, the person regularly engages in binge eating or purging behavior.

Bulimia Nervosa

1. Recurrent episodes of binge eating, characterized by both of the following:
   a. Eating in a discrete period of time (e.g., within any 2-hour period) an amount of food that is definitely larger than most people would eat during a similar period of time and under similar circumstances.
   b. A sense of lack of control over eating during the episode (e.g., a feeling that one cannot stop eating or control what or how much one is eating).
2. Recurrent inappropriate compensatory behavior in order to prevent weight gain, such as self-induced vomiting; misuse of laxatives, diuretics, enemas, or other medications; fasting; or excessive exercise.
3. The binge eating and inappropriate compensatory behaviors both occur, on average, at least twice a week for 3 months.
4. Self-evaluation is unduly influenced by body shape and weight.
5. The disturbance does not occur exclusively during episodes of anorexia nervosa.

Specify type:
Purging type: The person regularly engages in self-induced vomiting or the misuse of laxatives or diuretics.
Nonpurging type: The person uses other inappropriate compensatory behavior, such as fasting or excessive exercise, but does not regularly engage in self-induced vomiting or misuse of laxatives or diuretics.
A separate category of **Eating Disorders Not Otherwise Specified** covers the wider variety of conditions that does not conform exactly to these definitions of anorexia and bulimia.

Source: American Psychiatric Association: Diagnostic and Statistical Manual of Mental Disorders, 4th ed. Washington, D.C., American Psychiatric Association, 1994, pp. 544–545, 549–550.

entirely immune, but those in some sports appear to be at higher risk:

1. Appearance sports, such as gymnastics, figure skating, diving
2. Endurance sports, such as running, cross-country skiing
3. Weight category sports, such as rowing or crew, martial arts (judo, wrestling)

Triggers for such behavior include prolonged periods of dieting, frequent weight fluctuations, sudden increases in training volume, and traumatic events such as injury or loss of a coach.[10] Health risks include serious metabolic, endocrine, skeletal, and psychiatric problems, which will ultimately hinder rather than enhance athletic performance.

In the normal female adolescent and adult population, 1 percent are anorexic and 3 percent are bulimic. In athletes, the incidence is not known.

Diagnosis

1. Behaviors suggesting the condition: Weight loss, excessive preoccupation with food and weight, unexplained personality changes (depression, anxiety, self-criticism), wearing of baggy or layered clothing to conceal the body, excessive exercise beyond normal practice hours, unwillingness to eat with the team, disappearance to the restroom after meals, smell of vomitus on the breath.
2. Symptoms: Unusual or unexplained fatigue, sensation of bloating after eating, difficulty in concentrating, lightheadedness. Purging symptoms include sore throat, chest or abdominal pain, diarrhea, and constipation.
3. Physical findings: Low weight, dry hair and skin, brittle nails, bradycardia (less than 50 beats per minute), hypercarotenemia, cold cyanosed extremities, lanugo or baby-fine hair, parotid gland enlargement (chipmunk cheeks) in bulimics, Russell's sign (calluses on back

Table 18–2
Criteria for the Anorexic Athlete
("Anorexia Athletica")

Criteria	Degree
Weight loss (>5% of expected body weight)	+
Delayed puberty*	(+)
Menstrual dysfunction†	(+)
Gastrointestinal complaints	+
Absence of medical illness or affective disorder explaining the weight reduction	+
Distorted body image	(+)
Excessive fear of becoming obese	+
Restriction of food (<1200 kcal/day)	+
Use of purging methods‡	(+)
Bingeing	(+)
Compulsive exercise	(+)

Key: + = absolute criteria; (+) = relative criteria.
*No menstrual bleeding at age 16 (primary amenorrhea).
†Primary amenorrhea, secondary amenorrhea, oligomenorrhea.
‡Self-induced vomiting, use of laxatives and diuretics.
Source: Sundgot-Borgen J: Risk and trigger factors for the development of eating disorders in female elite athletes. Med Sci Sports Exer 26(4):414–418, 1994.

of hands from self-induced vomiting), erosion of dental enamel at the back of teeth (may be initially picked up by the dentist), face and extremity edema, postural hypotension.

Laboratory Tests

1. Complete blood cell count may show leukopenia, anemia, and thrombocytopenia.

2. Electrolytes—hyponatremia in women who overload with fluids, hypokalemia and hyperchloremic metabolic alkalosis from excessive vomiting, metabolic acidosis from laxative abuse.

3. Evidence of dehydration, renal compromise—elevation of blood urea nitrogen, creatinine.

4. Liver function tests show low albumin, high transaminases.

5. Thyroid function tests—T_3 often low from decreased peripheral conversion of T_4 to T_3.

6. Urinalysis—pyuria, hematuria, proteinuria, high pH.

7. Electrocardiogram—bradycardia, low-voltage, low inverted T-waves and prolonged Q-T interval.

8. Bone densitometry (DEXA) in women with significant menstrual dysfunction may show low bone density.

9. Upper GI or endoscopy in bulimic patients with esophageal bleeding.

Treatment

1. Multidisciplinary team: Primary care physician, coach, parents, athlete. It is also helpful to have a nutritionist, psychologist, exercise physiologist, strength trainer

2. Caring confrontation, focusing on concept of energy deficit, performance aspects of proper nutrition and training

3. Improvement in diet, nutritional counseling

4. Physician may need to restrict activities if weight loss continues or if ECG or electrolyte abnormalities continue to be present

5. Hospitalize if weight less than 30 percent of expected, or severe ECG abnormalities, hypotension, dehydration or electrolyte disturbance

6. Psychological assessment and ongoing therapy

Usual Course and Recovery

It is thought that 40 percent of patients will recover, 30 percent will recover but have relapses, and the remaining 30 percent will be chronically affected. Up to 10 to 18 percent can die from suicide or cardiac arrhythmias. Follow-up is important, as recurrence rate is high, particularly at a time of injury or retirement from competition.

Prevention of disordered eating depends on early detection and treatment and education regarding lean body mass, proper nutrition, and training practices. It is important to decrease emphasis on body size and composition and to discuss the inherent error in current methods of determining body composition.

Osteoporosis

Osteoporosis is a major health problem with significant costs to the individual and health care system. It is estimated that osteoporosis affects one of every two women over the age of 60 in the United States. Although vertebral and wrist fractures can be painful and disabling, a hip fracture is often the "beginning of the end" for an older woman. At the very least, her independence is compromised, and there is a substantial mortality rate (50 percent) in the year following a hip fracture.

Peak bone mass is determined by heredity, age, race, sex, use of cigarettes, consumption of alcohol and caffeine, nutritional and hormonal status, muscular strength, and body composition. Risk factors include menopause (surgical or natural), amenorrhea, and other hypoestrogenic states, inactivity or immobilization, prolonged corticosteroid use, hypothyroidism, and low dietary calcium intake. More than 90 percent of peak bone mass is present by the age of 18, but women can continue to add bone density up until the third decade of life. There is a crucial "window of opportunity," particularly during the adolescent years, to build up maximal bone density in order to arrive at the time of menopause with an optimal bone mass. It is therefore important to avoid long spells of amenorrhea by early diagnosis and treatment.

Bone mineral density can be measured to monitor the results of therapy. Dual energy x-ray absorptiometry (DEXA) is the most accurate technique, but there is recent interest in the use of a much smaller and more portable ultrasound machine that can be used on bones such as the calcaneus for screening purposes. This method assesses both bone density and structure, and is thought to have a good correlation with future risk of hip fracture.

The World Health Organization has classified osteoporosis[11] into four categories:

Normal: patients with a bone mineral density within 1 standard deviation of their predicted mean peak bone mass.

Osteopenia: patients with a bone mineral density between 1.0 and 2.5 standard deviations below their predicted mean peak bone mass.

Osteoporosis: patients with a bone mineral density lower than 2.5 standard deviations below their predicted mean peak bone mass.

Severe osteoporosis: those patients having a bone mineral density greater than 2.5 standard deviations below their predicted mean bone mass, plus one or more fragility fractures.

Weight-bearing exercise has an osteogenic effect on bone density, especially if begun during the time of rapid skeletal growth.[12] Higher impact activities such as gymnastics, volleyball, and basketball are associated with higher bone mass density than moderate-impact sports (running, soccer) and low-impact sports such as swimming. Exercise training cannot completely compensate for the lack of adequate estrogen and available dietary calcium. Lower bone mass is associated with late menarche and amenorrhea. It is thought that even cycles with shortened luteal phases and anovulation can result in decreased bone density, due possibly to a decrease in progesterone, which also has an effect on bone density. In postmenopausal women, exercise helps to increase bone mineral density or retard bone loss but, again, is not effective on its own.

CONTRACEPTION AND THE FEMALE ATHLETE

Oral contraceptives frequently are used to regulate the menstrual cycle or treat athletic amenorrhea as well as a method of birth control.

In general, therapy should begin with a combination pill, low-dose estrogen (30 or 35 μg of estradiol), or triphasic pill. In the majority of women, there is probably little effect on athletic performance. The numerous health benefits of contraceptive use likely far outweigh the risks and side effects. These benefits include regular predictable cycles, less menstrual bleeding, less iron deficiency anemia, and lower risk of benign breast disease, polycystic ovarian syndrome, sexually transmitted diseases, and ectopic pregnancies. In addition, there may be a protective effect against premature osteoporosis, especially when these hormones are prescribed to treat menstrual dysfunction.[13]

Oral contraceptives may be safely used in adolescents over the age of 16, or 3 years after puberty,[14] and up until menopause in the absence of any risk factors such as smoking or cardiovascular disease. Menstrual cycles can be manipulated around the time of important competition by continuing to take either the monophasic pill, or the highest dose of a triphasic preparation. Menstruation can usually be prevented for about 7 to 10 days, before breakthrough bleeding will occur. Another option is to progressively shorten the cycles of the pill, so that withdrawal bleeding occurs in the week prior to competition, and that most of the "synthetic" hormones have cleared from the system.

Other methods of birth control such as the diaphragm or condoms are less reliable and more user-dependent, but condoms do offer protection from sexually transmitted diseases. The intrauterine device (IUD) can cause heavy cramping periods, with an increased incidence of anemia. There are also progesterone-only forms of birth control, such as progestin-only pills, or alternate delivery systems such as subdermal implants (Norplant) or injectable Depo-Provera (medroxyprogesterone acetate). The latter is thought to potentially have a detrimental effect on bone density because of induction of amenorrhea.

EFFECTS OF HORMONES ON ATHLETIC PERFORMANCE

Any discussion of the effects of the female sex steroids on athletic performance is fraught with difficulty.[15] The female athlete is subject to a variety of shifting hormone patterns throughout puberty, her reproductive years, and into the menopause. During an ovulatory menstrual cycle, both estrogen and progesterone are initially low during the follicular phase, with estrogen then rising to its peak just prior to ovulation. In the luteal phase, secretion from the corpus luteum raises levels of estrogen and progesterone. If conception does not take place, hormonal concentrations gradually fall, and menstruation ensues.

The administration of exogenous hormones in the form of oral contraceptives or hormonal replacement therapy is further complicated by the variety of dosages and regimens. Suffice it to say that, for the majority of active women, neither the phase of the menstrual cycle, nor the administration of hormones should have any significant effect on the athlete's ability to participate in her chosen sport or recreation. For the elite athlete, for whom the difference between first and second place in competition means that any physiologic disadvantage is to be avoided if at all possible, more detailed counseling may be in order.

EXERCISE AND PREGNANCY

Pregnancy induces profound physiologic changes that may potentially affect athletic performance. There is a rise in resting respiratory rate, increased body temperature, and an increase in blood volume. Some studies have even suggested enhanced cardiorespiratory fitness following pregnancy, secondary to a "training effect."

In general, women with uncomplicated pregnancy can participate in activities at the same level as before they were pregnant. (It is not the appropriate time to begin training for a new sport.) In the first trimester, it is important to avoid situations in which overheating may occur, because the higher body temperatures that result from extreme exercise, saunas, and hot tubs, are thought (but have not conclusively been proved) to have a potential teratogenic effect on the fetus.

Concerns About Exercise During Pregnancy[16]

A number of factors may suggest a careful approach to exercising during pregnancy:

1. Exercise-induced hyperthermia, fetal heart rate changes (mainly due to redistribution of blood flow away from the maternal splanchnic circulation to the exercising muscles)
2. Birth weight changes (not necessarily a disadvantage)
3. Possible miscarriage (not supported by evidence)
4. Labor patterns—active stage of labor may be shorter, but there may be prolonged second-stage labor due to strong perineal musculature
5. Maternal injury—postural changes, shift in center of gravity, alteration of balance
6. Maternal weight gain, lower back pain, increased laxity of ligamentous structures

Absolute contraindications to exercise during pregnancy[17] include the following:

1. Clinically significant heart disease (ischemic or valvular)
2. Type I diabetes mellitus, peripheral vascular disease, thyroid disease, or uncontrolled hypertension, other serious systemic disorders (hepatitis, renal disease)
3. Incompetent cervix
4. Two or more spontaneous abortions in previous pregnancies
5. Placenta previa or bleeding in current pregnancy
6. Ruptured membranes or premature labor in current pregnancy

7. Toxemia or preeclampsia in current pregnancy

8. Very low proportion of body fat; eating disorder (anorexia, bulimia)

9. Multiple pregnancy

10. Evidence of fetal growth retardation in current pregnancy

Relative contraindications to exercise during pregnancy include:

1. History in previous pregnancies of premature labor, intrauterine growth retardation, preeclampsia, or toxemia

2. Significant anemia or iron deficiency (hemoglobin less than 10 g/dl)

3. Significant pulmonary disease (chronic obstructive pulmonary disease)

4. Mild valvular or ischemic heart disease, significant cardiac arrhythmia

5. Obesity or type II diabetes before pregnancy

6. Very low physical fitness level before pregnancy

7. Presence of twins (after 24 weeks' gestation)

8. Medications that can alter cardiac output or blood flow distribution

9. Breech in the third trimester

Recommendations for Exercise During Pregnancy

Exercise during normal pregnancy is beneficial, provided that sensible precautions are taken. The mother must be aware of maintaining nutritional status and adequate hydration. An exercise prescription is helpful and should note type, frequency, and intensity (depends on initial fitness) of exercise. Regular monitoring by the physician for intrauterine growth or medical problems is recommended. There is an excellent tool (the PARmed-X for pregnancy) that physicians can use in counseling their pregnant patients. It was developed in Canada by Dr. L.A. Wolfe and Dr. M. Mottola in conjunction with the Canadian Society of Exercise Physiology (CSEP) and Health Canada. It can be ordered from CSEP, 185 Somerset St. W., Suite 202, Ottawa, ON K2P 0J2; telephone (613) 234-3755, Fax (613) 234-3565.

Patients should be instructed to watch for warning signals before, during, and after exercise. Usually the mother can return to sports 2 to 6 weeks after a vaginal delivery, waiting slightly longer after a cesarean section (risk of wound dehiscence). High levels of circulating relaxin can lead to laxity of ligaments and increased soft-tissue and overuse injuries. Adequate breast support (well-fitting bra) is necessary, and lactation may be affected by exercise if sufficient calories are not consumed.

REFERENCES

1. American College of Sports Medicine Position Stand on Exercise and Women. Med Sci Sports Exerc 29(5):i–ix, 1997.
2. Barr SI, McKay HA: Nutrition, exercise, and bone status in youth. Int J Sport Nutrition 8:124–142, 1998.
3. American College of Sports Medicine Position Stand. The recommended quantity and quality of exercise for developing and maintaining cardiorespiratory and muscular fitness, and flexibility in healthy adults. Med Sci Sports Exerc 30(6):975–991, 1998.
4. Arendt L, Dick R: Knee injury patterns among men and women in collegiate basketball and soccer: NCAA data and review of literature. Am J Sports Med 23:694–701, 1995.
5. Staeger JM, Wigglesworth JK, Hatler LK: Interpreting the relationship between age of menarche and prepubertal training. Med Sci Sports Exerc 22:54–58, 1990.
6. American College of Sports Medicine Position Stand on the Female Athlete Triad: Disordered eating, amenorrhea and osteoporosis. Med Sci Sports Exerc 29(5):i–ix, 1997.
7. Loucks AB, Vaitukaitis J, Cameron JL, et al: The reproductive system and exercise in women. Med Sci Sports Exerc 24:S288–S293, 1992.
8. Johnson MD: Tailoring the preparticipation exam to female athletes. Physician Sports Med 20(7):61–72, 1992.
9. American Psychiatric Association Diagnostic and Statistical Manual, 4th ed. Washington, D.C., American Psychiatric Association, 1994.
10. Sundgot-Borgen, J: Risk and trigger factors for the development of eating disorders in female elite athletes. Med Sci Sports Exerc 26(4):414–418, 1994.
11. Kanis JA, Melton J III, Christiansen C, et al: The diagnosis of osteoporosis. J Bone Min Res 9:1137–1141, 1994.
12. Grimston SK, Willows ND, Hanley DA: Mechanical loading regime and its relationship to bone mineral density in children. Med Sci Sports Exerc 25(11):1203–1210, 1993.
13. DeCherney A: Bone-sparing properties of oral contraceptives. Am J Obstet Gynecol 174:15–20, 1996.
14. American Academy of Pediatrics, Committee on Sports Medicine: Amenorrhea in adolescent athletes. Pediatrics 84(2):394–395, 1989.
15. Lebrun CM: Effects of the different phases of the menstrual cycle and oral contraceptives on athletic performance. Sports Med 16:400–430, 1993.
16. Stevenson L: Exercise in pregnancy. Part 1: Update on pathophysiology. Can Fam Physician 43:97–104, 1997.
17. Stevenson L: Exercise in pregnancy. Part 2: Recommendations for individuals. Can Fam Physician 43:107–111, 1997.

Chapter 19 | The Mature Athlete

ROB JOHNSON, M.D.

The "graying" of the population of the United States mirrors that in other industrialized societies. Life expectancy at the previous turn of the century averaged about 51 years of age for women and about 48 years for men.[1] Conquering infectious disease and other improvements in illness care resulted in boosting the life expectancy to almost 79 years in women and 72 years in men by 1987. Remarkably, 20 percent of the population of the United States is expected to be over 55 years of age early in the twenty-first century. Longer life expectancy translates into more productive years following the traditional retirement age. Increased leisure time in the mature population has permitted more of the aging population to participate in recreational activities for both enjoyment and competition. This renewed interest in physical activity should translate into a healthier older population. Attendant with this change, the primary care practitioner must be equipped with the knowledge to counsel this group of athletes and physically active participants and to treat associated illness and infirmity.

The value of habitual physical activity has been at the forefront of our nation's health policy makers since the release of the Surgeon General's Report in July 1996.[2] In that document, we were encouraged to accumulate 30 minutes of physical activity throughout the day on most days of the week. The general mortality rate has been shown to decline steadily as the average person exercises to an energy expenditure between 500 calories per week (the equivalent of walking or running 5 miles a week) and 3500 calories per week (the equivalent of walking or running 35 miles per week).[3] Furthermore, those who exercised to an energy expenditure of 1000 calories a week had a 21 percent lower mortality rate than those who were sedentary (expending 300 calories on exercise per week).

Approaching the relationship of physical inactivity and disease from another perspective, a sedentary lifestyle doubles the risk of cardiovascular disease.[4] Moreover, those with low levels of cardiorespiratory fitness may see their relative risk of heart disease to be fivefold greater than for those of high fitness levels.[5] The good news, however, is that the greatest gains in health and longevity are possible in those who are able to alter their lifestyle and move from sedentary behavior to being moderately active, not necessarily to the highest fitness level.[5, 6]

Not only can regular activity reduce the mortality risk of cardiovascular disease, but it has been shown to modify the risk of other diseases and disease risk factors. Habitual physical activity has been shown to reduce body fat composition, lower blood pressure up to 10 mm Hg and actually lower the risk of ever developing hypertension, increase HDL (high density lipoprotein) levels up to 15 percent, improve insulin sensitivity (which reduces glucose intolerance), lower fibrinogen levels and decrease platelet aggregation (making the exercising individual "antithrombotic"), reduce the risk of both female and male osteoporosis, and finally, reduce the risk of colon cancer and reproductive cancers of both men and women.[4, 7]

Another group of mature athletes also surfaces, and with them, concern for other risks arises. This group comprises the competitive athletes. There have been some remarkable performances by "mature" athletes. Witness Al Oerter, who was an Olympic gold medalist in the discus for the first time in 1956 and represented the United States again in the 1988 Olympics at the age of 52. World age-group records in almost all events continue to improve. Age has become less of a physical limitation than it once was.

Each sport seems to have a different defining age for the term "masters" athlete. For instance, in long-distance running, a woman becomes a master at age 35 while a man reaches the master class at age 40. Among other competitive sports, these ages do not necessarily define the masters, or mature, athlete. Nevertheless, the risk of injury during training and competition may differ from that of the younger athlete.

If physicians are not already encouraging the mature population to begin or maintain a physical activity program, they must begin. This chapter is designed to highlight the effects of aging on essential body systems activities, outline the beneficial effects of activity on these same systems, discuss the health and injury risks, and suggest methods for safely prescribing exercise for the mature population.

EFFECTS OF AGING

One definition of aging suggests it is a phenomenon that leads to a progressive loss of adaptive capabilities and a decline in ability to function as in the past.[8] Decrements in physiologic function are an expected, but not necessarily accepted, phenomenon as the human body ages. A summary of these aging characteristics can be seen in Figure 19–1.[9] These changes must be considered in more detail to better understand the mature athlete. Throughout the discussion of the aging process, one must make a clear distinction between aging and disuse.[10]

Cardiovascular System

Maximum oxygen consumption ($Vo_{2\,max}$) represents a common measure of fitness. In general,

someone who remains physically active will see a decline in $Vo_{2\,max}$ that is one half of the decline in the sedentary person.[11] More specifically, the maximal aerobic capacity decreased by only 1.5 ml/kg/min in highly active individuals between the ages of 45 and 69 *if* they maintained their health and a high level of activity.[12] If the level of exercise was not continued, fitness losses were multiplied. A group of elite distance runners were tested 22 years after initial testing during their competitive years.[13] The group that remained the most highly trained showed a mere 6 percent decline per decade in $Vo_{2\,max}$. A second group, which remained slightly less active but fitness-trained, had a 10 percent per decade decrement, whereas a group that failed to continue training exhibited a 15 percent drop in $Vo_{2\,max}$ per decade. Clearly, fitness activities can thwart some of the age-related fitness decay.

Respiratory System

A variety of pulmonary alterations are related to the aging phenomenon.[14] These changes contribute to the decline in performance observed in the mature athlete.

Some of the flow-volume characteristics that are altered by aging include the following:

1. Decreased inspiratory flow caused by increased lung volume and shortening of the muscles of respiration.

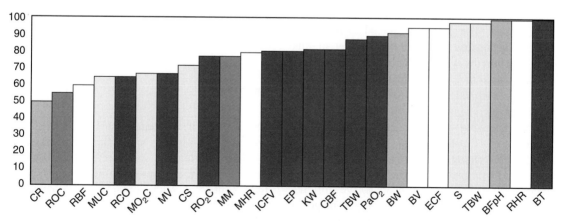

Figure 19–1. Changes in physiologic function that occur with aging. Values given are for the average 70-year-old subject as a percentage of values at age 35. Key: CR = Cardiac reserve. ROC = Reserve oxygen consumption. RBF = Renal blood flow. MUC = Maximum urinary concentration. RCO = Resting cardiac output. MO₂C = Maximum oxygen consumption. MV = Minute ventilation. CS = Cell solids. RO₂C = Resting oxygen consumption. MM = Muscle mass. MHR = Maximum heart rate. ICFV = Intracellular fluid volume. EP = Exchangeable potassium. KW = Kidney weight. CBF = Cerebral blood flow. TBW = Total body water. PaO₂ = Arterial oxygen tension. BW = Brain weight. BV = Blood volume. ECF = Extracellular fluid. S = Stature. TBW = Total body weight. BFpH = Body fluid pH. RHR = Resting heart rate. BT = Body temperature.

2. Maximum flow is diminished because of decreased respiratory muscle strength.

3. Loss of elastic recoil of the airway increases airway resistance, thereby decreasing expiratory flow rate.

In their entirety, these modifications result in a 17 percent decrease in expiratory flow and a decrease in forced expiratory volume (FEV_1) by 30 percent (32 ml/year) observed between the ages of 20 and 60.

Total lung capacity diminishes only slightly. Changes in lung volume that occur between the ages of 20 and 60 include a 7 percent drop in total lung capacity, an increase in residual volume of 37 percent, and a decrease in vital capacity of 19 percent (25 ml/year).

Between the ages of 20 and 60, the maximum voluntary ventilation falls by 31 percent. Pulmonary blood flow is altered by increasing pulmonary artery pressure, which doubles the arterial resistance. Finally, the diffusing capacity for pulmonary gas exchange drops by 40 percent, creating ventilation-perfusion mismatches.

Coupled with the reductions in maximum heart rate, the diminishing lung function serves as another significant limiting factor in athletic performance.

Bone

Osteoporosis is an age-related change in both men and women. The abrupt hormonal change that heralds menopause is an obvious marker of this phenomenon in women. The postmenopausal woman may lose 2 to 3 percent of her bone mass each year. Men exhibit a similar but more gradual bone density change. Typically, the remodeling process involving resorption and redeposition is slowed.[10]

Weight-bearing activity is widely known to slow the osteopenia of the postmenopausal woman. Women who had been active athletes when young maintained a distinct advantage in bone mineral density in their later years over sedentary counterparts, even if they failed to continue their high exercise levels.[15] Although less studied, a similar effect is presumed to occur in men. The stimulus of exercise causes the bone to model and remodel, enhancing the strength and slowing the inevitable osteopenic changes.

Muscle

Skeletal muscle changes that result from the aging process have been well studied. From age 30 to age 70, muscle mass decreased by 22 percent in women and 23 percent in men.[16] Functionally, this translates to improvement in both maximum isometric and dynamic strength up to age 30, maintenance of these strength parameters until age 50, followed by decline in both strength measures through age 70 with decrements measured from 24 to 36 percent.[17] After age 80, losses of muscle are accelerated, and cross-sectional area is reduced by as much as 40 percent.[18] Strength loss is thought to be related to the actual loss of mass rather than the loss of the capabilities of the contractile elements.

Muscle morphology undergoes rather interesting modifications. With age, there is a tendency to shift toward type I muscle fibers.[19] One study showed 39 percent type I fibers in the 20- to 29-year-old age group. At ages 60 to 65, 66 percent of the muscle fibers were type I.[20] Type I muscle fibers seem to resist the aging process quite effectively. Those type II fibers that do remain show substantial reduction in fiber size by as much as 26 percent.[21] More specifically, there has been a preferential atrophy of type IIb fibers compared to type IIa. Neuropathic changes are blamed for the loss of muscle fibers.[21] The metabolic capacity of the muscle fiber and the function of phosphagens and glycolytic enzymes are unchanged as part of the aging process.[21] It is also thought that the aging muscle may be more susceptible to fatigue than younger skeletal muscle.[22]

Cartilage

Changes within cartilage contribute to the aging process. The proteoglycan subunits of cartilage become smaller and lose some water content. These chemical changes result in diminished elasticity with a concomitant increase in vulnerability to injury.[23]

Tendons and Ligaments

Tendons and ligaments undergo similar loss of elasticity, making sprains and strains more likely.[23]

Nervous System

Aging of the nervous system results in a 37 percent decrease in the number of spinal motor neurons, with a 10 percent decline in nerve conduction velocity. The practical demonstration of these changes is slower reaction time, slower information processing, and consequently, increased time interval to mount a motor response to a sensed stimulus in athletic performance as well as daily activity.[23]

Movement Capability

Changes in the cardiovascular, skeletal, soft tissue, and nervous systems are responsible for a change in the capabilities of movement. The decline in maximum voluntary muscle contraction is accompanied by a reduced ability to maximally activate the muscle.[24] Although degradation in visual, vestibular, and somatosensory systems occurs with aging and is likely to affect coordination and postural stability, it is unlikely that these changes contribute significantly to falls. Rather, because most falls occur during locomotion, ascending and descending stairs, and transferring position, the weakening of the aging muscles is the likely culprit, especially in initiating the power and coordination necessary to execute recovery during any movement that results in loss of balance.

Flexibility

Soft tissue flexibility is a function of many of the soft tissue changes previously discussed. Flexibility decreases with age. This flexibility loss may reflect the adaptive response to disuse or, perhaps, the decreased connective tissue extensibility, prior injury, or the ravages of chronic disease.[23]

Thermoregulation

Going beyond the musculoskeletal system, aging has a profound affect on the thermoregulatory system. Study has shown greater passive core temperature lability in the elderly.[25] This is reflected physiologically by the onset of shivering and sweating responses at higher and lower temperatures, respectively. The magnitude of the reduction of responses beyond the thresholds implies a greater susceptibility to hyper- or hypothermia in the context of ambient temperature extremes complicated by exercise.

TRAINABILITY

What happens to the mature person who begins training at an advanced age? Can the older individual experience aerobic and strength gains as in the younger athlete?

Cardiovascular Training

Available information regarding cardiovascular training suggests that the gains are age-independent.[26] In studies of exercise programs ranging in length from 8 to 20 weeks, the response to training in the older exerciser resembles the response in the younger athlete. The level of training at which the older exerciser may start, however, is likely to be lower if there is a greater level of detraining. With regular training, the familiar exercise-related changes of increased blood volume, increased muscle glycogen, elevated aerobic enzyme activity, and increased number of mitochondria can be observed. After initiating an aerobic training program, the rate of decline in maximum oxygen consumption can be slowed by 5 percent per decade.[21] In fact, vigorous physical programs have produced increases in $Vo_{2\,max}$ from 20 to 30 percent over the starting fitness level. A study of 70- to 79-year-old men showed that their increases in $Vo_{2\,max}$ averaged 22 percent improvement.

Changes prompted by peripheral adaptations seem to be responsible for this improvement. Specifically, the responsible cellular changes are increased mitochondrial respiratory capacity, increased numbers of capillaries in the exercising muscle, and a transformation of muscle fibers from type IIb to type IIa fibers, altering the oxidative capacity of the muscle.[27, 28] Even though years of physical training may have been lost, initiating an exercise program at an advanced age can still reap many of the benefits associated with physical activity.

Strength Training

Strength training in older men and women has demonstrated the capability of these persons to rival, given the appropriate training stimulus, the strength gains of younger individuals.[21] More important, similar strength improvement has been seen in the frail elderly. These improvements are probably a result of an efficiency in recruiting additional motor units for the activity.[26] The practical result of strength training is the reduction in cardiovascular risk factors and maintenance of independent living.[29] For the insulin-resistant diabetic, strength training has shown increased insulin activity in the muscle with a resultant reduction in plasma insulin levels.[30]

Thus, the mature athlete or exerciser can achieve practical, measurable gains that clearly improve health and function. It is interesting that, for both strength and aerobic capacity, the mature athlete is as trainable as the younger athlete.

RISKS OF SPORT AND EXERCISE

Exertional Sudden Death

The most serious risk to the mature athlete is exertional sudden death due to latent or known cardiovascular disease. Exercise for this age group is the proverbial "two-edged sword." It can reduce the risk of heart disease. At the same time, it can kill those with heart disease.[31] Coronary artery disease is the number one cause of exertional sudden death in those over age 35. Of men who are just beginning exercise, it is estimated that 2 percent have silent coronary artery disease.[31] When counseling the beginning exerciser, the clinician must keep these figures in mind both for screening and for devising an exercise prescription that begins at an intensity low enough to minimize the risk. The actual risk of dying during exercise is minute. Epidemiologic studies of sudden exertional death have yielded a risk of jogging-related death as 1 death per 400,000 hours of the activity. Cross-country skiing has an estimated risk of 1 death in 600,000 hours, and recreational activity has a risk of 1 death for every 900,000 hours of leisure-time activities.[32] (Consider the individual who performs aerobic exercise 30 to 60 minutes five times per week. This exerciser accumulates only 130 to 260 hours per year.)

Physical fitness is protective against exertional sudden death. Siscovick, in his treatise on sudden death in athletes, has shown that everyone is at greater risk of dying during exercise.[33] The fit individual runs a risk of dying during exercise

five times the risk at rest. The sedentary person, however, has a risk of dying during exercise that is *fifty-six* times greater than the risk of dying while at rest.[33] Generally, the vigorous exerciser carries a risk only 40 percent of sedentary individuals of exertional sudden death. The obvious message here is: for those who never exercise, any vigorous activity places them in significant jeopardy.

The issue of screening for latent coronary artery disease is controversial. Astrand, one of the pre-eminent exercise physiologists, provides a most interesting view of this issue.[34] He suggests a medical examination for anyone in doubt about beginning an exercise program. Otherwise, he states, "In principle, however, there is less risk in activity than in continuous inactivity. In a nutshell, our opinion is that it is more advisable to pass a careful medical examination if one intends to be sedentary in order to establish whether one's state of health is good enough to stand the inactivity."[35]

In addition to a medical history and medical examination, the most commonly used test to evaluate someone prior to initiating an exercise program is the graded exercise test (GXT), or stress test. In the asymptomatic man or woman, the specificity and sensitivity of the GXT is poor. Low sensitivity implies that the test fails to accurately identify those who are at risk for exertional sudden death ("silent" heart disease), whereas the false-positive test may trigger expensive and inappropriate evaluation.[36] A review of the effectiveness of using the exercise stress test to screen asymptomatic individuals for heart disease demonstrated that only 21 percent of those with positive stress tests had angiographically proved significant coronary artery disease (more than 50 percent stenosis).[37] Consequently, most who die during exercise had a previously negative exercise stress test. Most who had positive stress tests did *not* have significant coronary artery disease: hence, the dilemma facing the clinician.

The American College of Sports Medicine has provided suggestions regarding the selection of those who should be considered candidates for exercise screening before beginning a moderately vigorous exercise program (Table 19–1).[38] Judicious application of these guidelines can minimize some of the sensitivity and specificity issues. Care must be used in applying and interpreting this screening.

Other experienced cardiologists suggest using the time to educate the patient rather than per-

Table 19-1
ACSM Guidelines for Exercise Testing and Participation

	Apparently Healthy		Higher Risk†		
	Younger*	Older	No Symptoms	Symptoms Present	With Disease‡
Medical examination and GXT					
Moderate exercise	No	No	No	Yes	Yes
Vigorous exercise	No	Yes	Yes	Yes	Yes

*Younger: men 40 years or younger, women 50 years or younger.

†Persons with two or more risk factors. Major coronary risk factors are hypertension (treated or untreated), cholesterol ($\geq$240 mg/dl), cigarette smoking, diabetes mellitus, family history of coronary or other atherosclerotic disease in parents or siblings prior to age 55.

‡Person with known cardiac, pulmonary, or metabolic disease

Note: Moderate exercise = exercise intensity 40–60% $VO_{2\,max}$ (slow progression, noncompetitive). Vigorous exercise = exercise intensity > 60% $VO_{2\,max}$.

Source: Eichner ER: Profile of the mature athlete. Adv Sports Med Fitness 1:1–21, 1988.

forming a GXT. Effective counseling can alert the exercise candidate to warning signs and symptoms of myocardial disease. Included in the educational session is information about a low-intensity program with appropriate increments in activity to achieve the benefits of exercise.

Thermal Injury

Hypothermia and hyperthermia also kill the exerciser. As mentioned earlier, the older athlete is less capable of handling the temperature extremes. Chronic disease and medications used to treat these diseases may further increase the thermal injury risk. Education and preventive efforts can help minimize the risks.

Musculoskeletal Injury

The earlier discussion of age-related changes to the cardiovascular system, muscle, bone, cartilage, tendons, ligaments, and movement capabilities serves as the basis for explaining injury proneness in the mature athlete. These changes allow for less margin of error in both training and competition. The safety margin of exercise is narrower than at younger ages.[39] A number of age-related microprocesses in bone and soft tissues set the stage for overuse and degenerative processes. Mineral loss in bone weakens it. Connective tissue and articular cartilage become rigid and stiff. Loss of compliance of the vasculature elevates the vascular resistance, which inhibits energy and oxygen transport to tissues. Thus, any damage to the tissues as a

result of overload requires a longer recovery period.

Most injuries occur during walking and jogging activities. In part, this is due to the high numbers of older athletes who practice these fitness activities.[40, 41] These injury rates varied from 14 to 57 percent incidence. As we age, the problems of degenerative changes in the musculoskeletal system and the effects of pre-existing injuries exact their toll. Prior study suggests as many as 36 percent of mature athletic injuries are a direct result of these changes.[41] Most activity-related injuries are attributed to the speed of movement.

Gender differences also exist. Data suggests women are injured more often than men.[40]

Injury data must, however, be placed in the proper perspective. Motor vehicle accidents account for 41 to 53 percent of all injuries in the older age groups. Sport and physical activity are responsible for only 8 to 21 percent of all reported injuries.[42]

A typical categorization of injuries related to sports and physical activity is to separate the acute injury from the overuse injury. As might be expected, overuse injuries have been observed to be more common in the older athlete.[43, 44] Further characterization of the overuse injury shows it to be more commonly a muscle strain of the lower extremity with a duration of recovery that tends to be longer than for a younger athlete with a similar injury.

The typical acute injury is usually caused by a fall, resulting in a sprain of a particular joint, usually in the lower extremity. Recovery from either acute or overuse injury seems to require about the same length of time. In competition in the 1985 World Masters Games, 32.4 percent of the men were treated for injury and 28.8 percent of the women sought treatment.[39] In a study of competitive orienteering, those competitors over the age of 50 required medical attention twice as often as the younger competitors.[45] Much of the information about injury in older athletes will change as more current data are gathered. Compared with the data from the mid-1980s, there are more mature athletes maintaining regular activity and sustaining highly competitive training programs and competition.

An interesting clinical sidelight to the study of injury in the older athlete has been the revelation that the older athlete tends to delay seeking a medical evaluation as compared to the younger athlete.[46] Complicating this medical delay is the chance of misdiagnosis or undertreatment by the clinician, who may lay the blame on the aging process rather than the physical training. This assumption results in lack of aggressive treatment and rehabilitation to return this athlete to the previous level of competitive function.

Diagnosis, treatment, and rehabilitation of the injured mature athlete should not differ from those in the younger athlete. Certainly, recovery may be slower and the level to which the athlete may elect to return are likely to differ.

Other than a few sports or multiparticipant events that have gathered injury data for the mature athlete, there is little information comparing injury frequency or injury type to the younger athlete.

Osteoarthritis

There is a widespread intuitive belief that those who remain athletically active have joints that readily reflect the ravages of long-term competition. But is there evidence to support this contention? The answer to this question is vitally important to the clinician who advises the mature adult to adopt a program of regular physical activity.

A group of runners ages 53 to 75 were studied over 6 years to determine if long-distance running over a number of years was associated with increased musculoskeletal pain.[47] When these runners were compared with control subjects, regular, vigorous running activity for many years was *not* associated with an increase in musculoskeletal

pain. More important, running activity was accompanied by a one third decrease in disability and a lower mortality rate. These same conclusions may not apply to those who have significant anatomic, biomechanical variants or those with prior lower extremity injuries, which increase the risk and rate of development of osteoarthritis.[48]

A general evaluation of physical disability compared runners to nonrunners.[49] Although 49 percent of runners reported some physical disability during the course of the study, 77 percent of the nonrunners reported physical disability. The best predictor of physical disability in this study was the presence of arthritis symptoms in both runners and nonrunners.

Generally, healthy joints do not see acceleration of degenerative changes. Unhealthy joints (prior injury or surgery or rheumatologic disease) are prone to more rapid degenerative changes. Consequently, the choice of fitness activity may have to reflect those physical limitations.

EXERCISE PRESCRIPTION FOR THE MATURE ATHLETE

The importance of habitual activity for adults and children has been firmly established. For those with many chronic diseases, exercise is a proven treatment modality or adjunctive therapy and must not be overlooked in the comprehensive management of these illnesses. Physical activity is a useful therapeutic modality in the following circumstances.[38]

Chronic obstructive pulmonary disease
Hypertension
Peripheral vascular disease
Diabetes mellitus (both type I and type II)
Obesity
Hyperlipidemias
Arthritis
End-stage renal disease
Organ transplants
Cancer
HIV-positive individuals

The goals of the exercise prescription[38] should be as follows:

1. Enhance physical fitness
2. Serve as a means of promoting health to re-

duce risk of developing disease or to reduce the risk of recurrence of disease or illness

3. Ensure safety of the participant

Developing an exercise program may be as simple as incorporating one's hobbies and interests and modifying some daily activities to include climbing stairs instead of using the elevator, walking rather than driving to the store, getting off the bus one stop early to walk the remaining distance to work, mowing the lawn, or performing other home maintenance duties.

Others will function better if they have a specific, well-ordered program to follow. A well-ordered exercise prescription should include instruction and guidance in regard to mode, intensity, frequency, duration of the exercise, and the rate of progression of the activity program.

The recommended mode involves any rhythmic or aerobic activity that employs the larger muscle groups and can be sustained over a prolonged time period. Popular aerobic activities include walking, biking, swimming, water aerobics, and running. Other recreational activities that incorporate any of these activities are ideal.

The intensity of the activity can range from 40 to 85 percent of the individual's $Vo_{2\,max}$ or 55 to 90 percent of the maximum heart rate or maximum predicted heart rate. For those less fit or previously sedentary, starting at the lower range (40 to 60 percent $Vo_{2\,max}$, 55 to 70 percent of the maximum predicted heart rate) is most prudent.

An appropriate duration for an activity is 15 to 60 minutes, which should include several minutes of warm-up and cool-down. The individual should perform the chosen activity(ies) three to five times per week. Daily activity is permitted for those who desire, but is not necessary to develop the health benefits of a regular program.

If there are no orthopedic, medical, or logistical problems, the program can be readjusted every 6 to 8 weeks, if desired. Generally, no progression should exceed an increase in quantity of 10 percent per week. When the activity schedule is changed, it is possible to alter either the mode, intensity, frequency, or duration.

Many other considerations enter the scheme and must be factored into the exercise prescription. These factors may include current or pre-existing medical or orthopedic conditions and medications for these conditions. Medications must be appraised in the context of adverse effects on exercise (such as propranolol, which may decrease effort and intensity of aerobic work) or adverse consequences of medications (such as diuretics increasing the risk of hypokalemia in the exercising individual, particularly the endurance athlete).

There is still a belief held by some medical practitioners that exercise is unnecessary as we age. The exact source of this attitude is uncertain. Perhaps it is unwarranted fear of injury or exertional sudden death or inadequacy of the clinician to properly advise the patient about exercise. Regardless, there is a role for exercise at every age. Benefits can be seen at any age. Encouragement— not discouragement—should be the clinical attitude.

Motivation and compliance issues remain obstacles for many people. By including an exercise history as part of the medical history during the annual or biannual examination of this population, a message is delivered regarding the importance. Educating the patient about minimum levels of activity that promote health benefits may remove barriers and misconceptions held by the sedentary individual. Goal-setting and scheduled follow-up counseling and trouble-shooting sessions enhance exercise compliance.

A final source of motivation is for the clinician to serve as a practicing role model for the role of exercise in promoting health.

SUMMARY

Studies from the Human Nutrition Research Center for Aging have shown ten biomarkers of aging that can be sustained by regular exercise.[50] These biomarkers synthesize and summarize the discussion of this chapter. They are as follows:

1. Muscle mass
2. Basal metabolic rate
3. Aerobic capacity
4. Cholesterol/HDL ratio
5. Bone density
6. Strength and flexibility
7. Body fat percentage
8. Glucose tolerance
9. Blood pressure
10. Body's ability to regulate thermal homeostasis

Much as it is true that "children are not small adults," the aging process requires that the mature athlete be approached differently from the young adult athlete. By understanding the physiologic changes associated with the aging process, managing the training and injuries of the older exercising population becomes more effective. Optimal management of this population will ensure they maximize their health.

REFERENCES

1. Seto JL, Brewster CE: Musculoskeletal conditioning of the older athlete. Clin Sports Med 10(2):401–429, 1991.
2. U.S. Department of Health and Human Services: Physical Activity and Health: A Report of the Surgeon General. Atlanta, U.S. Department of Health and Human Services, Centers for Disease Control and Prevention, National Center for Chronic Disease Prevention and Health Promotion, 1996.
3. Paffenbarger RS, Hyde RJ, Wing AL, et al: Physical activity, all-cause mortality, and longevity of college alumni. N Engl J Med 314:605–613, 1986.
4. Rauramaa R, Leon AS: Physical activity and risk of cardiovascular disease in middle-aged individuals. Sports Med 22(2):65–69, 1996.
5. Blair SN: Physical activity, physical fitness and health. Res Q Exerc Sport 64:365–376, 1993.
6. Lakka TA, Venalainen JM, Rauramaa R, et al: Relation of leisure-time physical activity and cardiorespiratory fitness to risk of acute myocardial infarction. N Engl J Med 330:1549–1554, 1994.
7. Paffenbarger RS: 40 years of progress: Physical activity, health and fitness. American College of Sports Medicine 40th Anniversary Lectures, 1994, pp. 93–109.
8. Kilborn A, Hartley LH, Saltin B, et al: Physical training in sedentary middle-aged and older men. Scand J Clin Lab Invest 24:315–322, 1969.
9. Berman R, Haxby JV, Pomerantz RS: Physiology of aging, part I: Normal changes. Patient Care 22:20–36, 1988.
10. Wilmore JH: The aging of bone and muscle. Clin Sports Med 10(2):231–244, 1991.
11. Heath GW, Hagberg JM, Ehsani AA, et al: A physiological comparison of young and older endurance athletes. J Appl Physiol 51:634–640, 1981.
12. Kasch FW, Boyer JL, Van Camp SP, et al: Effect of exercise on cardiovascular aging. Age Aging 22:5–10, 1993.
13. Trappe SW, Costill DL, Vukovich MD, et al: Aging among elite distance runners: A 22-year longitudinal study. J Appl Physiol 80(1):285–290, 1996.
14. Jones NL: The lung of the mature athlete. In Sutton JR, Brock RM (eds): Sports Medicine for the Mature Athlete. Indianapolis, Benchmark Press, 1986.
15. Etherington J, Harris PA, Nandie D, et al: The effect of weight-bearing exercise on bone mineral density: A study of ex-elite female athletes and the general population. J Bone Miner Res 11(9):1333–1338, 1996.
16. Flag JL, Lakatta EG: Role of muscle loss in age-associated reduction in $Vo_{2\,max}$. J Appl Physiol 65:1147–1151, 1988.
17. Larson L: Morphological and functional characteristics of the aging skeletal muscle in man. Acta Physiol Scand Suppl 457:1–36, 1978.
18. Vandervoort AA, Hayes KL, Belanger AY: Strength and endurance of skeletal muscle. Physiother Can 38:167–173, 1986.
19. Gollnick PD, Armstrong RB, Saubert CW, et al: Enzyme activity and fiber composition of human skeletal muscle. J Appl Physiol 34:1038–1044, 1972.
20. Larsson L, Karlsson J: Isometric and dynamic endurance as a function of age and skeletal muscle characteristics. Acta Physiol Scand 104:129–136, 1978.
21. Rogers MA, Evans WJ: Changes in skeletal muscle with aging: Effects of exercise training. Exerc Sports Sci Rev 21:65–102, 1993.
22. Davis CTM, Thomas DO, White MJ: Mechanical properties of young and elderly human muscle. Acta Med Scand Suppl 711:219–226, 1986.
23. Ting J: Running and the older athlete. Clin Sports Med 10(2):317–342, 1991.
24. Grabiner MD, Enoka RM: Changes in movement capabilities with aging. Exerc Sports Sci Rev 23:65–104, 1995.
25. Anderson GS, Meneilly GS, Mikjovic IB: Passive temperature lability in the elderly. Eur J Appl Physiol 73(3–4):278–286, 1996.
26. Stamford BA: Exercise and the elderly. Exerc Sports Sci Rev 16:341–379, 1988.
27. Gollnick PD, Armstrong RB, Saltin B, et al: Effect of training on enzyme activity and fiber composition of human skeletal muscle. J Appl Physiol 34:107–111, 1973.
28. Gollnick PD, Armstrong RB, Saubert CW IV, et al: Enzyme activity and fiber composition in skeletal muscle of untrained and trained men. J Appl Physiol 33:312–319, 1972.
29. Evans WJ: Reversing sarcopenia: How weight training can build strength and vitality. Geriatrics 51(5):46–47, 51–53, 1996.
30. Miller JP, Pratley RE, Goldberg AP, et al: Strength training increases insulin action in healthy 50–65-year-old men. J Appl Physiol 77(3):1122–1127, 1994.
31. Eichner ER: Profile of the mature athlete. Sports Med Fitness 1:1–21, 1988.
32. Eichner ER: The exercise hypothesis: An updated analysis. In Krakauer LJ, Anderson JL, Shephard RJ (eds): 1984 YearBook of Sports Medicine. Chicago, Year Book Medical Publishers, 1984, pp. 9–19.
33. Siscovick DS, Weiss NS, Fletcher RH, et al: The incidence of primary cardiac arrest during vigorous exercise. N Engl J Med 311:874–877, 1984.
34. Astrand PO: Exercise physiology of the mature athlete. In Sutton JR, Brock RM (eds): Sports Medicine for the Mature Athlete. Indianapolis, Benchmark Press, 1986.
35. Astrand PO, Rodahl K: Textbook of Work Physiology, 3rd ed. New York, McGraw-Hill, 1985, p. 608.
36. Johnson RJ: Assessing cardiac risk with the exercise test. Your Patient and Fitness 7(1):6–13, 1993.
37. Froechlicher VF, Maron B: Exercise testing and ancillary techniques to screen for coronary heart disease. Prog Cardiovasc Disease 14:261–274, 1981.
38. Blair SN, Painter P, Pate RR, et al (eds): Guidelines for Exercise Testing and Prescription. Philadelphia, Lea & Febiger, 1991.
39. Kallinen M, Markku A: Aging, physical activity and sports injuries. Sports Med 20(1):41–52, 1995.
40. Carroll JF, Pollock ML, Graves JE, et al: Incidence of injury during moderate- and high-intensity walking training in the elderly. J Gerontol 47:M61–M66, 1992.
41. Pollock ML, Carroll JF, Graves JE, et al: Injuries and adherence to walk/jog and resistance training programs in the elderly. Med Sci Sports Exerc 23:1194–2000, 1991.
42. Biener K, Buhlmann H: Sports behaviour and sports accidents in old age. Dtsch Z Sportmed 6:210–215, 1984.
43. Dehaven KE, Lintner DM: Athletic injuries: Comparison

by age, sport, and gender. Am J Sports Med 14:218–224, 1986.

44. Kallinen M, Alen M: Sports-related injuries in elderly men still active in sports. Br J Sports Med 28:52–55, 1994.

45. Korpi J, Haapanen A, Svohn T: Frequency, location, and types of orienteering injuries. Scand J Sports Sci 9:53–56, 1987.

46. Menard D, Stanish WD. The aging athlete. Am J Sports Med 17:187–196, 1989.

47. Fries JF, Singh G, Marfeld D, et al: Relationship of run-ning to musculoskeletal pain with age. A six-year longitu-dinal study. Arthritis Rheum 39(1):64–72, 1996.

48. Lohr DD: Does running exercise cause osteoarthritis? Md Med J 45(8):641–644, 1996.

49. Ward MM, Hubert HB, Shi H, Block DA: Physical disabil-ity in older runners: Prevalence, risk factors, and progres-sion with age. J Gerontol A Biol Sci Med 50(2):M70–M77, 1995.

50. Evans W, Rosenberg L: Biomarkers: The 10 Keys to Prolonging Vitality. New York, Fireside, 1991.

Chapter 20 | Risks of Exercise

JAMES MORIARITY, M.D.

The human body is designed for movement and the human spirit for competition. It seems ironic to speak of the risks of exercise when exercise is inherent to the human condition. Primary care physicians often represent the expert advisors who are consulted on matters of health, including the effects that exercise may impart, both good and bad, on a person's well-being. They are often asked to provide "permission" for exercise in the form of an athletic school physical, a health club release form, or an exercise prescription. Although physicians should never present barriers to exercise, they may need to channel a patient's enthusiasm into less physically stressful activities. At other times, they must deny permission to compete when the risk of competition poses a serious threat to the patient's health, and suggest instead a different, less dangerous activity. To give sound advice on the risks of exercise requires a methodology of evaluation.

To describe every risk for every sport is not the intention of this chapter. Nor will the special state of pregnancy and exercise be discussed (see Ch. 18). Rather, a methodology of evaluation of risk is outlined, along with examples of how this methodology applies. It is based on the following three components of an individual's ability to participate in an activity: (1) the physical demands of the sport, (2) the inherent risk of the sport, and (3) the physical condition of the patient (Table 20–1). Not until all three of these components are understood and assessed can an expert opinion on the risks of exercise be given and permission for participation be granted.

PHYSICAL DEMANDS OF SPORT: THE DIFFERENCE BETWEEN EXERCISE AND COMPETITION

The distinction between exercise and competition is necessary in assessing risk, particularly cardiovascular risk. Exercise is defined by the National Institutes of Health as a "planned, structured, and repetitive bodily movement done to improve or maintain one or more components of physical fitness."[1] Physical fitness is characterized by optimal cardiovascular endurance, musculoskeletal strength and flexibility, and desirable body composition.[2] The minimal quantity of exercise necessary to begin working toward physical fitness is an accumulation of 30 minutes of moderately intense physical activity on most (5 to 7) days of the week.[2] Moderate intensity correlates well with "somewhat hard" on the Borg scale of perceived exertion, 60 to 90 percent of maximal heart rate, or at the most precise, 50 to 85 percent of $VO_{2\,max}$.

Competition is a contest requiring certain physical attributes and skills. Competitive sport does not necessarily have as its goal improved physical fitness, and different sports require different levels of fitness as a factor for success. In competition, factors such as agility, speed, balance, coordination, and reaction time may be more important in determining the outcome of the contest than cardiovascular endurance, muscle fitness, or body composition, although in many sports such factors improve with higher levels of fitness. Competitive sport may be subdivided into low, moderate, or high levels of dynamic (lots of body movement) or static (lots of muscle straining) activities. Sports requiring high dynamic and high static components, such as rowing or boxing, require the highest level of physical conditioning. Sports with low dynamic and low static requirements, such as golf, require the least level of physical conditioning. This classification system is the framework for suggested activity in the

Table 20–1
Categories of Risk Factors in Exercise

1. Physical demands of the sport
2. Inherent risk of the sport
3. Physical condition of the athlete

Table 20-2
Dynamic and Static Demands of Selected Sports

	Low Dynamic	Moderate Dynamic	High Dynamic
Low static	Bowling, cricket, curling, golf	Baseball, softball, table tennis, doubles in tennis, volleyball	Badminton, cross-country skiing, field hockey, racquetball, cross-country running, soccer, tennis singles
Moderate static	Archery, diving, equestrian events	Fencing, field events, figure skating, football, rugby, sprinting	Basketball, ice hockey, lacrosse, middle distance running, swimming, team handball
High static	Field events (throwing), gymnastics, martial arts, weight lifting	Body building, downhill skiing, wrestling	Boxing, canoeing, cycling, rowing, speed skating

*Adapted from the 26th Bethesda Conference Guidelines, Classification of Sports, January 6–7, 1994, Bethesda, Maryland.

Bethesda Guidelines for athletes with cardiovascular abnormalities[3] (Table 20–2).

Cardiovascular risk for an athlete of any age increases as the inherent dynamic and static cardiovascular demands of the sport increases. It must be assumed that patients requesting permission to compete in these sports will do so with the *highest* (as opposed to moderate) level of intensity they are capable of. Therefore, athletes requesting permission for competition cannot be cleared for participation without a cardiovascular examination suitable to their age, and knowledge of risk factors.

In contrast, most patients seeking to exercise for the purpose of attaining health and fitness at a level of moderate intensity may be given permission to do so without pretesting or medical consultation.[4] Exceptions to this statement include those individuals with known coronary artery disease and men over 40 and women over 50 with multiple cardiovascular risk factors such as hypertension, smoking, hyperlipidemia, diabetes, and familial history of sudden death before age 60. For these individuals, exercise testing prior to initiation of an exercise program is recommended.

In general, exercising for health at moderate intensity carries a very low health risk for healthy individuals and does not require medical clearance or pretesting. Competitive sport, especially in the high static or dynamic ranges, implies high-intensity effort with greater cardiovascular risk and requires cardiovascular clearance appropriate for the patient's age and medical history.

THE INHERENT RISKS OF SPORT

The inherent risk of an activity is an epidemiologic figure that describes the number and type of injuries that can be expected to occur in participating athletes. Terms used to describe inherent risk include injuries per game, injuries per practice, injuries per exposure, missed practices, and missed games. Inherent risk may be described as the "endemic injury rate." The endemic injury rate for any sport is never zero.

Theoretically, the only way to change the endemic injury rate of a sport is by changing the playing equipment, tightening rule enforcement, or by modification of the rules. For example, collision with the goal post is a common cause of injury in soccer. According to one report, with the addition of protective padding to the goal post, the incidence of injury was reduced.[5] Likewise, in hockey facial injuries were reduced with the introduction of protective facemasks. Rule changes in football that penalize players for head-down tackling (spearing), together with an aggressive educational program, have reduced the number of catastrophic head and neck injuries. Tighter rule enforcement by reducing contact days and prohibiting shoulder pads in noncontact days has significantly lowered the spring practice injury rate in college football.

Conversely, equipment changes may sometimes increase injury rates. The increased use of metal bats in baseball has resulted in an increase in the velocity of batted balls. Likewise in ice hockey, the use of protective facemasks and headgear has, according to some coaches, increased the amount of "rough play" on the ice.

The inherent risk of injury in college athletes is of great interest to the NCAA Sports Sciences Committee. Since 1982, the NCAA has conducted an ongoing Injury Surveillance System (ISS) for 16 sports played by its member institutions. The ISS has provided information on a variety of injury parameters, including injuries in practice and in games, severity of injury, and injury requiring surgery.[6]

The ISS data yielded surprising results about the inherent injury rate of collegiate athletics. There is little surprise that football, specifically spring football, has the highest practice injury rate and that fall football has the highest game injury rate. But the highest percentage of injuries requiring surgery is in women's gymnastics, with women's basketball a close second (Table 20–3). The ISS was one of the first surveys to identify the increased risk of anterior cruciate ligament tear in women compared with that in their male counterparts. Many etiologic factors have been proposed, including femoral notch width, strength imbalances between hamstring and quadriceps muscle groups, and differences in myoneural firing patterns of the quadriceps and hamstring muscles.[7] Because of the consistently high injury rate in spring football, the number of contact days was reduced. Preliminary results seem to support the efficacy of this decision.

In the younger age groups, the greatest number of injuries can be expected to occur in the sports with the highest participation.[8] Not surprisingly, football and basketball predominate in the 15- to 24-year-old age group, and baseball and soccer top the list in the 5- to 14-year-old age group. Most injuries are mild musculoskeletal sprains and strains, but serious and fatal injuries do occur. Baseball alone accounts for 40 percent of all eye injuries in children aged 11 to 15 in the United States. Fatal blows to the head and chest from thrown and batted balls resulted in 183 deaths in children during the years 1973–1981. During the same years, 260 deaths occurred as a result of football participation. Most soccer fatalities that have occurred are a result of players striking the goalpost during competition. Wrestling, which ranks fourth overall in high school participation, ranks second to football in number of injuries requiring surgery.

Sudden death during exercise in an athlete from nontraumatic events is always a newsworthy event and usually elicits a discussion about the risk of exercise and sport. Most cases of sudden death are related to heart disease or defects, with a clear division according to age. Prior to age 35, athletes dying suddenly during exercise are found at autopsy to have had structural heart defects, with hypertrophic cardiomyopathy the predominant finding.[9] Past the age of 35, the predominant causative factor is coronary artery disease. Athletes need not have extensive, widespread coronary artery disease to be at risk of sudden death.

The actual incidence of sudden death during exercise is low. A 1980 study of joggers from the state of Rhode Island concluded that the risk of sudden death in otherwise healthy 30- to 65-year-old men was 1 death in 15,240 joggers per year.[10] A Seattle study arrived at similar numbers, with a calculated death rate during exercise of 1 in 18,000 per year for men aged 25 to 75.[11] These

Table 20–3
NCAA Injury Surveillance System 1996–1997

Sport	Injury Rate: Combined Practice and Game (Per 1000 Exposures)	Injuries Requiring Surgery (As a Percentage of All Injuries All Sports)	Injury Rate: (7 + Days Missed Practice) (Per 1000 Exposures)
Spring football	9.6	8.3%	4.1
Wrestling	9.6	6.1%	3.7
Women's gymnastics	9.3	8.9%	3.6
Women's soccer	8.5	5.5%	2.3
Men's soccer	8.1	4.9%	2.0
Football	6.5	6.7%	2.3
Men's lacrosse	5.7	5.2%	1.9
Men's basketball	5.7	5.8%	1.3
Ice hockey	5.7	4.1%	1.9
Women's basketball	5.6	8.7%	1.5
Men's gymnastics	5.4	6.1%	1.9
Field hockey	5.3	5.6%	1.2
Women's volleyball	4.8	4.9%	1.3
Women's lacrosse	4.2	4.1%	1.0
Women's softball	3.9	5.9%	1.2
Baseball	3.4	5.6%	1.1

Table 20–4
Sudden Death in College and High School Athletes

Sport	Participants High School/College	Deaths High School/College	Est. Death Rate Per Million High School/College
Football (men)	9,400,000	53	5.61
	680,000	14	20.28
Basketball (men)	5,100,000	28	5.48
	260,000	9	34.7
Soccer (men)	2,100,000	6	2.85
	250,000	1	4.06
Wrestling (men)	2,400,000	9	3.75
	100,000	0	0
Baseball (men)	4,100,000	5	1.22
	390,000	2	5.14
Track (men)	4,300,000	9	2.09
	270,000	1	3.67
All others (men)	4,100,000	11	2.7
Totals for men	33,000,000	115	6.6
	2,500,000	31	14.5
Women in all sports	18,000,000	11	1.16
	1,200,000	3	2.81

Source: Adapted from Van Camp S, et al: Nontraumatic Sports Death in College and High School Athletes. Med Sci Sports Exerc 27(5):641–643, 1995.

numbers apply to men without known coronary artery disease. The amount of vigorous exercise performed weekly was also correlated with death rates, with the conclusion that, although the risk of sudden death was transiently increased during vigorous exercise, the overall death rate in those who exercised regularly was much lower.

The incidence of sudden death in younger athletes of college and high school age has been investigated.[12] Data have been collected by the National Center for Catastrophic Sports Injury Research over a 10-year period in 16 sports. Death rates were described as the number of deaths per million athletes per year. Of the 160 total deaths reported, 146 were in males and 14 were in females, and the greatest number occurred among high school students (126 versus 34). Cardiac abnormalities were present in 72 percent of athletes with hypertrophic cardiomyopathy (HCM) predominant (51), followed by coronary artery anomalies (16), heat stroke (13), and exertional rhabdomyolysis with sickle cell trait (7). Football recorded the highest number of deaths (67), followed by basketball (37). The preponderance of males over females with sudden death is unexplained. Of the 14 female deaths, 5 were in basketball and 3 in swimming (Table 20–4).

EXERCISE RISK IN THE OLDER POPULATION

The inherent risk of sports and exercise injury in the older population is receiving greater attention as the general population ages. With the onset of the new millennium, 20 percent of the population will be 65 or older with nearly 1 in 8 people above the age of 85. The beneficial effect of regular exercise in the aging process is addressed at length by the American College of Sports Medicine.[13] See Chapter 19 for a discussion of exercise and the mature adult.

Most of the exercise-associated injuries in the older population are directly related to the degenerative aging process[14] (Table 20–5). The majority of the injuries are mild, respond well to a brief cessation of activity, and rarely preclude resumption of activity. Lower extremity muscles are the most common location of injury. Immobilization of an injured extremity is an iatrogenic risk of exercise and is especially hazardous in the elderly. Immobilization should be avoided if at all possible. The complications of joint immobilization include muscle atrophy, decreased range of

Table 20–5
Physiologic Changes in the Aging Process

Connective tissue loses pliability
Cartilage loses hydration
Blood vessels stiffen
Muscle repairs more slowly
Cardiac output declines
Muscle mass and motor neurons regress
Balance, coordination, and reaction time decrease

motion, and altered proprioception of the involved extremity.

Walking and jogging are popular forms of exercise with documented training benefit for young, middle-aged, and older adults. In three separate studies of three generations of walkers and joggers, Pollock was able to identify injury risk among the different age groups. Injury risk was defined as a stoppage or significant alteration of training for 1 week or longer. The average injury rates identified were 18 percent for young adults (ages 20 to 35), 41 percent for middle-aged adults (ages 49 to 65), and 57 percent for older adults (ages 70 to 79).[15] In the elderly population, three patterns of injury were described. First, almost all injuries occurred during the jogging phase of training. Second, most injuries involved the foot. Finally, most injuries occurred in the female participants. The conclusion of the investigation was that exercise regimens for the elderly should be modified to limit high-impact, high-intensity loading of the lower extremities, especially in women.

PHYSICAL CONDITION OF THE ATHLETE

The third component that determines risk of athletic participation is the physical condition of the athlete. Physical condition is assessed by a focused review of the athlete's family history, past medical history, review of systems, and physical examination with an eye toward uncovering any factor that may compromise the athlete's ability to safely compete. The examining physician should ideally be familiar with the physical and technical demands of the sport to make a valid recommendation.

Not every physical finding need be pathologic to disqualify or modify participation. For example, Tanner staging of young athletes has been suggested as a means of determining eligibility for participation in contact sports. Proponents of Tanner staging segregation cite an increased risk of injury to skeletally immature athletes. Opponents of Tanner staging claim insufficient data to justify segregation and also the harm that may occur from singling out a youngster as being less physically mature. What is known is that physeal injuries increase during the adolescent years as a result of

athletes attaining greater power and speed as they mature physically.

Another example of nonpathologic physical findings that may increase risk is neck and shoulder strength in football. Development of strong trapezius, sternocleidomastoid, and cervical musculature is an important deterrent to concussive head injury and cervical spine injury. In the author's institution, walk-on football athletes are required to participate in off-season weight training and attain a set standard of neck and shoulder strength before contact is allowed.

Many medical conditions may limit or preclude exercise and competition because of an increased, unacceptable risk. The presence of aortic stenosis with a significant gradient may disqualify an athlete from competition, even though he or she may feel perfectly normal. Likewise, the presence of retinal disease in insulin-dependent diabetic athletes may restrict the athlete to a specified intensity level of activity. Cervical disk disease is a contraindication to contact sports. The practicing physician should have at his or her disposal the generally accepted guidelines for activity in athletes with complicated medical conditions.[16–18]

The physical condition of the elderly patient is especially important in assessing the risk of exercise. Beginning with the feet and progressing to the head, there are many clues on history and physical examination that suggest potential danger (Table 20–6). Nevertheless, one must keep in mind that there is no medical condition that cannot benefit from some form of exercise. A common sense approach can match every patient with an activity that will provide years of enjoyment, safety, and health benefit.

Table 20–6
Physical Impairments That Increase the Risk of Exercise

Loss of visual acuity
Hearing loss
Vertigo/ataxia
Restricted cervical motion
Orthostatic hypotension
Degenerative joint disease
Cardiac arrhythmias
Loss of cardiac output
Chronic obstructive pulmonary disease (COPD)
Autonomic dysfunction
Osteoporosis
Peripheral neuropathy
Peripheral vascular disease

SUMMARY

To properly assess the risk of exercise, the physician must know three things: (1) the dynamic and static demands of the activity, (2) the inherent risk of the activity, and (3) the physical condition of the patient.

There is a difference between exercise and competition. Most individuals, regardless of age, who do not have risk factors for cardiovascular disease may engage in mild to moderately intense activities without medical supervision or pre-exercise testing. Those with risk factors should be cleared medically prior to beginning an exercise program. All competitive sport has inherent risk of injury, which may be modified by improved equipment, tighter rule enforcement, or a change in the rules.

Sudden death during exercise is rare. Structural heart disease is the most common cause of sudden death in individuals younger than 35 years old. Atherosclerotic heart disease is the most common cause of sudden death after the age of 35 years.

The physical condition of the athlete is correlated with the risk of exercise with special precautions necessary for elderly athletes. There is an appropriate exercise for every patient.

REFERENCES

1. Physical Activities and Cardiovascular Health. National Institute of Health Consensus Statement, Vol 13, No 3, Dec. 18–20, 1995, pp. 1–33.
2. Nieman D: The Exercise-Health Connection. Champaign, IL, Human Kinetics, 1997, p. 6.
3. 26th Bethesda Conference: Recommendations for Determining Eligibility for Competition in Athletes With Cardiovascular Abnormalities, Jan. 6–7, 1994. Printed as a supplement to Med Sci Sports Exerc, Vol 26, No 10, 1994.
4. NIH Consensus Statement: Physical Activity and Cardiovascular Risk, p. 10.
5. Janda D, Bir C, Wild B, et al: Goal post injuries in soccer. Am J Sports Med 23(3):340–345, 1995.
6. Benson M (ed): 1996–1997 NCAA Sports Medicine Handbook, 9th ed. 1996.
7. Arendt E, Dick R: Knee injury patterns among men and women in collegiate basketball and soccer. Am J Sports Med 23(6):694–701, 1995.
8. Rome E: Sports related injuries among adolescents: When do they occur and how can we prevent them? Pediat Rev 16(5):184–187, May 1995.
9. Maron B, Shirani J, Poliac LC, et al: Sudden death in young competitive athletes: Clinical, demographic, and pathological profiles. JAMA 276:199–204, 1996.
10. Thompson PD, Funk EJ, Carlson RA, Sturner WQ: Incidence of death during jogging in Rhode Island from 1975–1980. JAMA 247:2535–2538, 1982.
11. Siscovick D, Weiss N, Fletcher R, Lasky T: The incidence of primary cardiac arrest during vigorous exercise. New Engl J Med 311(14):874–877, 1984.
12. Van Camp S, Bloor C, Mueller F, et al: Nontraumatic sports death in high school and college athletes. Med Sci Sports Exerc 27(5):641–647, 1995.
13. ACSM Position Stand: Exercise and physical activity for older adults. Med Sci Sports Exerc 30(6):992–1006, 1998.
14. Kallineu M, Markku M: Aging, physical activity and sports injuries. Sports Med 20(1):41–52, 1995.
15. Pollock M, Carrol IF, Graves JE: Injuries and adherence to walk/jog and resistance training in the elderly. Med Sci Sports Exerc 23:1194–1200, 1991.
16. 26th Bethesda Guidelines. Recommendations for Determining Eligibility for Competition in Athletes with Cardiovascular Abnormalities. Supplement to Med Sci Sports Exerc 26(10), Oct 1994.
17. Head and Spine Trauma. Supplement to Med Sci Sports Exerc Vol 29(7), July 1997.
18. Devlin JT, Ruderman N: The Health Professional's Guide to Diabetes and Exercise. Alexandria, VA, American Diabetic Association, 1995.

Chapter *21* | The Athlete with Medical Problems

I *The Hypertensive Athlete*

MARK NIEDFELDT, M.D.

Hypertension is represented by systolic blood pressure (SBP) of 140 mm Hg or greater, diastolic blood pressure (DBP) of 90 mm Hg or greater, or taking antihypertensive medication. The objective for identifying and treating hypertension is to reduce the mortality and morbidity risks of cardiovascular disease.[1]

Hypertension often begins in young adulthood. Its incidence increases with age, affecting 5 to 10 percent of adults 20 to 30 years old and 20 to 25 percent of middle-aged adults.[2] Athletes are usually thought to be free of cardiovascular disease and hypertension owing to their apparent high level of fitness, and the overall incidence of hypertension in this group is approximately 50 percent less than in the general population.[3] However, athletes still should be screened for hypertension, and if the condition is diagnosed, they must be treated appropriately.

CLASSIFICATION OF HYPERTENSION

Hypertension tends to progress through stages. The Sixth Report of the Joint National Committee on Prevention, Detection, Evaluation, and Treatment of High Blood Pressure (JNC VI) divides hypertension into six classifications (Table 21–1). These classifications are for individuals who are not taking antihypertensive medications and have no acute illnesses. The classification is determined after two or more blood pressure readings at two or more visits following the initial screening. If the SBP and DBP fall into different categories, the higher category should be used.

Most athletes with hypertension will fall into the stage 1 or stage 2 level. The stage 1 level (140 to 159 mm Hg SBP, 90 to 99 mm Hg DBP), previously known as borderline hypertension, is

generally the earliest stage of hypertension. At this level, there is an increased heart rate (HR) and cardiac output (CO) with normal total peripheral resistance (TPR). The stage 2 level (160 to 179 mm Hg SBP, 100 to 109 mm Hg DBP) will exhibit a normal HR and CO with increased vascular resistance. In stage 3 hypertension (above 180/110 mm Hg), CO is depressed due to increased afterload and there is a further increase in vascular resistance.[4]

CLINICAL PATHOPHYSIOLOGY OF HYPERTENSION

Hypertension can be divided into two main categories—primary and secondary hypertension. Primary hypertension, in which no direct cause of hypertension is found, constitutes approximately 95 percent of cases.[5] Several different physiologic changes may occur. There may be abnormal neuroreflexes and sympathetic control of peripheral resistance, including sympathetic baroreceptor activation of the sympathetic nervous system along with increased circulating catecholamines and pressors such as angiotensin. There may also be abnormal renal and metabolic control of vascular volume and compliance mediated by changes in sodium balance, plasma volume, and the renin-angiotensin system. Endothelial mediators and both smooth muscle sodium and calcium balance are altered. Abnormal local smooth muscle and endothelial control of vascular resistance occurs with resultant structural changes within the vascular smooth muscle and alteration in arterial baroreceptor function, which result in sustained increases in systemic vascular resistance.[6]

Secondary hypertension is found in approximately 5 percent of cases. These patients tend to be younger adults with a rapid onset of severe

Table 21-1
Classification of Blood Pressure

| Category | Blood Pressure (mm Hg) | |
	Systolic	Diastolic
Optimal	<120	<80
Normal	<130	<85
High normal	130–139	85–89
Hypertension		
Stage 1	140–159	90–99
Stage 2	160–179	100–109
Stage 3	≥180	≥110

Source: Adapted from the Sixth Report of the Joint National Committee on Detection, Evaluation, and Treatment of High Blood Pressure (JNC-VI). Arch Intern Med 157:2413–2446, 1997.

hypertension, or those with hypertension that responds poorly to routine therapies. The most common cause of secondary hypertension is renal disease, either vascular or parenchymal.[5] In renal vascular disease increased renin stimulates the conversion of angiotensin I to angiotensin II, a potent vasoconstrictor. As a result, aldosterone is released and the kidneys retain sodium and water. In renal parenchymal disease, the damaged kidneys are unable to excrete excess sodium and water. The endocrine system is another main culprit in secondary hypertension. Adrenal gland malfunction can be responsible for pheochromocytoma, Cushing's syndrome, or primary aldosteronism. Hyperthyroidism can result in increased CO leading to increased SBP, whereas hypothyroidism can lead to increased DBP from increased peripheral resistance. Acromegaly from excess growth hormone can result in fluid volume excess, and the increased calcium of hyperparathyroidism leads to increased peripheral resistance. The estrogen in oral contraceptives can lead to hypertension in about 5 percent of women taking the medication for over 5 years.[6] Coarctation of the aorta, a vascular cause of secondary hypertension, should also be considered.

CLINICAL EVALUATION

The key in clinical evaluation is the proper measurement of blood pressure. The screening blood pressure should be performed in a standard measurement situation. This is often difficult to do with athletes, whose increased blood pressure is often first detected during a routine sports physical ex-

amination taking place outside a doctor's office. Measurements should be performed with the subject in a seated position with the arm supported at heart level following 5 minutes of rest. Any high reading should be measured again after waiting at least 2 minutes after the first reading. It is also important to use the appropriate blood pressure cuff size. The bladder in the cuff should encircle at least 80 percent of the arm. Many athletes will require a large cuff size. The cuff should be deflated at a rate of 2 to 3 mm Hg per second, and rapid deflation of the cuff should be avoided.[6]

The history should focus on cardiovascular and hypertension risk factors. Risk factors include male sex; postmenopausal state in women; race, with African-Americans affected more often than whites by about a 2:1 ratio and Asians affected the least; a family history of hypertension or cardiac disease in men under 55 years old and women under 65; diabetes mellitus; dyslipidemia; age over 60 years; and smoking.[1] Metabolic risk factors that increase the incidence of hypertension include obesity, glucose intolerance, and the previously mentioned endocrine disorders including adrenal dysfunction, hyperparathyroidism, hypo- or hyperthyroidism, pheochromocytoma, and sex hormone excess or decrease. Stress is a risk factor for hypertension. Chronic environmental or social stress may lead to higher circulating catecholamines and chronic neurogenic activation of the sympathetic nervous system.[7]

Behavioral factors related to increased hypertension include high sodium intake, excessive alcohol consumption, recreational drug abuse (especially cocaine and stimulants), smoking or chewing tobacco, and anabolic steroid use. Over-the-counter medications such as nonsteroidal anti-inflammatory drugs, caffeine, diet pills, and decongestants may lead to increased blood pressure. Some herbal remedies may also increase blood pressure, and the athlete should be questioned regarding the use of herbs and other supplements.

The physical examination focuses on ruling out secondary causes of hypertension and looking for end-organ damage. Funduscopic examination is performed to rule out hypertensive retinopathy. The neck is examined for carotid bruits, jugular venous distention, and enlargement of the thyroid gland. Cardiovascular examination focuses on abnormalities in rate, rhythm, cardiac size, murmurs, and extra heart sounds. Pulmonary examination looks for rales or bronchospasm. The abdominal examination seeks abdominal masses or bruits, and the examination of the extremities evaluates edema and peripheral pulses.

Laboratory studies are done to determine the presence of target organ damage or causes of secondary hypertension. These tests include complete blood count, sodium and potassium levels, blood urea nitrogen (BUN), creatinine level, fasting glucose level, total cholesterol and high density lipoprotein (HDL) cholesterol, urinalysis, and electrocardiogram. Other studies should be pursued if the clinician is suspicious of a secondary cause of hypertension.

TREATMENT OF HYPERTENSION

Nonpharmacologic Therapy

Nonpharmacologic treatment of hypertension has few to no side effects but depends on long-term adherence and lifestyle changes. Athletes are often more motivated than the general population to comply with recommendations. Lifestyle modifications are recommended as an adjunct for all hypertensive patients, but they are most appropriate for those with mild hypertension. These modifications cannot always keep athletes off medication, but they may reduce the medication dosage and thus the possibility of medication side effects.

Dietary sodium (Na$^+$) intake is linked to increased blood pressure. Response of blood pressure to sodium is variable, but in general African-Americans, older people, and diabetics seem to be more sensitive.[8] Seventy-five percent of sodium intake is derived from processed food. A reduction to 2.4 g per day of sodium in the diet can result in a significant decrease in blood pressure, thus reducing the dosage of medication needed in some cases.[1]

High dietary potassium (K$^+$) intake may protect against developing hypertension and improve blood pressure control.[9] This effect is especially evident in hypokalemic patients, but increased potassium may have some effect in normokalemic individuals.[1]

Increased calcium intake (1 to 2 g per day) may lower blood pressure in some individuals, especially in women who are calcium-deficient, but the overall effect is minimal.[10] Therefore, routine supplementation is not recommended for the purpose of reducing hypertension.[1]

A lower magnesium level may lead to higher blood pressure because magnesium is a vasodilator. Although there may be some benefit to supplementation in selected patients,[11] especially those whose magnesium has been depleted by use of diuretics, routine supplementation is not recommended.[1]

Excess body weight is correlated with increased blood pressure. Weight reduction of just 10 pounds reduces blood pressure in overweight people with hypertension.[12] It also seems to enhance the blood pressure–lowering effect of many medications.[13] Obesity increases the preload and afterload of the heart, which can affect athletic performance. A weight reduction diet plan should include a high-fiber diet with low saturated fat.[14]

Excess alcohol can cause resistance to antihypertensive therapy. Adults who drink should limit alcoholic beverage intake to the equivalent of two beers daily. Women and lighter weight individuals should consume no more than the equivalent of one beer daily.[1] Stimulants such as cocaine and ephedrine should be avoided. Athletes should also be counseled regarding the risk with anabolic steroid use for developing or exacerbating hypertension.

Relaxation techniques such as biofeedback, muscle relaxation, meditation, and stress management may have value as adjunct therapy in some patients.

Regular aerobic exercise adequate to achieve moderate fitness can lower blood pressure, enhance weight loss, and reduce mortality risk. Sedentary individuals have a 20 to 50 percent higher risk of developing hypertension as compared to more active peers.[15] Endurance exercise conditioning has been shown to lower SBP and DBP an average of 10 mm Hg in individuals with mild hypertension. It is difficult to tell if this benefit is a direct effect of exercise or secondary to weight loss, as many studies are either poorly designed or uncontrolled.[16] The effect of exercise on hypertension is even more dramatic in those whose hypertension is secondary to renal dysfunction.

Pharmacologic Therapy

Pharmacologic treatment of hypertension must be individualized and carefully monitored for potential side effects. In most cases, a low dose of the initial drug is given and titrated as needed while monitoring for side effects. Adherence is improved if a long-acting formulation taken once daily is used. Athletes will also need to monitor any effects of medications on their performance because some medications have a potential influence on exercise tolerance. The physician must be aware of the likely effects of antihypertensive medications on athletic performance. He or she should also be aware that the U.S. Olympic Committee (USOC) and the National Collegiate Athletic Association (NCAA) ban some medications.[17] It is important to remember that nonsteroidal anti-inflammatory drugs (NSAIDs) may decrease the action of several antihypertensives including diuretics, beta blockers, and angiotensin-converting enzyme (ACE) inhibitors.[18]

Diuretics

The diuretic antihypertensive drugs include both the thiazides and the loop inhibitors. Thiazides are often recommended as initial therapy for hypertension. Several randomized control trials have shown a decrease in mortality and morbidity rates using these agents. However, many of these studies have been done in elderly subjects. These medications decrease plasma volume, cardiac output, and systemic vascular resistance.[19] Possible side effects include hypovolemia, orthostatic hypotension, and urinary loss of potassium and magnesium. This can lead to muscle cramps, arrhythmias, and rhabdomyolysis in athletes, especially those practicing or competing in warm weather. Short-term increases in plasma cholesterol, glucose, and uric acid have also been noted.[20] Because of these effects, loop diuretics are inappropriate for use in the treatment of hypertension in athletes. The thiazide diuretics do not have effects as pronounced as the loop diuretics and are most useful as second-line therapy in salt-sensitive hypertensive athletes.[1] They should be used in small doses and possibly combined with a potassium-sparing agent. All diuretics are banned substances and cannot be used by athletes who are required to undergo drug testing.[17]

Angiotensin-Converting Enzyme Inhibitors

Angiotensin-converting enzyme (ACE) inhibitors cause the competitive inhibition of ACE in plasma and vascular smooth muscle that converts angiotensin I to angiotensin II.[5] These medications block the vasoconstriction and Na^+ retention caused by angiotensin II. There is an increase in

stroke volume, a slight decrease in heart rate, and a decrease in total peripheral resistance with the use of ACE inhibitors.[19] These antihypertensive agents have been shown to have beneficial effects in patients with heart failure, systolic dysfunction, or nephropathy, and they have been shown to reverse ventricular hypertrophy. This medication is also recommended for diabetics. In exercise, there is no major effect on energy metabolism, no impairment of maximum oxygen uptake ($Vo_{2\ max}$), and generally no deleterious effects on training or competition.[18] The major side effect is a dry, nonproductive cough and possible exacerbation of bronchospasm. There are also anecdotal reports of postural hypotension after intense exercise, but this can be eliminated by an adequate cool-down period following intense exercise. This class of antihypertensive drugs is excellent for mild to moderate hypertension and is often the first-line agent for hypertension in athletes. Effectiveness may be improved with addition of a low-dose diuretic either taken separately or in combination. The concomitant use of NSAIDs and ACE inhibitors may increase the potassium-sparing effect of the medication.[18] Women of childbearing age should use contraception when taking these medications because they are contraindicated during pregnancy.

The angiotensin II receptor blockers produce effects similar to those of the ACE inhibitors but avoid the most common side effect—dry cough. There are not sufficient data currently to document cardiac and renal protection. Therefore, these agents are generally recommended only for those who cannot tolerate the ACE inhibitors.[1]

Alpha Blockers

Alpha-1–receptor blockers competitively block postsynaptic alpha-1 arteriolar smooth muscle receptors. This class of antihypertensive agents decreases systemic vascular resistance with no reflex increase in heart rate or cardiac output. There can be a first dose effect, especially in the elderly. There are no major changes in energy metabolism during exercise and the $Vo_{2\ max}$ is preserved. Therefore, there are no major effects on training or sports performance.[18] These agents are useful in diabetic athletes who have hypertension and hypercholesterolemia because they will not exacerbate the other conditions.[6]

The central alpha agonists act on $alpha_2$ receptors in the brain stem to block central sympathetic stimulation. These medications are rarely used today. There is a minor decrease in heart rate and systemic vascular resistance at rest. The sympathetically mediated Na^+ retention is blocked. Side effects are significant and include mild to moderate drowsiness, dry mouth, and impotence. Rebound hypertension can occur with abrupt discontinuation of oral clonidine.[6] During exercise there are no major changes in energy metabolism, the $Vo_{2\,max}$ is preserved, and no major effect on training or sports performance is noted.[18]

Beta Blockers

Beta blockers may be either noncardioselective or cardioselective. The noncardioselective agents decrease heart rate by 20 to 30 percent. There is also a decrease in contractility of the heart. Systemic vascular resistance is increased, especially in the muscle and skin. Because lipolysis and glycogenolysis are inhibited, hypoglycemia may occur after intense exercise. Perceived exertion ratings are increased,[18] which may decrease compliance in athletes. An increased total cholesterol and decreased HDL cholesterol may be noted.[6]

The cardioselective agents have less effect on beta-2 vasodilatation, lipolysis, and glycogenolysis. However, the impairment of cardiac output and $Vo_{2\,max}$ is similar. During exercise there is a significant loss of $Vo_{2\,max}$ with decreased cardiac output and skeletal muscle flow. Well-trained athletes have a greater drop in $Vo_{2\,max}$ than do sedentary patients. Impairment of substrate mobilization causes earlier achievement of the lactate threshold and fatigue. Exercise-induced bronchospasm or asthma may be exacerbated, and athletes with these conditions should generally avoid these medications. Although there are fewer side effects with cardioselective agents, this class is not recommended in athletes unless an underlying condition exists that requires their use.[19]

When the combined alpha and beta blockers are used, the beta-blocker effects are greater than the alpha-blocker effects. There is a decreased systemic vascular resistance but less impairment of muscle blood flow and $Vo_{2\,max}$. These agents may be the best choice if beta blockade is necessary.[18] Beta blockers are banned by the USOC in precision events such as archery, shooting, diving, and ice skating.[17]

Calcium Channel Blockers

Calcium channel blockers inhibit calcium slow-channel conduction. This reduces calcium concentration in vascular smooth muscle cells. The result is decreased systemic vascular resistance with generalized vasodilatation.[18] These agents are effective in reversing ventricular hypertrophy. Dihydropyridines (i.e., amlodipine, nifedipine) can cause reflex tachycardia, fluid retention (pedal edema), and vascular headaches. The non-dihydropyridines (i.e., verapamil, diltiazem) can cause heart rate suppression and minor impairment of maximal heart rate, decreased left ventricular contractility, and constipation (verapamil).[1] During exercise there is no major effect on energy metabolism, and $Vo_{2\,max}$ is generally preserved.[19] There is the potential for competitive "steal" of muscle blood flow due to vasodilatation and earlier onset of lactate threshold.[4] In general, this class of antihypertensives is well tolerated and effective, especially in African-Americans.[1] These agents are often used as first-line agents in African-American athletes.

Summary of Therapy

In mild hypertension, nonpharmacologic interventions are employed for 6 months with frequent monitoring. If control is adequate, the athlete may continue lifestyle modifications. However, it is important to emphasize the need for long-term follow-up care and management. If control is inadequate, pharmacologic intervention is needed. Low-dose initial therapy consisting of ACE inhibitor, calcium channel blocker, or alpha blocker may be instituted. If beta blockade is needed, a combined beta and alpha blocker may be the best choice. Observe for 6 to 8 weeks. If the athlete is at the goal blood pressure, emphasize the need for long-term follow-up care and management.[1]

The physician may be able to reduce dosage or withdraw medication in a few cases after 6 to 12 months if excellent blood pressure control is maintained, as a small number of athletes may remain normotensive. If the athlete is not at goal blood pressure, the dosage of the initial medication may be adjusted, or a second medication may be added, usually a diuretic. A different medication may need to be substituted if significant side effects are noted.[1] Always be aware of NCAA or USOC regulations if the athlete is competing in events sponsored by either of these organizations.

When to Refer

Athletes with hypertension not responding to first- or second-line agents or those with severe end organ disease should be referred to a hypertension specialist. Patients with secondary hypertension may need referral for treatment and management of the underlying condition.

EXERCISE IN HYPERTENSIVE PATIENTS

During dynamic (aerobic) exercise several physiologic changes occur. This includes an increased cardiac output due to increases in heart rate, stroke volume, and contractility. Decreased vascular resistance occurs resulting in increased systolic blood pressure with little change in diastolic blood pressure. In the athlete with mild to moderate hypertension the normal increased cardiac output is accompanied by a higher vascular resistance, which results in increased SBP *and* DBP. In severe hypertension, along with the increased vascular resistance, decreased stroke volume leads to a lower cardiac output.[4]

Isometric exercise (heavy weightlifting) shows a different physiologic response. A rapid combined rise in systolic and diastolic pressure (pressor response) occurs with a reflex increased heart rate and resultant increased cardiac output. No change in vascular resistance is seen. In the hypertensive athlete, the relative increase in blood pressure is similar to that seen in the normotensive athlete, but the starting point is higher. Thus, the end blood pressure is higher than in normotensive individuals.[4] Presently, there are no good research data concerning the safety of isometric exercise in well-controlled hypertensives.

Return to Practice and Competition

The recommended mode, frequency, duration, and intensity of exercise are generally the same as those for nonhypertensive individuals. Hypertensive athletes should have their blood pressure controlled before returning to participation in vigorous sports because both dynamic and isometric exercise can cause remarkable blood pressure increases. The result is inefficient shunting of blood to the skin, increased core temperatures, and increased fluid and potassium losses, which can be major problems for athletes. Recommendations regarding athletic participation are based on the 26th Bethesda Conference guidelines.[21] Athletes with

high-normal blood pressure have no restrictions. Athletes with mild to moderate hypertension that is controlled at 140/90 mm Hg or less have no restriction for dynamic exercise. Physicians may choose to limit isometric training or sports in some cases. Athletes with uncontrolled blood pressure above 140/90 mm Hg should be limited to low-intensity dynamic exercise. This restriction also applies to athletes with controlled hypertension with end-organ involvement. These athletes should avoid isometric sports.

Athletes with severe hypertension with no end-organ involvement may be limited to low-intensity dynamic sports if the blood pressure is under adequate control. In athletes with secondary hypertension of renal origin, low-intensity sports are recommended. These athletes should avoid collision sports that could lead to kidney damage.

Key Points

- Hypertension can affect athletes despite their apparent high level of fitness.
- Because there is a wide range of therapeutic options, it is important for practitioners to individualize therapy based on the patient's age, sex, race, and activity level.
- Close follow-up is necessary to monitor for side effects that may impede performance; avoiding such side effects will lead to better compliances.
- Awareness of potential banned substances is essential.

REFERENCES

1. Joint National Committee on Detection, Evaluation, and Treatment of High Blood Pressure: The Sixth Report of the Joint National Committee on Detection, Evaluation, and Treatment of High Blood Pressure (JNC-VI). Arch Intern Med 157:2413–2446, 1997.
2. Gifford RW, Kirkendall W, O'Connor DT, Weidman W: Scientific Council Special Report: Office evaluation of hypertension. Circulation 79:721–731, 1989.
3. Lehmann M, Durr H, Meikelbach H, Schmid A: Hypertension and sports activity: Institutional experience. Clin Cardiol 13:197–208, 1990.
4. Lund-Johansen P: Hemodynamics in essential hypertension. Clin Sci 59:3435–3545, 1980.
5. Hanson P, Andrea BE: Treatment of hypertension in athletes. *In* DeLee JC, Drez D (eds): Orthopaedic Sports Medicine. Philadelphia, W.B. Saunders, 1994, pp. 307–319.

6. Kaplan NM: Clinical Hypertension, 6th ed. Baltimore, Williams & Wilkins, 1994.
7. Julius S, Nesbitt S: Sympathetic overactivity in hypertension. A moving target. Am J Hypertens 9(11):113S–120S, 1996.
8. Weinberger MH: Salt sensitivity of blood pressure in humans. Hypertension 27(pt 2):481–490, 1996.
9. Whelton PK, HE J, Cutler JA, et al: Effects of oral potassium on blood pressure: Meta-analysis of randomized controlled trials. JAMA 277:1624–1632, 1997.
10. Cappuccio FP, Elliot P, Allender PS, et al: Epidemiologic association between dietary calcium intake and blood pressure: A meta-analysis of randomized clinical trials. Ann Intern Med 124:825–831, 1996.
11. Stamler J, Caggiula AW, Grandits GA: Chapter 12: Relation of body mass and alcohol, nutrient, fiber, and caffeine intakes to blood pressure in the special intervention and usual care groups in the Multiple Risk Factor Intervention Trial. Am J Clin Nutr 65(suppl):338S–365S, 1997.
12. Trials of Hypertension Prevention Collaborative Research Group. Effects of weight loss and sodium reduction intervention on blood pressure and hypertension incidence in overweight people with high-normal blood pressure: The Trials of Hypertension Prevention, phase II. Arch Intern Med 157:657–667, 1997.
13. Neaton JD, Grimm RH Jr, Prineas RJ, et al: For the Treatment of Mild Hypertension Study Research Group. Treatment of Mild Hypertension Study: Final results. JAMA 270:713–724, 1993.
14. Appel LJ, Moore TJ, Obarzanek E, et al: For the DASH Collaborative Research Group. A clinical trial of the effects of dietary patterns on blood pressure. N Engl J Med 336:1117–1124, 1997.
15. Blair SN, Goodyear NN, Gibbons LW, Cooper KH: Physical fitness and incidence of hypertension in healthy normotensive men and women. JAMA 252:487–490, 1984.
16. Petrella LS: How effective is exercise training for the treatment of hypertension? Clin J Sports Med 8:224–231, 1998.
17. Olympic Committee, Division of Sports Medicine and Science, Colorado Springs, Drug Education and Control Policy, 1992.
18. Gifford RW: Antihypertensive therapy: Angiotensin-converting enzyme inhibitors, angiotensin II receptor antagonists, and calcium antagonists. Med Clin North Am 81(6):1319–1334, 1997.
19. Chick TW, Halperin AK, Gacek EM: The effect of antihypertensive medications on exercise performance: A review. Med Sci Sports Exerc 20:447–454, 1988.
20. Freis ED: Current status of diuretics, β-blockers, α blockers, and α-β blockers in the treatment of hypertension. Med Clin North Am 81(6):1305–1318, 1997.
21. 26th Bethesda Conference: Recommendations for determining eligibility for competition in athletes with cardiovascular abnormalities. J Am Coll Cardiol 24(4):845–899, 1994.

II *The Asthmatic or Allergic Athlete*

MARK NIEDFELDT, M.D.

Affecting 14 million to 15 million Americans, asthma is an obstructive disease of the airways characterized by airway inflammation and hyperreactivity.[1] The obstruction is initiated by inflammatory events in the airways, particularly the release of inflammatory mediators from mast cells, macrophages, and epithelial cells. The subsequent bronchial wall edema, mucus production, airway smooth muscle contraction, and hypertrophy influence the airflow obstruction.[2] The airway hyperreactivity is an exaggerated bronchoconstriction response to various stimuli including allergens, environmental irritants, viral respiratory infections, cold air, and exercise. It is well known that strenuous exercise can trigger bronchospasm, thus putting the asthma patient at risk for an exacerbation. Many individuals with asthma will find their symptoms to be worse when they exercise at high intensities, but many people with no other asthma symptoms may experience asthmatic symptoms when exercising. This is called exercise-induced

asthma (EIA). Patients with asthma obtain the same benefits as others from regular physical activity, including reduced risk of cardiovascular disease, diabetes, obesity, and other health problems. Exercise may also chronically reduce airway responsiveness, leading to fewer exacerbations, lowered use of medication, and less time lost from work and school.[3, 4] Thus, patients with asthma should be encouraged to exercise and to learn to adapt their treatment regimens accordingly. Asthma sufferers can compete at a very high level. The 1984 U.S. Olympic team had 26 of 597 athletes with documented asthma, and 67 athletes experienced EIA.[5] Forty-one athletes with asthma or EIA won medals at the Los Angeles Olympic Games.

EXERCISE-INDUCED ASTHMA

Exercise-induced asthma often goes unrecognized and undiagnosed.[6] The symptoms of EIA are often perceived to be part of the experience of normal vigorous exercise,[7] and denial of symptoms is common among young athletes.[2] Evenly distributed between the sexes and occurring at any age, EIA is present in 3 to 10 percent of the general population without asthma.[8] Up to 90 percent of people with asthma experience EIA during the course of their disease, and most asthmatics consider exercise a major precipitant of their asthma.[9–11] The condition is characterized by a transient increase in airway resistance following several minutes of exercise.[12] The obstruction is totally or partially reversible in response to therapy. In the 35 to 40 percent of patients with allergic rhinitis who experience EIA, precipitating factors include allergens, viruses, cold air, and air pollutants.[9–13]

Pathophysiology

Two main theories concerning the pathophysiology of EIA implicate water loss and thermal expenditure. The *water loss theory* hypothesizes that the loss of water throughout the bronchial mucosa into the exhaled air during exercise leads to local lung events and changes in osmolarity, pH, and temperature of the airway epithelium, which cause bronchospasm.[14] The *thermal expenditure theory* suggests that EIA is a direct result of heat transfer from the pulmonary vascular bed into the air during and after exercise.[15] Heat is lost during exercise, and rewarming following exercise causes dilatation and hyperemia of the bronchial vessels, which leads to EIA. It is generally believed that thermodynamic events within the airway during hyperpnea are related to the airway obstruction in EIA. Because of the hyperventilation during exercise, the upper airway is unable to bring inspired air to body temperature and 100 percent humidity. Heat and water are drawn from the respiratory tissue in order to warm and humidify the inspired air, resulting in respiratory tissue water loss and airway cooling.[16] However, the etiology of EIA is probably multifactoral, and the pathophysiology of the disease is not completely understood.

Clinical Evaluation

Patients generally present with the typical signs of asthma including wheezing, chest tightness, short-ness of breath, and coughing.[2] Questions should be raised regarding type of exercise: free running outdoors is more likely to produce asthmatic symptoms than treadmill running, stationary biking, or swimming. The physician should inquire about increased symptoms at higher workloads and environmental factors such as cold, dry air, air pollution, smoke, and allergens because these factors can influence the severity of EIA as well.[6]

Maximal bronchoconstriction generally occurs 3 to 15 minutes after exercise ceases.[17] A refractory period follows the acute exacerbation and is generally present for 1 to 3 hours after exercise. Increased bronchospasm can occur 3 to 9 hours later and is referred to as the late response.[18] During exercise, the athlete may complain of coughing, wheezing, dyspnea, or chest discomfort. Complaints of decreased or limited endurance are common as well. Symptoms often vary by season or outdoor temperature. In some cases the athlete has been forced to discontinue, decrease, or alter the exercise regimen because of symptoms. Minimal problems are noted with swimming or during exercise in warm, humid environments. Sometimes the only complaints may be of vague gastrointestinal discomfort, nausea, or headache.[6] Chest pain is a common complaint in children.[19]

The diagnosis of EIA is often made on history alone, because the physical examination is often normal.[6] The pharynx should be examined for mucus, indicating postnasal drainage. Nasal examination may reveal erythema, congestion, and enlarged turbinates, and percussion of the sinuses may elicit tenderness. Chest examination should include auscultation of the lungs to assess the presence of prolonged expiratory phase, wheeze, or cough with inspiration.[2]

Testing

If the athlete reports possible symptoms but the history is atypical, pulmonary function testing at rest can be performed. Pulmonary function testing results showing FEV_1 and FEV_1/FVC values below 80 percent of predicted values indicate obstructive airway disease. Active patients often have lung function results well above the normal predicted values, so a drop that is still in the acceptable range may represent a bronchospastic problem for the patient. Bronchoprovocative testing is sensitive for hyperreactive airways.[11] The methacholine challenge test can be used. Some laboratories use cold, dry air for bronchoprovocation. Exercise testing involves determining baseline lung function before exercise followed by 6 to 10 minutes of strenuous exercise at 85 to 90 percent of the predicted maximal heart rate. Forced expiration is then measured at 5- to 10-minute intervals following exercise for a total of 15 to 30 minutes. Postexercise decreases of 10 to 20 percent in FEV_1 indicate mild EIA, 20 to 40 percent in moderate, and over 40 percent is severe EIA.[20] Exercise challenge is less sensitive than methacholine challenge but is highly specific for EIA. Positive results provide verification that the disease is present. Peak flows may be used in the field and by the athlete to monitor progress with treatment or to aid in diagnosis.

A trial of a short-acting beta-2 agonist 15 to 30 minutes prior to exercise is a cost-effective first step: if there is clear benefit, exercise challenge testing is unnecessary. The exercise challenge test can be helpful in some cases to demonstrate to patients the benefit of medication for their symptoms and may reduce the use of unnecessary medications in patients with an unclear history.[2]

Treatment

Education

Educating the patient about asthma and EIA and the appropriate treatment regimen is important. The athlete needs to recognize triggers of the asthma. This can help the athlete control the condition. By understanding the process of EIA, the athlete can use the refractory period to advantage. The proper use, timing, and dosage of medications along with monitoring by peak flows is essential for optimal control of asthmatic symptoms.

Nonpharmacologic Therapy

The nonpharmacologic treatment of EIA can include activity and condition modification. A warm-up can be incorporated into the exercise program so the refractory period can be used as the exercise time. This warm-up period should incorporate subthreshold exercise.[6] For example, a recreational jogger can begin by stretching and walking followed by slow jogging for the first 8 to 10 minutes. A cool-down period following exercise will allow a gradual rewarming of the airways, lessening the chance of postexercise

symptoms. Improved physical conditioning may reduce the need for medication and decrease the incidence of asthma attacks. Short bursts of activity have been shown to decrease EIA, so athletes may want to choose a sport incorporating this type of activity.[21] Warm, humid air will decrease the symptoms of EIA. Indoor swimming is a good exercise for athletes with EIA because they avoid the allergens found in the outside air, and the exercise is done in a warm, humid environment. Wearing a facemask during cold, dry conditions helps humidify the air and reduce symptoms in athletes who must compete outdoors.

Pharmacologic Therapy

The goals of pharmacologic treatment are to prevent the onset of asthma episodes and treat breakthrough episodes. Most patients can be successfully managed with either single or combination therapy. Peak flows can be used by the patient to monitor symptoms and institute preventive measures when needed.

Beta Agonists Beta agonists are the drugs of choice for preventing isolated EIA and for on-demand treatment of asthma exacerbations. Short-acting beta agonists are the most effective agents for preventing EIA.[22] These agents reverse contraction of bronchial smooth muscle and are very effective bronchodilators. The short-acting inhaled beta agonists should be administered 15 minutes before exercise. The effect of these medications usually lasts 2 to 6 hours. Salmeterol is a long-acting beta agonist that can protect against EIA for up to 12 hours, but it cannot be used as a rescue medication because of its long onset of action.[2] Therefore, patients should also have a short-acting beta agonist available. The effect of the short-acting beta agonist may be blunted by the long-term use of salmeterol.[23] Tolerance can be reduced by the use of salmeterol once daily.[24] This medication is especially useful during school hours in children over age 12. Because the protective effects of salmeterol against EIA may wane over time, additional or alternative therapy may be required in patients with breakthrough symptoms.

Current guidelines for management begin with administration of a short-acting inhaled beta agonist 15 minutes before exercise followed by a 15-minute warm-up period of stretching and low level exercise and a 15-minute rest period prior to intense exercise. If symptoms develop during exercise, two puffs of the short-acting beta agonist may be repeated.[11]

Cromolyn Cromolyn sodium may also be administered for the treatment of EIA prior to exercise. Although the mechanism of action of cromolyn sodium in EIA is unknown, it does inhibit both the early and late phase responses, probably through inhibition of mast cell mediator release and an alteration in calcium influx.[2] It is most effective in patients with normal pulmonary function test results.

Nedocromil Sodium Nedocromil sodium is an inhaled anti-inflammatory agent that has been found to inhibit EIA as well as cromolyn sodium when administered before exercise.[25] Some physicians use cromolyn or nedocromil as first-line therapy,[6] but these medications seem to be most effective in combination with a beta agonist for those athletes who do not have an adequate response to a beta agonist alone.[2] The dosage may be increased to four puffs prior to exercise.[6]

Ipratropium Bromide Ipratropium bromide is an atropine derivative that has bronchodilating effects and can be added to the pre-exercise treatment regimen of athletes with EIA that is inadequately controlled with a combination of a beta agonist and cromolyn or nedocromil.[6]

Corticosteroids Inhaled corticosteroids reduce airway inflammation and bronchial hyperreactivity and are often used in maintenance therapy for chronic asthma. Their use may improve effectiveness of inhaled beta agonists in decreasing effects of EIA.[11]

Theophylline Oral theophylline is used in the treatment of chronic asthma and has been used in the treatment of EIA. It is generally used for patients who do not respond to inhaled beta agonists. Theophylline has a slow onset of action, and even rapid-release forms require 1 to 2 hours for onset, making this medication less useful in the athletic setting.

Leukotriene Modifiers Leukotriene modifiers such as montelukast, zafirlukast, and zileuton show promise for treating patients who have known allergic triggers including environmental allergens, exercise, and cold. Leukotrienes are known mediators of asthma and affect the airways by decreasing ciliary activity and increasing mucus secretions and venopermeability; they are potent bronchoconstrictors. Once-daily doses of the leukotriene modifiers block the early and late bronchoconstrictor responses to antigen challenge and have demonstrated protection against EIA.[26]

When to Refer

Referral to an allergist or pulmonologist may be indicated if the patient's asthma is controlled poorly, multiple allergic triggers are present, or in severe cases.

Return to Practice and Competition

Prior to the athlete's returning to strenuous training or competition, the asthma should be well controlled as indicated by peak flows or FEV_1 above 80 percent. Athletes may need to skip exercise sessions or practices on days when they are wheezing, when allergies are troubling, or when peak flows indicate a decline in lung function. Upper respiratory infections often cause an exacerbation in asthmatic symptoms and may require alterations in the athlete's training regimen.

The athlete may be encouraged to participate in a sport that has less potential for exacerbation of asthma or EIA symptoms. Sporting activities more likely to cause EIA include running, cycling, soccer, basketball, and cross-country skiing. Sporting activities less likely to cause EIA include kayaking, swimming, aerobics, dancing, gymnastics, downhill skiing, playing goalie in soccer, and playing defense in a team sport.

Key Points

- Asthma is an obstructive disease of the airways initiated by inflammatory events.
- Asthma symptoms tend to worsen during exercise.
- Many people without asthma experience asthmatic symptoms while exercising. This is called exercise-induced asthma.
- Asthmatics can benefit from exercise and athletic participation.
- The pathophysiology of exercise-induced asthma is probably multifactoral.
- In exercise-induced asthma, maximal bronchospasm occurs 3 to 15 minutes after exercise and is followed by a 1- to 3-hour refractory period.
- Pulmonary function testing is often unnecessary unless the history is atypical. If performed, FEV_1 and FEV_1/FVC are less than 80 percent of predicted values.

● Education about asthma, avoiding triggers, and proper pharmacologic management are key in maintaining athletic performance.

EXERCISE-INDUCED ANAPHYLAXIS

Exercise-induced anaphylaxis is characterized by a sensation of warmth, pruritus, cutaneous erythema, urticaria, upper respiratory obstructive symptoms, and occasionally vascular collapse. Risk factors include a history or family history of atopy, hypersensitivity to certain foods (shellfish, nuts, and celery), and either hot and humid or cold weather conditions.[13]

Clinical Evaluation

Exercise-induced anaphylaxis occurs exclusively with exercise. Clinical features include a flushing sensation, pruritus, gastrointestinal complaints such as vomiting, and throat tightness or choking. Diffuse large urticarial wheals, angioedema, bronchospasm, and hypotension may occur.[27, 28] These symptoms may also progress to anaphylaxis. Angioedema, with painful swelling of the face, extremities, and oral cavity, may also occur.

Symptoms generally begin within 5 minutes of starting exercise and typically abate between 30 minutes to 4 hours after exercise. Moderate-to-hard exercise usually precipitates the symptoms. Laboratory tests are rarely helpful for exercise-induced anaphylaxis and cholinergic urticaria.

Treatment

Initial treatment is to stop exercise and move to a cool place. An injection of diphenhydramine should be given if possible. If symptoms progress to wheezing, throat tightness, or lightheadedness, patients should receive an injection of epinephrine and be transported to an emergency department for further monitoring. Following treatment and resolution of symptoms, a nonsedating antihistamine can be prescribed and the patient discharged with injectable epinephrine.[13, 28]

When symptoms are more advanced, injectable epinephrine may need to be repeated in 15 to 20 minutes. The acute treatment of anaphylaxis follows the ABC (*a*irway, *b*reathing, *c*irculation) protocol and requires transportation to an emergency department as soon as possible.

Most patients will recover in a few minutes with cessation of exercise, cooling, and antihistamine treatment. Patients who experience anaphylaxis should be referred to an allergist. They should wear a medical alert bracelet documenting the condition. Patients should be advised to exercise in the cool part of the day with a partner who is aware of their condition. Precipitant foods should be avoided. If symptoms develop, the athlete should stop exercising and seek a cool place. If symptoms do not abate, an antihistamine should be administered. If symptoms progress to lightheadedness, hives, throat tightness, or wheezing, epinephrine should be administered immediately and the patient should be transferred to a medical facility.

When to Refer

Any patient who experiences anaphylaxis should be evaluated by an allergist.

Key Points

● The clinical features of exercise-induced anaphylaxis often include a flushing sensation, pruritus, gastrointestinal complaints, and throat tightness or choking. Diffuse, large urticarial wheals, angioedema, bronchospasm, and hypotension may also occur.
● Symptoms begin within 5 minutes of exercise.
● Treatments include cessation of exercise, diphenhydramine, and possibly epinephrine.

REFERENCES

1. Cypcar D, Lemanske RF: Asthma and exercise. Clin Chest Med 15(2):351–368, 1994.
2. Rupp NT: Diagnosis and management of exercise-induced asthma. Physician Sportsmed 24(1):77–87, 1996.
3. Cochrane LM, Clark CJ: Benefits and problems of a physical training programme for asthmatic patients. Thorax 45(5):345–351, 1990.

4. Szentagothai K, Gyene I, Szocska M, et al: Physical exercise program for children with bronchial asthma. Pediatr Pulmonol 3(3):166–172, 1987.
5. Voy RO: The US Olympic Committee experience with exercise-induced bronchospasm, 1984. Med Sci Sports Exerc 18(3):328–330, 1986.
6. Storms WW, Joyner DM: Update on exercise-induced asthma: (a) report of the Olympic Exercise Asthma Summit Conference. Physician Sportsmed 25(3):45–55, 1997.
7. Rupp NT, Brudno DS, Guill MF: The value of screening for risk of exercise-induced asthma in high school athletes. Ann Allergy 70(4):339–342, 1993.
8. McCarty P: Wheezing or breezing through exercise-induced asthma. Physician Sportsmed 17(7):125–130, 1989.
9. Anderson SD: Issues in exercise-induced asthma. J Allergy Clin Immunol 76(6):763–772, 1985.
10. Anderson SD: Exercise-induced asthma: The state of the art. Chest 87(suppl):191S–195S, 1985.
11. Mahler DA: Exercise-induced asthma. Med Sci Sports Exerc 25(5):554–561, 1993.
12. Spector SL: Update on exercise-induced asthma. Ann Allergy 71(6):571–577, 1993.
13. Kobayashi RH, Mellion MB: Exercise-induced asthma, anaphylaxis, and urticaria. Prim Care 18(4):809–831, 1991.
14. Anderson SD, Daviskas E: An evaluation of the airway cooling and rewarming hypothesis as the mechanism for exercise-induced asthma. *In* Holgate ST (ed): Asthma, Physiology, Immunopharmacology, and Treatment: Fourth International Symposium. London, Academic Press, 1993.
15. McFadden ER, Gilbert IA: Vascular responses and thermally induced asthma. *In* Holgate ST (ed): Asthma, Physiology, Immunopharmacology, and Treatment: Fourth International Symposium. London, Academic Press, 1993.
16. McFadden ER: Hypothesis: Exercise-induced asthma as a vascular phenomenon. Lancet 335:880–883, 1990.
17. Brundo DS, Wagner JM, Rupp NT: Length of postexercise assessment in the determination of exercise-induced bronchospasm. Ann Allergy 73(3):227–231, 1994.
18. McFadden ER: Exercise and asthma (editorial). N Engl J Med 317:502–504, 1987.
19. Wiens L, Sabath R, Ewing L, et al: Chest pain in otherwise healthy children and adolescents is frequently caused by exercise-induced asthma. Pediatrics 90(3):350–353, 1992.
20. Eggleston PA: Methods of exercise challenge. J Allergy Clin Immunol 73(5 pt 2):666–669, 1984.
21. Reiff DB, Choudry NB, Pride NB, et al: The effect of prolonged submaximal warm-up exercise on exercise-induced asthma. Am Rev Respir Dis 139(2):479–484, 1989.
22. AAP issues statement of exercise-induced asthma in children. Am Fam Physician 40(4):314, 316, 1989.
23. Grove A, Lipworth BJ: Bronchodilator subsensitivity to salbutamol after twice daily salmeterol in asthmatic patients. Lancet 346:201–206, 1995.
24. Simons FE, Gerstner TV, Cheang MS: Tolerance to the bronchoprotective effect of salmeterol in adolescents with exercise induced asthma using concurrent inhaled glucocorticoid treatment. Pediatrics 99(5):655–659, 1997.
25. deBenedictis FM, Tuteri G, Bertotto A, et al: Comparison of the protective effects of cromolyn sodium and nedocromil sodium in the treatment of exercise-induced asthma in children. J Allergy Clin Immunol 94(4):684–688, 1994.
26. O'Byrne PM, Israel E, Drazen JM: Antileukotrienes in the treatment of asthma. Ann Intern Med 127:472–480, 1997.
27. Briner WW, Sheffer A: Exercise-induced anaphylaxis. Med Sci Sports Exerc 24(8):849–850, 1992.
28. Briner WW: Physical allergies and exercise: Clinical implications for those engaged in sports activities. Sports Med 15(6):365–373, 1993.

III *The Diabetic Athlete*

JAMES MORIARITY, M.D.

There are currently 14 million diabetic patients in the United States. Most are cared for by primary care physicians. The discovery of insulin by Banting and Best in 1921 liberated many juvenile onset diabetics from ketoacidosis and certain death. The arrival of the sulfonylurea agents provided a means of treatment for adult onset diabetes. With the advent of the portable glucose scanners, diabetic patients have been able to achieve a greater degree of blood glucose control than was ever thought possible.

Until recently, the concept of an insulin-dependent diabetic patient regularly achieving success in athletics was impractical except in unusual circumstances. Now, with the successes of such notable diabetic athletes as Ron Santo, Wade Wilson, Bobby Clarke, Jonathan Hayes, and Curt Fra-

ser, those with insulin-dependent diabetes mellitus (IDDM) have role models for emulation on the playing fields. Most diabetic patients, as well as those not diabetic, will never achieve the athletic success of these individuals. Many, however, will desire to be as recreationally active, competitive, and fit as they are able.

The trials, tribulations, and ultimate victories of athletes and nonathletes has been championed by the American Diabetes Association and the International Diabetic Athletes Association (IDAA).[1] These two organizations provide physicians and athletes with invaluable information for the conduct of exercise in diabetes. As an example, in the 1992 New York City Marathon, the IDAA, in cooperation with the official medical staff, sponsored a support station for runners with diabetes.[2] Twenty runners with IDDM utilized the support stations, and 13 agreed to complete a postrace questionnaire. All the diabetic runners finished the marathon. The average prerace blood sugar level was 11.9 mM (209 mg/dl), and the average postrace blood sugar level was 5.9 mM (106 mg/dl). The average reduction in daily dose of insulin for the race day was 38 percent. None of the runners experienced any adverse affects.

Physicians will be increasingly challenged to provide information, encouragement, and in some cases permission for diabetic athletes to compete. In addition, the benefit of exercise in the prevention and treatment of diabetes has been advocated. The primary care physician must be aware of the risks, benefits, and methods used in exercise as a treatment modality in order to counsel wisely.

DEFINITIONS

Diabetes mellitus is defined as "a group of metabolic diseases characterized by hyperglycemia resulting from defects in insulin secretion, insulin action, or both."[3] Diagnostically, diabetes mellitus is stated to occur when one of three criteria is fulfilled:

1. Symptoms of diabetes plus a random glucose concentration above 200 mg/dl
2. Fasting glucose concentration over 126 mg/dl
3. Two-hour glucose concentration above 200 mg/dl during an oral glucose tolerance test

Impaired glucose tolerance is that gray area between the designations "normal" and "diabetes" and is often referred to as the prediabetic state. Criteria used to describe this condition are as follows:

1. Fasting glucose concentration over 110 mg/dl but below 126 mg/dl
2. Two-hour glucose level above 140 mg/dl but below 200 mg/dl[3]

Diabetes mellitus is classified as type 1 or type 2, depending on the need for insulin therapy.

Type 1, or Insulin-dependent diabetes mellitus (IDDM), is defined as the need for nearly continuous use of insulin to prevent hyperglycemia and ketosis in an individual who weighs less than 125 percent of their ideal weight.[4] IDDM is characterized by absolute insulin deficiency with loss of both basal insulinemia and postprandial rise in insulin secretion. Inheritance of IDDM seems to be through a genetically recessive trait, with contributions from both parents necessary for phenotypic expression. Risk of developing IDDM for offspring in whom one parent has IDDM ranges from 2.5 to 6.1 percent. When both parents have IDDM, the range increases to 10 to 25 percent.[5] Approximately 1 million or 1 in 500 children under the age of 18 have IDDM.

Although the onset of IDDM is most common in the young, 7 percent of newly diagnosed insulin-dependent patients are over the age of 30.[5] The risk of developing IDDM varies by race. In Japan, where there is a low incidence of diabetes in both young and adults, the incidence is 0.8 per 100,000 population per year. In Finland, the incidence is much higher, with 28 per 100,000 individuals developing IDDM each year.[6]

Type 2, or non–insulin-dependent diabetes mellitus (NIDDM), is defined as a fasting blood sugar level greater than 140 mg/dl or a 2-hour postprandial blood sugar level greater than 200 mg/dl in response to a 75-g oral glucose challenge (WHO criteria). Unlike IDDM, in which there is an *absolute* lack of insulin, NIDDM is characterized by a *relative* lack of basal and postprandial insulin in response to a glucose load. Even though patients with NIDDM are classified as "individuals who survive without insulin," it is estimated that 30 percent of adults with NIDDM take injectable insulin.[7] The prevalence of NIDDM in the U.S. ranges from 2.8 to 5 percent of the adult population.[8, 9] Worldwide, there is great variation in the prevalence of NIDDM among different population groups.

PREDISPOSING FACTORS

A number of factors are related to the development of NIDDM, including age, family history, android-type obesity, lack of physical activity, and impaired glucose tolerance.[10–14]

The onset of NIDDM is age-related. Between the ages of 50 and 89, the prevalence of NIDDM increases to 12 to 16 percent of the population. If this subgroup is further stratified by decade and sex, the prevalence rate increases with each decade, and men consistently have a higher prevalence rate than women.[15]

Family history and obesity are the two strongest predisposing factors for the development of

NIDDM.[11] A concordance rate of 60 to 90 percent for NIDDM in identical twin studies points to genetic transmission.[12] The association of NIDDM with hypertension, hypertriglyceridemia, and android-type obesity has been called ''the deadly quartet'' because of the strong association of these factors with early death from cardiovascular disease.[16] Obesity has been linked with NIDDM in 80 percent of cases and has well-known clinical association with impaired glucose intolerance. Lack of physical activity not only correlates with the onset and maintenance of obesity but also may be an independent risk factor for the development of NIDDM by virtue of the ''thrifty genotype'' hypothesis. This evolution theory postulates that hunter-gatherers exposed to recurrent periods of ''feast-famine cycles'' developed compensatory insulin resistance (a finding in NIDDM) as a means of averting famine-induced hypoglycemia—a genetic trait that is unmasked in modern people with lack of physical activity.[13]

EFFECT OF DIABETES MELLITUS ON EXERCISE

The ability of the human organism to balance its varied energy reserves with the demands of energy-requiring activities ranging from sleeping and reading to dancing and sprinting is an engineering marvel worthy of reverent examination. Pivotal to the orchestration of this physiologic symphony is insulin.

Simply stated, the three main energy fuels in the body are carbohydrate, fat, and to a limited degree protein located in reservoirs in the liver, muscle, and adipose tissue. Carbohydrate is stored as glycogen in the liver and muscle and released in the circulation for muscle use as glucose. Fat is stored as triglyceride in adipose tissue and released to the circulation as free fatty acids for oxidative metabolism in muscle mitochondria and as glycerol for gluconeogenesis use by the liver. Protein is stored as muscle tissue and released as amino acid substrates for gluconeogenesis in the liver. Insulin has the unique ability to regulate the usage of all three fuel reservoirs.

During periods of inactivity and noneating, glucose need by muscle is minimal, circulating insulin is low, and blood glucose is stable. The basal insulinemia present suppresses any further glucose production via glycogenolysis, gluconeo-genesis, and lipolysis to the extent that stable glycemia is maintained.

Following food intake, insulin boluses from pancreatic islet cells are secreted into the portal system and actively promote glucose disposal by stimulating glucose uptake in the liver and storage as glycogen. Additionally, these insulin boluses inhibit any glucose release by the liver by blocking hepatic glycogenolysis and gluconeogenesis. Postprandial insulin further promotes protein synthesis and fat storage in adipocytes. At the muscle level, normoglycemia is maintained through insulin-mediated uptake of glucose at the cell membrane. Intracellular glucose transporters carry glucose molecules within the muscle for storage as muscle glycogen. In normal as well as diabetic individuals, muscle glycogen synthesis is the principal pathway of glucose disposal.[17]

During exercise, insulin secretion is suppressed. Glucose production from hepatic glycogenolysis and gluconeogenesis is allowed to proceed, stimulated by the counterregulatory hormones glucagon, epinepherine, and cortisol. A ready source of hepatic-derived glucose becomes available for use. Lipolysis, also stimulated by the counterregulatory hormones, provides a steady source of free fatty acids for muscle oxidative phosphorylation and glycerol for hepatic gluconeogenesis. The net effect is the maintainance of stable blood glucose levels.

Ironically, and crucially, muscle uptake of glucose is *increased* 20-fold during exercise despite the marked *decrease* in circulating insulin.[18] This non–insulin-mediated increase in glucose uptake with exercise is often referred to as *increased insulin sensitivity*. In actuality, the increased uptake of glucose is the consequence of muscle contraction that, independent of insulin, increases the number of glucose transporters both at the cell membrane and in the intracellular space.[18, 19] Additionally and independently of insulin, exercise stimulates muscle glycogen synthetase activity.[17] Exercise-induced increases in glucose transport and glycogen synthetase activity persist up to 48 hours beyond the duration of the exercise period, enhancing the removal of glucose from the blood stream (i.e., improving insulin sensitivity) and facilitating intramuscular storage of glycogen for use at a later time. Thus, insulin activity is essential to the close regulation of blood sugar, hepatic glucose output, free fatty acid storage and release, protein metabolism, and muscle uptake and storage of glucose.

IN IDDM, there is an absolute deficiency of insulin. Without clinical replacement, metabolic control is lost and ketoacidosis ensues. Although it is relatively simple to administer insulin, replacement therapy is not physiologic and cannot mirror the tight glucose regulation of endogenous insulin.

In NIDDM, insulin secretion is present but insufficient to control blood glucose. Even though basal insulin and postprandial insulin levels are increased over nondiabetic control subjects, patients with NIDDM continue to experience hyperglycemia. Debate exists as to whether NIDDM is a disorder of insulin resistance, islet cell dysfunction, or a combination of both.[13] Three major metabolic disturbances are found in patients with NIDDM:

1. Impairment in insulin production and release by pancreatic beta cells
2. Reduced sensitivity to insulin in muscle, liver, and fat tissues
3. Excessive hepatic glucose production in the basal state[20]

Insulin resistance in muscle is a condition found in both IDDM and NIDDM. This resistance is thought to stem from a decrease in the number of glucose transporters in the intracellular membrane. Insulin receptor sites do not appear to be reduced in number. Also contributing to insulin resistance in muscle is the finding that both IDDM and NIDDM patients have reduced blood flow to exercising muscle.[21] This reduction is independent of duration of diabetes or the age of the patient. Reduction of regional blood flow may in part account for the lower $Vo_{2 max}$ seen in patients with diabetes compared with age-matched control subjects. An important feature is that the non–insulin-mediated glucose uptake brought on by exercise is not impaired in diabetic patients.

Hepatic insulin resistance is an important contributing factor to the development of diabetes and loss of glucose control. Laboratory studies have demonstrated loss of hepatocyte responsiveness to insulin in downregulating glycogenolysis and gluconeogenesis activity.[22] In type 2 diabetes, increased hepatic glucose output is a major contributor to fasting hyperglycemia with augmented gluconeogenesis a greater culprit than glycogenolysis. Exercise induction of hepatic glucose output by increases in glucagon and epinephrine activity further exacerbates worsening glycemic control in insulin-deficient individuals.

Insulin resistance in adipose tissue results in a failure of the adipocyte to suppress triglyceride breakdown, releasing large amounts of free fatty acids and glycerol for conversion to glucose in the liver. The well-known association of obesity with NIDDM and impaired glucose tolerance (fasting blood sugar level between 115 and 140 mg/dl) is likely to have as its root cause a genetic defect in the metabolism of fat involving the beta-3 receptor on visceral fat cells.[23]

In summary, glucose homeostasis is a tightly controlled metabolic function with insulin playing the predominant role. In order for exercise to safely progress, insulin secretion must be suppressed for enhancement of glycolytic activity in the muscle, lipolysis in the adipocyte, and glucose production by the liver. Exercise imparts to muscle the ability to take up glucose in the absence of insulin. Exercise-facilitated glucose uptake in muscle remains for up to 48 hours following a single episode of exercise. Diabetes is characterized by an absolute or relative lack of insulin coupled with insulin resistance in liver, muscle, and fat. Although insulin can be replaced by injection, the process is not physiologic and glucose homeostasis can be difficult to maintain. Excessive hepatic glucose output is a major contributor to hyperglycemia in diabetes. Also, the capacity for exercise to impart increased insulin sensitivity to muscle is not diminished in the diabetic condition.

EXERCISE IN THE PREVENTION AND TREATMENT OF DIABETES

One of the most convincing arguments for the importance of regular daily exercise is the role exercise plays in the prevention of diabetes. Several studies have examined the beneficial role of exercise as it relates to impaired glucose tolerance, previously known as "prediabetes."[11, 24, 25] The prevalence of impaired glucose tolerance in the adult population is twice that of NIDDM and is a strong predictor for eventual diabetes. Regular exercise has been shown to reduce overall glucose levels by 12 percent after 3 months, and these levels are sustainable over a 21-month follow-up.

In a most convincing study, University of Pennsylvania alumni between the ages of 39 and 68 were evaluated for the risk of developing NIDDM in correlation with level of physical activity.[11] There was a steady decline in the incidence of NIDDM with increasing levels of physical activity. The protective effect of exercise was independent of an association with hypertension, obesity, or family history. Indeed, those alumni with the greatest risk factors for diabetes—namely, obesity and family history—benefited the most from increasing levels of physical activity. From the calculations of the study, it was determined that every 500 kcal of energy expenditure from exercise *per week* imparted a 6 percent reduction in the age-adjusted risk of NIDDM (Fig. 21–1). For the average individual, 500 kcal can be expended in 1 hour of continuous jogging, biking, or swimming.

Exercise has also been shown to be beneficial in the treatment of diabetes.[26–29] A study performed on 652 NIDDM patients (one third taking insulin, one third taking oral agents, and one third on no medications) resulted in improved fasting glucose, improved lipid studies, weight loss, and reduced blood pressure after an intensive 26-day intervention program. Of the patients taking insulin and oral medications, 39 percent and 71 percent were able to discontinue their medication.[27]

Improvement in insulin sensitivity with exercise is not confined to NIDDM. Soon after the discovery of insulin in 1921, R.D. Lawrence recorded the reduced need for insulin following exercise in patients requiring insulin. For many years, this was thought to be secondary to the accelerated absorption of insulin from exercising muscle, or the result of delayed gastric emptying accompanying exercise. Using sophisticated investigative techniques, researchers have been able to compare glucose uptake at constant insulin infu-sion rates with insulin decline at constant glucose infusion rates, clearly demonstrating that exercise does result in improved insulin sensitivity in the insulin-dependent patient.

Exercise in patients with diabetes confers the same lipid-lowering effects and cardiovascular protection as in nondiabetics. Increases in triglycerides, total cholesterol, and LDL cholesterol are common in diabetes and contribute greatly to the increased incidence of major athersclerotic disease. Improvements in lipid parameters with exercise lowers cardiovascular morbidity and mortality rates. Exercise in diabetic patients does not raise HDL cholesterol levels to the extent that it does in nondiabetic patients.

Athletes with diabetes demonstrate the same cellular increases in glycolytic and oxidative enzyme concentrations with physical training as control subjects. Glycogen storage in muscle is markedly decreased in sedentary diabetics, and training restores and enhances glycogen synthetase activity to restore muscle glycogen levels.[17] $VO_{2\ max}$ in diabetic individuals is reduced at baseline levels relative to control subjects but does demonstrate increases with training. This finding may be the result of reduced blood flow to exercising muscle seen in diabetic patients.[21] Increases in capillarization in skeletal muscle seen with training is less apparent in diabetics with longer duration of disease.

DIABETES AND TIGHT GLUCOSE CONTROL

The Diabetes Control and Complications Trial Research Group study published in 1993 clearly

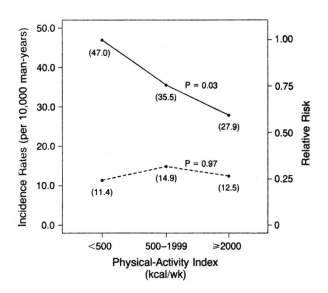

Figure 21–1. Incidence rates for the development of NIDDM compared with average caloric expenditure per week from physical activity. *Solid line* is incidence rate for high-risk patients with positive family history of diabetes, obesity, or hypertension. The *dashed line* is the incidence rate for low-risk patients. (With permission from Helmrich S, Raglund D, Leung R, Paffenbarger R: Physical activity and reduced occurrence of non-insulin dependent diabetes mellitus. N Engl J Med 325:147–152, 1991. Copyright 1991 Massachusetts Medical Society.)

demonstrated the beneficial effects of tight glucose control in the development and progression of complications in type I diabetes.[30] The United Kingdom Prospective Diabetes Study begun in 1977 is expected to confirm similar beneficial affects of tight glucose control in NIDDM.[32] Because of the importance of the findings in the DCCT study, the American Diabetes Association revised the standard of care recommendations for patients with diabetes to include an emphasis on tighter glucose control.[31] Intensive treatment of IDDM is defined as three or more subcutaneous injections of insulin daily, or continuous infusion of insulin via an insulin pump. Nonintensive treatment is defined as 1 or 2 daily insulin injections.[32] With better glycemic control, glycosolated hemoglobin levels are lower.

One of the frequently asked questions of medical practitioners is, Will increased exercise improve glucose control? In contrast to NIDDM, in which exercise is unquestionably beneficial in the control of blood glucose, there are no convincing data to suggest a similar benefit in IDDM. The increased insulin sensitivity bequeathed to regular exercisers with IDDM is in part counterbalanced by an increased need for additional calories and its risk of attendant hyperglycemia. Nevertheless, exercise has many desirable benefits for patients with IDDM, even if better glucose control is not one of them. Exercise placed within the big picture of lifestyle goes well beyond the benefit of blood sugar levels.[33]

Intensive therapy of diabetes mellitus is not inexpensive, nor is it without risk. The estimated annual cost to patients participating in intensive control regimens ranges from $3800 to $8800.[34] Hypoglycemic episodes are three times more likely in intensively controlled patients than those more traditionally treated. Some argue that the ADA guidelines for the care of NIDDM are long, costly, and difficult to implement in the primary care setting.[8] From an epidemiologic perspective, macrovascular disease is the leading cause of death in NIDDM, and cessation of cigarette smoking, if applicable, is the single most important recommendation for improving the mortality rate. A graph on the relative impact of various interventions on 10-year mortality rates in diabetic and nondiabetic men is presented in Figure 21–2.[35]

Despite the recent emphasis on tight glucose control in the treatment of both IDDM and NIDDM, diet, exercise, and weight reduction when appropriate remain the cornerstones of treatment in NIDDM. Early treatment with oral agents or insulin in NIDDM may lessen the central role of lifestyle modification. A 3- to 4-month trial of dietary counseling coupled with a regular exercise regimen to improve insulin sensitivity and glucose utilization is a reasonable first step in the management of a newly diagnosed or poorly controlled NIDDM patient. Lack of improvement in glycosolated hemoglobin with lifestyle changes reflects the need for oral agents or insulin.

RISKS OF EXERCISE

Just as the benefits of exercise in diabetes are well documented, so are the risks of exercise. The systemic nature of diabetes places multiple organ systems in harm's way. With proper evaluation and care, some degree of exercise is possible in all patients with diabetes, regardless of attendant complications. There are, however, contraindications to strenuous exercise (defined as exercise above 75 percent $Vo_{2\,max}$ or 80 percent of maximum heart rate) in diabetic patients with the following problems[36]:

1. Poor blood sugar control
2. Proliferative retinopathy
3. Microangiopathy
4. Neuropathy
5. Nephropathy
6. Cardiovascular disease

Athletes with IDDM or NIDDM requesting permission to participate in strenuous exercise should be screened carefully for the preceding secondary complications of diabetes. If these are present, strenuous physical activity may not be recommended. However, some degree of exercise is possible. The Clinical Practice Recommendations 1998 published by the ADA[31] has clear guidelines for exercise recommendations.

The most immediate and common problem associated with exercise and diabetes is the development of hypoglycemia. Symptomatic hypoglycemia occurs on the average once or twice a week in most IDDM patients. Disabling hypoglycemia may afflict up to 25 percent of IDDM in a given year.[37] This is especially relevant to patients attempting tight control. Hypoglycemia as a consequence of exercise may occur during or shortly after exercise or may be delayed 8 to 16 hours after conclusion of exercise. Too much insulin,

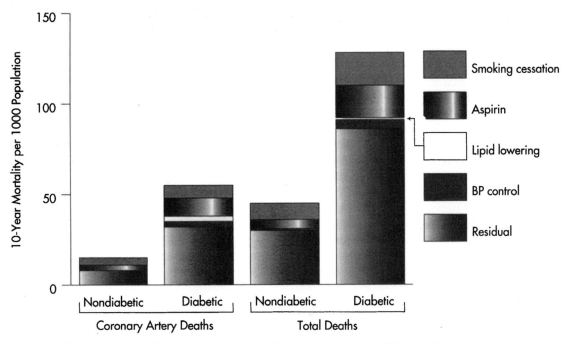

Figure 21–2. Relative impact of various interventions on 10-year mortality rates in diabetic and nondiabetic men between the ages of 35 and 57. (With permission from Peters AL, McCullough DK, Hayward RA, et al: Case one: Too little too late—Delayed diagnoses of NIDDM. Clin Outcomes Management 1(2):9–26, 1994.)

too little food, too much exercise, and failure to time peak insulin activity with availability of food all contribute to exercise-induced hypoglycemia. Symptomatic hypoglycemia is relatively simple to treat unless the athlete is physically unable to ingest sugar-containing fluids or foods. Sports such as long-distance solo swimming, scuba diving, race care driving, and technically difficult rock climbing may pose difficulty to the treatment of hypoglycemia.

Asymptomatic hypoglycemia, or "hypoglycemic unawareness,"[37] is characterized by the diabetic athlete's loss of autonomic-induced warning signals of impending hypoglycemia. Adrenergic signals of hypoglycemia include palpitations, tremor, and anxiety. Cholinergic signals include sweating, hunger, and paresthesias. With increasing duration of diabetes, autonomic activity may be lost.

Other causes of hypoglycemia unawareness in patients and athletes with diabetes are defective counterregulatory responses of glucagon and epinephrine to falling glucose levels from failing pancreatic and adrenal tissue, and a heightened tolerance of brain tissue to function in dangerously low glucose levels before cognitive impairment signals the patient or others that hypoglycemia is present.[37] Hypoglycemic unawareness is also found in intensive insulin treatment programs in which overall plasma glucose levels are lower. Athletes with hypoglycemic unawareness must be especially careful in their conduct of exercise.

PREPARTICIPATION EVALUATION

Preparticipation evaluation of patients with diabetes is done for two reasons: (1) because the patient seeks permission to participate in organized competition and (2) for the purpose of beginning an exercise program for fun or therapeutic benefit.

There is no organized competitive sport that is without the participation of diabetic athletes. The ADA and the International Diabetic Athletes Association are two organizations that encourage and provide help to diabetic athletes in their pursuit of athletic excellence. Prior to the strong work of these two organizations, patients with diabetes were often discouraged from pursuing the pleasure and self-satisfaction of competitive sports. The principal differences between competitive and therapeutic exercise are the risk of physical injury and impairment from the activity, the intensity and duration of training required to prepare for and sustain the activity, and the likelihood that the patient will be able to maintain the selected activity for many years.

Speaking strictly from a health-benefit conservative point of view, diabetic patients—especially those in the pediatric age group—should be encouraged to pursue athletic activities that are lifelong, primarily aerobic, that permit limited contact, and that have predictable, low to moderate training intensity. Speaking from a more liberal, empowerment point of view, patients with uncomplicated diabetes should not be restrained or discouraged from competing in any sport. Obviously, each case must be individualized based on patient, parent, physician, and in some cases coaching and administration comfort in anticipating the needs of the athlete.

The preparticipation evaluation of a patient with diabetes should proceed in a logical and comprehensive manner.

1. The first step in a preparticipation evaluation is to ensure that the minimal levels of care of the athlete are being met. The ADA has published standards of care for patients with diabetes (Table 21–2).[38] The preparticipation examination should not function as a substitute for ongoing medical care.

2. The second step is a history and physical examination that evaluates the specific requirements of the sport and the physical capabilities of the patient. This is no different from those in any other athlete seeking permission to compete (Table 21–3).

3. The physician must make a diligent search for diabetic complications that may influence the type of exercise or sport permitted; specifically, such complications include retinopathy, nephropathy, cardiovascular disease, and neuropathy.

4. It is important to have a discussion with the patient and family about the anticipated changes in insulin dosage, dietary needs, strat-

Table 21–2
Standards of Care for Patients with Diabetes Mellitus

Nature of Intervention	Recommended Frequency		Treatment Goal
	Patients on Insulin	**Patients not on Insulin**	
HbA$_{1c}$ evaluation	Quarterly	As often as needed to achieve and maintain near-normal blood glucose levels (usually quarterly)	Keep at or below 8%
Evaluation of FPG concentration	As often as needed	As often as needed (usually 4–6 times/year)	Keep at or below 140 mg/dl
Fasting lipid profile (total cholesterol, HDL, LDL, triglycerides)	Initially—subsequent frequency depends on results and treatment	Initially—subsequent frequency depends on results and treatment	LDL ≤ 130 mg/dl (no CHD) LDL ≤ 100 mg/dl (with CHD)
Urine protein evaluation	Yearly	Yearly	Negative
Determination for microalbuminuria	Yearly (if urine protein negative)	Yearly (if urine protein negative)	Negative
Office visit for diabetes (to include weight, blood pressure, foot examination)	Quarterly	Quarterly to semiannually	Education Management of diabetes and lipid disorders Early detection and treatment of complications
Telephone follow-up	As needed—sometimes weekly	As needed—sometimes weekly	Adjustment of insulin doses and encouragement to comply with regimen
Self-monitoring of blood glucose	Daily—preprandially and before bedtime (snack) ideal (regimen based on patient's needs)	As needed, based on patient preference	As close to normal as possible, based on patient circumstances
Ophthalmology referral	Yearly	Yearly	Early treatment and detection of diabetic retinopathy

HbA$_{1c}$ = glycosylated hemoglobin; FPG = fasting plasma glucose; HDL = high-density lipoprotein; LDL = low-density lipoprotein; CHD = coronary heart disease.

Source: Peters AL, et al: Case one: Too little too late—delayed diagnosis of NIDDM. J Clin Outcomes Management 1:9–26, 1994.

Table 21–3
Components of a Preparticipation Physical Examination for Patients with Diabetes

Height, weight, waist-to-hip ratio, and if possible, body fat percentage
Ophthalmoscopic examination
Pulse rate and regularity
Blood pressure determination, with orthostatic measurements
Chest auscultation
Cardiac examination
Palpation and auscultation of carotid, abdominal, and femoral arteries
Palpation and inspection of lower extremities for edema and presence of arterial pulses
Foot examination
Neurologic examination
Absence or presence of xanthoma and xanthelasma
Orthopedic or other medical conditions that would limit exercise or require special consideration
Laboratory tests (if not recently performed and clinically indicated), including fasting blood glucose, glycosylated hemoglobin, fasting serum lipids and lipoproteins, serum creatinine, urinalysis, thyroid function tests, resting ECG, exercise ECG, pulmonary studies, and review of results of previous pertinent tests (e.g., coronary angiography, echocardiographic studies, nuclear medicine studies)

Source: Gordon N: The exercise prescription. *In* Ruderman N, Devlin JT (eds): The Health Professional's Guide to Diabetes and Exercise. Alexandria, VA, American Diabetes Association, 1995, pp. 71–89. Adapted with permission from the American College of Sports Medicine and from the American Diabetes Association.

egies to avoid hypoglycemia, and necessity for increased glucose monitoring.

Cardiovascular disease is the leading cause of morbidity and mortality in diabetes. The association of silent myocardial infarction and diabetes is well known. Exercise treadmill testing is recommended for all diabetic patients over 35 years of age and for IDDM patients on insulin longer than 15 years. Increased blood pressure response to exercise in normotensive patients with NIDDM is often exaggerated and can be assessed by treadmill evaluation. Decreasing serial measurements of exercise capacity can give clues to impaired left ventricular function and incipient diabetic cardiomyopathy.[39-41] Treadmill testing can also determine correlations between target heart rate, blood pressure, and perceived level of exertion that can give diabetic patients clues to self-determination of set limits.

Diabetic retinopathy increases in incidence with advancing duration of diabetes.[42] Retinopathy is aggravated by increases in intraocular pressure,

pressure against weakened capillaries, and decreased oxygen tension. Exercises that increase vascular pressure and reduce oxygen tension may worsen retinopathy. It is recommended that exercising blood pressure (or correlated heart rate) in patients with proliferative retinopathy never exceed a systolic maximum of 170 mm Hg (180 mm Hg for background retinopathy). Treadmill evaluation is a useful technique to establish these limits. Diligent monitoring of blood pressure is necessary in patients with proliferative disease.

Autonomic neuropathy can influence a variety of organ systems integral to the performance of exercise (Table 21–4). Alterations in cardiovascular neural control can result in increased heart rates at rest, blunted heart rate response to exercise, hypotensive or hypertensive responses to exercise, or postexercise hypotension. Many bedside techniques to evaluate cardiac autonomic neuropathy have been described (Table 21–5). Exercise testing is a valuable tool to evaluate the response to exercise.

Extremity evaluation—especially of the foot—is an important screening requirement for the determination of suitable exercise regimens. Weight-bearing exercises in patients with impaired protective sensation of the foot are contraindicated. Evaluation for signs of peripheral arterial

Table 21–4
Complications of Autonomic Neuropathy that May Affect Exercise

Resting tachycardia and decreased maximal responsiveness
Decreased heart rate variability
Orthostasis/hypotension with exercise
Exaggerated blood pressure responses with supine position and exercise
Loss of diurnal blood pressure variation
Cardiovascular and cardiorespiratory instability
Abnormal systolic ejection fractions at rest/exercise
Abnormal diastolic filling rates/times at rest/exercise
Poor exercise tolerance
Failure of pupil adaptation to darkness
Gastroparesis and diabetic diarrhea
Hypoglycemia
Decreased hypoglycemia awareness
Hypoglycemia unresponsiveness
Heat intolerance due to defective sympathetic thermoregulation and sweating (prone to dehydration)
Susceptibility to foot ulcers and limb loss due to disordered regulation of cutaneous blood flow
Incontinence

Source: Vinik AI: Neuropathy. *In* Ruderman N, Devlin JT (eds): The Health Professional's Guide to Diabetes and Exercise. Alexandria, VA, American Diabetes Association, 1995, pp. 181–198.

Table 21-5
Office Evaluation of Cardiovascular Autonomic Function

Test	Method/Parameters
Resting heart rate	>100 beats/min is abnormal.
Beat-to-beat heart rate variation	With the patient at rest and supine (no overnight coffee or hypoglycemic episodes), breathing 6 breaths/min, heart rate monitored by ECG or Q-Med device, a difference in heart rate of >15 beats/min is normal and <10 beats/min is abnormal, R-R inspiration/R-R expiration >1.17 (abnormal <1.0).
Heart rate response to standing	During continuous ECG monitoring, the R-R interval is measured at beats 15 and 30 after standing. Normally, a tachycardia is followed by reflex bradycardia. The 30:15 ratio is normally >1.03.
Heart rate response to Valsalva maneuver	The subject forcibly exhales into the mouthpiece of a manometer to 40 mm Hg for 15 sec during ECG monitoring. Healthy subjects develop tachycardia and peripheral vasoconstriction during strain and an overshoot bradycardia and rise in blood pressure with release. The ratio of longest R-R to shortest R-R should be >1.2.
Systolic blood pressure response to standing	Systolic blood pressure is measured in the supine subject. The patient stands and the systolic blood pressure is measured after 2 min. Normal response is a fall of <10 mm Hg, borderline is a fall of 10–29 mm Hg, and abnormal is a fall of >30 mm Hg.
Diastolic blood pressure response to isometric exercise	The subject squeezes a handgrip dynamometer to establish a maximum. Grip is then squeezed at 30% maximum for 5 min. The normal response for diastolic blood pressure is a rise of >16 mm Hg in the other arm.
ECG Q-T/Q-T_C intervals	The Q-T_C should be <440 msec.

Source: Vinik AI: Neuropathy. *In* Ruderman N, Devlin JT (eds): The Health Professional's Guide to Diabetes and Exercise. Alexandria, VA, American Diabetes Association, 1995, pp. 181–198.

disease and peripheral neuropathy should be done. Signs and symptoms of peripheral artery disease are listed in Table 21–6. Peripheral neuropathy, including sensory loss, can be evaluated by measuring tendon reflexes, vibratory sensation, and touch sensation using a Semmes-Weinstein 5.07 monofilament over pressure-sensitive areas of the foot.[44]

Nephropathy will develop in one third of

Table 21-6
Signs and Symptoms of Peripheral Arterial Disease

Intermittent claudication
Cold feet
Nocturnal pain
Rest pain
Nocturnal and rest pain relieved with dependency
Absent pulses
Blanching on elevation
Delayed venous filling after elevation
Dependent rubor
Atrophy of subcutaneous fatty tissue
Shiny appearance of skin
Loss of hair on foot and toes
Thickened nails, often with fungal infection
Gangrene

Source: Levin M: The diabetic foot. *In* Ruderman N, Devlin JT (eds): The Health Professional's Guide to Diabetes and Exercise. Alexandria, VA, American Diabetes Association, 1995, pp. 137–151.

IDDM patients and in a considerable number of patients with NIDDM.[45] Antihypertensive control and tight glucose control are the two most important parameters in preventing the onset of diabetic nephropathy. There is no evidence that light to moderate exercise will hasten the onset of nephropathy or worsen existing nephropathy in normotensive diabetic patients in good control. Intense daily exercise and its effect on glomerulopathy is less understood.

In diabetic patients without proteinuria at rest, exercise may induce proteinuria following an exercise bout.[45] The excreted protein is of glomerular origin and likely the result of increased filtration fraction within the glomerulus. There is no convincing evidence that suggests that exercise-induced proteinuria in diabetic subjects predicts future nephropathy. When screening diabetic patients for albuminuria, care should be taken that samples are taken in the early morning before exercise.

In diabetic patients with microalbuminuria, exercise transiently increases protein excretion proportional to the observed increase in blood pressure.[45] Again, the protein is of glomerular origin. Whether the observed correlation with exercise-induced hypertension is cause or effect is not clear. It is not known if the transient increase in protein excretion brought on by exercise is deleterious to the kidney. Exercise in these individuals is not contraindicated.

Diabetic patients with overt albuminuria at rest already exhibit decreased glomerular filtration and exaggerated pressor response to exercise. There are currently no guidelines either recommending or discouraging exercise in these individuals.[45]

In the special case of patients on dialysis or following renal transplant, a cautious and conservative approach is recommended in preparing an exercise program. In spite of the significant obstacles to be overcome, exercise can improve these patients' sense of well-being and improve their ability to perform activities of daily living.[46]

THE PHARMACOLOGY OF INSULIN AND ITS RELATIONSHIP TO EXERCISE

In the United States, approximately 1.1 million people require injectable insulin to sustain life (IDDM) and an additional 1.8 million people require injectable insulin to control hyperglycemia (NIDDM).[7] If exercise in these individuals is to progress safely, a thorough understanding of the pharmacologic properties of insulin and insulin agonists is necessary.

Insulin was discovered and investigated in 1921 by Banting, Best, Macleod, and Collip and first administered experimentally to Leonard Thompson in 1922. By July 1922, Eli Lilly and Company was producing large amounts of porcine insulin for research use, and by 1923 it produced insulin commercially. Krogh and Hagedorn began European production of insulin in 1923 from the Nordisk-Novo laboratories. In the mid-1930s Hagedorn was able to alter the chemical structure of insulin and prolong its action by adding protamine to delay its absorption. Scott and Fisher of the Connaught Laboratories achieved a similar affect by incorporating zinc into the chemical structure. Protamine zinc combinations and NPH (neutral protamine Hagedorn) insulins were commercially available along with the "regular insulins" for combination therapy by the 1940s. Long-acting insulin was introduced by Novo-Nordisk in the 1950s as lente insulin, which was insulin with zinc and no protamine. Short-acting, intermediate-acting, and long-acting insulins were now available for clinical use.[47]

The 1970s brought the arrival of monocompo-

nent insulins (free of proinsulin and immunogenic peptides). Beef insulin differs from human insulin by two amino acids and pork by one amino acid. At this point, all insulin was still of animal (beef and pork) origin. The first human analogue insulin was derived from the enzymatic cleavage and amino acid substitution of pork insulin. Currently, human insulin is all made from recombinant, genetic engineering and is stoichiometrically identical to human insulin[48] (Table 21–7).

An exciting development in the field of insulin pharmacology is the development of Lys/Pro insulin.[49] Lys/Pro insulin is an analogue of human insulin in which the only difference from human insulin is the reversal of the Lys and Pro sequence at the B_{28} and B_{29} positions. This small alteration prevents the individual insulin molecules from aggregating together, thus facilitating more rapid absorption from tissue deposits after injection. Lys/Pro insulin has a rapid onset of action (approximately 30 minutes), more rapid peak of action, and is entirely gone in 4 hours.[50] These qualities are highly desirable for a rapid-acting insulin and make Lys/Pro an ideal candidate for mealtime insulin use. Novo-Nordisk is currently investigating a long-acting insulin analogue that will possess qualities ideal for use as a basal insulin.[49]

The most efficient method for achieving metabolic control in diabetes is to simulate normal endogenous insulin secretion.[49] Normal insulin secretion in nondiabetic individuals consists of basal and food-stimulated components. Basal insulin primarily inhibits hepatic glucose production, whereas food-stimulated or prandial insulin stimulates glucose disposal. The metabolic half-life of endogeneous insulin is 5 to 7 minutes.[51] Endogenous insulin, unlike injected insulin, is secreted into the portal circulation, where it must first pass through the liver. Injected insulin is absorbed over a variable period of time and circulates first through the peripheral circulation. Choice of insulin preparation should be matched to the patient's lifestyle and activity level with the intent of providing both adequate basal insulinemia and suitable prandial insulinemia.[48]

Human insulins and animal insulins have similar but not identical properties[48] (Table 21–8). The differences are small for short-acting insulins, moderate for intermediate-acting insulins, and greatest for long-acting insulins. Human insulin is more hydrophilic (soluble) than animal insulin and therefore has faster absorption, earlier peak activity, and shorter duration of action.

Table 21–7
Insulins Available in the United States

Formula	Manufacturer	Dose
Short-Acting (Usual Onset 0.5–2.0 h; Usual Duration 3–6 h)		
HUMAN		
Humulin regular	Lilly	U-100
Novolin R (regular)	Novo Nordisk	U-100
Velosulin human (regular)	Novo Nordisk	U-100
Novolin R Penfill (regular)	Novo Nordisk	U-100
PORK		
Iletin II regular	Lilly	U-100, U-500
Purified pork R (regular)	Novo Nordisk	U-100
Regular	Novo Nordisk	U-100
BEEF/PORK		
Iletin I (regular)	Lilly	U-100
Intermediate-Acting (Usual Onset 3–6 h; Usual Duration 12–20 h)		
HUMAN		
Humulin L (lente)	Lilly	U-100
Humulin N (NPH)	Lilly	U-100
Novolin L (lente)	Novo Nordisk	U-100
Novolin N (NPH)	Novo Nordisk	U-100
Novolin N Penfill (NPH)	Novo Nordisk	U-100
BEEF		
NPH	Novo Nordisk	U-100
Lente	Novo Nordisk	U-100
PORK		
Iletin II Lente	Lilly	U-100
Iletin II NPH	Lilly	U-100
Purified pork lente	Novo Nordisk	U-100
Purified pork N (NPH)	Novo Nordisk	U-100
BEEF/PORK		
Iletin I Lente	Lilly	U-100
Iletin I NPH	Lilly	U-100
Long-Acting (Usual Onset 6–12 h; Usual Duration 16–36 h)		
HUMAN		
Humulin U (ultralente)	Lilly	U-100
BEEF		
Ultralente	Novo Nordisk	U-100
Premixed Combinations		
HUMAN		
Humulin 50/50 (50% NPH, 50% regular)	Lilly	U-100
Humulin 70/30 (70% NPH, 30% regular)	Lilly	U-100
Novolin 70/30 (70% NPH, 30% regular)	Novo Nordisk	U-100
Novolin 70/30 Penfill	Novo Nordisk	U-100
Novolin 70/30 Prefilled	Novo Nordisk	U-100

Source: Clinical Education Series; Medical Management of Insulin-Dependent Diabetes Mellitus. Alexandria, VA, American Diabetes Association, 1995.

Table 21-8
Properties of Human and Animal Insulin

Insulin	Onset (Hours)	Peak (Hours)	Effective Duration (Hours)	Maximum Duration (Hours)
Animal				
Regular	0.5–2.0	3–4	4–6	6–8
NPH	4–6	8–14	16–20	20–24
Lente	4–6	8–14	16–20	20–24
Ultralente	8–14	Minimal	24–36	24–36
Human				
Regular	0.5–1.0	2–3	3–6	4–6
NPH	2–4	4–10	10–16	14–18
Lente	3–4	4–12	12–18	16–20
Ultralente	6–10	None	18–20	20–30

Source: Clinical Education Series: Medical Management of Insulin-Dependent Diabetes Mellitus. Alexandria, VA, American Diabetes Association, 1995.

Short-acting animal and human insulins have some differences in absorption rate, with human insulin being absorbed slightly faster, making it more suitable for prandial use. Regular and NPH insulins may be mixed without consequences, but regular and lente insulin mixed and allowed to sit over a few minutes will result in a slower absorption of the regular insulin.

Intermediate insulins have greater differences. Human insulins are consistently absorbed more rapidly than animal insulins and have a more rapid onset of action and shorter duration of activity. Among the human insulins, NPH has a more rapid onset of action than lente (zinc insulin).

Long-acting insulins have the greatest variability. Bovine ultralente insulin has the longest duration of activity (36 hours) and is virtually peakless, making it an attractive insulin for basal insulinemia. Its long duration of action, however, increases the likelihood of insulin overlap and resulting hypoglycemia. Human ultralente has a similar duration of action, but unlike its bovine counterpart, it shows a small peak activity at 8 hours with decreasing effectiveness after 18 hours. In practice, human ultralente may likewise be considered a peakless insulin, although twice-daily injections of human ultralente may be needed to achieve basal insulinemia. Human ultralente also does not mix well with regular insulin in the same syringe, changing absorption and duration of action for both insulins.

Multiple premeal injections of regular insulin coupled with basal ultralente offers patients more flexibility in meal timing and exercise planning. This manner of insulin administration is often referred to as "a poor man's insulin pump." Twice-daily injections of intermediate and regular insulins can result in excellent glycemic control but restrict the user to a more predictable meal and exercise schedule.

Storage temperature of insulin has an effect on its potency. This may be important for athletes engaged in outdoor activities when temperature fluctuations are likely to occur. Insulin should be protected from freezing temperatures and direct exposure to heat[52] (Table 21–9).

Insulin can be administered in a variety of

Table 21-9
Effects of Temperature on Insulin Storage

Temperature	Effect
<2°C (36°F; risk of freezing)	Short-acting insulin (soluble): usually no damage, but change to a new vial as soon as possible Long- or intermediate-acting insulin: probable loss of biologic activity; change to a new vial as soon as possible
2–8°C (36–46°F)	Ideal storage temperature
8–30°C (46–86°F)	No significant effect on insulin activity for 1 month
30–45°C (86–113°F)	Acceptable for very short periods (days); loss of biologic activity possible

Note: Check all insulins regularly for clumping or precipitation.

Source: Grimm JJ: Mountain hiking. *In* Ruderman N, Devlin JT (eds): The Health Professional's Guide to Diabetes and Exercise. Alexandria, VA, American Diabetes Association, 1995, pp. 299–302.

methods.[53] Subcutaneous injection with a disposable needle is the most common method. "Insulin pens" offer convenience for travelling, day-long competitions and are available in regular and mixtures. Continuous subcutaneous insulin infusion pumps provide a continuous infusion of basal insulin and allow the user to adjust mealtime boluses. Implantable insulin pumps with closed loop sensors that can automatically adjust insulin release to measured blood sugars are still largely experimental.

Multiple factors can influence insulin absorption including site and depth of injection, skin temperature, vascularity, and exercise.[53, 54] It is difficult clinically to control all these variables. Much has been written about the accelerated absorption rates of insulin injected subcutaneously over exercising muscles as opposed to a "neutral site," such as the abdomen. Although there are differences in absorption rates, they are not consistently present, nor is there strong evidence to say they are a cause of hypoglycemia. What does seem to be consistent is that insulin injected subcutaneously is absorbed more quickly over underlying exercising muscle, and that massage or heat applied to the injection site will increase absorption rates. The athlete should understand that injection site absorption may be influenced by exercise and that alterations in glucose levels may be affected.

Inadvertent injection of insulin intramuscularly rather than subcutaneously definitely has a more rapid onset of action and should be avoided before exercise. This circumstance can be avoided by grasping the injection site with a pinch technique and injecting at an oblique angle, rather than perpendicular to the skin, and by using shorter needles (less than 8 mm).

STRATEGIES FOR CONTROLLING BLOOD SUGAR LEVELS DURING EXERCISE

Long before there were physicians advocating the benefits of exercise, there were diabetic patients exercising and learning, through the process of trial and error, methods to control their insulin, meal planning, and intensity of training. To paraphrase an often quoted line, "The best laboratory for the study of diabetic athletes is the playing fields of our nation." The finest teachers of physicians continue to be their patients, and physicians should listen and learn from their experience.

Portable glucose monitors have greatly aided the diabetic in monitoring glucose levels. There can be no substitute for frequent glucose readings during the initiation of an exercise program, changes in training programs, or in prolonged competition.

A diabetic athlete who begins exercise in a well-controlled state (blood sugar 100 to 200 mg/dl, no ketones) will experience little difficulty in completing activity lasting up to an hour. Muscle demands for glucose will be met by stored muscle glycogen and available liver glycogen. If the athlete has timed the activity to avoid peaking levels of injected insulin, there will be a steady or declining level of insulin and a rising level of glucagon ready to liberate glucose to hungry exercising muscle.

An athlete who begins exercise in a poorly controlled state (blood sugar above 250 mg/dl, plus ketones) risks worsening hyperglycemia and eventual ketosis. Peripheral glucose uptake will be impaired by the relative or absolute lack of insulin, and hepatic glycogenolysis and gluconeogenesis from unopposed glucagon activity will add to the already high levels of circulating glucose.

Finally, a diabetic athlete who begins exercise with a glucose level greater than 100 mg/dl or during a time of peaking insulin activity risks hypoglycemia. As the demands of exercise deplete muscle glycogen and blood sugar begins to fall, the liver is called on to release its supply. If the athlete's insulin levels are relatively high, glucagon is inhibited, and glycogenolysis and gluconeogenesis and release of glucose supplies cannot take place.

Therefore, the goal of a diabetic athlete should be to time the exercise period to coincide with steady or falling levels of insulin. This information is best obtained by pre-exercise measurement of blood glucose, knowledge of insulin duration, and elapsed time from the last meal. Pre-exercise evaluation of blood sugar determines if exercise may safely proceed.

1. If hypoglycemic (blood sugar below 80 to 100 mg/dl), eat a snack of at least 10 to 20 g of carbohydrate.

2. If hyperglycemic (blood sugar above 250 mg/dl), delay exercise, check ketones, and administer insulin if necessary.

3. If normoglycemic (blood sugar between 100 and 250 mg/dl), proceed with exercise.

For well-controlled diabetic athletes, mild to moderate exercise lasting less than 30 minutes can be safely performed without alterations in insulin dose or food intake. If there is concern about hypoglycemia, 10 to 20 g of carbohydrate in a snack is effective in preventing postexercise hypoglycemia[55] (Table 21–10).

For well-controlled diabetic athletes planning an exercise activity lasting greater than 30 minutes, some alteration in insulin or food intake may be necessary if exercise is to proceed safely and postexercise hypoglycemia prevented. This can be accomplished in two ways. Either insulin can be reduced or food intake increased prior to and after exercise. Sometimes it is necessary to do both.

For exercise of longest duration, some adjustments in insulin and food intake are necessary. In addition, blood sugar levels should be measured every 30 to 60 minutes during the activity, and carbohydrate (30 to 60 g in divided portions during each hour) must be consumed during the competition.[56] Postcompetition feeding to replace liver and muscle glycogen stores will serve to provide energy for the next competition or training activity and aid in the prevention of delayed onset hypoglycemia.

Insulin adjustments in anticipation of exercise depends on the duration and intensity of the planned exercise and the particular insulin regimen utilized by the patient. The following insulin recommendations assume that the individual athlete is in acceptable pre-exercise capillary blood glucose ranges (Table 21–11).

Nutritional support and planning is crucial to the success of athletes. In athletes with diabetes, nutrition is vital for both success and safety. A training diet complete with adequate amounts of carbohydrate, protein, vitamins, and fluid is no less important and deserves just as much emphasis in athletes with diabetes as nondiabetic athletes. In addition, athletes with diabetes must use food as a means of preserving safe levels of blood glucose and "feeding their insulin."

Training diets differ in caloric amounts based on body size and activity. For individuals training 1 hour per day, 5 to 6 g of carbohydrate per kilogram of body weight is needed per day to restore liver and muscle glycogen levels. This requirement increases to 8 g per kg for training longer than 2 hours and 10 g per kg for long endurance activities.[56] For athletes with diabetes, restoration of hepatic glycogen levels is essential to avoid exercise-induced hypoglycemia and delayed-onset hypoglycemia. In addition to the usual pre-exercise or precompetition meal taken 3 to 4 hours before, athletes with diabetes may benefit from a small amount of carbohydrate (10 to 20 g)

Table 21–10
Examples of 15-Gram Carbohydrate Portions

Starches (About 15 g Carbohydrate and 80 kcal)

8 animal crackers	½ English muffin	4 rye crisp, each 2 in. × 3½ in.
½ bagel (1 oz)	3 graham crackers, each 2½ in.	6 saltine crackers
2 crisp bread sticks, each 4 in. × ½ in. (⅔ oz)	pretzels (¾ oz)	2–4 wafers of no-fat-added, whole wheat crackers, such as Finn, Kavli, Wasa (¾ oz)

Fruits (About 15 g Carbohydrate and 60 kcal)

Raw Fruit	*Dried Fruit*	*Fruit Juice*
1 apple, 2 in. across	4 apple rings	½ cup apple juice or cider
½ banana, 9 in. long	7 apricot halves	⅓ cup cranberry juice cocktail
½ medium grapefruit	2½ medium dates	½ cup grapefruit juice
15 small grapes	1½ figs	⅓ cup grape juice
1 nectarine, 2½ in. across	3 medium prunes	½ cup orange juice
1 orange, 2½ in. across	2 tablespoons raisins	½ cup pineapple juice
1 small pear		
2 plums, each 2 in. across		

Low-Fat Milk Products (About 12 g Carbohydrate and 90 kcal)

1 cup skim milk	1 cup 1%-fat milk
1 cup ½%-fat milk	8 oz plain nonfat yogurt

Source: Gordon NF: Diabetes: Your Complete Exercise Guide. Champaign, Human Kinetics Publishers, 1993.

Table 21–11
Insulin Adjustments to Exercise

Once-Daily Regimen

Morning exercise lasting >45 min:
Decrease regular insulin by 25% for mild to moderate activity
Decrease regular insulin by 35% for moderate activity
Decrease regular insulin by 50% for strenuous activity (athletes in training)
Afternoon or evening exercise lasting >45 min:
Decrease NPH/lente by 15% for mild to moderate activity
Decrease NPH/lente by 20% for moderate activity
Decrease NPH/lente by 25% for strenuous activity (athletes in training)

Twice-Daily Regimen

Morning exercise lasting >45 min:
Decrease morning regular insulin as above
Early afternoon exercise lasting >45 min:
Decrease morning NPH insulin as above
Evening exercise lasting >45 min:
Decrease supper NPH and regular insulin as for once-daily insulin

More Than Twice-Daily Injections

Premeal regular insulin can be decreased for exercise occurring postprandially (from 25–50% decrements depending on the intensity and duration)
Bedtime or morning NPH or ultralente should be decreased only for very prolonged and intense exercise (tournaments, marathons, etc.) occurring at any time of the day

Continuous Subcutaneous Insulin Infusion

Premeal boluses should be decreased as above for postprandial exercise
For light exercise, the basal rate can be maintained
For moderate or intense exercise, the basal rate should be discontinued for the duration of exercise taking into account that a moderate amount of subcutaneous insulin remaining in the infusion site (3–5 U) will be absorbed.

For Unanticipated Exercise

Insulin doses cannot be modified, thus hypoglycemia can be prevented by extra food
Mild to moderate exercise = 1 fruit exchange every 30–45 min
Moderate exercise = 1 starch + 1 protein before exercise + 1 fruit every 30–45 min during exercise
Strenuous exercise = 2 starches + 1 protein before exercise + 1–2 fruit(s) every 30–45 min during exercise

Source: Clinical Education Series. Medical Management of Insulin-Dependent Diabetes Mellitus. Alexandria, VA, American Diabetes Association, 1995.

taken 15 to 30 minutes prior to exercise.[55] There is a natural tendency to overeat in anticipation of exercise, and care must be taken to match the snack with the actual calories required.

Delayed hypoglycemia occurring 1 to 12 hours postexercise can afflict diabetic athletes who have failed to ingest adequate carbohydrate necessary for muscle and liver glycogen replenishment. Exercise of prolonged duration requires that the athlete replenish depleted glycogen stores in liver and muscle. This is best accomplished within 4 hours after conclusion of the exercise or competition. Carbohydrates moderately high in glycemic index (see Table 21–12) are recommended. Athletes subjected to multiple daily training regimens or competitions are at higher risk for the development of hypoglycemia and will most likely do better with multiple small doses of short-acting insulin and reduced long-acting insulin. It is important for patients beginning exercise programs or those altering training schedules to test blood sugar frequently in the hours following exercise. For this reason also, it may be prudent to avoid late evening training regimens, or if there is late

competition to provide box lunches for the bus ride home.

Carbohydrates can be classified by their glycemic index (Table 21–12). Glycemic index is a measurement of a particular food's absorption from the gut, conversion to glucose, and appearance in the blood stream relative to that of glucose or white bread. Foods high in glycemic index are closer in composition to simple sugars and foods with low glycemic indexes more akin to complex carbohydrates. Diets composed of carbohydrates of low glycemic index are correlated with better glucose control in NIDDM[57] and IDDM. Others have stated that the glycemic character of the carbohydrate is ameliorated by the presence of fat and protein accompanying the meal.[58]

As mentioned previously, exercise of prolonged duration requires supplementation of carbohydrate in a range of 30 to 60 g per hour. There are a variety of commercial products on the market that contain carbohydrate in varying amounts. A listing of many of the products along with their respective nutrient contents is listed in Tables 21–13 to 21–15.

Table 21–12
Glycemic Index of Selected Food Products

Food	Glycemic Index	Food	Glycemic Index
BREADS		BREAKFAST CEREALS	
White	100	Cornflakes	119
Whole wheat	99	All-Bran	73
Rye	58	Shredded wheat	97
CEREAL PRODUCTS		FRUIT	
Rice (white)	83	Apple	53
Rice (brown)	96	Banana	79
Spaghetti	66	Grapefruit	36
		Grapes	62
VEGETABLES		Orange	66
Potato (instant)	116	Orange juice	67
Potato (new, boiled)	81	Pear	47
Potato (Russett, baked)	135	Raisins	93
Potato (sweet)	70	SUGARS	
Frozen peas	74		
Sweet corn	87	Glucose	138
DRIED LEGUMES		Sucrose	86
		Fructose	30
Baked beans	60	DAIRY PRODUCTS	
Kidney beans	54	Skim milk	46
Dried green peas	56	Yogurt	52
Red lentils	43	Ice cream	52
Soybeans (dried)	22		

Note: Mean glycemic indices adjusted so that white bread = 100.
Source: Bantle JP: The dietary treatment of diabetes mellitus. Med Clin North Am 72:1291, 1988.

EXERCISE PRESCRIPTION

Exercise prescriptions for patients with diabetes are similar to nondiabetic patients (Table 21–16). It is important to remember that the improvements in insulin resistance and the non–insulin-mediated glucose uptake that exercise affords diminishes after 48 hours. Daily, or at least every other day, exercise is recommended to sustain this benefit.

Second, exercise is not a treatment for poorly controlled insulin-dependent diabetes and should not be used with the intention of improving gly-

Table 21–13
Nutritional Analysis of Fluid Replacement Beverages

Beverage	Portion	Calories	Carbohydrate (g)	Sodium (mg)	Potassium (mg)	Carbohydrate Concentration (%)
All Sport Body Quencher	8 fl oz	70	20	55	55	8
Exceed Energy Drink Powder	2 Tbsp + 8 fl oz water	70	17	50	45	7
Gatorade Thirst Quencher	8 fl oz	50	14	110	30	6
PowerAde Thirst Quencher	8 fl oz	70	19	55	30	8
Soft drinks	8 fl oz	110–130	27–32	9–30	Trace	10–13
Fruit juice	8 fl oz	120–180	30–45	0–15	61–510	12–18

Source: Franz MJ: Nutrition, exercise, and diabetes. *In* Ruderman N, Devlin JT (eds): The Health Professional's Guide to Diabetes and Exercise. Alexandria, VA, American Diabetes Association, 1995, pp. 99–108.

Table 21-14
Nutritional Content of High-Carbohydrate Beverages

Beverage	Serving Size	Calories	Carbohydrate (g)	Sodium (mg)	Carbohydrate Concentration (%)
Exceed High Carbohydrate Drink Powder	6 Tbsp + 8 fl oz water	230	59	115	24
GatorLode	12 fl oz	283	71	95	20
Carbo Energizer	8 fl oz	237	59	130	25
Carbo Powder	16 fl oz	339	85	100	18

Source: Franz MJ: Nutrition, exercise, and diabetes. *In* Ruderman N, Devlin JT (eds): The Health Professional's Guide to Diabetes and Exercise. Alexandria, VA, American Diabetes Association, 1995, pp. 99–108.

Table 21-15
Nutritional Content of Selected Food Supplements

Supplement	Serving Size	Calories	Carbohydrate, g (% Total Calories)	Protein, g (% Total Calories)	Fat, g (% Total Calories)
Beverages					
Ensure	8 fl oz	250	34 (54)	9 (14)	9 (32)
GatoPro	8 fl oz	360	58 (65)	16 (18)	7 (17)
Sport Shake	8 fl oz	310	45 (58)	11 (13)	10 (29)
Sustacal	8 fl oz	240	33 (55)	14.5 (24)	5.5 (21)
Bars					
Exceed Sports Bar	1 bar (2.8 oz)	280	53 (76)	12 (17)	2 (7)
Power Bar	1 bar (2.25 oz)	225	42 (75)	10 (16)	2.5 (9)
Tiger Sport Ultimate	1 bar (2.3 oz)	230	40 (69)	11 (19)	3 (12)

Source: Franz MJ: Nutrition, exercise, and diabetes. *In* Ruderman N, Devlin JT (eds): The Health Professional's Guide to Diabetes and Exercise. Alexandria, VA, American Diabetes Association, 1995, pp. 99–108.

Table 21-16
Components of the Exercise Prescription

Screening

Search for vascular and neurologic complications, including silent ischemia

Exercise ECG in patients with known or suspected CAD, >30 years of age with IDDM, with IDDM for >15 years, or >35 years of age with NIDDM

Exercise Program

Type: Aerobic

Frequency: 3–5 times/week

Duration: 20–60 min

Intensity: 50–74% of maximal aerobic capacity

Energy expenditure: Modulate type, frequency, duration, and intensity to attain an energy expenditure of 700–2000 calories/week

Timing: Time participation so that it does not coincide with peak insulin absorption

Avoid Complications

Warm up and cool down

Careful selection of exercise type and intensity

Patient education

Proper footwear

Avoid exercise in extreme heat or cold

Inspect feet daily and after exercise

Avoid exercise when metabolic control is poor

Maintain adequate hydration

Monitor blood glucose if taking insulin or oral hypoglycemic agents, and follow guidelines to prevent hypoglycemia

Compliance

Make exercise enjoyable

Convenient location

Positive feedback from involved medical personnel and family

ECG = electrocardiogram; CAD = coronary artery disease; IDDM = insulin-dependent diabetes mellitus; NIDDM = non–insulin-dependent diabetes mellitus.

Source: Gordon N: The exercise prescription. *In* Ruderman N, Devlin JT (eds): The Health Professional's Guide to Diabetes and Exercise. Alexandria, VA, American Diabetes Association, 1995, pp. 69–83.

cemic control. Poorly controlled IDDM is a contraindication to exercise and should be corrected before exercise is advocated.

Third, the type of exercise recommended in IDDM should be matched with the type of insulin regimen the patient is currently using. Athletes and patients with unpredictable exercise habits, intense training regimens, or involved in long endurance activities will not do well in insulin programs that permit little flexibility.

Finally, physicians should actively encourage individuals with strong risk factors for developing NIDDM (obesity and positive family history) to begin exercise programs. The elapsed time from onset of NIDDM and diagnosis is 4 to 7 years[59] with many patients presenting with complications at the time of diagnoses. Exercise is truly one of the best therapeutic modalities for persons at risk for diabetes.

REFERENCES

1. Thurm U, Harper P: I'm running on insulin: Summary of the history of the International Diabetes Athletes Association. Diabetes Care 15(15):1811–1813, 1992.
2. Grimm JJ, Muchnick S: Type I diabetes and marathon running. Diabetes Care 16(12):1624, 1993.
3. Report of the Expert Committee on the Diagnosis and Classification of Diabetes Mellitus. Supplement 1, Clinical Practice Recommendations 1998. Diabetes Care 21:S5, Jan. 1998.
4. Harris M, Robbins D: Prevalence of adult onset IDDM in the U.S. population. Diabetes Care 17(11):1337–1340, 1994.
5. Ginsberg-Fellner F: Genetic counseling in type I diabetes. *In* Lebovitz H (ed): Therapy for Diabetes Mellitus and Related Disorders, 2nd ed. Alexandria, VA, American Diabetes Association, 1994, pp. 4–10.
6. Campaigne BN, Lampman RM: Exercise in the Clinical Management of Diabetes. Champaign, Human Kinetics, 1994, p. 2.
7. Galloway JA: New directions in drug development: Mixtures analogues, modeling, Human insulin: A decade of experience and future developments. Supplement. Diabetes Care 16(3):1209–1240, 1993.
8. Kerr C: Improving outcomes in diabetes: A review of the outpatient care of NIDDM patients. J Fam Pract 40(1):63–74, 1995.
9. Gordon NF: Diabetes: Your Complete Exercise Guide. Champaign, Human Kinetics, 1993.
10. Jackson RA: Mechanisms of age-related glucose intolerance. *In* Halter J, Christensen N (eds): Diabetes Mellitus in Elderly People. Diabetes Care 13(2):9–20, 1990.
11. Helmrich S, Raglund D, Leung R, Paffenbarger R: Physical activity and reduced occurrence of non-insulin dependent diabetes mellitus. N Engl J Med 325:147–152, 1991.
12. Yki-Jarvinen H: Pathogenesis of non-insulin dependent diabetes mellitus. Lancet 343:91–94, 1994.
13. Zimmet PZ: Hyperinsulinemia—How innocent a bystander? Human insulin: A decade of experience and future developments. Supplement. Diabetes Care 16(3):56–70, 1993.

14. Campaigne BN, Lampman RM: Exercise in the Clinical Management of Diabetes. Champaign, Human Kinetics, 1994, pp. 4–7.
15. Singard DL, Sinsheimer P, Barrett-Connor EL, McPhillips JB: Community-based study of prevalence of NIDDM in older adults. Diabetes mellitus in elderly people. Diabetes Care 13(2):3–9, 1990.
16. Kaplan NM: The deadly quartet: Upper body obesity, glucose intolerance, hypertriglyceridemia, and hypertension. Arch Intern Med 149:1514–1520, 1989.
17. Shulman GI, Rothman DL, Jue T, et al: Quantitation of muscle glycogen synthesis in normal subjects, and subjects with no insulin dependent diabetes by ^{13}C nuclear magnetic resonance spectroscopy. N Engl J Med 322:223–228, 1990.
18. Schwartz RS: Exercise Training in Treatment of Diabetes Mellitus in Elderly Patients. Diabetes Care 13(2):77–86, 1990.
19. Campaigne BN, Lampman RM: Exercise in the Clinical Management of Diabetes. Champaign, Human Kinetics, 1994, p. 40.
20. Campaigne BN, Lampman RM: Exercise in the Clinical Management of Diabetes. Champaign, Human Kinetics, 1994, p. 5.
21. Menon R, Grace A, Burgoyne W, et al: Muscle blood flow in diabetes mellitus. Diabetes Care 15(5):693–695, 1992.
22. DeFronzo RA, Simonson D, Ferranninni E: Hepatic and peripheral insulin resistance: A common feature of type 2 (non insulin dependent) and type I (insulin dependent) diabetes mellitus. Diabetologica 23:313–319, 1982.
23. Sherman C: Gene that regulates fat is linked to type II diabetes. Fam Pract News 12/1/95, p. 5.
24. Bourn D, Mann J, McSkimming, et al: Impaired glucose tolerance and NIDDM: Does a lifestyle intervention program have an effect? Diabetes Care 17(11):1311–1319, 1994.
25. Long SD, O'Brien K, MacDonald KG, et al: Weight loss in severely obese subjects prevents the progression of impaired glucose tolerance to type II diabetes. Diabetes Care 17(5):372–375, 1994.
26. Rasmussen O, Lauszus F, Hermansen K: Effects of postprandial exercise on glycemic response in IDDM subjects: Studies at constant insulinemia. Diabetes Care 17(10):1203–1205, 1994.
27. Barnard RJ, Jung T, Inkeles S: Diet and exercise in the treatment of NIDDM: The need for early emphasis. Diabetes Care 17(12):1469–1472, 1994.
28. Campaigne BN, Lampman RM: Exercise in the Clinical Management of Diabetes. Champaign, Human Kinetics, 1994, pp. 124–125.
29. Schneider S, Ruderman N: Exercise and NIDDM. Council on Exercise. Diabetes Care 13(7):785–790, 1990.
30. The Diabetes Control and Complications Trial Research Group: The Effect of Intensive Treatment of Diabetes on the Development and Progression of Long-Term Complications in Insulin-Dependent Diabetes Mellitus. N Engl J Med 329:977–986, 1993.
31. American Diabetes Association: Standards of medical care for patients with diabetes mellitus. Diabetes Care 21:S23–S32, Jan. 1998.
32. Peterson KA, Smith CK: The DCCT findings and standards of care for diabetes. Am Fam Physician 52(4):1092–1126, 1995.
33. Cunningham LN: Comparison of the acute and long term effects of exercise on glucose control in type I diabetes. Diabetes Spectrum pp. 224–225, 1988.
34. Ginsberg BJ, Mazze R: Clinical consequences of the diabetes control and complications trial. N Engl J Med 91:221–224, 1994.
35. Peters AL, McCullough DK, Hayward RA, et al: Case

one: Too little too late—Delayed diagnoses of NIDDM. J Clin Outcomes Management 1(2):9–26, 1994.

36. Campaigne BN, Lampman RM: Exercise in the Clinical Management of Diabetes. Champaign, Human Kinetics, 1994, p. 141.

37. Cryer PE: Hypoglycemia unawareness in IDDM. Human insulin: A decade of experience and future developments. Diabetes Care 16(3):40–47, 1993.

38. American Diabetes Association: Standards of medical care for patients with diabetes mellitus. Diabetes Care 17:616–623, 1994.

39. Raev DC: Which left ventricular function is impaired earlier in the evolution of diabetic cardiomyopathy: An echocardiographic study of young type I diabetic patients. 17(7):633–640, 1994.

40. Ferraro S, Perrone-Filardi P, Maddalena G, et al: Comparison of left ventricular function in insulin- and non-insulin-dependent diabetes mellitus. Am J Cardiol 71:409–414, 1993.

41. Blake GA, Levin SR, Koyal SN: Exercise induced hypertension in normotensive patients with NIDDM. Diabetes Care 13(7):799–801, 1990.

42. Aiello LA, Cavallerano J, Aiello LP, Bursell SE: Retinopathy. *In* Ruderman N, Devlin JT (eds): The Health Professional's Guide to Diabetes and Exercise. Alexandria, VA, American Diabetes Association, 1995, pp. 145–151.

43. Vinik AI: Neuropathy. *In* Ruderman N, Devlin JT (eds): The Health Professional's Guide to Diabetes and Exercise. Alexandria, VA, American Diabetes Association, 1995, pp. 181–198.

44. Levin M: The diabetic foot. *In* Ruderman N, Devlin JT (eds): The Health Professional's Guide to Diabetes and Exercise. Alexandria, VA, American Diabetes Association, 1995, pp. 137–151.

45. Mogensen CA: Nephropathy: Early. *In* Ruderman N, Devlin JT (eds): The Health Professional's Guide to Diabetes and Exercise. Alexandria, VA, American Diabetes Association, 1995, pp. 163–174.

46. Braden GL: Nephropathy: Advanced. *In* Ruderman N, Devlin JT (eds): The Health Professional's Guide to Diabetes and Exercise. Alexandria, VA, American Diabetes Association, 1995, pp. 175–180.

47. Bliss M: The history of insulin. Human insulin: A decade of experience and future developments. Diabetes Care 16(3):4–7, 1993.

48. Heinemann L, Richter B: Clinical pharmacology of human insulin. Human insulin: A decade of experience and future developments. Diabetes Care 16(3):8, 1993.

49. Galloway JA: New directions in drug development: Mixtures, analogues, modeling. Human insulin: A decade of experience and future developments. Diabetes Care 16(3):16–23, 1993.

50. Tucker M: Insulin analogue offers better control, fewer hypoglycemic episodes. Family Pract News, Vol 24, Oct. 1, 1994, p. 39.

51. Zinman B: Insulin regimens and strategies for IDDM. Human insulin: A decade of experience and future developments. Diabetes Care 16(3):24–28, 1993.

52. Grimm JJ: Mountain hiking. *In* Ruderman N, Devlin JT (eds): The Health Professional's Guide to Diabetes and Exercise. Alexandria, VA, American Diabetes Association, 1995, pp. 299–302.

53. Saudek CD: Future developments in insulin delivery systems. Human insulin: A decade of experience and future developments. Diabetes Care 16(3):122–131, 1993.

54. Berger M: Adjustment of insulin therapy. *In* Ruderman N, Devlin JT (eds): The Health Professional's Guide to Diabetes and Exercise. Alexandria, VA, American Diabetes Association, 1995, pp. 115–122.

55. Nathan DN, Madnek S, Delahanty L: Programming preexercise snacks to prevent post-exercise hypoglycemia in intensively treated insulin-dependent diabetics. Ann Intern Med 4:483–486, 1978.

56. Franz MJ: Nutrition, exercise, and diabetes. *In* Ruderman N, Devlin JT (eds): The Health Professional's Guide to Diabetes and Exercise. Alexandria, VA, American Diabetes Association, 1995, pp. 99–108.

57. Brand JC, Colagiuri S, Crossman S, et al: Low glycemic index foods improve long-term glycemic control in NIDDM. Diabetes Care 14(2):95–102, 1991.

58. Bantle JP: The dietary treatment of diabetes mellitus. Med Clin North Am 72(6):1285–1300, 1988.

59. Harris MI, Klein R, Welborn TA, Kneuman MW: Onset of NIDDM occurs at least 4–7 years before clinical diagnoses. Diabetes Care 15:815–819, 1992.

IV *The Athlete with Heart Disease*

MARK NIEDFELDT, M.D.

Most competitive athletes involved in high-intensity activities are young and without heart disease. As athletes age, however, different types of cardiac problems may become manifest. As the population ages, we are seeing older athletes participating in strenuous activities, and masters competitions have lengthened the time of competition for older athletes. This section outlines some of the recommendations regarding cardiovascular abnormalities in athletes and provides exercise recommendations and guidelines for disqualifica-

tion. For further information, the reader should refer to the guidelines for participation in competitive athletics for patients with cardiovascular abnormalities described in the 26th Bethesda Conference Report.[1]

CORONARY HEART DISEASE

The most frequent cause of exercise-related events and sudden death in adults is atherosclerotic coronary artery disease. The incidence of cardiac events is also increased during vigorous physical activity.[2, 3] The prevalence of atherosclerotic coronary artery disease and the incidence of coronary events increase with advancing age.[1] Patients with coronary heart disease vary a great deal in their clinical status, and consideration should be given to the extent of coronary artery disease, left ventricular dysfunction, myocardial ischemia, and the presence of cardiac arrhythmias. Many of these patients have additional medical problems including hypertension, peripheral vascular disease, valvular heart disease, chronic obstructive pulmonary disease, and diabetes mellitus.

Most athletes with coronary heart disease have reduced maximal oxygen uptake and exercise tolerance.[4] The stroke volume is decreased due to myocardial ischemia or damage previously caused by infarction.[5] Heart rate is also decreased, most likely partially due to enhanced vagal tone as well as other unknown mechanisms.[4] Patients with angina have a decreased exercise tolerance because of discomfort, which often occurs at a highly reproducible exertion level.[6] These patients are often deconditioned because they or their doctors have restricted their activity. Beta-adrenergic blockers given after myocardial infarction may limit exercise capacity in some cases.[4] A coronary artery vasospastic component may be present; when it is, it may contribute to exercise-induced ischemia in some cases.[7] This condition is most frequently seen in coronary sites previously damaged by atherosclerosis.[8]

Exercise offers many benefits for patients with coronary heart disease. Patients with angina often experience some of the greatest benefits. These patients show increases in effort tolerance following exercise training, as exercise training reduces submaximal heart rate at any given activity level, delaying the onset of symptoms.[9] Coronary perfusion may be improved in some exercising patients by an unknown mechanism.[10] Exercise training in postmyocardial infarction patients has resulted in decreased total cholesterol, low-density lipoprotein, and triglycerides and increased high-density lipoprotein levels.[11] Depression has also been lessened in postmyocardial infarction patients who are active in an exercise program.[12] The weight loss associated with exercise also helps control risk factors for coronary heart disease such as obesity and diabetes.[13] Cardiac rehabilitation programs have been shown to reduce fatal cardiovascular events and total mortality rate by 20 to 25 percent.[14]

Exercise Recommendations

Patients with coronary heart disease require a complete medical history, physical examination, and exercise test prior to starting an exercise program.[15] Any abnormalities should be fully investigated. Patients with unstable angina, severe aortic stenosis, uncontrolled cardiac arrhythmias, or decompensated congestive heart failure should postpone exercise training until their conditions are controlled.[16] Many patients may need to begin with a supervised exercise program that is specifically designed for their needs and based on the severity of their symptoms. Patients should be reevaluated every 2 to 3 months after beginning an exercise program.[16]

The exercise prescription is individualized on the basis of functional capacity and includes both formal exercise sessions and everyday physical activities. It is based on the traditional prescription for developing a training effect in healthy people.[17] As a general rule, 20 to 60 minutes of continuous or intermittent (minimum of 10 minutes) large muscle group aerobic activity is appropriate 3 to 5 days a week. This activity may be performed starting at 55 percent of maximal heart rate (220 minus age). Those who are quite unfit may start at a lower intensity level (40 to 50 percent of maximal heart rate).[4] Progression is slow and gradual, with monitoring of symptoms as intensity and duration of activities are increased.

Return to Practice and Competition

When testing shows athletes to be at mildly increased risk, they can participate in low dynamic and low-to-moderate static competitive sports, but they should avoid intensely competitive situations. These athletes have normal or near normal left ventricular systolic function at rest (ejection fraction above 50 percent), normal exercise tolerance for age as demonstrated during exercise testing, absence of exercise-induced ischemia or arrhythmias, and absence of hemodynamically significant stenosis in all major coronary arteries (if angiography is performed).[1] Athletes in this category who are engaging in competitive sports should undergo reevaluation of their risk stratification at least annually. Those found to be at increased risk should generally be restricted to low-intensity competitive sports, and should have a medical reevaluation every 6 months with exercise testing at least yearly.[1]

CARDIAC ARRHYTHMIAS

Arrhythmias are common in athletes. Many findings interpreted as abnormal using strict criteria are actually normal in athletes. Arrhythmias that cause extreme bradycardia or tachycardia are likely to cause severe symptoms in the athlete. During extreme bradycardia, the heart rate is insufficient to perfuse the body regardless of stroke volume. In excessive tachycardia, the stroke volume is severely decreased due to the shortened time spent in diastole, and cardiac output is again decreased.

Arrhythmias normally associated with training include sinus bradycardia, wandering atrial pacemaker, and sinus pauses. Escape rhythms are frequently noted, including abnormal atrial focus, junctional rhythm, and idioventricular rhythm along with AV conduction delays, especially the first-degree and type 1 second-degree (Wenckebach) blocks. Premature ventricular complexes are also frequently noted on electrocardiography.

General evaluation of arrhythmias includes history of prodrome, syncope, presence of possible arrhythmia, medication usage (including over-the-counter drugs), inciting events, or family history of heart disease, syncope, or sudden death. The physical examination focuses on the cardiovascular system. Initial testing includes an electrocardiogram (ECG). Exercise testing and monitoring through a 24-hour ambulatory ECG may be helpful in some cases. If structural heart disease is suspected, echocardiogram is the test of choice.

Return to Practice and Competition

Participation recommendations for athletes with cardiac abnormalities are often drawn from the 26th Bethesda Conference,[1] which was sponsored by the American College of Sports Medicine and the American College of Cardiology. Recommendations for eligibility are determined by type of cardiac abnormality, severity of the abnormality, and the physiologic demands of the sport. The more common serious rhythm disturbances are reviewed here, but the reader is referred to the Bethesda guidelines for further detail.

Atrial Fibrillation

Atrial fibrillation often occurs in association with coronary artery disease or hypertension. Evaluation should include an exercise test comparable to the intended athletic activity. If athletes with atrial fibrillation and no structural heart disease maintain a ventricular rate comparable to an appropriate sinus tachycardia during physical activity while receiving no therapy or medical therapy, they may participate in all competitive sports.[1] Athletes who require anticoagulation should not participate in sports with danger of bodily collision.

Wolff-Parkinson-White Syndrome

Athletes should have a 12-lead ECG, a 24-hour ECG recording during athletic activity, exercise test, and echocardiogram to exclude associated cardiovascular abnormalities. Athletes over age 20 with no history of palpitations or tachycardia and no evidence of structural cardiac abnormalities may participate in all competitive sports. Athletes with syncope or near syncope in addition to an arrhythmia should not participate in competitive sports until they have been adequately treated and symptom-free for over 6 months. Athletes with episodes of associated atrial fibrillation or flutter with a resultant heart rate over 240 beats per minute are restricted to low-intensity exercise. Many of these patients are considered for radiofrequency ablation of the accessory pathway.[18]

Premature Ventricular Complexes

Athletes with premature ventricular complexes (PVCs) and no structural heart disease who do not have an increase in PVCs or any symptoms during exercise or exercise testing can participate in competitive sports. Athletes with structural heart disease can participate in low-intensity competitive sports only, regardless of whether they are being treated or not.[1]

Ventricular Tachycardia

Athletes with nonsustained or sustained ventricular tachycardia should not compete in any sports for at least 6 months after the last episode. The athlete may return to competition if there are no clinical recurrences, no structural heart disease is present, and ventricular tachycardia is not reproducible during exercise. If structural heart disease is present, only low-intensity activities are permitted.

Ventricular Flutter and Ventricular Fibrillation

Athletes with no recurrences after 6 months of treatment may engage in low-intensity sports.

Atrioventricular Block

Asymptomatic athletes who show no evidence of structural heart disease and have a first-degree AV block that does not worsen with exercise may participate in all competitive sports. A type 1 second-degree (Wenckebach) AV block can be present in otherwise healthy, well-trained athletes.[19] Athletes with no structural abnormalities or worsening of the block during exercise may participate in all competitive sports. Those with structural abnormalities or worsening of the block with exercise require further evaluation. Athletes with a type 2 second-degree (Mobitz) AV block or an acquired complete heart block should be treated with permanent pacemaker placement before resuming any athletic activity.

Congenital Long Q-T Interval Syndrome

The diagnosis of long Q-T syndrome may be complex and requires not only a measurement of the Q-T interval but also a history of symptoms, family history, and ECG changes, such as T-wave alterations or abnormal configuration.[20] These athletes are at risk for sudden death with activity and should be restricted from all competitive sports.[1]

SUDDEN CARDIAC DEATH

Sudden death in young athletes often receives much attention. It is quite shocking for an apparently healthy young athlete to die suddenly, often on the playing field. Although these deaths are devastating, they are extremely rare, considering the vast numbers of young athletes participating in sporting activities.

The incidence of sudden death in young athletes (less than age 30) is approximately 10 to 25 individuals per year in organized high school and college athletics. The numbers are hard to compile because there is no national registry. The overall incidence is often thought to be approximately 1 per 200,000 to 300,000 student athletes per academic year.[21] The rate of sudden death related to exercise is reported to be 1 per 15,000 for apparently healthy adult male athletes.[22] To prevent one death, one individual needs to be identified and protected out of a group of approximately 250,000 athletes.

The causes of sudden death are varied. Most cardiovascular lesions provide few or no premonitory signs and symptoms and are unlikely to be diagnosed during life. Most of the athletes who succumb to sudden death are males with structural, usually congenital, heart disease. Only about 10 percent of deaths occur in females.[21, 23] Reasons for this discrepancy include fewer cardiac lesions, less participation in sports, less intensive training, and lack of participation in sports more liable to lead to cardiac death, such as football.[24] Hypertrophic cardiomyopathy (HCM) is responsible for approximately one third of cases of sudden death in young athletes.[21, 23] This familial disease is identifiable by echocardiography in about 0.2 percent of the general population. In HCM, sudden death often occurs in the context of moderate to severe exertion. Most who die from this condition are young and asymptomatic. The risk of death in an individual with HCM is difficult to stratify, as there are many mechanisms that may be responsible for the fatal arrhythmia and cardiac collapse. HCM is an important cause of sudden death in African-American male athletes, although it is less frequently reported in hospital-based tertiary care programs. This may be due to limited access to specialty care in African-American communities.

The second most common cause of sudden death in young athletes is congenital malformations of the coronary arteries; the most important of these is anomalous origin of the left main coronary artery from the right sinus of Valsalva.

In adults over age 35, the most common cause of sudden death during athletics is atherosclerotic coronary artery disease.[25]

Myocarditis is an uncommon cause of sudden death and is generally caused by a virus, usually Coxsackievirus B.[26] Myocarditis is suspected clinically on the basis of fatigue, exertional dyspnea, syncope, palpitations, arrhythmias, or acute congestive heart failure in the presence of left ventricular dilatation. It is associated with evidence of ventricular dysfunction or ST-T changes on ECG. An endomyocardial biopsy may be required for diagnosis.[1] Athletes judged as probably having myocarditis should be withdrawn from all competitive sports and should spend 6 months convalescing after the onset of clinical manifestations. Prior to return to competitive training, their cardiac status should be evaluated. The athlete should be allowed to return when ventricular function and cardiac dimensions have returned to normal and clinically relevant arrhythmias are absent on ambulatory monitoring.[1]

Preparticipation Screening

Detecting pre-existing cardiovascular abnormalities that have the potential to cause sudden death is an important objective of the preparticipation examination. However, the traditional history and physical examination detect only approximately 3 percent of abnormalities that eventually result in sudden death in high school and college athletes.[23] Echocardiography has been suggested for use as part of the preparticipation examination, but it has shown a low yield of identifiable cardiovascular disease.[27] Currently the American Heart Association has not recommended noninvasive testing such as electrocardiography or echocardiography as part of preparticipation physical examinations. Even with noninvasive testing, no large-scale screening process can detect all important cardiovascular abnormalities in all athletes.[28]

A history and physical examination should be performed in high school and college-age athletes before they participate in organized high school and college athletics. The American Heart Association currently recommends repeated screening every 2 years, although other groups recommend only interim history and blood pressure screening, with further physical examination performed if problems are noted during the history or blood pressure screening.[29] The preparticipation screening history should include questions regarding a family history of premature sudden death or heart disease, a personal history of heart murmur, hypertension, early fatigue, syncope, exertional dyspnea or chest pain, and if the athlete is a child, parental verification of the history. The physical examination includes auscultation of the heart, seeking to identify any murmurs with the patient in both supine or sitting and standing position, checking

femoral pulses, looking for stigmata of Marfan's syndrome, and blood pressure measurement.[28]

For athletes over the age of 35, a history and physical examination should include personal history of risk factors and family history of premature ischemic heart disease. If coronary artery disease is suspected on the basis of risk factor profile (i.e., two or more risk factors other than age or gender or a single but marked abnormal factor), exercise stress testing should be considered in men older than 40 and women older than 50.[28]

Exercise Recommendations

As mentioned earlier, the 26th Bethesda Conference report and the American Heart Association screening recommendations have provided expected standards of care. It is recommended that these guidelines be followed for participation recommendations.

Key Points

- Exercise offers many benefits for patients with coronary heart disease including delay of onset of symptoms, decreased risk factor profile, and reduction in fatal cardiovascular events.
- Arrhythmias are common in athletes because there are several arrhythmias normally associated with training.
- Atherosclerotic coronary artery disease is the most frequent cause of exercise-related cardiac events and sudden death in adults.
- Most young athletes with sudden death are males with structural heart disease, mainly hypertrophic cardiomyopathy.
- No screening test can detect all important cardiovascular abnormalities in athletes.
- Participation recommendations for athletes with cardiac abnormalities are often drawn from the 26th Bethesda Conference.

REFERENCES

1. 26th Bethesda Conference: Recommendations for determining eligibility for competition in athletes with cardiovascular abnormalities. J Am Coll Cardiol 24(4):845–899, 1994.

2. Willich SN, Lewis M, Lowel H, et al: Physical exertion as a trigger of acute myocardial infarction. N Engl J Med 329:1684–1690, 1993.
3. Mittleman MA, Maclure M, Tofler GH, et al: Triggering of acute myocardial infarction by heavy physical exertion: Protection against triggering by regular exertion. N Engl J Med 329:1677–1683, 1993.
4. American College of Sports Medicine Position Stand. Exercise for patients with coronary artery disease. Med Sci Sports Exerc 26(3):i–v, 1994.
5. Clausen JP: Circulatory adjustments to dynamic exercise and effects of physical training in normal subjects and in patients with coronary artery disease. *In* Sonnenblick EH, Lesch M (eds): Exercise and Heart Disease. New York, Grune & Stratton, 1977, pp. 39–75.
6. Lazarus B, Cullinane E, Thompson PD: Comparison of the results and reproducibility of arm and leg exercise tests in men with angina pectoris. Am J Cardiol 47:1075–1079, 1981.
7. Yasue H, Omote S, Takizawa A, et al: Circadian variations of exercise capacity in patients with Prinzmetal's variant angina: Role of exercise-induced coronary artery spasm. Circulation 59:938–948, 1979.
8. Gordon JB, Ganz P, Nabel EG, et al: Atherosclerosis influences the vasomotor response of epicardial coronary arteries to exercise. J Clin Invest 83:1946–1952, 1989.
9. Clausen JP, Tm-Jensen J: Heart rate and arterial blood pressure during exercise in patients with angina pectoris: Effects of training and of nitroglycerin. Circulation 53:436–442, 1976.
10. Franklin BA: Exercise training and coronary collateral circulation. Med Sci Sports Exerc 23:648–653, 1991.
11. Tran ZV, Brammell HL: Effects of exercise training on serum lipid and lipoprotein levels in post-MI patients. A meta-analysis. J Cardiopulm Rehabil 9:250–255, 1989.
12. Emery CF, Pinder SI, Blumenthal JA: Psychological effects of exercise among elderly cardiac patients. J Cardiopulm Rehabil 9:46–53, 1989.
13. National Obesity Consensus Conference. Ann Intern Med 100:888–900, 1985.
14. Oldridge NB, Guyait GH, Fischer ME, et al: Cardiac rehabilitation after myocardial infarction: A combined experience of randomized clinical trials. JAMA 260:945–950, 1988.
15. American College of Sports Medicine: ACSM's Guidelines for Exercise Testing and Prescription, 5th ed. Media, PA, Williams & Wilkins, 1995, pp. 177–193.
16. Fletcher GF, Froelicher VF, Hartley LH, et al: Exercise standards: A statement for health professionals from the American Heart Association. Circulation 82:2286–2322, 1990.
17. American College of Sports Medicine Position Stand. The recommended quantity and quality of exercise for developing and maintaining cardiorespiratory and muscular fitness, and flexibility in healthy adults. Med Sci Sports Exerc 30(6):975–991, 1998.
18. Leitch JW, Klein GJ, Yee R, et al: Prognostic value of electrophysiology testing in asymptomatic patients with Wolff-Parkinson-White pattern. Circulation 82:1718–1723, 1990.
19. Bjorstad H, Storstein L, Meen HD, et al: Ambulatory electrocardiographic findings in top athletes, athletic students and control subjects. Cardiology 84:42–50, 1994.
20. Garson A Jr, MacDonald D II, Fournier A, et al: The Long QT syndrome in children: An international study of 287 patients. Circulation 87:1866–1872, 1993.
21. Van Camp SP, Bloor CM, Mueller FO, et al: Nontraumatic sports death in high school and college athletes. Med Sci Sports Exerc 27:641–647, 1995.
22. Siscovick DS, Weiss NS, Fletcher R, et al: The incidence of primary cardiac arrest during vigorous exercise. N Engl J Med 311:874–877, 1984.
23. Maron BJ, Shirani J, Poliac LC, et al: Sudden death in young competitive athletes: Clinical, demographic, and pathologic profiles. JAMA 276:199–204, 1996.
24. Maron BJ: Cardiovascular risks to young persons on the athletic field. Ann Intern Med 129:379–386, 1998.
25. Waller BF, Roberts WC: Sudden death while running in conditioned runners age 40 years or over. Am J Cardiol 45:1292–1300, 1980.
26. Maron BJ, Shiriani J, Mueller FO, et al: Cardiovascular causes of "athletic field" deaths: analysis of sudden death in 84 competitive athletes. Circulation 88(Suppl I):I–50, 1993.
27. Fuller CM, McNulty CM, Spring DA, et al: Prospective screening of 5,615 high school athletes for risk of sudden cardiac death. Med Sci Sports Exerc 29:1131–1138, 1997.
28. Maron BJ, Thompson PD, Puffer JC, et al: Cardiovascular preparticipation screening of competitive athletes: A statement for health professionals from the Sudden Death Committee (clinical cardiology) and Congenital Cardiac Defects Committee (cardiovascular disease in the young), American Heart Association. Circulation 94:850–856, 1996.
29. McGrew CA: Insight into the AHA scientific statement concerning cardiovascular preparticipation screening of competitive athletes. Med Sci Sports Exerc 30(10):S351–S353, 1998.

V The Athlete with Chronic Obstructive Pulmonary Disease

MARK NIEDFELDT, M.D.

The incidence of chronic obstructive pulmonary disease (COPD) is extremely low in athletes. However, chronic lung diseases in the category of COPD are becoming more common in the United States. Many patients with COPD can benefit from an exercise program. This section describes optimal treatments for patients with COPD and gives an overview of pulmonary rehabilitation.

COPD is present in 14 to 20 million people in the United States, and its prevalence is steadily increasing, especially in women. It is the fourth leading cause of death, and is second among causes of chronic disability. The overall cost of caring for COPD patients is estimated at $40 billion annually.[1] The cost of long-term oxygen alone is estimated at $1.6 billion. Most of the money spent caring for a patient with COPD is spent in the last year of life.[2] It is important for physicians to maximize patients' functional capacity by optimizing their medication regimen, which, along with pulmonary rehabilitation, can help patients to maintain or increase their level of independence and activity.

COPD is a spectrum of chronic bronchitis, emphysema, and associated partially reversible asthmatic components that limit bronchial airflow. COPD may be thought of as accelerated lung aging, with the patient losing lung capacity at a faster than normal rate. The natural course of the disease is progressive deterioration.

The overwhelming cause of COPD is tobacco smoke, which causes an accelerated decline in forced expiratory volume (FEV_1). Over 15 percent of smokers will progress to COPD. Most of these smokers will have a 20 pack-year (1 pack per day for 20 years) or greater history of smoking. Passive or "second-hand" smoke also increases the symptoms of COPD. Approximately 1 percent of patients may have α_1-antitrypsin deficiency, which can accelerate lung damage.[3] COPD patients also are at higher risk of developing several forms of lung cancer independent of their tobacco exposure.[4]

CLINICAL EVALUATION

COPD progresses gradually from no symptoms to periods of mild symptoms, often misinterpreted as natural aging. The patient often initially notices dyspnea when engaging in a physical challenge such as stair climbing. As the disease progresses, lower levels of exertion cause respiratory distress. Continued progression leads to constant dyspnea, even at rest. The avoidance of activity leads to physical deconditioning, which causes increased dyspnea both at rest and with activity, and a vicious circle develops. The patient experiences chest tightness, wheezing, cough with frequent purulent secretions, claustrophobia, depression, anxiety, and insomnia. Other organ systems decompensate from tissue hypoxia and malnutrition.[3] Malnutrition is associated with severe COPD and

is caused by increased caloric demands from the work of breathing along with a decreased appetite. Patients with low body weight have been found to have higher mortality and morbidity rates. They also experience more dyspnea and reduced exercise capacity due to a reduction in both peripheral muscle mass and diaphragmatic muscle mass that follows decreased calorie intake and malnutrition.[5]

Acute exacerbations of bronchitis are common in the latter stages of COPD and are characterized by airway inflammation, infection, purulent mucous blockage, and airway remodeling. *Hemophilus influenzae, Streptococcus pneumoniae,* and *Moraxella catarrhalis* frequently colonize patients. These bacteria are responsible for about 70 percent of disease exacerbations.[3]

TREATMENT

COPD is basically a self-inflicted disease. The most important first step is to stop the self-destruction by stopping smoking. Second-hand smoke should be avoided.[6] Other bronchial irritants such as dust, molds, paints, and solvents should also be avoided.

Patients with chronic lung diseases are at increased risk of serious complications and exacerbations from influenza infection and should receive the influenza vaccine yearly. Pneumococcal vaccine is also recommended for this population as a preventive measure.[3]

Medications

Medication strategy must be viewed over the long term. Physicians and patients must plan for both disease progression and frequent exacerbations. A stepwise and systematic approach has been recommended for adding and deleting medications.

Ipratropium bromide suppresses vagally medicated airway smooth muscle contraction and reduces mucus secretion. It is as effective and lasts longer than beta agonists but is slower in onset. Ipratropium also diminishes sputum production without altering viscosity. It is well tolerated when taken regularly and has not demonstrated attenuation. It is often used as a first-line agent in the treatment of COPD. It is not intended for use as a rescue medication.[7]

Short-acting beta agonists, such as albuterol, are bronchodilators used for intermittent relief of symptomatic bronchospasm and bronchial edema. These medications are typically used on an as-needed basis because recent studies have shown that regular use leads to developing tolerance.[8] The long-acting beta agonist salmeterol is available for suppressing nocturnal symptoms. Salmeterol is not intended as a rescue medication because of its slower onset and longer duration of action. Beta agonists are especially helpful when administered prior to an exercise session.[9]

Theophylline is a weak bronchodilator that moderately increases the strength of contraction of both respiratory and other muscles. It promotes collateral ventilation and mucociliary clearance, and it may have an anti-inflammatory effect. Theophylline also tends to prevent morning dyspnea.[10] The problem with theophylline is that its toxicity range overlaps its therapeutic range, and blood levels need to be monitored. Theophylline is mainly used in patients who are unable to adhere to a regimen of inhaled medications.

Corticosteroids have been utilized for both short-term exacerbation rescue and long-term maintenance. The short-term (i.e., 5 to 7 days) use of high-dose oral steroids for acute exacerbations can bring dramatic relief of symptoms at minimal risk of side effects. Inhaled steroids are the choice when long-term maintenance therapy is needed because of the side effects of long-term oral corticosteroids.[11]

Antibiotics are used during exacerbations in response to early signs the patient may exhibit, such as worsening dyspnea and purulent sputum. Initially, patients may respond to older antibiotics, but after several exacerbations, newer antibiotics may be needed.

Supplemental oxygen can be of great benefit to a subset of patients. The parameters are generally a pulse oximetry reading of less than 88 percent or a PaO_2 less than or equal to 55 mm Hg at rest. Some patients may need oxygen only during exertion. It is also helpful during meals for patients who experience oxygen desaturation while eating and may improve appetite.[2]

Pulmonary Rehabilitation

The primary goal of rehabilitation is to restore the patient to the highest possible level of independent function and reduce disability from disease. This is accomplished by helping patients to increase their activity through exercise training and to re-

duce and gain control of their symptoms. Major objectives of pulmonary rehabilitation are to control, alleviate, and, if possible, reverse the symptoms and pathophysiologic processes leading to respiratory impairment to improve the quality and prolong the length of the patient's life.[12] Pulmonary rehabilitation has been shown to improve exercise capacity, improve quality of life, decrease dyspnea, and decrease the number of hospitalizations.[13, 14] Most pulmonary rehabilitation programs are multidisciplinary, using the skills of several areas including physical therapists, respiratory therapists, exercise physiologists, dietitians, and psychologists for the benefit of the patient. Prior to starting a pulmonary rehabilitation program, the patient should have the disease under maximal medical control.

Exercise training builds endurance and strength while effectively reducing dyspnea and raising the patient's tolerance for activity. This helps the patient gain confidence, relieves anxiety, and increases the patient's ability to tolerate activities of daily living.[14] The exercise prescription for COPD patients should be individualized. The mode of exercise can be any mode of aerobic exercise training that involves large muscle groups. Walking is highly recommended because it is the basis of movement and activities of daily living. Alternative modes that can be used include cycling and rowing. The arm ergometer is included in many exercise programs because it may help increase arm endurance and decrease dyspnea during upper extremity use. It may also have a direct effect on ventilation. The frequency of exercise is based on individual needs. The recommended minimum goal for exercise frequency is 3 to 5 days per week. Individuals with lower functional capacity may require daily exercise training for optimal improvement. There is no consensus as to the optimal intensity of exercise training. Patients are often started at a level approximately 50 percent of maximal exertion. This corresponds to a level of moderate on the perceived exertion scale. At this level adherence will be maximized, especially with new exercisers. COPD patients often should be supervised during early exercise sessions so that the intensity or mode of exercise can be adjusted appropriately. The minimum goal for exercise duration is 20 to 30 minutes of continuous activity. At the beginning of the exercise program, the patient may not be able to achieve this goal. Therefore, intermittent exercise may need to be used initially until the patient can sustain prolonged exertion.[15] Weight training has also been shown both to increase strength in the exercised muscle groups and to increase general endurance.[16]

Many pulmonary rehabilitation programs will also use ventilatory muscle training, teach breathing techniques, and provide educational and psychological support programs for patients and their families.

When to Refer

The advanced COPD patient may need to be referred to a pulmonologist for optimization of the treatment regimen if exacerbations are severe or increasing in frequency. Referral is also generally needed for the patient to engage in a pulmonary rehabilitation program.

Return to Practice and Competition

The goal of most patients with COPD is simply to return to or maintain their activities of daily living.

Key Points

- Patients with COPD can benefit from a comprehensive exercise training program which can increase their ability to tolerate activities of daily living, reduce anxiety, and decrease dyspnea.
- The medical management of COPD should be optimized prior to starting a pulmonary rehabilitation program.
- The primary goal of pulmonary rehabilitation is to restore the patient to the highest possible level of independent function and reduce disability from disease.

REFERENCES

1. Celli BR, Snider GL, Heffer J, et al: Standards for the diagnosis and care of patients with COPD. Am J Respir Crit Care Med 152(suppl 5):S78–S121, 1995.
2. Odonohue WJ Jr, Plummer AL: Magnitude of usage and cost of home oxygen therapy in the United States. Chest 107:301–302, 1995.
3. Tiep BL: Disease management of COPD with pulmonary rehabilitation. Chest 112:1639–1656, 1997.
4. Anthonisen NR, Connett JE, Kiley JP, et al: Effects of smoking intervention and the use of an inhaled anticholinergic bronchodilator on the rate of decline of FEV_1: The Lung Health Study. JAMA 292:1427–1505, 1994.
5. Ferreira IM, Verreschi IT, Nery LE, et al: The influence of 6 months of oral anabolic steroids on body mass and respiratory muscles in undernourished COPD patients. Chest 114:19–28, 1998.
6. American Thoracic Society. Cigarette smoking and health: Official statement of the American Thoracic Society. Am J Respir Crit Care Med 153:825–833, 1996.
7. Rennard SI, Serby CW, Ghafouri M, et al: Extended therapy with ipratropium is associated with improved lung function in patients with COPD: A retrospective analysis of data from seven clinical trials. Chest 110:62–70, 1996.
8. Georgopoulos D, Wong D, Anthonisen NR: Tolerance to beta$_2$-agonists in patients with chronic obstructive pulmonary disease. Chest 97:280–284, 1990.
9. Belman MJ, Botnick WC, Shin JW: Inhaled bronchodilators reduce dynamic hyperinflation during exercise in patients with chronic obstructive respiratory disease. Am J Respir Crit Care Med 153:967–975, 1996.
10. Kidney J, Dominguez M, Taylor PM, et al: Immunodulation by theophylline in asthma: Demonstration by withdrawal of therapy. Am J Respir Crit Care Med 151:1907–1914, 1995.
11. Decramer M, Stas KJ: Corticosteroid induced myopathy involving respiratory muscles in patients with chronic obstructive pulmonary disease or asthma. Am Rev Respir Dis 93:800–802, 1992.
12. ACCP/AACVPR Pulmonary Rehabilitation Guidelines Panel. Pulmonary rehabilitation: Joint AACP/AACVPR evidence-based guidelines. Chest 112:1363–1396, 1997.
13. Reardon J, Awad E, Normandin E, et al: The effect of comprehensive outpatient pulmonary rehabilitation on dyspnea. Chest 105:1046–1052, 1994.
14. Ries AL, Kaplan RM, Limberg TM, et al: Effects of pulmonary rehabilitation on physiologic and psychosocial outcomes in patients with chronic obstructive pulmonary disease. Ann Intern Med 122:823–832, 1995.
15. American College of Sports Medicine. ACSM's Guidelines for Exercise Testing and Prescription, 5th Ed. Media, PA, Williams & Wilkins, 1995, 194–205.
16. Simpson K, Killian K, McCartney N, et al: Randomized controlled trial of weightlifting exercise in patients with chronic airflow limitation. Thorax 4770–4775, 1992.

VI Seizure Disorders and Athletics

MARK NIEDFELDT, M.D.

Physicians who treat athletes are mainly concerned with three types of seizures: exercise-induced seizures, seizures that result from a violent injury during athletic performance, and seizures resulting from disorders such as epilepsy. This section reviews seizure disorders in general as well as in the athletic arena.

A seizure is a transient disturbance of cerebral function due to an abnormal paroxysmal neuronal discharge in the brain. It is the result of a shift in the normal balance of excitation and inhibition within the central nervous system.[1] The normal and properly functioning brain is capable of having a seizure under certain circumstances, and individuals have differing degrees of susceptibility to seizures. People can develop chronic seizure disorders, most often following penetrating head trauma.

Epilepsy, defined as two or more unprovoked seizures, describes a condition in which a person has recurrent seizures due to a chronic underlying process.[2] Epilepsy is common, developing in approximately 1 to 2 percent of the population of the United States.[1] The seizures tend to be episodic, and there may be months or even years between seizures, depending on circumstances or precipitating factors. Epilepsy has several causes. Idiopathic epilepsy usually presents with the onset of seizures between the ages of 5 and 20 years but may start later in life. No specific cause can be found and no other neurologic abnormality can be identified. Symptomatic epilepsy, on the other hand, may be caused by congenital abnormalities and perinatal injuries, metabolic disorders or changes (i.e., hypoglycemia, alcohol withdrawal), trauma (especially in young adults), tumors and other space-occupying lesions (middle to later life), vascular disease (older age group), degenerative disorders, and infectious disease (i.e., meningitis, brain abscess).[1]

CLASSIFICATION OF SEIZURES

Seizures are divided into groups on the basis of the region of the brain affected. Those affecting only part of the brain are known as partial sei-

zures. Partial or focal seizures arise from a restricted region of the cerebral cortex. The initial clinical and electroencephalographic (EEG) manifestations of partial seizures show that only a restricted part of one cerebral hemisphere has been activated. The manifestations of a partial seizure depend on the area of the brain involved. Partial seizures are subdivided into simple seizures, during which consciousness is preserved; complex seizures, during which consciousness is impaired; and partial seizures with secondary generalization, which lead to tonic, clonic, or tonic-clonic seizures. Seizures arising from all regions of the cerebral cortex simultaneously are known as generalized seizures. Generalized seizures and their manifestations are instantaneous and show widespread involvement.[2]

Partial Seizures

In partial seizures, the seizure behavior observed depends on the region of the cerebral cortex initially involved in the paroxysmal discharge. The behavior or experience may involve the sensory, motor, affective, autonomic, or visual neural systems.

Simple partial seizures present without obvious alteration of consciousness and may be manifested by focal motor symptoms such as convulsive jerking or somatosensory symptoms such as tingling that can spread to other parts of the limb or body, depending on their cortical representation. In some instances, special sensory symptoms such as light flashes or buzzing indicate involvement of visual, auditory, olfactory, or gustatory regions of the brain. There may also be autonomic symptoms or signs. When psychic symptoms occur, they are usually accompanied by impairment of consciousness, but the sole manifestations of some seizures are phenomena such as dysphasia, dysmnestic symptoms (i.e., déjà vu, jamais vu), affective disturbances, illusions, or structured hallucinations.

Complex partial seizures are characterized by focal seizure activity accompanied by a transient impairment of the patient's ability to maintain normal contact with the environment. These seizures may cause impaired consciousness and are frequently preceded by auras. The patient is often amnestic for the actual seizure episode. These seizures can be preceded, accompanied, or followed by the psychic symptoms, automatisms, or some of the other symptoms mentioned for simple seizures.

A *partial seizure with secondary generalization* can be difficult to distinguish from a generalized seizure. Often bystanders identify only the dramatic tonic-clonic activity. A thorough history will reveal a localized occurrence or pending aura, which identify a simple partial seizure. Often, the diagnosis can be made only through careful EEG analysis.

Generalized Seizures

Absence (petit mal) seizures are characterized by sudden, brief lapses of consciousness, sometimes with mild clonic, tonic, or atonic components; autonomic components (enuresis); or accompanying automatisms. Onset and termination of events are abrupt, with the episode often lasting only a few seconds. For example, the patient may miss a few words during conversation or break off in mid sentence for a few seconds. The patient is often unaware of these lapses, which can occur hundreds of times daily. Unexplained "daydreaming" and decline in school performance often initiate the investigation. Absence seizures almost always begin in childhood and frequently cease by the age of 20 years. However, other forms of generalized seizures occasionally replace them.

Atypical absence seizures may present with more marked changes in muscular tone. Attacks may have a more gradual onset and termination and more obvious motor signs than typical absence seizures. This type of seizure is often associated with structural abnormalities of the brain and may accompany other neurologic dysfunctions such as mental retardation.

Myoclonic seizures consist of single or multiple myoclonic jerks and are commonly associated with metabolic disorders, degenerative CNS disease, and anoxic brain injury. *Tonic-clonic (grand mal) seizures* are characterized by sudden loss of consciousness. The patient becomes rigid, falls to the ground with arrested respiration, and may become cyanotic. Contraction of the muscles of

respiration and the larynx account for the typical moan. The jaw also contracts and the tongue may be bitten. This tonic phase usually lasts for less than a minute and is followed by a clonic phase lasting for 2 to 3 minutes, which consists of jerking of the body musculature due to alterations in contraction and relaxation of the body musculature. This is followed by a stage of flaccid coma. Postictally, the patient is unresponsive and limp. Bowel or bladder incontinence may occur during this stage along with headache, disorientation, confusion, drowsiness, nausea, soreness of the muscles, or a combination of these symptoms. Some patients have vague premonitory symptoms that should be distinguished from the aura of partial seizures. Variants of the grand mal seizure include pure tonic or clonic seizures. *Atonic seizures* (epileptic drop attacks) are associated with known epileptic syndromes and present with a sudden loss of postural muscle tone lasting 1 or 2 seconds. There may be a brief loss of consciousness, heightening the danger of head injury, but there is no postictal confusion.

CLINICAL FINDINGS

If a patient presents immediately following a seizure, the primary concern is monitoring vital signs, providing respiratory and cardiac support, and initiating treatment if the seizures resume. If the patient presents later, the evaluation focuses on the history of the event. Often the clinical and laboratory findings are normal and the diagnosis is made strictly from the history. The history should be obtained from the patient and, if possible, any observers of the event. If this is the patient's first seizure, it is necessary to determine whether the patient indeed had a seizure, the underlying cause of the event, appropriate treatment for any underlying illness, and whether anticonvulsant medications are needed.

If the patient has a history of seizures, the history focuses on precipitating events and adequacy of anticonvulsant treatment.[3] Specific questions should focus on loss of consciousness, focality, warning signs (aura), incontinence, tongue biting, psychic phenomena (déjà vu, jamais vu, paranoid or hostile feelings), and any hallucinations. The clinician should inquire about prodromal symptoms such as headache, mood alterations, lethargy, and myoclonic jerking, which may have alerted the patient to an impending seizure hours before it occurred. These symptoms are separate from the aura that precedes a generalized seizure by a few seconds or minutes and is actually a part of the seizure, arising locally from a restricted region of the brain. In most patients, seizures are unpredictable and are independent of ongoing activities, but they will occasionally occur at a particular time or in relationship to certain precipitants. Common precipitants are lack of sleep, missed meals, stress, menstruation, alcohol ingestion or withdrawal, and illicit use of drugs. Fever, flashing lights, music, or reading may provoke a seizure in susceptible individuals. The patient or observers should also describe the postictal state if possible. Questions should be asked regarding presence of drowsiness, disorientation, and loss of bowel or bladder continence.

The physical examination includes a search for infection or systemic illness. Signs of head trauma or alcohol and illicit drug ingestion may be present. All patients require a complete neurologic evaluation including mental status, visual fields, and motor and sensory testing. The presence of lateralized or focal signs postictally suggests that the seizure may have a focal origin.[1]

The initial laboratory investigation attempts to rule out the common metabolic causes of seizures: electrolytes, glucose, calcium, magnesium, liver and renal function tests, and complete blood cell count should be ordered. A syphilis screen and toxin screen of the blood or urine should be performed in high-risk groups. Lumbar puncture is indicated if there is any suspicion of meningitis or encephalitis and is mandatory in any patient infected with the human immunodeficiency virus (HIV). These tests help exclude various causes of seizures and provide a baseline for treatment.[2]

EEG is performed to support the diagnosis of epilepsy and may help classify the seizure disorder. This evaluation is important to determine the most appropriate anticonvulsant treatment.

Computed tomography (CT) or magnetic resonance (MR) imaging is indicated for patients with focal neurologic symptoms or signs, focal seizures, or EEG findings of a focal disturbance. MR imaging has been shown to be superior to CT in identification of cortical lesions causing seizures. This type of evaluation should also be performed in patients with clinical evidence of a progressive disorder and in those presenting with seizures after the age of 30, as the chance of neoplasm is increased in these groups. A chest radiograph may also be taken in these patients, as the lungs are a common site for primary or secondary neoplasms. Positron emission tomography (PET) and single photon emission computed tomography (SPECT) are functional imaging studies that can be used to evaluate certain patients, especially those with medically refractive seizures.

DIFFERENTIAL DIAGNOSIS

Transient ischemic attacks (TIAs) are distinguished from partial seizures by their longer duration, lack of spread, and symptomatology. TIAs lead to loss of motor or sensory function, and seizures lead to convulsive jerking or paresthesias. *Rage attacks* are usually situational and lead to goal-directed aggressive behavior. *Panic attacks* can be difficult to distinguish from simple or complex partial seizures unless there is evidence of psychopathologic disturbances between attacks and unless the attacks have a clear relationship to external circumstances.

Generalized seizures can be confused with several conditions as well. *Syncopal episodes* usually occur in relation to postural change, emotional stress, instrumentation, pain, or straining and are typically preceded by pallor, sweating, nausea, and malaise. The loss of consciousness is accompanied by flaccidity. Recovery is rapid with recumbency, and there is no postictal headache or confusion. Serum creatine kinase is elevated for 3 hours after a tonic-clonic seizure but is normal after syncope.[1] *Cardiac dysrhythmias* causing cerebral hypoperfusion are more common in older patients with known vascular disease who lose consciousness. Prodromal symptoms are usually absent. If the attacks are related to activity and a systolic murmur is noted on physical examination, aortic stenosis may be present. Holter or event monitoring may be necessary in some cases. *Brain stem ischemia* causing loss of consciousness can be caused by basilar artery migraine and vertebrobasilar vascular disease. Loss of consciousness is preceded or accompanied by other brain stem signs. A *pseudoseizure* simulating epileptic seizure denotes both hysterical conversion reaction and malingering. Many of these patients have true seizures as well or a family history of epilepsy. The pseudoseizures tend to occur at times of emotional stress. These attacks superficially resemble tonic-clonic seizures, but generally there is no tonic phase. Asynchronous thrashing of the limbs and goal-directed behavior (shouting, swearing) often occurs. Postictally, there are no changes in behavior, neurologic findings, or EEG tracings. The serum prolactin level increases dramatically between 15 and 30 minutes following a tonic-clonic convulsion in most patients, and this can help distinguish real events from false ones.[2]

TREATMENT

Drug treatment is prescribed with the goal of preventing further attacks and is usually continued until there have been no seizures for at least 3 years. The drug initiated for treatment depends on the type of seizure to be treated. The dosage of the drug is increased gradually until seizures are controlled, blood levels reach the upper limit of the therapeutic range, or side effects prevent further increases. If seizures continue despite treatment at the maximal tolerated dose, a second drug is added and its dose increased until blood levels are in the therapeutic range. At this point, the first drug may be withdrawn gradually. It is necessary to monitor complete blood cell counts and liver function tests while patients are taking anticonvulsant medications.[4] Exercise does not affect the metabolism anticonvulsant medications, and no special precautions are needed in prescribing anticonvulsants for athletes.[5] However, some side effects of anticonvulsant drugs are more problematic for athletes. Many anticonvulsants may cause ataxia, dizziness, sedation, or incoordination which may obviously cause problems during athletic participation (Table 21–17).

Special Concerns

Alcohol withdrawal seizures are tonic-clonic seizures which may occur within 48 hours of withdrawal of alcohol after a period of high or chronic intake. Treatment with anticonvulsants is generally not required because this type of seizure is generally self-limited.

Exercise-induced seizures occur during exercise or in the immediate postexercise period. This type of seizure is infrequent and may be associated with the metabolic disturbances that occur during prolonged exercise such as a marathon or triathlon. Any athlete who has a new-onset seizure during exercise should have a complete neurologic evaluation. An exercise EEG may be needed, especially if the baseline EEG is normal. This diagnosis should be considered in the assessment of any athlete experiencing exercise-induced syncope.[6]

Posttraumatic seizures may occur immediately after impact or within the first 24 hours of head trauma. Early seizures occur within the first week and often are accompanied by prolonged posttraumatic amnesia (over 24 hours), depressed skull fracture, or acute intracranial hematoma. Late seizures occur within the first year and are often caused by depressed skull fracture, acute intracranial hematoma, or early epilepsy.

Tonic-clonic *status epilepticus* is a medical emergency and refers to continuous seizures or repetitive discrete seizures with impaired consciousness in the interictal period lasting 15 to 30 minutes. Poor adherence to anticonvulsant drug regimen is the most common cause, but status epilepticus is also seen following head trauma, metabolic disturbances, drug toxicity, or with CNS infection. The mortality rate may be as high as 20 percent, and the incidence of neurologic and mental sequelae is high. The prognosis depends on the length of time between the onset of status epilepticus and the start of effective treatment. Initial management includes maintenance of the airway and 50 percent dextrose IV. If seizures continue, 10 mg of diazepam IV is given over 2 minutes and repeated in 10 minutes if there is no response. Phenytoin (20 mg/kg) is given IV at a rate of 50 mg/min. Do not administer in a glucose-containing solution because it will precipitate. Electrocardiographic monitoring should be in place to follow the cardiac arrhythmias that can be caused by phenytoin. In some institutions fosphenytoin, which is converted into phenytoin, is used at the same dose at a rate of 150 mg/min. Fosphenytoin can be given in any solution. These medications can be repeated at 5 to 10 mg/kg if the seizures continue after the initial dose. If the seizures continue, phenobarbitol is then given at a dose of 20 mg/kg IV at a rate of 50 to 100 mg/min. This can be repeated at 5 to 10 mg/min. Patients who are still seizing after this treatment are admitted to an ICU, and coma is induced.[4]

When to Refer

After an initial seizure the patient should be referred to a neurologist for an EEG Any patient with refractory seizures or with poorly controlled

Table 21–17
Commonly Used Anticonvulsant Drugs

Generic Name	Trade Name	Indication	Therapeutic Range	Adverse Effects
Phenytoin	Dilantin	Generalized tonic-clonic, partial	10–20 µg/ml	Nystagmus, ataxia, incoordination, sedation, confusion, gum hyperplasia, lymphadenopathy, hirsutism, osteomalacia, skin rash, hepatotoxicity
Carbamazepine	Tegretol	Generalized tonic-clonic, partial	4–12 µg/ml	Ataxia, dizziness, diplopia, vertigo, nausea, vomiting, aplastic anemia, hepatotoxicity
Valproic acid	Depakane, Depakote	Generalized tonic-clonic, absence, myoclonic	50–150 µg/ml	Ataxia, sedation, tremor, hepatotoxicity, thrombocytopenia, weight gain, nausea, vomiting, transient alopecia
Phenobarbitol	Luminol	Generalized tonic-clonic, partial	10–40 µg/ml	Ataxia, sedation, confusion, dizziness, depression, skin rash
Primidone	Mysoline	Generalized tonic-clonic, partial	4–12 µg/ml	Ataxia, sedation, nystagmus, vertigo, nausea, vomiting, irritability
Febamate	Felbatol	Partial	Not established	Insomnia, dizziness, sedation, headache, anorexia, nausea, vomiting, hepatotoxicity, aplastic anemia; only approved for second-line therapy, blood counts must be performed every 2–4 weeks
Gabapentin	Neurontin	Partial	Not established	Sedation, ataxia, dizziness, fatigue; no known significant drug interactions
Lamotrigine	Lamictal	Partial	Not established	Dizziness, sedation, ataxia, headache, skin rash, visual disturbances
Ethosuximide	Zarontin	Absence, myoclonic	40–100 µg/ml	Ataxia, fatigue, headache, nausea, vomiting, anorexia, skin rash, bone marrow suppression
Clonazepam	Klonopin	Absence, myoclonic	10–70 ng/ml	Ataxia, sedation, lethargy, anorexia

Source: Adapted from Willmore LJ, Ferrendelli JA: Epilepsy. *In* Dale DC, Federman DD (eds): Scientific American Medicine. New York, Scientific American, 1998, 11:XII:1–15; Lowenstein DH: Seizures and epilepsy. *In* Fauci AS, et al (eds): Harrison's Textbook of Internal Medicine, 14th ed. New York, McGraw-Hill Book Co., 1998, pp. 2311–2325; Brodie MJ, Dichter MA: Antiepileptic drugs. N Engl J Med 334:168–175, 1996.

seizures should be referred for a neurology consultation.

Return to Practice and Competition

Athletes with epilepsy may participate in sports. Epileptics are not at increased risk for having seizures during exercise. In fact, the risk of seizure is decreased during exercise.[7] This may be due to the release during exercise of β-endorphins, which tend to inhibit seizures.[8] Regular physical exercise has not been shown to adversely affect pharmacokinetics of antiepileptic drugs.[9] Epileptics whose seizures are under excellent control (no seizures in the past year) or who have been seizure-free for 2 years off medication may be allowed to participate in selected collision and contact

sports.[10] Several factors must be weighted in deciding whether to permit participation in sports, including the risk of death or severe injury if a seizure occurs during sports participation, preexisting brain injury or dysfunction, and potential effects of anticonvulsants on athletic performance. Swimming is often singled out as a sport to avoid for many epileptics. However, swimming is acceptable provided that there is close supervision, preferably by a trained lifeguard who has been informed of the participant's condition.[3]

Key Points

- The normal brain is capable of having a seizure under certain circumstances.

- Partial seizures affect only part of the brain and manifestations depend on the area of the brain involved; generalized seizures affect the entire brain and are characterized by sudden, brief losses of consciousness, sometimes with clonic, tonic, or atonic components.
- Exercise-induced seizures occur during exercise or in the immediate postexercise period and may be associated with metabolic disturbances from prolonged exercise.
- Athletes with epilepsy may participate in sports and are not at increased risk for having a seizure during exercise.
- If seizures are under excellent control, some athletes may be allowed to participate in some collision or contact sports.

REFERENCES

1. Willmore LJ, Ferrendelli JA: Epilepsy. *In* Dale DC, Federman DD (eds): Scientific American Medicine. New York, Scientific American, 1998, pp. 1–15.
2. Lowenstein DH: Seizures and epilepsy. *In* Fauci AS, et al. (eds): Harrison's Textbook of Internal Medicine 14th ed. McGraw-Hill Book Co. New York, 1998, pp. 2311–2325.
3. Cantu R: Epilepsy and athletics. Clin Sports Med 17(1): 61–69, 1998.
4. Brodie MJ, Dichter MA: Antiepileptic drugs. N Engl J Med 334:168–175, 1996.
5. Nakken KO, Bjorholt PG, Johannessen SI, et al: Effect of physical training on aerobic capacity, seizure occurrence, and serum levels of antiepileptic drugs in adults with epilepsy. Epilepsia 31:88–94, 1990.
6. Ogunyemi A, Gomex MR, Klass DW: Seizures induced by exercise. Neurology 38:633–634, 1988.
7. Eriksen HR, Ellertsen B, Gronningsaeter H, et al: Physical exercise in women with intractable epilepsy. Epilegia 35:1256–1264, 1994.
8. van Linschoten R, Backx FJG, Mulder OGM, et al: Epilepsy and sports. Sports Med 19:9–19, 1990.
9. Gates JR: Epilepsy and sports participation. Phys Sports Med 19:98–104, 1991.
10. American Academy of Pediatrics Committee on Children with Handicaps: Sports and the child with epilepsy. Pediatrics 72:884–885, 1983.

VII The Role of Exercise and Athletics in Anxiety and Depression

MARK NIEDFELDT, M.D.

Exercise is increasingly seen as a remedy for depression and anxiety disorders in the entire population. Exercise can complement traditional treatments such as psychotherapy and medications in patients who are displaying symptoms of depression and anxiety and can also be preventive in those who do not have an illness. This section addresses the diagnosis and treatment of depression and anxiety disorders as well as the role of exercise in the management of these disorders.

Depression is the most common psychiatric diagnosis in the primary care setting. Lifetime incidence of depression is estimated to be approximately 5 percent for men and 10 percent for women.[1] An estimated 15 percent of those with severe depression will commit suicide.[2] This is especially alarming because 80 percent of those suffering from depression can be treated successfully.[3] Only about one third of people suffering from depression seek medical or psychiatric care:

most of those who seek help are seen by primary care physicians.[4] Depression may also increase vulnerability to other disease.[5] In the elderly, depression is responsible for more hospitalizations than any other disorder except cardiovascular disease, and it leads to increased mortality and morbidity rates.[6]

Although depression is fairly well recognized in women and older people, it may not be recognized as readily in athletes of either sex. Many athletes face enormous pressures from coaches, teammates, parents, and fans. If the athlete does not have adequate coping mechanisms, depression may develop. Overtraining in athletes may also lead to symptoms of depression and a decrease in performance.[7]

Anxiety and panic disorders affect up to 3 to 5 percent of the population.[8] The generalized anxiety disorder usually has its initial manifestations between the ages of 20 to 35 years with a slight predominance of women affected. A panic attack is a discrete period of intense fear or discomfort occurring in an unusual way. Most attacks last less than 1 hour.[9] Panic disorder is characterized by four unexpected intense, short-lived attacks of severe anxiety accompanied by significant physiologic disturbances in 1 month followed by at least 1 month of persistent fear of having another attack.[8] It is most often first seen before age 25, tends to be familial, and has a 2:1 female-to-male ratio. Women may be especially vulnerable during the premenstrual period.[10] Many patients with these disorders undergo work-ups for other medical problems prior to the diagnosis being made. Both anxiety and panic disorders can lead to depression, suicide, and substance abuse in an attempt to self-medicate. Anxiety and panic attacks may occur in athletes. The symptoms can range from mild "butterflies" or hyperventilation to full-blown panic attacks. Performance anxiety is not considered abnormal unless it progresses to a panic attack.

CLINICAL EVALUATION

Depressed patients often exhibit several diagnostic symptoms. These symptoms include depressed mood, loss of interest in activities, weight loss or gain, sleep disturbance, fatigue, guilt, poor concentration, decreased ability to think or concentrate, and recurrent thoughts of suicide or death.[8] These symptoms may cause significant distress or functional impairment. In athletes, a common complaint is fatigue. The patient may present as tired, nervous, irritable, or angry. Physical examination may find little or no physical pathology, but if any physical problem is present, the patient is often preoccupied with his/her illness and the symptoms are often out of proportion to the severity of the illness.[11]

Symptoms of the anxiety disorders include apprehension, irritability, and hypervigilance along with somatic complaints generally attributable to the autonomic nervous system: tachycardia, hyperventilation, palpitations, sweating, and tremor. Gastrointestinal complaints are also common. These symptoms are long-lasting and persistent for at least 1 month.[8]

Laboratory testing can be done to rule out other diseases that may mimic anxiety and depression, including hyperthyroidism, hyperparathyroidism, pheochromocytoma, seizure disorders,

cardiac arrhythmias, and vestibular dysfunction. Thyroid function studies, complete blood cell count, and chemistry panel will help rule out occult disease. An electrocardiogram may help rule out any cardiac arrhythmia or ischemia in patients over age 45.

TREATMENT

The mainstays of treatment of depression have traditionally been pharmacotherapy, psychotherapy, especially outpatient psychotherapy including cognitive behavior therapy and interpersonal therapy, and electroconvulsive therapy (ECT) in resistant cases. This chapter will not discuss ECT but will cover the promising role of exercise in managing depression and anxiety disorders.

Pharmacotherapy

The main focus of pharmacotherapy at the time of this writing is selective serotonin reuptake inhibitors (SSRIs). This class of medications has an advantage over other classes of drugs owing to a lower side-effect profile, especially on the cardiac and central nervous systems. Generally, the SSRIs are the drugs of choice for exercising patients with depression. These medications are also being used for anxiety disorders, including panic disorder. This class appears to have no negative effects on cardiac conduction or cardiac output. Common side effects include nausea and diarrhea, which are often self-limited.[12] Although some patients may also experience insomnia, this is usually self-limited.[13] Patients do not develop dependency on SSRIs. Venlafaxine (Effexor) appears to have a side-effect profile similar to the SSRIs.[14]

The tricyclic antidepressants have been used for years in the treatment of depression, anxiety, and panic disorders. However, these medications have anticholinergic side effects, such as dry mouth, which may be annoying to exercising individuals. They may also be dangerous for athletes because of repolarization effects when the heart rate is increased.[15] There does not seem to be any decrease in cardiac output from tricyclics, but a modest self-limiting increase in heart rate may be noted. Dizziness or orthostatic hypotension may occur, so patients must be aware of possible dehydration.[2] Sedation and fatigue along with tremor and myoclonus are also seen, which may be particularly distressing to patients who participate in precision sports. Urinary retention and constipation are common, as is weight gain. If a tricyclic antidepressant needs to be used, desipramine and nortriptyline produce the fewest side effects.[16]

Benzodiazepines are used in the treatment of anxiety. Patients can become dependent in less than 2 weeks on medications in this class, although the low-potency benzodiazepines may have less abuse potential. The major side effects are sedation and psychomotor impairment. Some patients may also experience fatigue, ataxia, amnesia, or slurred speech. These side effects lessen as tolerance develops.

Psychotherapy

Psychotherapy for depression and anxiety may focus on several areas including behavioral, cognitive, assertive, relaxation, mental imaging, and desensitization therapies. Therapy may define the stresses that precipitate the disorder, the patient's self-esteem level, and support systems.

Exercise

Exercise as remedy for depression and anxiety has recently drawn increased attention. Exercise has many advantages over traditional therapies. It is relatively inexpensive, can be done by most patients, and has fewer side effects than most medications.[17] Activity level has been shown to be inversely correlated to various measures of depressive symptoms, independent of the effects of education and physical health status.[18] This correlation is especially strong in women over age 40. Women who report low physical activity levels are especially vulnerable to high levels of depressive symptoms.[19] Increased physical activity is associated with higher perceived levels of meaningfulness of life and better subjective health in the elderly. Patients generally report less anxiety, more energy, and better life satisfaction.[20] Many of the positive effects of exercise on depression may stem from the social interaction that takes place in many exercise programs.[17]

When exercise is compared to psychotherapy, there is often no difference between patients who receive therapy versus those in the exercise group, although there may be even greater benefits if the techniques are combined.[17] Exercise seems bene-

ficial regardless of the type, with resistance exercise appearing to be as effective as aerobic exercise. However, people participating in aerobic exercise show improved conditioning and other cardiovascular benefits as well.[21]

Exercise has also been compared to tricyclic antidepressants and may be as effective as these medications in the treatment of depression.[22] To date, no study has been completed comparing SSRIs and exercise. The degree in improvement in fitness does not seem to correlate to the improvement in depressive symptoms. Patients with minimal fitness gains often exhibit the same psychological improvement as patients who achieve greater gains in fitness.[17]

Exercise may improve depressive symptoms by both biologic and psychological mechanisms. The best known of the major biological mechanisms is the release of endogenous endorphins.[23] These substances have a morphine-like action that reduces pain and induces a state of euphoria. However, high levels of exercise intensity (over 85 percent of maximal oxygen uptake) are necessary to release these substances.[24] Exercise also increases the neurotransmission of some or all of the major brain monoamines, including norepinephrine, dopamine, and serotonin.[25] Depression is often associated with impaired transmission of these substances due to problems in production, transfer, reuptake, and breakdown. Exercise improves transmission of monoamines, which may improve mood. Regular exercise may also lead to increased adrenal steroid reserves, which will be available to counter stress. A final postulated biologic mechanism is based on the theory that temperature changes in the brain stem are thought to cause a more relaxed state. Therefore, the increase in body temperature during exercise may have a short-term tranquilizing effect. This theory is not widely accepted, however.[26]

Psychological mechanisms have also been offered. Depression may be a response to a perceived loss of control. Exercise can provide a sense of mastery and allow patients to regain control of their body and life. Exercise also provides a diversion from unpleasant situations or stressful stimuli.[27] The social interaction of an exercise program may be beneficial, as many depressed individuals tend to isolate themselves. Overall, the perception of fitness may be more important than the actual fitness itself because the perception of fitness has been more closely correlated with increased functioning than actual fitness.[17]

Exercise has also been shown to be helpful in treatment of anxiety for many of the reasons previously mentioned. A specific theory regarding the efficacy of exercise in treatment of anxiety is based on the fact that anxiety and exercise have many similar physical symptoms. Both cause increased perspiration, heart rate, and blood pressure. Because anxiety is associated with emotional and physical distress, the absence of emotional distress during exercise may increase psychological function.[28]

The Exercise Prescription

The type of exercise program chosen will depend on the person's health, level of fitness, and interests. An awareness of potential side effects of medications when exercising is crucial. Exercises that use the large muscle groups are recommended. Sedentary individuals need to begin slowly. Realistic goal setting is important because goals must be attainable. Short-term goals are more realistic than long-term goals. It is important for the patient to experience early success. This will keep them motivated to strive for future goals.[17] The physician needs to set up a program that will allow the patient to progress at a reasonable pace. It is often helpful to have the patient enroll in an organized exercise program such as those offered at recreational departments, YMCAs, or athletic clubs. These programs can help give the patient the social component of exercise that can be beneficial as well as a structured program that may reduce the possibility of injury and attrition. Once short-term goals are met, the physician can help the patient progress to a more idealistic exercise prescription. In the elderly or in many sedentary individuals, emphasis may be placed on non–weight-bearing or minimal weight-bearing activities to avoid injury. Exercise in water, stationary cycling, and walking are excellent activities for this population. The most common reason for cessation of an exercise program is injury. Most injuries are of the overuse type and are often avoidable.[29]

The goal exercise prescription will involve exercise three to five times a week for 30 to 40 minutes plus 5 to 10 minutes each of warm-up and cool-down activities. The main exercise should be performed at 60 to 70 percent of maximal heart rate. The exercise itself should be challenging but not self-defeating. Resistance exercise can be included in the exercise prescription, but aerobic exercise should be the mainstay of the program so patients can also gain cardiovascular benefits.[30]

When to Refer

Referral to a counselor, therapist, psychologist, or psychiatrist for psychological therapy may be a good adjunct for many patients with anxiety or depression. Patients who are resistant to first-line pharmacologic treatments may need referral to a psychiatrist for medication prescription or adjustments.

Key Points

- Depression and anxiety disorders are common in the general population, and most of these patients present initially to their primary care physician.
- Athletes are not immune from depression and anxiety disorders.
- Selective seratonin reuptake inhibitors (SSRIs) tend to have the lowest side effect profile for active individuals.
- Exercise may be as useful as other treatment modalities in treating depression.
- It is important for patients to experience early success in their exercise program in order to adhere to the program.

REFERENCES

1. Kessler RC, McGonagle KA, Zhao S, et al: Lifetime and 12-month prevalence of DSM-III-R psychiatric disorders in the United States: results from the National Comorbidity Survey. Arch Gen Psychiatry 51:8–19, 1994.
2. Artal M: Exercise against depression. Phys Sportsmed 26(10):55–60, 1998.
3. Potter WZ, Rudorfer MV, Manji H: The pharmacologic treatment of depression. N Engl J Med 325(9):633–642, 1991.
4. Martinsen EW: Physical activity and depression: Clinical experience. Acta Psychiatr Scand 377(suppl):23–27, 1994.
5. Wells KB, Stewart A, Hays RD, et al: The functioning and well-being of depressed patients. JAMA 262:914–919, 1989.
6. Barefoot JC, Schroll M: Symptoms of depression, acute myocardial infarction, and total mortality in a community sample. Circulation 93(11):1976–1980, 1996.
7. Morgan WP, Costill DC, Flynn MG, et al: Mood distur-

bance following increased training in swimmers. Med Sci Sports Exerc 20(4):408–414, 1988.

8. American Psychiatric Association: Diagnostic and Statistical Manual of Mental Disorders, 4th ed. Washington, DC, American Psychiatric Association, 1994.

9. Rubin A, Chassay CM: When anxiety attacks: Treating hyperventilation and panic. Phys Sportsmed 24(12):54–65, 1996.

10. Garssen B, Buikhuisen M, van Dyck R: Hyperventilation and panic attacks. Am J Psychiatry 153(4):513–518, 1996.

11. Smith AM, Stuart MJ, Weise-Bjornstal DM, et al: Competitive athletes: Preinjury and postinjury mood state and self-esteem. Mayo Clin Proc 68:937–947, 1993.

12. Cookson J: Side-effects of antidepressants. Br J Psychiatry 163(suppl 20):20–24, 1993.

13. Settle EC: Antidepressant side-effects: Issues and options. J Clin Psychiatry Monogr 10(1):48–61, 1992.

14. Feighner JP: The role of venlafaxine in rational antidepressant therapy. J Clin Psychiatry 55(suppl A):62–68, 1994.

15. Roose SP, Glassman AH: Cardiovascular effects of tricyclic antidepressants in depressed patients with and without heart disease. J Clin Psychiatry Monogr 7:1–13, 1989.

16. Weinstein RS: Panic disorder. Am Fam Physician 52(7):2055–2063, 1995.

17. Moore KA, Blumenthal JA: Exercise training as an alternative treatment for depression among older adults. Alt Therapies 4:48–56, 1998.

18. Stephens T: Physical activity and mental health in the United States and Canada: Evidence from four population surveys. Prev Med 17:35–47, 1988.

19. Farmer ME, Locke BZ, Moscicki EK, et al: Physical activity and depressive symptoms: The NHANES I epidemiologic follow-up study. Am J Epidemiol 128:1340–1351, 1988.

20. Ruuskanen JM, Ruoppila I: Physical activity and psychological well-being among people aged 65–84 years. Age Aging 24:292–296, 1995.

21. Doyne EJ, Ossip-Klein DJ, Bowman ED, et al: Running versus weight lifting in the treatment of depression. J Consult Clin Psychol 55:748–754, 1987.

22. Martinsen EW, Medhus A, Sabdvik L: Effects of aerobic exercise on depression: A controlled study. Br Med J 291:109, 1985.

23. Casper RC: Exercise and mood. World Rev Nutr Diet 71:58–62, 1993.

24. Nicoloff G, Schwenk TL: Using exercise to ward off depression. Phys Sportsmed 23(9):44–58, 1995.

25. Ransford CP: A role for amines in the antidepressant effects of exercise: A review. Med Sci Sports Exerc 14:1–10, 1982.

26. Morgan WP, O'Connor PJ: Exercise and mental health. *In* Dishman RK (ed): Exercise Adherence: Its Impact on Public Health. Champaign, IL, Human Kinetics, 1988, pp. 91–121.

27. Bahrke MS, Morgan WP: Anxiety reduction following exercise and meditation. Cognit Ther Res 2:323–333, 1978.

28. Breus MJ, O'Connor PJ: Exercise-induced anxiolysis: test of the "time out" hypothesis in high anxious females. Med Sci Sports Exerc 30(7):1107–1112, 1998.

29. Pollock ML, Carroll JF, Graves JE, et al: Injuries and adherence to walk/jog and resistance training programs in the elderly. Med Sci Sports Exerc 23:1194–1200, 1991.

30. Pollack ML, Gaesser GA, Butcher JD, et al: The recommended quantity and quality of exercise for developing and maintaining cardiorespiratory and muscular fitness, and flexibility in healthy adults. Med Sci Sports Exerc 30(6):975–991, 1998.

VIII *The Athlete with Infectious Disease*

MARK NIEDFELDT, M.D.

EXERCISE AND THE IMMUNE SYSTEM

Athletes with concurrent illnesses present special problems for the physician. The standard medical advice in many situations is rest, which may be difficult for many athletes. Guidelines for return to activity should be based on current understanding of the disease and the demands of the athlete's activity. They should also consider the immune system, as exercise may affect bone marrow and lymphoid tissue, leukocytes, antibodies, complement, cytokines, and interferons, which function to recognize, entrap, and destroy invading microbes and tumor cells.[1]

EXERCISE IN PATIENTS WITH INFECTIONS

Athletes and active people may be at greater risk of contracting infectious diseases because of increased exposure. Athletes are often in close contact with other participants; transmission may occur through direct contact, airborne droplets from heavy respiration or coughing, or contact with contaminated objects such as towels, mats, or water bottles.

Fever

Althetes will often ask their physician whether they can exercise when they have a fever. Although a low-grade fever does not cause any problems, a significant fever over 100.4°F (38°C) has a definite effect on exercise. In the respiratory system, airway resistance increases, and diffusion capacity and ratio of alveolar ventilation to pulmonary gas exchange decrease.[2] In the cardiovascular system, heart rate and O_2 consumption increase, whereas blood pressure, peripheral resistance, and resultant maximal workload decrease.[3] Muscles experience premature fatigue and lessening of strength.[4] A higher set point in the hypothalamus puts the athlete at greater risk for dehydration and heat illness. Overall, febrile athletes have impaired endurance, strength, coordination, and concentration, which can lead to injury.[2, 4] Therefore, athletes should generally avoid strenuous activity when their temperatures rise above 100.4°F (38°C).

Viral Respiratory Infections

The common cold is the most prevalent infection in athletes. Rhinoviruses account for 25 to 30 percent of colds, especially in the early fall and mid to late spring months, and coronaviruses are more common in midwinter. Other clinically important viruses include influenza, parainfluenza, and respiratory syncytial viruses. These viruses have multiple strains, so immunity often does not develop.[5] The incubation period is usually 24 to 48 hours. Transmission is person to person either by air or direct contact, making athletes belonging to teams—especially those who travel and are housed together—especially susceptible. Winter athletes are at no increased risk from exposure to the elements.

Clinical Evaluation

The symptoms of a viral respiratory infection are well known. Rhinorrhea, sneezing, mild malaise, and scratchy throat are present. Maximal symptoms on days 2 to 4 of the infection correlate with maximal communicability. Cough and hoarseness may begin later. Total symptomatic time is usually about 1 week, but up to 25 percent of cases last 2 weeks.[5] Some athletes, particularly those with a history of asthma, may develop a bronchospasm that may be exacerbated with exercise, especially in cold, dry conditions.

Treatment

Mild to moderate upper respiratory infections generally do not require interruption of exercise schedules. Althletes with bronchospasm may need to use an inhaler and avoid cold, dry air. Fluids, throat lozenges, and warm saline gargles can be used to relieve symptoms, whereas antipyretics can relieve fever and myalgias. Nasal congestion can be treated with topical or oral decongestants.[6] It is important to remember that the U.S. Olympic Committee (USOC) bans many cold remedies, including over-the-counter medications and cough suppressants such as the topical decongestant phenylephrine and the oral medications pseudoephedrine and phenylpropanolamine. Most of the same medications are acceptable to the National Collegiate Athletic Association (NCAA). Both the USOC and the NCAA ban cough suppressants containing codeine.

Gastroenteritis

Most cases of common gastroenteritis are viral, caused by either rotavirus or Norwalk agent.[7] The diarrhea is generally self-limited, and most patients require only oral hydration. Diarrhea may also be caused by bacteria (traveler's diarrhea). The most common agents are *Campylobacter jejuni,* Salmonella, Shigella, and *E. coli.* Protozoan agents include *Giardia, Entamoeba histolytica,* and Cryptosporidium.[7] These agents can often be avoided by eating only fully cooked meats, and when in foreign countries, avoiding dairy products, lettuce and other raw produce, and tap water.

Treatment

Mild to moderate gastroenteritis requires only supportive treatment with fluids and antidiarrheals. Athletes may participate as long as they are well hydrated and the diarrhea is becoming less frequent. However, more severe cases may lead to dehydration and electrolyte imbalance. Therefore, exercise is not recommended in these cases, especially in warm weather. Kaopectate, an adsorbent that improves stool form, is useful if there is any doubt as to the etiology of the diarrhea. Other antidiarrheals such as loperamide (Imodium) and diphenoxylate hydrochloride (Lomotil) are antimotility agents and should be avoided in suspected bacterial or protozoal infections. Bacterial and protozoal infections can be diagnosed through stool evaluation and are treated with the appropriate antibiotic.

Human Immunodeficiency Virus

The concern of transmission of the human immunodeficiency virus (HIV) during competition has caused many athletes, coaches, parents, athletic trainers, and physicians to contemplate the risks and frequency of blood exposure during athletic competition. When Earvin "Magic" Johnson disclosed in November 1991 that he was infected by the human immunodeficiency virus, the issue rose to the forefront of media and general public attention. Blood exposure during athletic contests is no longer viewed as a sign of toughness but is now viewed as a danger to the other athletes.[8]

Overview

HIV is a retrovirus transmitted through sexual contact or exposure to infected blood or blood products. It infects the CD^{4+} T lymphocytes, leading to gradual deterioration of the body's immune system, increased susceptibility to opportunistic infection, and acquired immune deficiency syndrome (AIDS). With the development of new sensitive tools for monitoring HIV replication in infected people, the risk for disease progression and death can be assessed accurately, and the efficacy of anti-HIV therapies can be determined directly. The ability of more potent drugs to inhibit HIV replication has made it possible to design therapeutic strategies involving combinations of anti-retroviral drugs that accomplish prolonged and near-complete suppression of detectable HIV replication in may HIV-infected people.[9] The more sensitive and reliable measurements of plasma viral load have been demonstrated to be powerful predictors of a person's risk for progression to AIDS and time to death. HIV RNA levels indicate the magnitude of HIV replication and its associated rate of CD^{4+} T-cell destruction, while CD^{4+} T-cell counts indicate the extent of HIV-induced immune damage already suffered.[10]

HIV is present in all body fluids and has been transmitted through blood, semen, vaginal secretions, organ transplants, and breast milk. The most common mechanisms of transmission are sexual intercourse and shared needles. There is no evidence of transmission through saliva, tears, body contact, or sweat.[11]

To date there are no known cases of HIV transmission during sports activities, despite the fact that HIV-positive athletes are continuing to compete. In 1993, 11 such athletes competed in NCAA-sanctioned sporting events.[12] Magic Johnson returned to NBA and Olympic competition. The estimate of risk of HIV transmission during professional football is estimated to be less than 1 in 85 million game contacts.[13] There have, however, been two reports of transmission during bloody fistfights outside the athletic arena.[14, 15] There has also been a report of a body builder who contracted HIV by sharing contaminated needles while injecting anabolic steroids.

In general, athletes are at more risk for HIV infection off the field, engaging in high-risk behaviors. Preventing transmission in athletes consists mainly of education regarding sexual practices and sharing needles. Any exposed skin wounds should be securely covered with bandages or wraps to prevent leakage of blood or serous fluid during the sporting activity. Blood on the skin of an injured athlete and other participants should be washed off immediately with soap and water or a premoistened towelette. The wound should then be properly dressed with an occlusive dressing. Small amounts of dried blood on uniforms or equipment do not constitute a risk for transmission of blood-borne pathogens. Nonabsorbent surfaces exposed to blood should be cleaned with a solution of bleach and water. Athletic trainers and physicians should use disposable gloves when blood is present on athletes or their clothing.[17]

Treatment

Infection with HIV is always harmful, and true long-term survival free of clinically significant immune dysfunction is unusual. Regular, periodic measurements of HIV RNA levels and CD^{4+} T-cell counts are necessary to determine the risk for disease progression and to determine when to initiate or modify antiretroviral treatment regiments. Maximum achievable suppression of HIV replication should be the goal of therapy, using potent combination antiretroviral therapy. The drugs need to be used in combination according to optimal schedules and dosages, and the therapy must be individualized for the patient.[9] Even when the viral loads are below detectable limits, people with HIV infection are still considered infectious. They should continue to avoid behaviors that are associated with transmission of HIV.

There is no medical or public health basis for routine screening of athletes for HIV infection. Athletes need not be excluded from participation in a sports activity solely because they are infected with HIV. Physicians should counsel an HIV-infected athlete about the disease, its course, and the mode of transmission to minimize exposure to any competitors or teammates. The athlete may be encouraged to avoid contact and collision sports due to the risk of possible blood exposure.

Hepatitis B Virus

Hepatitis B virus (HBV) is present in higher concentrations in blood and is more stable in the environment than HIV. There is one reported incident of HBV transmission during sports. The source of the outbreak of hepatitis B among sumo wrestlers in Japan in 1980 was an asymptomatic wrestler who positive for hepatitis B surface antigen and hepatitis B e antigen. The hepatitis B e antigen is associated with higher circulating levels of virus and greater infection rate. Sumo wrestlers have most of their body exposed, and the infected wrestler, who had many scars on his extremities, often bled from injuries while wrestling.[18]

There is no medical or public health basis for routine screening of athletes for HBV infection. The remainder of counseling is the same as for HIV. Athletes with HBV infection need not be excluded from competition but may be encouraged to avoid contact or collision sports.

Currently, most infants and youngsters in the United States are vaccinated against hepatitis B. This should provide protection for the future generation of athletes. Vaccination consists of a series of three injections and is currently recommended for teenagers who were not immunized as children.

Infectious Mononucleosis

Infectious mononucleosis is an acute viral infection most frequently caused by the Epstein-Barr virus (EBV). EBV is a double-stranded DNA virus from the herpesvirus family. Most people are infected with EBV at some point in their lifetime. In younger children the illness is often subclinical, but in young adults the disease tends to be more severe. The virus is reactivated only in immuno-compromised or transplant patients. Other infrequent causes of mononucleosis are cytomegalovirus, HIV, *Toxoplasma gondii,* and human herpesvirus type 6.[19]

EBV is transmitted through direct contact with infected saliva or, rarely, infected blood products or bone marrow. Transmission probably requires prolonged contact with infected oral secretions. The virus is excreted for months, and carriers are often asymptomatic. The incubation period is between 3 and 7 weeks. There is no need to quarantine affected patients.[20]

Clinical Evaluation

The overt illness is most common in adolescents and young adults. A prodome consisting of malaise, fatigue, and low-grade headache lasts 3 to 5 days and is usually followed by a sore throat. Anorexia, chills, nausea, abdominal discomfort, myalgias, and arthralgias may occur. The acute phase of the infection lasts between 1 and 3 weeks and most patients fully recover within 6 to 8 weeks.[21]

Physical findings include a severe pharyngitis that may be exudative with palatal petechiae. Lymphadenopathy can be generalized but typically involves the posterior cervical chain. Splenomegaly is usually present by the second week. Other less common findings include hepatomegaly, jaundice, a rubella-like rash, and periorbital edema.[22]

Heterophil IgM antibody testing (Monospot) confirms the diagnosis of mononucleosis. The sensitivity and specificity of this test is 85 percent and 97 percent, respectively.[19] IgM antibodies to EBV viral capsid antigen antibodies can be detected early in the infection through immunofluorescence. A modest leukocytosis usually occurs during the acute phase with more than 10 percent atypical lymphocytes. Liver function tests may be elevated two- to threefold, and platelet count may be mildly reduced.[20, 22]

Complications are rare but may include autoimmune hemolytic anemia, airway obstruction, Guillain-Barré syndrome, encephalitis, and hepatitis. In exercise and athletics, splenomegaly and the potential for splenic rupture are major concerns. This rare complication has no relation to the severity of mononucleosis or elevation of laboratory values. Trauma is a risk factor for splenic rupture, but most ruptures happen during normal activities of daily living.[19]

Treatment

Treatment is generally supportive. Warm saline or anesthetic (lidocaine) gargles are helpful for pharyngitis. Bacterial pharyngitis is sometimes present and should be treated appropriately, avoiding ampicillin or amoxicillin, which may produce a rash in patients with mononucleosis. Acetaminophen is given for fever or malaise. Corticosteroids have been used but are mainly utilized in patients with airway obstruction secondary to tonsillar hypertrophy.[19] Corticosteroids do not decrease spleen size or the risk of splenic rupture. Antiviral medications such as acyclovir are used in immunocompromised patients but have no role in uncomplicated mononucleosis. Splenic rupture can be diagnosed by ultrasound or computed tomography (CT).

Return to Practice and Competition

The return to activity, especially athletic activity, is a difficult issue, with splenic rupture being the major concern. The most dangerous period for patients with splenomegaly is 4 to 21 days after the initial onset of symptoms. Patients without splenomegaly may gradually return to activity as tolerated starting 2 weeks after onset of symptoms. In patients with splenomegaly, serial ultrasounds or CT scans may be performed starting 3 weeks after onset of symptoms and repeated every 1 to 2 weeks to document decrease in spleen size. Athletes may return to contact sports within 4 weeks if no splenomegaly is noted on physical examination or radiologic study.[22]

Influenza

Typical influenza illness is characterized by abrupt onset of fever, myalgia, sore throat, and nonproductive cough. Influenza can cause severe malaise lasting several days, which differentiates it from other respiratory illnesses. If the patient has either primary influenza pneumonia or secondary bacterial pneumonia, the illness can be more severe. Influenza continues to cause major epidemics of respiratory disease. During epidemics, acute illness and complications generate a high rate of

physician visits and may necessitate hospitalization even of previously healthy children and adults.[23]

In the United States, two measures are available to reduce the impact of influenza. The first is immunoprophylaxis with an inactivated (i.e., killed virus) vaccine. Vaccinating people at high risk prior to the influenza season each year is the most effective measure for reducing the impact of influenza.[24] Each year's influenza vaccine contains three virus strains (usually two type A and one type B) representing the influenza viruses that are likely to circulate in the United States during the upcoming winter. The vaccine is made from highly purified, egg-grown viruses that have been made noninfectious (inactivated). Influenza vaccine rarely causes systemic or febrile reactions. The antibody titers resulting from the vaccine are protective against illnesses caused by strains similar to those in the vaccine or the related variants. If people develop influenza illness despite vaccination, the vaccine can be effective in preventing lower respiratory tract involvement or other secondary complications. When vaccine and circulating viruses are well matched, influenza vaccine has been shown to prevent illness in approximately 70 to 90 percent of healthy people under age 65.[23]

Because influenza vaccine contains only killed viruses, it cannot cause influenza. The most frequent side effect is soreness at the vaccination site. Occasionally fever, myalgia, and other symptoms follow vaccination, usually in young children or other people with no prior exposure to the antigens in the vaccine. These symptoms usually last 1 to 2 days. In healthy young adults the influenza vaccine is not associated with higher rates of systemic symptoms as compared to placebo. People may be hypersensitive to vaccine components. Vaccination carries a theoretical risk for increased incidence of Guillain-Barré syndrome, but this seems to apply mainly to those with a history of the syndrome.[25]

Athletes who participate in winter sports are often encouraged to have a flu vaccine to minimize the disruption of activities during epidemics. College students who reside in dormitories should be encouraged to have the flu vaccine. The optimal timing of vaccine is between October and mid-November. Influenza activity generally peaks between late December and early March.[23]

Two antiviral agents have activity specifically against influenza A viruses: amantadine hydrochloride and rimantadine hydrochloride. These agents interfere with the replication cycle of type A influenza viruses. When administered prophylactically to healthy adults before and throughout the flu season, these drugs are 70 to 90 percent effective in preventing illness.[26] However, chemoprophylaxis is not a substitute for vaccination except in those unable to be vaccinated due to hypersensitivity to vaccine. They can also reduce the severity and duration of signs and symptoms of influenza A illness when administered within 48 hours of illness onset. Due to possible induction of amantadine or rimantadine resistance, treatment should be discontinued as soon as clinically warranted, usually after 3 to 5 days of treatment or within 24 to 48 hours after the disappearance of symptoms and signs.[23] Both medications can cause mild central nervous system (CNS) and gastrointestinal side effects in young healthy adults. However, the incidence of CNS side effects is higher with amantadine. Concurrent administration of antihistamines or anticholinergic drugs may increase the incidence of adverse CNS side effects with amantadine, while rimantadine has no significant reactions with other medications. Recommended dosage of both medications is 100 mg twice daily.[26]

COMMON SKIN INFECTIONS

Dermatophytes

Dermatophytes are fungi that thrive only in nonviable skin (stratum corneum, hair, and nails). The areas mainly affected in athletes are the groin, body, and feet.

Tinea of the groin, tinea cruris (jock itch), often develops in the summer months owing to sweating or wearing wet clothing and in the winter owing to wearing several layers of clothing. Men are affected much more frequently than women are. Distribution is in intertriginous areas, especially the groin, thigh, and buttocks. The lesions tend to be bilateral and begin in the crural fold. A plaque forms and advances out onto the thigh. Involvement of the scrotum is unusual. Scaling is present along the active border of the lesions; within the borders, skin appears red-brown. Moist lesions may be contaminated with Candida organisms or bacteria.[27]

Tinea corporis (ringworm) appears on the face, trunk, and extremities. Lesions begin as flat,

scaly spots that develop a raised border, extending out in all directions. The advancing border tends to be scaly and erythematous, most often with central clearing. Vesicles or papules may be present. Predisposing factors include warm, humid environment, tight clothing, and direct contact with an infected individual.[27]

Tinea pedis (athlete's foot) is found typically between the toes, especially the third and fourth web spaces or along the arch of the foot. The usual presentation is vesicles or bullae in the web space with maceration and erosion present in more severe cases. The lesions often spread to the dorsal and plantar surfaces of the foot. Secondary infections often occur. Erythematous lesions are often seen on the plantar surface. Itching may be mild to intense, especially when footwear is removed.[27]

Treatment

Tinea cruris responds to most antifungal creams, including miconazole, clotrimazole, and terbinafine. Although lesions generally respond quickly, creams should be applied twice a day for at least 10 days.[28] Loose cotton or wicking clothing and talcum powder may also be helpful. Oral agents may sometimes be used in extensive or refractory cases: fluconazole once a week for 4 weeks, griseofulvin daily for 2 to 6 weeks, ketoconazole daily for 2 weeks, terbinafine daily for 2 weeks, or itraconazole daily for 1 to 2 weeks.[27]

Tinea corporis responds to most antifungal creams as well. The cream should be applied twice a day for 2 weeks or 1 week after resolution of the lesions. Oral agents may be chosen if there is extensive involvement at the same dosage used for tinea cruris. Exposed lesions need to be completely cleared or completely covered prior to return to play in contact sports.[29]

Tinea pedis limited to the web space responds to most topical antifungal agents. The older agents (e.g., clotrimazole) require twice a day use for at least 4 weeks. Nonadherence to this long regimen is the reason for recurrence and treatment failure in many cases. Terbinafine achieves cure in 1 week in many cases.[30] Econazole nitrate is useful in severely macerated web spaces owing to its activity against several types of bacteria.[31] Wearing wider shoes and placing lamb's wool between the toes prevents recurrence. Powders applied directly to the feet can also absorb moisture and prevent recurrence. Oral agents are useful in extensive cases, especially those involving large areas of the sole of the foot. Griseofulvin is used for 6 to 12 weeks, fluconazole once a week for 3 to 4 weeks, itraconazole daily for 4 weeks, or terbinafine daily for 6 weeks.[27]

Impetigo

Impetigo originates as a small vesicle or pustule that ruptures to expose a red, moist base. A honey-colored crust accumulates as the lesion expands outward. There is little surrounding erythema. Satellite lesions appear beyond the periphery. The lesions are not painful and are otherwise asymptomatic. The most common areas of infection are the skin around the nose and mouth and the limbs. Untreated cases may last for weeks. The infecting agent is a beta-hemolytic streptococcus that cannot invade intact skin. The infection is usually initiated by minor trauma to the skin and is aggravated by scratching. The lesions are often then contaminated with staphylococci. Warm, moist climate and poor hygiene are often precipitating factors.[27]

Treatment

Impetigo may resolve spontaneously. Mupirocin ointment (Bactroban) may be used on small lesions, but this local treatment is not effective for evolving lesions.[32] Crusts should be removed prior to applying mupirocin ointment. Bathing using an antibacterial soap may help prevent recurrences at distant sites if local treatment is chosen. Oral therapy for 5 to 10 days with dicloxacillin, cephalexin, or erythromycin induces rapid healing. Azithromycin for 5 days is also effective, and the regimen may be easier to adhere to owing to once-daily dosing.[33] Patients may return to contact sports when lesions are completely healed.[27]

Herpes Gladiatorum

Cutaneous herpes can be found in athletes involved in contact sports and is transmitted by direct skin-to-skin contact. Outbreaks have been reported mainly in wrestlers and rugby players.[34] The lesions tend to be clusters of vesicles, generally of uniform size, on a pink base. These lesions tend to crust over and heal in a few days. It is important to recognize and exclude from competition athletes with this skin condition to prevent transmission.

Treatment involves the use of antiviral agents such as acyclovir or famciclovir. Athletes susceptible to recurrent bouts may be placed on suppressive therapy during the competition season. No contact sports or activities should be allowed until lesions have resolved.[27]

Key Points

- Exercise may affect several parts of the immune system.
- Athletes should generally avoid strenuous activity when their body temperatures rise above 100.4°F (38°C).
- Physicians should be aware of USOC and NCAA regulations when prescribing symptomatic treatment for viral respiratory infections.
- Athletes with HIV and HBV may participate in competitive athletics but should be counseled regarding their disease, its course, and the modes of transmission.
- Athletes with infectious mononucleosis may return to contact sports within 4 weeks if there is no evidence of splenomegaly on physical examination or radiologic study.
- Flu vaccine is the most effective measure for reducing the impact of influenza.
- Exposed lesions of tinea corporis, impetigo, or herpes gladiatorum must be completely healed or covered prior to return to play.

REFERENCES

1. Eichner ER: Infection, immunity, and exercise. Phys Sprortsmed 21(1):125–135, 1993.
2. Friman G, Wright JE, Ilback NG, et al: Does fever or myalgia indicate reduced physical performance capacity in viral infections? Acta Med Scand 217(4):353–361, 1985.
3. Montague TJ, Marrie TJ, Bewick DJ, et al: Cardiac effects of common viral illnesses. Chest 94(5):919–925, 1988.
4. Roberts JA: Viral illnesses and sports performance. Sports Med 3(4):298–303, 1986.
5. Hilding DA: Literature review—the common cold. Ear Nose Throat J 73:639–647, 1994.
6. Bryant BG, Lombardi TP: Selecting OTC products for coughs and colds. Am Pharm 33:19–24, 1993.
7. Blacklow NR, Greenberg HB: Viral gastroenteritis. N Engl J Med 325(4):252–264, 1991.
8. Johnson RJ: HIV infection in athletes. Postgrad Med 92:73–80, 1992.
9. Lipsky JJ: Antiretroviral drugs for AIDS. Lancet 348:800–803, 1996.

10. Mellors JW, Nunoz A, Giorgi JV, et al: Plasma viral load and CD⁴⁺ lymphocytes as prognostic markers of HIV-1 infection. Ann Intern Med 126(12):946–954, 1997.
11. Mast EE, Goodman RA, Bond WA, et al: Transmission of blood-borne pathogens during sports: Risk and prevention. Ann Intern Med 122:283–285, 1995.
12. American Medical Society for Sports Medicine, American Academy of Sports Medicine: Human immunodeficiency virus and other blood-borne pathogens in sports. Clin J Sports Med 5(3):199–204, 1995.
13. Brown LS, Drotman DP, Chu A, et al: Bleeding injuries in professional football: Estimating the risk for HIV transmission. Ann Intern Med 122:271–274, 1995.
14. Ippolito G, Del Poggio P, Arici C, et al: Transmission of zidovudine-resistant HIV during a bloody fight. JAMA 272:433–434, 1994.
15. O'Farrell N, Tovey SJ, Morgan-Capner P: Transmission of HIV-1 infection after a fight. Lancet 339:246, 1992.
16. Sklarek HM, Mantovani RP, Erens E, et al: AIDS in a bodybuilder using anabolic steroids. N Engl J Med 311(26):1701, 1984.
17. Mast EE, Goodman RA: Prevention of infectious disease transmission in sports. Sports Med 24(1):1–7, 1997.
18. Kashiwagi S: Outbreak of hepatitis B in members of high school wrestling club. JAMA 248:213–214, 1982.
19. Peter J, Ray CG: Infectious mononucleosis. Pediatr Rev 19(8):276–279, 1998.
20. Maki DG, Reich RM: Infectious mononucleosis in the athlete: Diagnosis, complications, and management. Am J Sports Med 10(3):163–173, 1982.
21. Straus SE, Cohen JI, Tosato G, et al: Epstein-Barr virus infections: Biology, pathogenesis, and management. Ann Intern Med 118:45–58, 1993.
22. Eichner ER: Infectious mononucleosis: recognition and management in athletes. Phys Sportsmed 15(12):61–72, 1987.
23. ACIP: Prevention and control of influenza. MMWR 47(No. RR-6):1–26, 1998.
24. Nichol KL, Lind A, Margolis KL, et al: The effectiveness of vaccination against influenza in healthy, working adults. N Engl J Med 333:889–893, 1995.
25. Nichol KL, Lind A, Margolis KL, et al: Side effects associated with influenza vaccination in healthy working adults. A randomized, placebo-controlled trial. Arch Intern Med 156:1546–1550, 1996.
26. Douglas RD: Drug therapy: Prophylaxis and treatment of influenza. N Engl J Med 322:443–450, 1990.
27. Habif TF: Clinical Dermatology: A Color Guide to Diagnosis and Therapy, 3rd ed. St Louis, MO, Mosby-Year Book, 1996.
28. Panagiotidou D, Kousidou T, Chaidemenosi G, et al: A comparison of itraconazole and griseofulvin in the treatment of tinea corporis and tinea cruris: A double-blind study. J Int Med Res 20(5):392–400, 1992.
29. Stiller MJ, Klein WP, Dorman RI, et al: Tinea corporis gladiatorum: An epidemic of *Trichophyton tonsorans* in student wrestlers. J Am Acad Dermatol 27(4):632–633, 1992.
30. Berman B, Ellis C, Leyden J, et al: Efficacy of a 1-week, twice-daily regimen of terbinafine 1% cream in the treatment of interdigital tinea pedis. Results of placebo-controlled, double-blind, multicenter trials. J Am Acad Dermatol 26(6):956–960, 1992.
31. Kates SG, Myung KG, McGinley KJ, et al: The antibacterial efficacy of econazole nitrate in interdigital toe web infections. J Am Acad Dermatol 23(4):243–246, 1990.
32. McLinn S: A bacteriologically controlled, randomized study comparing the efficacy of 2% mupirocin ointment (Bactroban) with oral erythromycin in the treatment of patients with impetigo. J Am Acad Dermatol 22(5 part 1):883–885, 1990.
33. Daniels R: Azithromycin, erythromycin, and cloxacillin in the treatment of infections of skin and associated soft tissues. European Azithromycin Study Group. J Int Med Res 19(6):433–445, 1991.
34. Belongia EA, Goodman JL, Holland EJ, et al: An outbreak of herpes gladiatorum at a high-school wrestling camp. N Engl J Med 325(13):906–910, 1991.

Chapter 22 | Joint Aspiration and Injection

L. TYLER WADSWORTH, M.D.

Therapeutic injection is among the most rewarding procedures a physician can perform for a patient. One of the most powerful ways to gain the confidence of a patient is to relieve pain. Many of the common corticosteroid-responsive conditions that confront the primary care physician occur in anatomic locations that are easily accessible. Although rarely the only treatment for a given condition, judicious use of corticosteroid therapy can hasten patient recovery, enhance compliance with rehabilitation, or help a patient recover from a difficult injury.

Joint aspiration has both diagnostic and therapeutic uses. There is no adequate substitute in the evaluation of an acute painful atraumatic joint effusion. In addition to providing fluid for laboratory and microscopic analysis, joint aspiration can improve pain and range of motion and remove infectious microorganisms and destructive lysosomal enzymes. The gold standard in diagnosis of the acute painful joint effusion is analysis of the synovial fluid. The appearance of the fluid is important. Clear or straw-colored fluid is typically not associated with infection or inflammation, although gonococcal and tubercular effusions may be clear or straw-colored. Turbid-appearing, green, yellow, bloody, or gray synovial fluid generally indicates infection or inflammation. Gram stain and culture, blood cell count and differential count, and microscopic analysis for uric acid, calcium pyrophosphate, or hydroxyapatite crystals are the most useful tests.

Therapeutic corticosteroid injection can be used for several purposes. The most common indications are control of inflammation in inflammatory and degenerative arthritis, reduction of swelling that may threaten neurovascular structures (carpal tunnel syndrome, Baker's cyst), and reduction of pain. In some situations, anesthetic injection can be administered as a diagnostic test. Referred pain from subacromial bursitis can on occasion be confused with radicular pain; relief in response to injection into the subacromial space would make radiculitis less likely. Trigger point injection can provide both diagnostic and therapeutic assistance in treatment of soft tissue conditions.

One of the keys to success with any of these techniques described here is to start with a relaxed patient. A calm, confident demeanor does much to reassure the patient. A thorough discussion of the potential risks of the specific procedure should be carried out up front, when the procedure is initially proposed. A casual comment such as, "By the way, I might possibly puncture your lung," just before the procedure does little to relax the patient. No matter how many times you have done this procedure, this is often the first time for this patient. Other patients may have been hastened through the procedure by hurried physicians who gave little attention to patient comfort. Spending a few extra minutes with an anxious patient makes the procedure go better for the patient *and* the physician. Describe the procedure to the patient beforehand, and explain what is being done during the procedure. A rare patient may request to be left "out of the loop," but most appreciate knowing what to expect.

RISKS, COMPLICATIONS, AND CONTRAINDICATIONS

Several risks and complications should be considered by the physician and patient before proceeding with joint aspiration or corticosteroid injection. Infection is extremely rare, on the order of one infection per 20,000 to 50,000 injections when sterile technique is used. "Postinjection flare" is the most common complication, occurring in 1 to

2 percent of patients. This is likely a reaction to the microcrystalline steroid suspension and is self-limited. There may be increased pain beginning 6 to 12 hours after the injection, usually subsiding within 48 hours. If pain persists past 72 hours, or is accompanied by fever or other systemic symptoms, the patient should be evaluated for infection.

Although there is little systemic absorption of intra-articular corticosteroids, diabetic patients may rarely experience difficulty with glycemic control, and some individuals experience facial flushing related to systemic absorption.

Collagen atrophy and tendon rupture is also quite rare, and can be avoided with careful technique. First, injection into tendons should be avoided. The appropriate target for injection of tendonopathies is the synovial sheath or paratenon. Most cases of tendon rupture have occurred after multiple injections. Skin atrophy is another uncommon complication, which can occur when injecting steroid within 5 mm of the skin surface. It is important to avoid this in individuals with dark pigmentation, as skin atrophy will often result in total loss of pigmentation in the affected area.

The other area of concern is the potential adverse effect on articular cartilage in weight-bearing joints. For this reason, it is reasonable to limit corticosteroid injection into any specific weight-bearing joint to three injections per year. In some situations, it may be reasonable to exceed this limit, although caution is advised and referral should be considered.

Several contraindications should also be considered. Injecting through a periarticular infection such as cellulitis would potentially seed the joint with infectious microorganisms and should be avoided. Likewise, care must be taken when there is evidence of sepsis or bacteremia to avoid spreading blood-borne pathogens into the joint. Of course, when the joint is believed to be the source of infection, aspiration is indicated, but injection should be avoided. The presence of anticoagulation or coagulopathy is also a relative contraindication to intra-articular and soft tissue injection because of the risk of intra-articular hemorrhage and hematoma formation.

Presence of an intra-articular fracture is also a relative contraindication to joint aspiration, and an absolute contraindication to corticosteroid injection. Of course, some fractures are diagnosed by joint aspiration, particularly occult tibial pla-

teau fractures. Aspiration of a prosthetic joint should be left to the orthopaedist.

GENERAL PRINCIPLES

Sterile technique is important. Sterile disposable needles and syringes should be used. The skin should be prepared with povidone/iodine, 70 percent isopropyl alcohol, or other antibacterial soap. A wide prepared area allows more room for palpation of the area, in case the needle needs to be reinserted. Sterile gloves should also be used, and universal precautions should be observed. When a joint is to be aspirated and then injected, or when a large effusion is anticipated, a sterile hemostat will allow the physician to stabilize the needle while the syringes are exchanged. The practice of using a preinjection local anesthetic varies among practitioners. In many cases, injection of an anesthetic is just as painful as performing the injection. When a large effusion is anticipated, which may require leaving the needle in the joint for up to a few minutes, injecting with a local anesthetic may be advisable. In other cases, a reasonable compromise is found in the use of sterile skin refrigerants, such as ethyl chloride. Unlike injected anesthetics, these can be administered without significant pain, and typically provide adequate anesthesia for more superficial injections.

A variety of corticosteroids is available for joint injection. Table 22–1 lists commonly used injectable corticosteroids, their relative potency, and duration of action. Shorter-acting steroids have the advantage of a faster onset of action, although systemic absorption tends to be more of a problem with the shorter-acting preparations. Celestone Soluspan is a unique agent that contains two esters of betamethasone, one of which peaks in approximately 48 hours, the other peaking at approximately 2 weeks. This agent provides a combination of acute and long-term pain relief and has a low incidence of postinjection flare. Dexamethasone acetate is another frequently used long-acting corticosteroid. Most of the injections described in this chapter can be administered with a combination of corticosteroid and local anesthetic. The anesthetic agent is useful in determining if the appropriate target was injected. More than 50 percent pain relief after an injection generally indicates successful administration of the injection.

Controversy exists as to the ideal agent for

Table 22-1
Commonly Used Injectable Corticosteroids

Corticosteroid	Preparation Strength (mg/ml)	Relative Potency (mg hydrocortisone/ml)	Onset	Duration
Hydrocortisone acetate (Hydrocortone)	50	50	Slow	Long
Triamcinolone hexacetonide (Aristospan)	20	100	Slow	Long
Dexamethasone sodium phosphate (Decadron)	4	100	Rapid	Short
Dexamethasone acetate (Decadron-LA)	8	200	Rapid	Long
Methylprednisolone acetate (Depo-Medrol)	20, 40, 80	100, 200, 400	Rapid	Intermediate
Betamethasone acetate and betamethasone sodium phosphate (Celestone Soluspan)	6	150	Rapid	Long

trigger point injection. A well-designed study by Garvey et al. indicated no significant difference between several treatment modalities including dry needling, local anesthetic, and local anesthetic with corticosteroid injection into myofascial trigger points. It is possible that the mechanical stimulation of trigger points is responsible for the long-term effectiveness of this procedure. A local anesthetic is useful for diagnostic purposes, as a good pain response indicates the likelihood that the injected trigger point is contributing to the patient's pain.

SPECIFIC TECHNIQUES

The specific diagnoses addressed here are described elsewhere in this book in detail. The focus of this chapter is on the technical aspects of ad-ministering the injection. Emphasis is on reviewing the local anatomy and landmarks, positioning of the patient, describing the technique, and appropriate dosing of corticosteroid and anesthetic. Corticosteroid dosages are based on the usual dosage ranges for betamethasone (Celestone Soluspan 6 mg/ml), methylprednisolone acetate (Depo-Medrol 40 mg/ml), or dexamethasone acetate (Decadron-LA 8 mg/ml). The PDR contains dosing information for specific locations. Many joints are accessible by approaches not mentioned in this chapter. The most consistent and reliable techniques are described.

Subacromial Space

Indications Subacromial impingement syndrome, subacromial/subdeltoid bursitis, supraspinatus tendonitis.

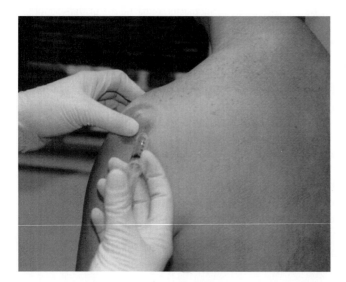

Figure 22-1. Injection into the subacromial bursa.

Landmarks The acromial process of the scapula, the acromioclavicular joint, and the humeral head.

Technique (Fig. 22–1) Injection into the subacromial space is most safely and comfortably done from a posterolateral approach with the patient sitting. The target is large and accessible, and injection is typically well tolerated. The arm should be relaxed in a dependent position; this allows gravity to slightly open the subacromial space. The posterior angle of the acromial process is easily palpable, even in obese individuals. The posterior edge of the acromion is palpated with the thumb, and the acromioclavicular joint is palpated with the index finger. The skin is entered below the posterior acromion, with the needle angled toward the acromioclavicular joint to enter the subacromial space. Typically, if bony resistance is felt, it is the acromion; the operator should withdraw slightly, move the needle inferiorly (not changing the angle), and make another gentle pass with the needle. Insertion depth is 2.5 to 3.5 cm (1 to 1½ inches).

Needle Size and Dosage A relatively large dose of anesthetic can be administered into the subacromial space; many physicians believe this disrupts the adhesions that are typically seen during arthroscopy. One to 2 ml of steroid with 6 to 10 ml of anesthetic is the recommended dose. When a large volume is injected, using a 22-guage needle is much more efficient than injecting up to 10 ml through a smaller needle. A 1½-inch needle is recommended to ensure entry into the subacromial space.

Acromioclavicular Joint

Indications Acromioclavicular arthrosis, degenerative change.

Landmarks The clavicle, the acromial process of the scapula, the acromioclavicular (AC) joint. The acromioclavicular joint is superficial; a smaller target, but quite accessible. The acromioclavicular joint is felt as an enlargement at the distal end of the clavicle. Confirmation of the joint location can be felt by applying inferior stress to the distal clavicle while palpating the AC joint. The distal clavicle will move slightly, but the acromion does not, giving a reliable indication of the precise location of the joint space.

Technique (Fig. 22–2) The patient may be seated or supine, although the seated position is preferred for ease of administration. This injection can be administered from the front, with the needle directed posteriorly, or from above, with the needle directed inferiorly. An insertion depth of 1 to 1.5 cm (⅜ to ½ inch) is adequate to enter the joint unless the patient is extremely obese.

Needle Size and Dosage A ½- to 1-inch 25-gauge needle is appropriate; 0.5 ml each of anesthetic and corticosteroid are prepared; 0.5 to 1 ml of this suspension can be injected. If the joint becomes distended, resistance is felt; do not force the remainder of the suspension into the joint.

Glenohumeral Joint

Indications Inflammatory or degenerative arthritis; diagnostic aspiration.

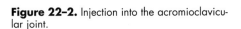
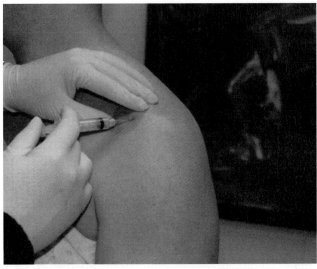

Figure 22–2. Injection into the acromioclavicular joint.

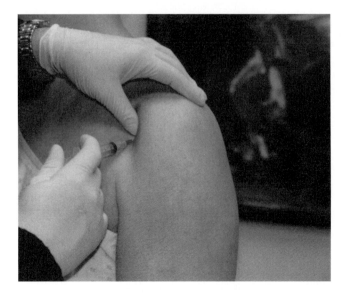

Figure 22–3. Glenohumeral joint: anterior approach to injection.

Landmarks Coracoid process humeral head, the acromial process of the scapula.

Technique: Anterior (Fig. 22–3) The patient may be seated or supine, although the seated position is preferred for ease of administration. The coracoid process is palpated inferomedial to the AC joint. The glenohumeral joint is palpable just inferior to the coracoid. Passively internally and externally rotate the patient's arm to confirm the location of the glenohumeral joint. The skin is entered just inferior to the coracoid, with the needle directed posteriorly or posteriorly and *slightly* superiorly, advancing the needle 2 to 3 cm (¾ to 1¼ inch).

Posterior (Fig. 22–4) The entry point is the same as that for injection into the subacromial space. The posterior angle of the acromial process is palpated. Instead of aiming the needle toward the acromioclavicular joint, and needle is directed toward the coracoid process. The posterior edge of the acromion is palpated with the thumb, and the coracoid process is palpated with the index or middle finger. The skin is entered below the posterior acromion, with the needle angled toward the coracoid process to enter the glenohumeral joint. Depth of penetration should be 2.5 to 3.5 cm (1 to 1½ inches).

Needle Size and Dosage For aspiration, 20-gauge, 1½-inch needle is the minimum recommended size; 18-gauge is preferred. A 5- to 20-ml syringe is recommended. For injection, a 25-gauge 1½-inch needle is recommended. One

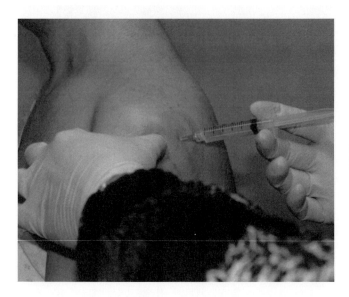

Figure 22–4. Glenohumeral joint: posterior approach to injection.

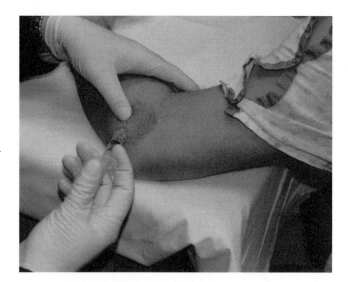

Figure 22-5. Injection for lateral epicondylitis.

to 2 ml of steroid can be mixed with 2 to 5 ml of anesthetic.

Lateral Humeral Epicondyle

Indications Lateral epicondylitis, epicondylalgia.

Landmarks Lateral humeral epicondyle, radial head. The radial nerve crosses the proximal radius at the radial neck.

Technique (Fig. 22–5) The patient may be seated or supine. The point of maximal tenderness in the common extensor tendon is palpated, usually at or slightly distal to the lateral epicondyle. The skin is entered at an oblique angle; the goal is to infiltrate the soft tissues overlying the extensor aponeurosis, with care taken to avoid injecting less than 5 mm from the skin. Several passes should be made with the needle, pausing to aspirate before injecting. Spread the injection through the point of maximal tenderness. Dysesthesias toward the thumb and index finger can indicate trauma to the posterior interosseus nerve; if this occurs, the needle should be withdrawn and redirected before corticosteroid is administered.

Needle Size and Dosage A 25-gauge 1- to 1½-inch needle is recommended; 0.5 to 1 ml of steroid should be mixed with 2 to 3 ml of anesthetic.

Medial Humeral Epicondyle

Indications Medial epicondylitis, epicondylalgia.

Landmarks Medial humeral epicondyle, ulnar nerve.

Technique (Fig. 22–6) The technique is similar to that for lateral epicondyle injection. The

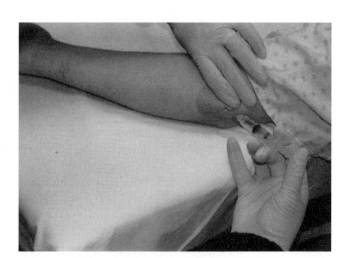

Figure 22-6. Injection for medial epicondylitis.

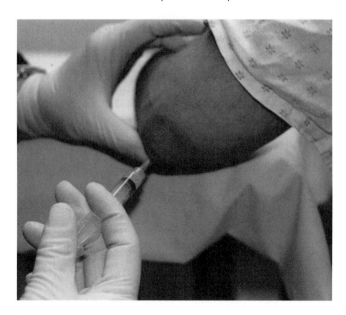

Figure 22–7. Injection into the olecranon bursa.

point of maximal tenderness is palpated in the common flexor tendon, typically just distal to the medial epicondyle. Care must be taken to avoid injecting the ulnar nerve. The skin is entered at an oblique angle and the soft tissues overlying the common flexor tendon infiltrated. Make several passes with the needle, fanning the injection over the point of tenderness, remembering to aspirate before injecting.

Needle Size and Dosage A 25-gauge 1- to 1½-inch needle is recommended; 0.5 to 1 ml of steroid should be mixed with 2 to 3 ml of anesthetic.

Elbow Joint

Indications Inflammatory or degenerative arthritis; diagnostic aspiration.

Landmarks Lateral humeral epicondyle, radial head, and radial nerve. The radial head can be palpated just distal to the lateral humeral epicondyle with the elbow flexed 90 degrees. The anterior and posterior borders of the radiohumeral joint can be palpated as the patient pronates and supinates the forearm, and the joint space becomes more readily apparent. The radiohumeral joint and the trochlear joint of the humerus and ulna share an articular cavity.

Technique The patient should be seated, with the elbow flexed 90 degrees. Enter the skin perpendicularly at the joint space to a depth of 1 to 1.5 cm (⅜ to ½ inch).

Needle Size and Dosage A ½- to 1-inch 25-gauge needle is appropriate; 0.5 to 1 ml each of anesthetic and corticosteroid are prepared. One to 2 ml of this suspension can be injected.

Olecranon Bursa

Indications Olecranon bursitis.

Landmarks Olecranon process of the ulna.

Technique (Fig. 22–7) When inflamed, the location and position of this bursa become obvious as a fluid-filled mass posterior to the olecranon. It is easily palpated and entered from a posterior position, with the needle aimed toward the olecranon process of the ulna. As much fluid as possible should be aspirated.

Needle Size and Dosage For aspiration, 20-gauge 1-inch needle is the minimum recommended size; 18-gauge is preferred. A 5- to 20-ml syringe is recommended; 0.5 ml of corticosteroid with a similar amount of anesthetic can be injected after aspiration.

First Dorsal Compartment of the Wrist (de Quervain's Tenosynovitis)

Indications De Quervain's stenosing tenosynovitis.

Landmarks The "anatomic snuff box," bordered anteriorly by the first dorsal compartment of the wrist (abductor pollicis longus and extensor pollicis brevis tendons) and posteriorly by the extensor pollicis longus tendon. The tendons are

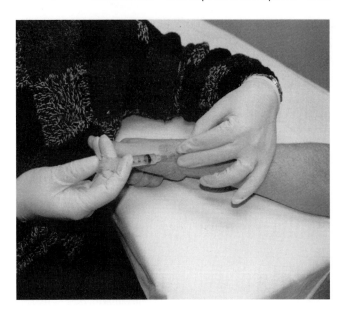

Figure 22–8. Injection into the first dorsal compartment of the wrist to relieve the pain from de Quervain's tenosynovitis.

more readily apparent with the thumb abducted. The volar aspect of the snuffbox is the first dorsal compartment; the dorsal aspect of the snuffbox is the extensor pollicis longus.

Technique (Fig. 22–8) The patient may be seated or lying supine. The point of maximal tenderness is identified, typically in the area of the radial styloid. The tendons are palpated with the thumb, or between the fingers of the nondominant hand. The needle is inserted bevel-up, directed at an oblique cephalad angle, nearly parallel to the tendons. When an increase in resistance is felt, usually at a depth of 5 to 8 mm (¼ to ⅜ inch), aspirate, and if there is no blood return, gently push the plunger. If there is resistance, the tip of the needle may be in the tendon. The needle should be withdrawn slightly; aspirate again, and

inject. The injected solution should be seen filling the tendon sheath like a balloon. Pain relief is typically dramatic and rapid.

Needle Size and Dosage A ½- to 1-inch 25-gauge needle is recommended; 0.5 ml each of anesthetic and corticosteroid are prepared; 0.5 to 1 ml of this suspension can be injected.

Wrist Joint

Indications Inflammatory or degenerative arthritis; diagnostic aspiration.

Landmarks Dorsal tubercle of the radius, proximal carpal row, and extensor carpi radialis.

Technique (Fig. 22–9) The patient may be seated or lying supine. With the wrist in a slightly flexed position, the dorsal tubercle of the radius

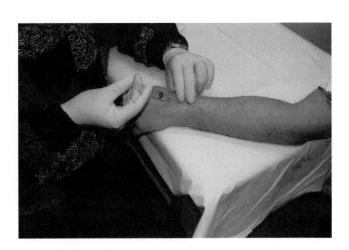

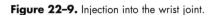

Figure 22–9. Injection into the wrist joint.

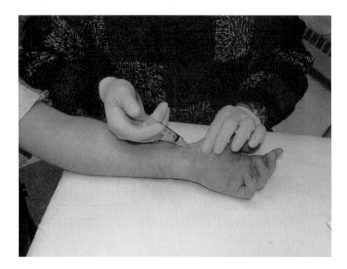

Figure 22–10. Injection into the wrist to relieve the pain due to carpal tunnel syndrome.

and the extensor carpi radialis tendon should be palpated. The wrist should be entered perpendicularly or with slight proximal angulation just distal to the dorsal tubercle and ulnar to the extensor carpi radialis tendon. Insert the needle to a depth of 1 to 1.5 cm (⅜ to ½ inch).

Needle Size and Dosage A 25-gauge 1- to 1½-inch needle is sufficient. A dose of 0.5 to 1 ml of steroid and 1 to 2 ml of local anesthetic may be injected.

Carpal Tunnel

Indications Carpal tunnel syndrome.

Landmarks Palmaris longus and flexor carpi radialis tendons; distal wrist crease; median nerve.

Technique (Fig. 22–10) The patient may be seated or lying supine. The needle is inserted at the distal wrist crease just radial to the palmaris longus tendon, at a 45-degree angle toward the middle finger, to a depth of 1 to 1.5 cm (⅜ to ½ inch). The needle may be felt to "pop" through the dense transverse carpal ligament. The patient is instructed to report any pain or paresthesias into the palm or fingertips during needle placement. If this occurs, the needle should be withdrawn and angled laterally before reinsertion.

Needle Size and Dosage A 25-gauge 1- to 1½-inch needle is sufficient. A dose of 0.5 to 1 ml of steroid and a similar dose of local anesthetic may be injected.

Flexor Tendon Sheath (Trigger Finger)

Indications Trigger finger.

Landmarks Flexor tendons; superficial pal-

mar arch of ulnar artery. The involved tendon can be most easily palpated by having the patient make an "O" with the involved finger and thumb.

Technique (Fig. 22–11) The patient may be seated or supine. The symptoms are typically caused by a thickening of the flexor tendons being entrapped just proximal to the MP joints. The injection should be just proximal to the metacarpal head at the level of the distal palmar crease. The technique is similar to injection into the first dorsal compartment of the wrist. The needle is inserted bevel-up, directed at an oblique angle parallel with the tendon toward the fingertips or arm. When an increase in resistance is felt, usually at a depth of 5 to 8 mm (¼ to ⅜ inch), and if there is no blood

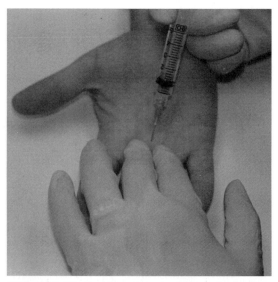

Figure 22–11. To relieve the pain of trigger finger, injection is made into the flexor tendon sheath.

return, the plunger should be gently pushed. If there is resistance, the tip of the needle may be in the tendon. Withdraw slightly, aspirate again, and inject. The injected solution can frequently be felt filling the tendon sheath by the patient, and a fluid wave may be observed. Pain relief is typically dramatic and rapid.

Needle Size and Dosage A ½- to 1-inch 25-gauge needle is appropriate; 0.5 ml each of anesthetic and corticosteroid are prepared; 0.5 to 1 ml of this suspension can be injected.

Metacarpophalangeal Joints

Indications Inflammatory or degenerative arthritis; diagnostic aspiration.

Landmarks Metacarpal head, base of proximal phalanx, extensor tendon.

Technique (Fig. 22–12) The patient may be seated or lying supine. The extensor tendon is easily palpated with the finger fully extended. For injection, the finger should be slightly flexed, or traction placed by an assistant. At the level of the joint space, the needle is inserted either medially or laterally under the extensor tendon to a depth of 5 to 8 mm (¼ to ⅜ inch).

Needle Size and Dosage A ½- to 1-inch 25-gauge needle is recommended; 0.5 ml each of anesthetic and corticosteroid are prepared; 0.5 to 1 ml of this suspension can be injected.

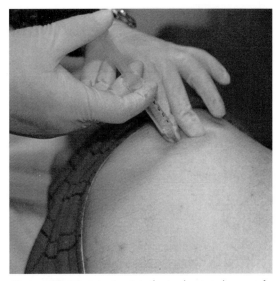

Figure 22–13. Injection into the trochanteric bursa, inferior view.

Trochanteric Bursa

Indications Trochanteric bursitis.

Landmarks Greater trochanter of the femur.

Technique (Figs. 22–13 and 22–14) The patient should lie prone or in a lateral decubitus position, with the involved side up. The point of maximal tenderness is palpated, typically in the posterior superior aspect of the greater trochanter. The skin should be entered just posterior to this area, with the needle directed slightly anteriorly

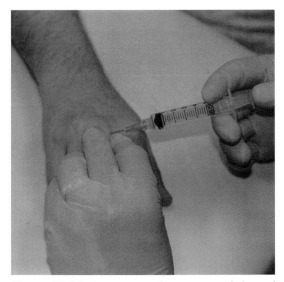

Figure 22–12. Injection into the metacarpophalangeal joint.

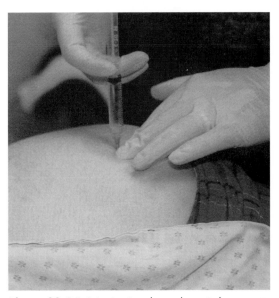

Figure 22–14. Injection into the trochanteric bursa, anterior view.

toward the area of tenderness. Depth of penetration largely depends on the size and obesity of the patient. Persons of average size typically require a depth of insertion of 2.5 to 3.5 cm (1 to 1½ inches). Several passes may be made with the needle, depositing a few milliliters of the solution each time, close to the trochanter.

Needle Size and Dosage A 22-gauge 1½-inch needle is the minimum length used to reach the trochanteric bursa in most patients. Some authors recommend using a 3½-inch needle to assure that the greater trochanter is reached. One to 2 ml of steroid can be mixed with 5 to 10 ml of anesthetic.

Knee Joint

Indications Inflammatory or degenerative arthritis; diagnostic aspiration.

Landmarks Patella, patellar tendon, medial femoral condyle, medial joint line, lateral joint line, lateral femoral condyle.

Technique: Supine (Fig. 22–15) Aspiration is performed more easily with the patient supine. The knee should be fully extended or slightly flexed, resting on a rolled towel. A medial or lateral approach may be used, although the medial approach typically is accomplished more easily because of the lateral tilt of the patella, and will be described here. The groove between the medial border of the patella and the medial femoral condyle should be located. The joint should be entered at or just distal to the level of the midpatella, but not below the level of the medial joint line. Place the needle an appropriate distance posterior to the medial border of the patella to accommodate

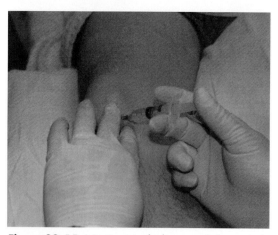

Figure 22–15. Injection into the knee, medial approach, while patient is supine.

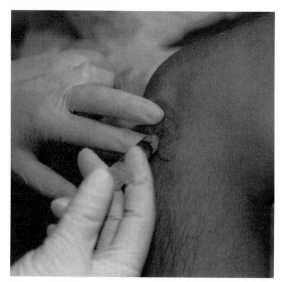

Figure 22–16. Injection into the knee, medial approach, while patient is seated.

the thickness of the patella. The needle should be directed toward the center of the knee joint, posteriorly and laterally, and inserted to a depth of 2 to 3 cm (¾ to 1¼ inches). Tangential patellar x-rays taken before the procedure can give an idea of the optimal angle of entry for this approach.

Seated When aspiration is not necessary, injection can easily be administered with the patient seated with the knee flexed 90 degrees.

Lateral Approach The ideal point of entry is slightly inferior and lateral to the origin of the patellar tendon at the level of the joint line. The needle is directed toward the center of the knee, medially, posteriorly, and slightly cephalad, and inserted to a depth of 2 to 3 cm (¾ to 1¼ inches).

Medial Approach (Fig. 22–16) The point of entry is slightly inferior and medial to the origin of the patellar tendon at the level of the joint line. The needle is directed toward the center of the knee, laterally, posteriorly, and slightly cephalad, and inserted to a depth of 2 to 3 cm (¾ to 1¼ inches).

Needle Size and Dosage For aspiration, 20-gauge 1½-inch is the minimum recommended size; 18-gauge is preferred. A 10- to 20-ml syringe is recommended. For injection, a 25-gauge 1½-inch needle is recommended. One to 2 ml of steroid can be mixed with 2 to 3 ml of anesthetic.

Pes Anserine Bursa

Indications Pes anserine bursitis.

Landmarks Medial aspect of the proximal tibia, sartorius, gracilis, and semitendinosus tendons.

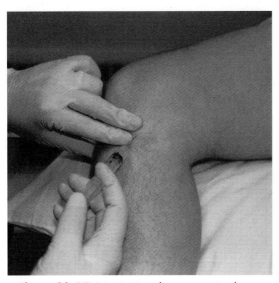

Figure 22–17. Injection into the pes anserine bursa.

Technique (Fig. 22–17) The patient should be seated on the examination table, with the knee flexed 90 degrees. The point of maximal tenderness is palpated medial to the tibial tuberosity at the insertion of the sartorius, gracilis, and semitendinosus tendons. The objective is to slip the needle between the tendons and the tibia. The skin should be entered lateral to the point of maximal tenderness, with the needle angled posteriorly and medially. Depth of insertion is approximately 5 to 10 mm (¼ to ⅜ inch). If the needle contacts the periosteum, the patient will experience pain. Withdraw the needle very slightly, aspirate, and

inject. Likewise, it is important not to inject the tendons themselves; if resistance is felt with injection, withdraw, redirect the needle, aspirate, and inject.

Needle Size and Dosage A 25-gauge 1- to 1½-inch needle is recommended. Inject 0.5 to 1 ml of steroid with 1 to 2 ml of anesthetic.

Medial (Tibial) Collateral Ligament Bursa

Indications Medial (tibial) collateral ligament bursitis ("no name, no fame" bursitis).

Landmarks Medial collateral ligament, medial joint line. The medial collateral ligament can be most easily palpated with the leg crossed, ankle over knee. The bursa is between the superficial and deep layers of the medial (tibial) collateral ligament.

Technique (Fig. 22–18) The patient should be seated on the examination table with the knee flexed 90 degrees. The point of maximal tenderness in the medial collateral ligament should be palpated. The skin should be entered anterior to the point of maximal tenderness, with the needle angled posteriorly and slightly laterally. Insert the needle to a depth of 1 to 1.5 cm (⅜ to ½ inch) and inject. If resistance is felt to injection, withdraw, change the angle of the needle, and reinsert. It is important not to inject the ligament or the medial meniscus.

Needle Size and Dosage A 25-gauge 1- to

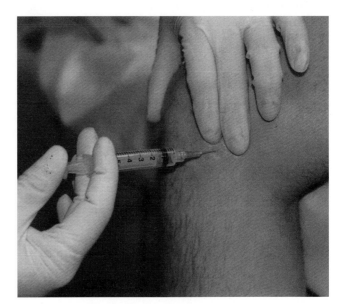

Figure 22–18. Injection into the medial collateral ligament bursa.

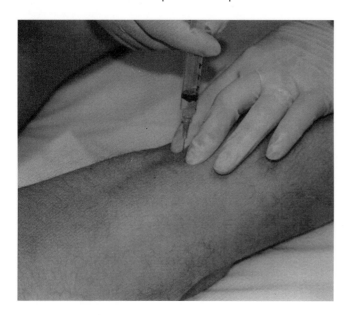

Figure 22–19. Injection into Baker's (popliteal) cyst.

1½-inch needle is recommended. Inject 0.5 to 1 ml of steroid with 1 to 2 ml of anesthetic.

Popliteal (Baker's) Cyst

Indications Painful popliteal (Baker's) cyst.

Landmarks Semimembranosus tendon, popliteal artery, and tibial nerve. A popliteal cyst can usually be observed most easily with the patient standing or lying prone. The cyst typically arises between the semimembranosus and medial head of the gastrocnemius.

Technique (Fig. 22–19) The patient should be lying prone. The cyst should be palpated, just lateral to the semimembranosus tendon at or slightly below the level of the joint line. Palpate the popliteal artery in order to avoid this structure. The needle should be inserted perpendicular to the skin. Usually, a decrease in resistance is felt as the needle enters the cyst typically at a depth of 1.5 to 3 cm (⅝ to 1½ inches). Aspiration confirms appropriate placement of the needle. As much fluid should be aspirated as possible, followed by injection.

Needle Size and Dosage For aspiration, 20-gauge 1-inch needle is the minimum recommended size; 18-gauge is preferred. A 10- to 20-ml syringe is recommended; 0.5 to 1 ml of corticosteroid can be injected with 1 to 2 ml of anesthetic.

Iliotibial Band Bursa

Indications Iliotibial band friction syndrome, bursitis.

Landmarks Lateral femoral epicondyle, iliotibial band.

Technique The patient should be seated with the knee flexed 90 degrees. The point of maximal tenderness is palpated where the iliotibial band crosses the lateral femoral epicondyle, proximal to the lateral joint line. The intent is to inject between the iliotibial band (ITB) and the epicondyle. The skin is entered anterior to the ITB and point of maximal tenderness, and the needle is angled posteriorly and slightly medially. The needle is inserted to a depth of 5 to 10 mm (¼ to ⅜ inch). If the needle contacts the periosteum, the patient will experience pain. Withdraw the needle very slightly, aspirate, and inject. Additionally, it is important not to inject the ITB itself, if resistance is felt with injection, withdraw, redirect the needle, aspirate, and inject.

Needle Size and Dosage A 25-gauge 1- to 1½-inch needle in recommended. Inject 0.5 to 1 ml of steroid with 1 to 2 ml of anesthetic.

Ankle Joint

Indications Inflammatory or degenerative arthritis; diagnostic aspiration.

Landmarks Lateral malleolus, anterior border of distal tibia, talar dome.

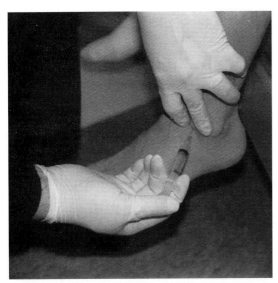

Figure 22–20. Proper insertion of the needle into the ankle joint for injection or aspiration.

Technique (Fig. 22–20) The patient should be seated with the leg in a dependent position. The angle between the distal tibia and the anterior border of the lateral malleolus should be palpated. The operator should flex and extend the ankle to feel the talar dome move beneath the tibia. The skin should be entered medial to the lateral malleolus, with the needle aimed posteriorly or slightly posteromedially toward the center of the joint. The needle should be inserted to a depth of 1 to 1.5 cm (⅜ to ½ inch), deeper if the patient is obese or if there is significant lower extremity edema.

Needle Size and Dosage For aspiration, a 20-gauge 1- to 1½-inch needle is the minimum recommended size; 18-gauge is preferred. A 10-ml syringe is recommended. For injection, a 25-gauge 1½-inch needle is recommended. One to 2 ml of steroid can be mixed with 2 to 3 ml of anesthetic.

Ankle Anterior Synovium

Indications Anterior synovial pinch syndrome.

Landmarks Lateral malleolus, anterior border of distal tibia, talar dome.

Technique (Fig. 22–21) The patient may be seated or lying supine. The area of tenderness in the angle between the lateral malleolus and distal tibia should be palpated. Palpable synovitis should be present in this area, as compared with the uninvolved side. The skin is entered just medial

to the lateral malleolus, angled medially and slightly posteriorly. The objective is to infiltrate the synovium and joint capsule in this area rather than to perform an intra-articular injection. The needle is inserted to a depth of approximately 1 cm (⅜ inch). Several passes may be made as the soft tissues in this area are infiltrated. The operator should be sure to aspirate before injecting.

Needle Size and Dosage A 25-gauge 1- to 1½-inch needle in appropriate; 0.5 to 1 ml of corticosteroid should be injected with 2 to 3 ml of local anesthetic.

Plantar Fascia

Indications Plantar fasciitis.

Landmarks Medial calcaneal tuberosity, medial calcaneal branch of posterior tibial nerve.

Technique (Fig. 22–22) The patient should be lying prone with the foot hanging off the examination table. Because an approach from the plantar aspect of the foot requires the needle to pass through the subcalcaneal fat pad, an approach from the medial aspect is advisable. The point of maximal tenderness is palpated at the origin of the plantar fascia on the medial calcaneal tuberosity. The needle is inserted on the medial aspect of the heel, aimed toward the point of maximal tenderness. Depending on the size of the patient, insert the needle 1.5 to 2.5 cm (⅝ to 1 inch). Do not inject the plantar fascia or medial calcaneal branch of the posterior tibial nerve. If pain is felt radiating across the heel or into the arch, or if

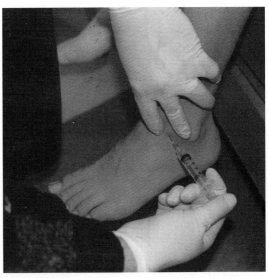

Figure 22–21. Injection into the anterior ankle synovium.

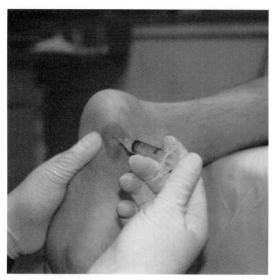

Figure 22–22. Injection into the plantar fascia.

there is resistance when the plunger is pressed, withdraw, change the angle slightly, and reinsert.

Needle Size and Dosage A 25-gauge 1- to 1½-inch needle is recommended. Inject 1 ml of steroid with 1 to 2 ml of anesthetic.

First Metatarsophalangeal Joint

Indications Inflammatory or degenerative arthritis; diagnostic aspiration.

Landmarks Metatarsal head, base of proximal phalanx, extensor hallucis longus tendon.

Technique (Fig. 22–23) The patient should be supine. Distract the joint with the nondominant hand, or have an assistant do this. At the level of the joint space, the needle is inserted either medially or laterally under the extensor tendon to a depth of 5 to 8 mm (¼ to ⅜ inch).

Needle Size and Dosage A ½- to 1-inch 25-gauge needle is recommended; 0.5 ml each of anesthetic and corticosteroid are prepared; 0.5 to 1 ml of this suspension can be injected.

Morton's Neuroma

Indications Morton's neuroma.

Landmarks Metatarsal heads, common digital (interdigital) nerves.

Technique (Figs. 22–24 and 22–25) The operator should palpate the point of maximal tenderness between the metatarsal heads of the involved toes and the transverse metatarsal ligament. The neuroma is typically between and slightly plantar to the metatarsal heads. The needle should be inserted into the web space between the involved metatarsal heads. Insert the needle to the level of the metatarsal head, typically 1.5 to 2.5 cm (⅝ to 1 inch).

Needle Size and Dosage A 25-gauge 1- to 1½-inch needle is appropriate; 0.5 to 1 ml of corticosteroid should be injected with 2 to 3 ml of local anesthetic.

Myofascial Trigger Points

Indications Diagnosis and treatment of myofascial trigger points.

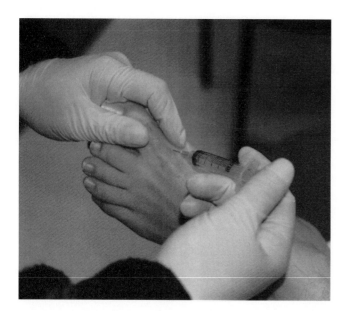

Figure 22–23. Needle insertion into the first metatarsophalangeal joint for injection or aspiration.

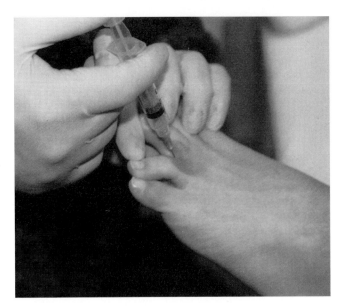

Figure 22–24. Injection for Morton's neuroma.

Landmarks Dependent on location of trigger points. A detailed knowledge of underlying organs and local neurovascular bundles is imperative.

Technique (Fig. 22–26) Myofascial trigger points, such as those often found in the trapezius of other periscapular muscles, are often palpable as fusiform firm nodules running parallel to the fibers in a muscle. The nodule may be trapped between the fingers of the nondominant hand. The skin is entered obliquely with the tip of the needle angled toward the center of the trigger point. Sometimes, a "twitch response" is noted, in which the muscle twitches when the trigger point

is entered. The trigger point and surrounding muscle is anesthetized, using a four-quadrant approach. Advance the needle into the trigger point, aspirate and inject. Withdraw the needle close to the skin, change the angle, and insert again to inject the soft tissues in all directions. Depth of insertion depends on the involved muscle and underlying organs.

Needle Size and Dosage A 25- to 27-gauge 1½-inch needle is recommended; 1 to 5 ml of anesthetic should be injected, depending on the size of the trigger point and the involved muscle.

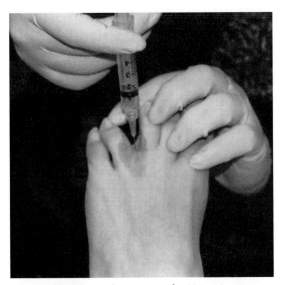

Figure 22–25. Another injection for Morton's neuroma.

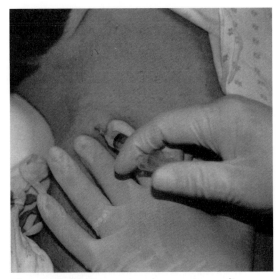

Figure 22–26. Injection into the trapezius to relieve myofascial trigger point.

SUGGESTED READINGS

Garvey TA, Marks MR, Wensel SW: A prospective randomized double-blind evaluation of trigger-point injection therapy for low-back pain. Spine 14(9):962–964, 1989.

Kerlan RK, Glousman RE: Injections and techniques in athletic medicine. Clin Sports Med 8(3):541–560, July 1989.

Klippel JH, Weyand CM, Wortmann RL: Primer on the Rheumatic Diseases, 11th ed. Atlanta, GA, Arthritis Foundation, 1997.

Pfenninger JL: Injections of joints and soft tissues: Part I. General guidelines. Am Fam Physician 44(4):1196–1202, 1991.

Pfenninger JL: Injections of joints and soft tissues: Part II. Guidelines for specific joints. Am Fam Physician 44(5):1690–1701, 1991.

Index

Note: Page numbers in *italics* indicate illustrations; those followed by t indicate tables.

ISBN 0-7216-7871-8